Vitamin C in Health and Disease

ANTIOXIDANTS IN HEALTH AND DISEASE

Series Editors

LESTER PACKER, PH.D.
University of California
Berkeley, California

JÜRGEN FUCHS, PH.D., M.D.
Johann Wolfgang Goethe University
Frankfurt, Germany

1. Vitamin A in Health and Disease, *edited by Rune Blomhoff*
2. Biothiols in Health and Disease, *edited by Lester Packer and Enrique Cadenas*
3. Handbook of Antioxidants, *edited by Enrique Cadenas and Lester Packer*
4. Handbook of Synthetic Antioxidants, *edited by Lester Packer and Enrique Cadenas*
5. Vitamin C in Health and Disease, *edited by Lester Packer and Jürgen Fuchs*

Additional Volumes in Preparation

Lipoic Acid in Health and Disease, *edited by Jürgen Fuchs, Lester Packer, and Guido Zimmer*

Flavonoids in Health and Disease, *edited by Catherine Rice-Evans and Lester Packer*

Related Volumes

Vitamin E in Health and Disease: Biochemistry and Clinical Applications, *edited by Lester Packer and Jürgen Fuchs*

Free Radicals and Oxidation Phenomena in Biological Systems, *edited by Marcel Roberfroid and Pedro Buc Calderon*

Vitamin C in Health and Disease

edited by

Lester Packer
University of California
Berkeley, California

Jürgen Fuchs
Johann Wolfgang Goethe University
Frankfurt, Germany

 MARCEL DEKKER, INC.   NEW YORK · BASEL · HONG KONG

Library of Congress Cataloging–in–Publication Data

Vitamin C in health and disease / edited by Lester Packer, Jürgen Fuchs.
    p. cm.— (Antioxidants in health and disease ; 5)
    Includes index.
    ISBN 0-8247-9313-7 (hardcover : alk. paper)
    1. Vitamin C—Health aspects. I. Packer, Lester. II. Fuchs,
Jürgen. III. Series.
    [DNLM: 1. Ascorbic Acid—physiology. 2. Ascorbic Acid—
therapeutic use. 3. Ascorbic Acid—chemistry. W1 AN884 v.5 1997
/ QU 210 V8363   1997]
    615'.328—dc21
    DNLM/DLC
    for Library of Congress
                                                                    97-7703
                                                                       CIP

The publisher offers discounts on this book when ordered in bulk quantities. For more information, write to Special Sales/Professional Marketing at the address below.

This book is printed on acid-free paper.

Marcel Dekker, Inc.
270 Madison Avenue, New York, New York 10016

Current printing (last digit):
10 9 8 7 6 5 4 3 2 1

PRINTED IN THE UNITED STATES OF AMERICA

Series Introduction

In June of 1992, 17 international researchers in the field of free radical and antioxidant biology and preventive medicine met at the village of Saas Fee, Switzerland, and drew up the Saas Fee Declaration to recognize the importance of prevention in medicine and health. Since then, hundreds of researchers from around the world have signed the declaration:

Saas Fee Declaration
On the significance of antioxidants in preventive medicine.

1. The intensive research on free radicals of the past 15 years by scientists worldwide has led to the statement in 1992 that antioxidant nutrients may have major significance in the prevention of a number of diseases. These include cardiovascular and cerebrovascular disease, some forms of cancer and several other disorders, many of which may be age-related.

2. There is now general agreement that there is a need for further work at the fundamental scientific level, as well as in large-scale randomized trials and in clinical medicine, which can be expected to lead to more precise information being made available.

3. The major objective of this work is the prevention of disease. This may be achieved by use of antioxidants which are natural physiological substances. The strategy should be to achieve optimal intakes of these antioxidant nutrients as part of preventive medicine.

4. It is quite clear that many environmental sources of free radicals exist, such as ozone, sunlight, and other forms of radiation, smog, dust, and other atmospheric pollutants. The optimal intake of antioxidants provides a preventive measure against these hazards.

5. There is a great need for improvement in public awareness of the potential preventive benefits of antioxidant nutrient intake. There is overwhelming evidence that the antioxidant nutrients such as vitamin E, vitamin C, carotenoids, alpha-lipoic acid and others are safe even at very high levels of intake.

6. Moreover, there is now substantial agreement that governmental agencies, health professionals, and the media should promote information transfer to the general public, particularly when evidence exists that benefits for human health and public expenditure are overwhelming.

This declaration arose from the overwhelming evidence now available indicating that antioxidants play a critical role in wellness, health maintenance, and the prevention of chronic and degenerative diseases. Antioxidants neutralize free radicals that are generated during normal metabolism and during exposure to environmental insult. Free radicals play a role in most major health problems of the industrialized world, including cardiovascular disease, cancer, and disorders of aging.

Some antioxidants are quite familiar as vitamins or vitamin-forming compounds: vitamin E, vitamin C, and the carotenoids, including beta-carotene. These antioxidants must be constantly replenished through the diet. Others, such as ubiquinols and the thiol antioxidants, including glutathione and lipoic acid, are manufactured by the body, but the levels of many of these can be bolstered through dietary supplementation. Until recently, it was thought that each antioxidant played its role in isolation from the others. But work in several laboratories indicates that there is a dynamic interplay among the systems. For example, when vitamin E neutralizes a free radical in a membrane, it becomes itself a relatively harmless free radical, which decomposes. However, vitamin C can regenerate vitamin E from the vitamin E radical, in effect "recycling" vitamin E. Vitamin E becomes a radical in the process, but it, too, can be recycled by interacting with other antioxidant systems. It has been shown that these interactions occur in the test tube, and nutritional supplementation studies support this idea for the whole organism. Thus, a picture is emerging of a complex interplay among the defense systems, with the various antioxidant cycles acting to prevent cell damage and disease. Our knowledge is far from complete but these findings already have implications in terms of recommendations for supplementation.

Hence, it seems particularly appropriate to offer this series at the present time. Never has the demand for knowledge about antioxidants been greater, and never has the potential for treating disease and improving health been clearer. The series highlights natural antioxidants and artificial antioxidants that mimic natural systems.

Lester Packer
Jürgen Fuchs

Preface

The story of discoveries about vitamin C—from the recognition that the lack of fresh fruits and vegetables in long sailing voyages led to scurvy to its characterization and establishment of biological requirements—is a fascinating saga. We owe much to the sea captains who kept accurate logs of their sailing voyages; to physiologists and historians of the subject; and to the pioneering discoveries on its chemical nature by Albert Szent-Györgyi and others. Interest in vitamin C has grown as our understanding of its biological mode of action has slowly expanded. It was even championed by the late Linus Pauling, who popularized its health aspects and generated interest in further research on vitamin C with respect to health and disease.

This volume represents an effort to bring together the best work that has been carried out on vitamin C from a number of different directions. Part I provides a thorough history of scurvy and vitamin C, from early sea voyages to its isolation, characterization, and synthesis; Part II follows with a discussion of its chemistry and biochemistry, as well as its transport. Especially important in the chemistry of vitamin C are its redox properties, and Chapters 4–6 expand on reactions of the vitamin C radical, redox cycling of vitamin C, and its regeneration. In addition, both antioxidant and prooxidant properties of vitamin C are covered (Chap. 3), as well as protein glycation by its oxidation products (Chap. 7).

These chemical mechanisms set the stage for Part II, which is concerned with the physiology and biomedical aspects of vitamin C. Chapters 9–19 include discussion of effects due to its role in collagen synthesis and protein hydroxylation, especially important in aging, and its effects on the oxidation of LDL and consequently on atherosclerotic disease, one of the major pathologies of aging in industrialized nations. In addition, the action of vitamin C in minimizing oxidative damage products of DNA, and its effects in various cells and tissues, including cells of the immune system (and its action in viral and immunodeficiency disease), the lens, the lung, and skin are examined.

Finally, Part IV of this volume deals with the effects of vitamin C at the level of health and disease. Chapters 20–29 discuss its metabolism, and establishment of human nutritional requirements and safety, both areas of concern for those who advocate the use of supplemental amounts of vitamin C. Epidemiological studies of vitamin C and its effects on, for example, cardiovascular, infectious, periodontal, and skin diseases, cancer, and cataracts, reveal a potential role for its use in prevention. Also examined are vitamin C's effects on the consequences of negative lifestyle habits such as cigarette smoke exposure and alcohol consumption.

This volume comes at an important time and represents a new and comprehensive treatment of this important topic. We have especially attempted to address areas of current pioneering research. Thus we express our gratitude for the advice and suggestions of a number of our colleagues who helped us to approach contributors who are experts in their fields and could provide the most up-to-date knowledge of vitamin C.

Lester Packer
Jürgen Fuchs

Contents

III. PHYSIOLOGY AND BIOMEDICAL ASPECTS

Contributors

Olav Alvares, BDS, M.S., Ph.D. Associate Professor, Department of Periodontics, University of Texas Health Science Center, San Antonio, Texas

Bruce N. Ames University of California, Berkeley, California

Karl E. Arfors Department of Experimental Medicine, Pharmacia AB, Uppsala, Sweden

Adrianne Bendich, Ph.D., F.A.C.N. Assistant Director, Human Nutrition Research, Hoffmann–La Roche, Inc., Paramus, New Jersey

Wolf Bors Institut für Strahlenbiologie, GSF Research Center Neuherberg, Oberschleissheim, Germany

Lou Ann S. Brown, Ph.D. Associate Professor, Department of Pediatrics, Emory University, Atlanta, Georgia

Garry R. Buettner Free Radical Research Institute, The University of Iowa, Iowa City, Iowa

Betty Jane Burri, Ph.D. Research Chemist, Western Human Nutrition Research Center, USDA, San Francisco, California

Mei-Ling Cheng, M.S. Research Associate, School of Medicine Technology, Chang Gung Medical College, Kwei-san, Tao-yuan, Taiwan

Daniel Tsun-Yee Chiu, Ph.D. Professor, Graduate Institute of Basic Medical Sciences, Chang Gung Medical College, Kwei-san, Tao-yuan, Taiwan

Ching K. Chow, Ph.D. Professor, Department of Nutrition and Food Science, University of Kentucky, Lexington, Kentucky

Roy M. Colven, M.D. Department of Medicine, University of Washington, Seattle, Washington

Carroll E. Cross, M.D. Professor, Department of Medicine and Physiology, University of California, Davis, California

Douglas J. Darr, Ph.D. Director, Technology Development, North Carolina Biotechnology Center, Research Triangle Park, North Carolina

C. K. Dorey Jean Mayer USDA Human Nutrition Research Center on Aging, Tufts University, Boston, Massachusetts

Jason P. Eiserich, Ph.D. Research Assistant, Department of Medicine, University of California, Davis, California

James E. Enstrom, Ph.D. School of Public Health, University of California, Los Angeles, California

Balz Frei, Ph.D. Associate Professor, Whitaker Cardiovascular Institute, Boston University School of Medicine, Boston, Massachusetts

Jürgen Fuchs, Ph.D., M.D. Department of Dermatology, Johann Wolfgang Goethe University, Frankfurt, Germany

Barry Halliwell, D.Sc. International Antioxidant Research Center, King's College, University of London, London, England

Steve Harakeh, Ph.D. Virology and Immunodeficiency Program, Linus Pauling Institute, Palo Alto, California

Gary E. Hatch, Ph.D. Research Pharmacologist, Pulmonary Toxicology Branch, U.S. Environmental Protection Agency, Durham, North Carolina

Harri Hemilä, Ph.D. Department of Public Health, University of Helsinki, Helsinki, Finland

Robert A. Jacob Western Human Nutrition Research Center, USDA, San Francisco, California

Raxit J. Jariwalla, Ph.D. Virology and Immunodeficiency Program, Linus Pauling Institute, Palo Alto, California

Ritva Järvinen, Ph.D.   Department of Clinical Nutrition, University of Kuopio, Kuopio, Finland

Dean P. Jones   Professor, Department of Biochemistry, Emory University, Atlanta, Georgia

Che-Hun Jung, Ph.D.   Research Associate, Department of Biochemistry, Michigan State University, East Lansing, Michigan

Paul Knekt, Ph.D.   Department of Health and Disability, National Public Health Institute, Helsinki, Finland

Hans-Anton Lehr, M.D., Ph.D.   Institute of Pathology, Johannes Gutenberg University, Mainz, Germany

Vincent M. Monnier, M.D.   Professor, Institute of Pathology, Case Western Reserve University, Cleveland, Ohio

Ulrich Moser   Roche Vitamines and Fine Chemicals, Basel, Switzerland

Etsuo Niki, Ph.D.   Professor, Research Center for Advanced Science and Technology, University of Tokyo, Tokyo, Japan

Noriko Noguchi   Research Center for Advanced Science and Technology, University of Tokyo, Tokyo, Japan

Thomas Nowell   Jean Mayer USDA Human Nutrition Research Center on Aging, Tufts University, Boston, Massachusetts

Kristiina Nyyssönen   Research Institute of Public Health, University of Kuopio, Kuopio, Finland

Martin Obin   Tufts University, Boston, Massachusetts

Beryl J. Ortwerth, Ph.D.   Professor and Director of Research, Department of Ophthalmology, Mason Eye Institute, University of Missouri, Columbia, Missouri

Lester Packer, Ph.D.   Professor, Department of Molecular and Cell Biology, University of California, Berkeley, California

Markku T. Parviainen   Research Institute of Public Health, University of Kuopio, Kuopio, Finland

Charlotte L. Phillips, Ph.D.   Assistant Professor, Departments of Biochemistry and Child Health, University of Missouri, Columbia, Missouri

Sheldon R. Pinnell, M.D.   Chief, Division of Dermatology, and J. Lamar Callaway Professor of Dermatology, Duke University Medical Center, Durham, North Carolina

Maurizio Podda, M.D.   Department of Dermatology, Johann Wolfgang Goethe University, Frankfurt, Germany

Richard C. Rose, Ph.D.   Department of Physiology and Biophysics, Finch University of Health Sciences, Chicago Medical School, North Chicago, Illinois

Rainer K. Saetzler   Department of Physiology, Temple University, Philadelphia, Pennsylvania

Jukka T. Salonen, M.D., Ph.D., M.Sc.P.H.   Professor and Director, Research Institute of Public Health, University of Kuopio, Kuopio, Finland

Howerde E. Sauberlich, Ph.D.   Professor, Department of Nutrition Sciences, University of Alabama at Birmingham, Birmingham, Alabama

Allen Taylor, Ph.D.   Director, Laboratory for Nutrition and Vision Research, Jean Mayer USDA Human Nutrition Research Center on Aging, Tufts University, Boston, Massachusetts

Constance S. Tsao, Ph.D.   Director, Department of Nutrition, Biochemistry, and Cancer Research, Linus Pauling Institute, Palo Alto, California

Albert van der Vliet, Ph.D.   Department of Internal Medicine, University of California, Davis, California

William W. Wells, Ph.D.   Professor, Department of Biochemistry, Michigan State University, East Lansing, Michigan

Matthew Whiteman, B.Sc.   International Antioxidant Research Center, King's College, University of London, London, England

John X. Wilson   Department of Physiology, University of Western Ontario, London, Ontario, Canada

Alan Anthony Woodall, Ph.D.   Department of Molecular and Cell Biology, University of California, Berkeley, California

Heather N. Yeowell, Ph.D.   Associate Research Professor, Division of Dermatology, Department of Medicine, Duke University Medical Center, Durham, North Carolina

Vitamin

C in
Health
and
Disease

1

A History of Scurvy and Vitamin C

HOWERDE E. SAUBERLICH
University of Alabama at Birmingham, Birmingham, Alabama

INTRODUCTION

Vitamin C: Generic descriptor for all compounds exhibiting qualitatively the biological activity of ascorbic acid (J Nutrition 1987; 117:7–15)

L-Ascorbic acid: 2,3-Didehydro-L-threo-hexano-1,4-lactone

Scurvy: A condition due to deficiency of ascorbic acid (vitamin C) in the diet and marked by weakness, anemia, spongy gums, a tendency to mucocutaneous hemorrhages, and a brawny induration of the muscles of the calves and legs (*Dorland's Medical Dictionary*, 26th ed. Philadelphia: Saunders, 1981).

This definition of scurvy could have been selected from descriptions published several centuries ago. For example, Chapin A. Harris defined scurvy in his 1849 book *A Dictionary of Dental Science* as a "disease characterized by spongy gums, offensive breath, livid spots on the skin, great general debility, and a pale, bloated countenance" (1).

Records and writings that relate to the history of scurvy are extensive. This is understandable in view of the enormous tragedy and misery that vitamin C deficiency has inflicted upon humankind over many centuries.

The conquest of scurvy represents a pinnacle in the history of nutrition. In the following pages, only a very brief and broad overview of the history of scurvy can be presented. However, the disastrous consequences of scurvy can still be appreciated. The literature cited can provide guidance to those interested in pursuing the subject further.

EARLY HISTORY OF SCURVY

Early writings describe diseases with features that would suggest the presence of scurvy as we now know it (2,3). Such descriptions appeared in the Thebes Ebers papyrus of about 1500 B.C., in the texts of Susruto the Indian surgeon about 400 B.C., in writings in the fifth

1

century of Hippocrates, in the records of the Roman Pliny the Elder in the first century (23–79 A.D.), and in documents of Chang Chi of China of about 200 A.D. (4–7). Evidence from records of ancient Mesopotamia suggest that the disease referred to as *bu' sanu* may have been scurvy (8).

The fifth century Babylonian Talmud describes a disease called *tzafdinah* (9). Gum bleeding was the major symptom. *Tzafdinah* has been translated as scurvy in modern Hebrew dictionaries as well as in the classic English version of the Talmud. Whether tzafdinah represents true scurvy has been questioned and may represent an ailment such as tooth abscess or pyorrhea.

A Norse report of scurvy is found in *Torstein the White's Saga* of the tenth century. During a voyage from Iceland to Norway, Torstein was afflicted with *skyrbyjugr* (10).

In 1227 Gilbertus de Aguila recognized, from his experience of a voyage to Palestine, clinical scurvy and "advised [voyagers] to carry an ample supply of apples, pears, lemons and muscatels as well as other fruits and vegetables" (11). With such effective advice, one may ask, Why did it take seven hundred years to conquer this disease? In part this delay may have been due to the lack of communication of this knowledge and the failure of its acceptance by the medical establishment.

Yet during the next five hundred years scurvy took a tremendous toll on sea travelers (2,6). Over a million seamen may have died from scurvy during the seventeenth and eighteenth centuries (12). Since scurvy was a scourge of navies, many of the early references to the disease were noted in the nautical records.

The records of Richard Hakluyt in 1589 provide the first appearance of the term *scurvy* in an English publication (2). He was on an expedition from England in 1582 led by Edward Fenton that was forced to return home because of severe storms in the Straits of Magellan. He wrote that when in sight of home two men died of the "skurvie." In 1541, the Dutch physician Joan Echtius called the disease *scorbutus* (10); he had latinized the Danish word *scorbuck*. Other early terms were *scarby* and *scorby*. Similar names for apparently the same disease have been used in other countries. The Swedish used *sckorbjugg*; the Danish *skorbug*; the Saxons *scorbie*; the Germans *scharbock*, *schorbock*, or *schorbuyck*.

EARLY LONG-DISTANCE SEA EXPLORATION

Early long-distance explorations by sea were conducted primarily by the Portuguese and Spanish (2). The earlier voyages were made close to shorelines and were short in duration and therefore scurvy was not observed. However, by the early 1440s, technological developments in the compass and design of larger ships permitted sailors to venture on longer voyages from Western Europe. The inducement was to find sea routes to the Far East for trade in silk and spices. Such routes would avoid the hazardous overland trade routes then controlled by Muslim Arabs. From that time on, scurvy made its appearance among sailors.

Vasco da Gama

For example, Vasco da Gama left Lisbon, Portugal, in 1497, with four ships and a crew of about 140 people. After about 6 months at sea they rounded the Cape of Good Hope of South Africa. Shortly thereafter they encountered scurvy, a disease unknown to these sailors. Fortunately, Moorish traders in the area were able to provide the sailors with oranges and the sailors recovered. On their return from the Far East, the illness reappeared while they were sailing across the Arabian Sea. Records state that 30 men died and only 7 or 8 were fit to navigate each ship.

Christopher Columbus

At about this time Christopher Columbus endeavored to reach the Indies by going west in the hopes of finding a shorter passage. Although this experienced Genoese sailor was denied support by Portugal, he sought help for his endeavor in England and elsewhere. Finally, after years of disappointment, Columbus found favor and needed support in Spain from King Ferdinand and Queen Isabella. This favor changed the course of history, not only in the New World but worldwide. Although Columbus made four voyages to the New World, he and his crew were apparently spared of scurvy. Only on his second voyage is there a suggestion in the physician's account that mild scurvy was present on arrival in the Caribbean area. Columbus's voyage to the New World took only 34 days, hence the absence of scurvy.

Ferdinand Magellan (1480-1521)

Although born in Portugal, Magellan sailed under the flag of Spain as he had fallen into a problem with the Portuguese royalty. Magellan was an experienced navigator. He left Seville, Spain, on August 10, 1519, with five ships and a contingent of 237 sailors. During his circumnavigation of the world Magellan lost 76 of his men to scurvy. Records suggest that their eating the wild celery of Patagonia prevented a greater loss of men during the long Pacific section of their journey.

Unfortunately, Magellan did not complete the first trip around the world. He became involved in a tribal war in the Philippines and was killed. Only one of his five original vessels continued on and completed the global trip. The sole surviving ship, *Victoria*, under the command of Juan Sebastian del Cano, arrived in Seville on September 6, 1522, with only 31 crew members left.

Records of the voyage of Magellan were maintained by a chronicler aboard, Antonio Pigafetta, an Italian volunteer. Despite the loss of ships and personnel, the journey was considered a success. The surviving ship took back a treasure of spices that more than paid for the cost of the journey.

Only a few of the numerous sailing expeditions conducted during the period of 1450 to 1750 by the Portuguese, Spanish, English, French, and Dutch have been noted. Accounts of many more expeditions, with extensive documentation, have been provided by Kenneth Carpenter (2). Those interested in medical history will find this book most interesting. Additional fascinating documents on historical aspects of scurvy are available (7,11,13–28); particularly informative is the series of reports by Carey P. McCord (7,21–30). Aside from famine, scurvy is probably the nutritional deficiency disease that has caused the most deaths and suffering in recorded history.

OTHER EXPEDITIONS (1500–1700)

The Spanish voyages stimulated other sea ventures. The first British expedition to the New World was to explore the Newfoundland coast. This was led by John Cabot in 1497. The voyage was also short, with no reference to serious illness. In 1601, John Guy, who participated in the first colonization of Newfoundland, stated that turnips were "exceedingly good for the scarby, by trial it hath recovered many of our sick men."

However, the French expedition under Jacques Cartier in 1535 to explore further New-foundland and the Saint Lawrence River was not so fortunate. They stayed too long and strayed too far, some as far as present day Montreal. As a result, it was necessary for them to winter over near the present site of Quebec. From mid-November until mid-April 1536, their ships were frozen in. By mid-February, virtually every one of the 110 men suffered severely from scurvy. According to tradition, a friendly Indian, Bon Agava, showed Cartier how to prepare a concoction from the bark and leaves of a tree, probably white cedar (*Thuja occidentalis*). Although the men disliked the taste of the drink, their recovery after its use was almost miraculous. Despite this experience, during the next 100 years, numerous French expeditions to this area continued to suffer from outbreaks of scurvy.

After the discoveries of Cartier in the New World, the king of France granted a charter to Cartier to explore and colonize the area in 1540. In May 1541, Cartier left France with five ships and sailed to a location near Quebec. These colonists apparently avoided scurvy, perhaps through the use of scurvy-protective greens. In 1542, Roberval from France arrived near Quebec with 200 settlers. Although saved from starvation by fish obtained from the Indians, many apparently developed and died from what appeared to be scurvy.

Other attempts were made in 1604 to colonize New France. An expedition under the command of Pontgrove, Poutrincourt, and de Monts established a fort on an island in the mouth of the St. Croux River of Nova Scotia. That winter, all of the 79 colonists developed scurvy, of which 36 died. Champlain, who founded the city of Quebec in 1608, also encountered scurvy. During the first winter in Canada, 18 of his 28 settlers apparently died of scurvy.

Sir Francis Drake in his circumnavigation in 1577–1580 in the *Golden Hind* relied on fresh provisions and fruits at every anchorage possible. For example, a stop was made near San Francisco, California. Any of the sailors with scurvy was rapidly restored to health by these stops (11). Although Drake had no deaths during the voyage, his men repeatedly were weakened and sick from scurvy. However, they were able to find places en route to obtain supplies before they reached a crisis point. Thus, for instance, on the way back to England, on the west coast of Africa, Drake found "oysters and plenty of lemons, which gave us good refreshing."

Other expeditions during the late 1500s and 1600s were not always so fortunate. The English sea captain Sir Peter Hawkins stated in the 1590s, "He was able, in the course of twenty years, in which he had been employed at sea, to give an account of 10,000 mariners consumed by the scurvy" (31).

Although the curative ability of oranges and lemons was recognized, few expeditions made any plans to carry them as preventives. On the voyages to the East Indies, the English East India Company provided instruction to include "lemon water" in the supplies. How well these instructions were followed is uncertain. The quality and quantity of the lemon juice could not be relied on to be effective in preventing outbreaks of scurvy in the ships. Thus, the journal for the voyage in 1696 states that the men were "falling down upon the scurvy" and when approaching Table Bay (Capetown), "most of our men were down sick and by then we had buried thirty men."

EARLY ENGLISH SETTLEMENTS IN THE UNITED STATES

The first English settlement in the United States was made in 1606 at Jamestown, Virginia (30). These settlers and those to follow encountered problems similar to those endured by the French colonists. Starvation, scurvy, and diseases were constantly endured. The James-town colony was about to be abandoned. Of the 500 colonists who had arrived by August

1609, only 60 remained alive in May 1610. Soon thereafter, Lord Delaware, the new governor of the colony, arrived with food and supplies and Jamestown was not abandoned. By 1630 the settlement had become stabilized and the population slowly increased. Food was now more varied and plentiful and scurvy was no longer the scourge it had been earlier in the Virginia colonies. Captain John Smith in 1626 recommended the juice of lemons for scurvy in his seaman's manual (11).

Other early colonies in America suffered to varying degrees from scurvy (30). Pilgrims arrived in New England in December 1620. With the cold upon them and with meager food supplies and poor shelter, 44 of the approximately 100 colonists died during the period of December through March, many from scurvy. With spring the survivors were able to plant and harvest sufficient foodstuffs and the following winter (1621–1622) the thankful Plymouth Colony was free of scurvy; thus the origin of Thanksgiving Day, a national holiday in the United States.

The Puritan group of about 2000 arrived in 1630 at Charlestown, Massachusetts, under the leadership of John Winthrop. Many landed ill with scurvy and suffered through the winter, when there were many deaths. Governor Winthrop apparently was aware of the value of lemon juice and scurvy grass and requested that his wife carry a quantity with her when she joined him in Charlestown.

COMMERCIAL TRADING COMPANIES

British East India Company

From the year 1600 and on, several commercial trading companies were established. The first major company was the British East India Company, chartered by Queen Elizabeth on December 31, 1600. Captain Lancaster was the commander of the first voyage of the British East India Company, which sailed from England in February 1601 (25). Lancaster, during his return from his voyage to the East Indies, encountered severe scurvy among his crew. He stopped in St. Helena to reprovision his ship and observed the miraculous effects of lemons and oranges in curing his men of scurvy. He returned to England from the East Indies in 1603 with a rich cargo of spices but with a loss of 105 deaths from scurvy. John Woodall (1569–1643) served as the first surgeon general for the East India Company. Woodall was aware of the benefits of using lemon juice in the prevention and treatment of scurvy (2,12). In his medical book he wrote that "the use of the juyce of Lemmons is a precious medicine and well tried, being sound and good, let it have the chiefe place, for it will deserve it" (12,25). Unfortunately, this advice was little heeded. Throughout the next 200 years, the trading ships were plagued with scurvy. The British East India Company ceased to exist in June 1874.

Hudson's Bay Company

The Hudson's Bay Company was established in 1670 primarily to enhance fur trading. Expeditions that wintered over in the Hudson's Bay encountered scurvy. For the most part, the cases of scurvy were mild and prevented by the ample consumption of fresh fish and game. The Hudson's Bay Company was still in operation as of 1971.

Dutch East India Company

The Dutch East India Company was established in 1602 to participate in the spice trade (25). The company had great interest in the health of its personnal. Even vegetable gardens to grow various greens were maintained on the ships. The Dutch had also learned of the value of oranges and lemons as protection against scurvy. In addition, the ships usually carried sauerkraut. Despite these actions, scurvy was encountered on the long voyages from Europe to the Indies. Its severity resulted in the establishment of a fort by the Dutch in 1654 at the Cape of Good Hope. The fort provided provisions for the Dutch East India Company's fleet en route to the East Indies. Homeward bound ships again stopped at the fort for supplies. The Dutch East India Company went out of existence in 1798.

Only a few of the many voyages of the sixteenth to eighteenth centuries have been noted. But most voyages were accompanied by scurvy, often with disastrous effects. Many of these voyages have been recounted by Carpenter (2), McCord (22–25), and others (11).

SEA SCURVY IN THE 1700S

The 1600s was a period of empire building by Spain, Portugal, Britain, and Holland. As a result, strong navies were built to extend exploration, expand empires, and develop and defend far-flung colonies.

The British Navy up until 1700 served primarily to guard the British coast and approaching shipping. Consequently, voyages were not long and hence avoided scurvy. When war was declared against Spain in 1739, long sea voyages became important and the ravages of scurvy appeared among the British sailors. Very tragic was the voyage of Commodore George Anson, who was instructed to capture the Spanish treasure galleon that crossed the Pacific each year carrying silver from Acapulco, Mexico, to the Philippines. He started with seven ships and a crew of 961 officers and men. However, only one ship and 145 men returned to England in 1744. Scurvy claimed the great majority of the rest. The survivors did, nevertheless, succeed in capturing the treasure galleon.

Tragic was the lack of provisions on the ships that could have served as sources of vitamin C. The British Navy held the view that lemons caused enteritis and that when in tropical areas the "crew should eat very little of them since they are the commonest cause of fevers and obstruction of vital organs."

John Wesley, founder of Methodism, published in 1745 his *Primitive physic*, representing a manual of remedies. The manual listed a number of antiscorbutics, including lemon juice, goose grass juice, nettle juice, scurvy grass, cresses, and orange juice (32). Another treatment was the use of turnips; as we now know, turnips are a fairly good source of vitamin C.

CAPTAIN JAMES COOK (1728–1779)

Captain Cook conducted three circumnavigations of the world. The first voyage started in 1768 with an extensive mapping of the coasts of New Zealand and Australia that provided claims to the lands for Great Britain. Fortunately Cook was familiar with the work of James Lind (discussed in the next section) and adopted his principles. Cook was insistent that his crews be provided orange and lemon juice and that at every opportunity during their voyages fresh fruit and vegetables be obtained. Consequently he was able to navigate during this three-year voyage on the *Endeavor*, a small ship with a crew of 70, with no loss of personnel due to scurvy (2,33–35).

Cook's second voyage with two ships (*Resolution* and *Adventure*) was to the South Pole area. Cook on the *Resolution* had only one case of scurvy during a period of 117 days at sea. In contrast, the companion ship, *Adventure*, under the direction of Captain Furneaux, encountered a serious incidence of scurvy, which was treated by landing on the New Zealand coast. After continuing at sea for another 6 weeks, scurvy was again encountered on the *Adventure* but not on the *Resolution*. When they reached Tahiti, "many were so weak they were unable to get on deck without assistance" (2). With the availability of fruits and coconuts, the men soon recovered. Cook's concern about providing antiscorbutic supplies permitted him to return home in 1776 without the loss of a single person to scurvy.

On his third voyage, begun in 1778, Cook discovered the Hawaiian Islands (Sandwich Islands). From there he sailed to the Alaska area, but he returned to Hawaii because of the icepack he encountered. As a result of an unnecessary altercation with the Hawaiian natives, he was killed at Kealakaku Bay in Hawaii in 1779.

JAMES LIND (1716–1794)

In 1739, James Lind, at the age of 23 years, joined the Royal Navy (Fig. 1). In 1746, after completing his apprenticeship, he was a full surgeon on the H.M.S. *Salisbury*, which had a crew of 350 (31,31a). In 1746 and again the following year, serious outbreaks of scurvy occurred on the ship. During the second outbreak, Lind carried out his famous experiment on scurvy (31,31a). This experiment represents the first controlled trial in clinical nutrition and probably in any area of clinical science. He had available a group of 12 scorbutic sailors who were placed in the hold of the ship and maintained on the same diet. Two men were

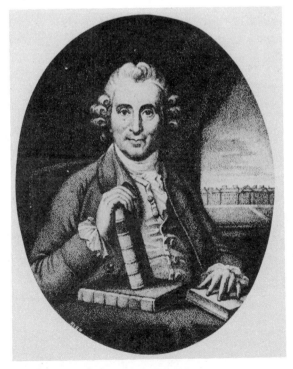

Figure 1 James Lind (1716–1791).

allocated to each of six different treatments for a period of 14 days. The condition of the two sailors who daily received two oranges and one lemon for 6 days was much improved. The other treatments failed. Unfortunately at the time Lind's experiment received little attention. He left the Navy disappointed in 1748 and returned to Edinburgh, where he was granted the doctor of medicine degree. In 1753, he published his famous book, *A Treatise of the Scurvy* (31). Lind was of the opinion that the first description of scurvy was that of the disease affecting the French Army that spent the winter of 1249–1250 in Egypt fighting the Saracens.

A few excerpts from James Lind's *A Treatise of the Scurvy*, published in 1753, allow an appreciation of the details and manner he employed in his experiments "of the prevention of scurvy" (31,36) (Fig. 2). Lind wrote: "On the 20th of May, 1747, I took twelve patients in the scurvy, on board the *Salisbury* at sea"—. "Two others had each two oranges and one lemon given them everyday. These they eat with greediness, at different times, upon an empty stomach. They continued but six days under this course, having consumed the quantity that could be spared"—. "The consequence was, that the most sudden and visible good effects were perceived from the use of the oranges and lemons; one of those who had taken them, being at the end of six days fit for duty"—. "The other was the best recovered of any in his condition; and being now deemed pretty well, was appointed nurse to the rest of the sick."

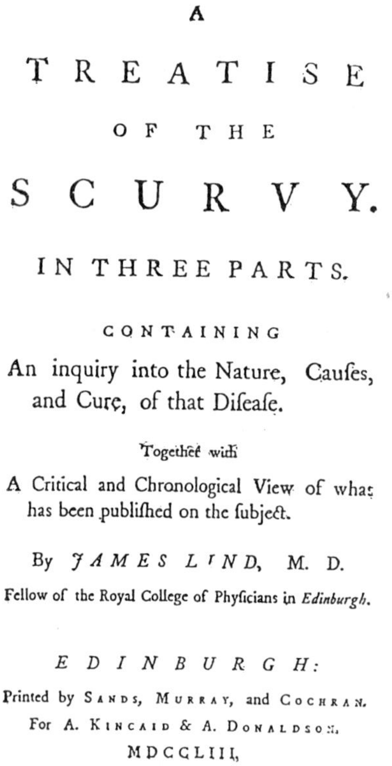

A

T R E A T I S E

O F   T H E

S C U R V Y.

IN THREE PARTS.

CONTAINING

An inquiry into the Nature, Caufes, and Cure, of that Difeafe.

Together with

A Critical and Chronological View of what has been publifhed on the fubject.

By *JAMES LIND*, M. D.

Fellow of the Royal College of Phyficians in *Edinburgh*.

EDINBURGH:

Printed by SANDS, MURRAY, and COCHRAN.
For A. KINCAID & A. DONALDSON.
MDCCLIII.

Figure 2 Title page to James Lind's *A Treatise of the Scurvy*.

James Lind described scurvy as follows (4,31):

In the early stages, patients do not look very sick, but are listless, perhaps a little pale, and have an aversion to exercise. They still eat well, but in a few days develop universal lassitude, stiffness, and feebleness of the knees, some difficulty breathing, itchy gums, and rough, dry skin splattered with bluish and reddish spots. These hemorrhages vary from the size of a lentil to a handsbreadth, mostly on the legs, less on the arms and trunk, and rarely on the head or face. The gums, however, bleed readily and become first soft and spongy and then putrid and rotten. The breath is foul, and the teeth fall out. The legs swell, at first only in the evening, but later all the time. Ulcers appear on the thighs, coated with blood and gore, and will not heal. Broken bones will not mend and even old, healed wounds may break apart. The patients are now susceptible to whatever infection is going around, often diarrhea. Many joints, but especially the knees, are very painful and greatly swollen with blood. Patients now have abdominal pain, cannot eat, are jaundiced and swollen all over, breathe with pain and labor, and may die suddenly. It is not easy to conceive a more dismal and diversified scene of misery.

Lind revised his treatise in 1772. He held the theory that scurvy was a disease that was initiated partly by cold, moist air and partly by diet; diet alone could not produce it. But another 150 years passed before it was established that the absence of a compound in the diet was the cause of scurvy. Dr. James Lind died in 1794 at 78 years of age. A year later, 1795, the British Admiralty adopted the use of citrus foods in the prevention of scurvy largely as the result of the efforts of Sir Gilbert Blane (37,38).

SIR GILBERT BLANE (1749–1832)

Sir Gilbert Blane was appointed as physician to the British Fleet in 1781. He spent time at sea and personally observed the casualty rate of scurvy in the fleet. Blane stated that "scurvy, one of the principal diseases with which seamen are afflicted, may be infallibly prevented, or cured, by vegetables and fruit, particularly oranges, lemons or limes" (37,38). Sir Gilbert Blane stated that the eradication of scurvy enabled a fleet of the same striking force to be maintained at sea with half the number of men and ships. The fleet concept had been of one sailor at sea contracting scurvy and one sailor on land recovering from scurvy. Disappointed likewise because his advice was ignored, Blane returned to civilian life and became the physician to the household of the prince of Wales. Because of this position and status, his views about the use of fruit in the cure of scurvy were being recognized. In 1795, Blane became commissioner to the Sick and Hurt Board. Thereupon, the board authorized that lemon juice in the amount of 0.75 ounce/day be a regular issue of the fleet. Nearly 50 years after the clinical trial of Lind, scurvy was essentially eliminated from the British Navy. Sir Gilbert Blane has been referred to as a father of naval medical science.

However, the use of lemon juice by the British fleet came into question. In 1875, an evaporated form of lemon juice (referred to as ROB) and West Indian lime juice were substituted for lemon juice. The vitamin C was destroyed in the preparation of the ROB and the limes contained less than one-third the ascorbic acid of oranges and lemons. As a result, scurvy again appeared regularly among the British sailors. Then Lord Lister stated before the Royal Academy that limes and vegetables were ineffective as antiscorbutics.

JOHN CLAIBORNE

John Claiborne was the first American to publish a document on scurvy (39). His essay was presented on May 22, 1798, in fulfillment of requirements for his medical degree from the

University of Pennsylvania. Claiborne provides a detailed description of the signs and symptoms of scurvy. Although he was familiar with the work of Lind, he gave little credence to the idea that diet was involved; rather, he was supportive of the concept that scurvy was a fever, therefore, an infection.

INFANTILE SCURVY (BARLOW'S DISEASE)

Although scurvy was described in children in 1650, no further reports appeared until over 200 years later (40–42). Scurvy in children appears somewhat different from that in adults. The child is in pain and screams with the slightest touch or movement. Swelling may occur about the knees with thickening of some bones (43).

In 1859 and 1862, Moeller of Kaliningrad described two children with "acute rickets." One child had swollen gums, "very nearly like a complete scorbutic state" (40). However, Moeller dismissed scurvy and considered the children to be suffering from "acute rickets." In 1883, Barlow of London described "acute rickets" as probably a combination of rickets and scurvy, with scurvy essential and rickets variable (44). In further studies, Barlow described in detail the clinical and pathological manifestations of infantile scurvy as well as its cause and means of treatment (42,43).

Barlow recognized that periosteal hemorrhage which resulted in deep-seated swellings in the limbs and intense pain occurred in children with scurvy. Barlow successfully treated scorbutic children with fresh cow's milk, juice of raw beef, and 2 teaspoonfuls of orange juice daily. Consequently, infantile scurvy is often referred to as Barlow's disease. Sir Thomas Barlow died in 1945 at the age of 100 years. Those interested in his accomplishments are referred to the articles by Aspin (45) and Lomax (46).

Frölich showed that raw milk normally contains enough of the antiscorbutic substance to provide complete protection from scurvy (47). He demonstrated that pasteurization of milk, if not properly conducted, could destroy the antiscorbutic substance and lead to infantile scurvy.

In 1914, Hess and Fish (48,49,49a) wrote,

> We must mention the very interesting and suggestive studies of Funk. This author had coined the word "vitamins" for substances which are essential to the health and life of the body, and the lack of which produces a group of diseases which he has termed the "avitaminosen," including beriberi, scurvy, pellagra and rickets. They are essential to life, although present in very small amounts. Such is the definition which Funk gives of the substances which he considers play an important and even vital part in nutrition.

Hess and Fish in their treatment of cases of infantile scurvy accepted the views of Funk (48,49). They stated, "There is no physiologic reason why orange juice should not be given in small quantities to an infant a few weeks of age."

During World War I, when fresh fruits and vegetables became scarce, a marked increase in infantile scurvy occurred, notably in Russia, Germany, and Austria (50). The incidence was particularly high in children of age 8 to 10 months (42). In 1919, Harden and associates prepared concentrates of the antiscorbutic substance in lemon juice. The preparations were used successfully to treat scorbutic children (41,51,52).

In 1955, Parson was the first physician to administer ascorbic acid (vitamin C) to a patient with infantile scurvy (53). The ascorbic acid was obtained from Albert Szent-Györgyi. The administration of a total of 450 mg of ascorbic acid over a period of 2 weeks was successful in treating the child. With the introduction of orange juice and other preparations of vitamin C in infant feeding, the occurrence of infantile scurvy has become rare. Nevertheless, cases of infantile scurvy continue to occur, primarily as a result of poor nutrition education.

SCURVY ON LAND

Early a belief was held that "sea scurvy" was different from "land scurvy" (54), although Lind in his Treatise (31) did not agree with this assumption. Lemon and other citrus fruits were recognized as the therapies of sea scurvy, but land scurvy was considered to be responsive to other treatments. In the sixteenth century, treatment for land scurvy employed preparations from specific "antiscorbutic" plants, which included scurvy grass (*Cochlearia officinalis*), water cress (*Nasturtium officinalis*), and brooklime (*Veronica beccabunga*) (54). Scurvy grass has been reported to contain an average of 60 mg ascorbic acid/100 g of fresh weight (54). Water cress contained somewhat more (83 mg/100 g), and brooklime had somewhat less (45 mg/100 g) (54). Food composition tables list the vitamin C content for the following foods (55,56):

Food item	Vitamin C content, mg/100 g
Willow (leaves)	465
Lemon juice	53
Lime juice	37
Orange juice	50
Watercress	68
Scurvy grass (stems and seedpods)	111
Alpine bearberry (berries)	52
Cabbage, raw, green	46
Turnips greens, cooked	60
Dandelion (leaves)	66

Scurvy on land was usually associated with military actions, sieges, and famines (7). Hippocrates (460–370 B.C.) noted a large number of men in an army with pains in the legs and gangrene of the gums associated with the loss of teeth. Although not established conclusively, the condition would suggest the presence of scurvy.

The Crusaders suffered greatly from pestilence and scurvy. Often they fell to siege and were subjected to starvation accompanied by scurvy. Thus the Third Crusade of 1189 under King Richard the Lion Hearted of England, King Philip II of France, and Emperor Frederick Barbarossa of Germany fell to siege and the consequences of scurvy. A similar fate befell the Fifth Crusade (1216–1220) and the Seventh Crusade (1249–1254).

Many other sieges and military disasters occurred in subsequent years. Lind in his Treatise of the Scurvy describes the siege of Thorn in Hungary in 1703 (31), which lasted 5 months and resulted in approximately 5000 deaths from scurvy in the besieged garrison. A considerable number of civilians also died of scurvy. Outbreaks were common in the Russian armies during the eighteenth century.

In 1734, the Hungarian Army was struck with scurvy, presumably because of a lack of fresh fruits and vegetables in the diet of the common soldiers. Officers who had green vegetables available seldom experienced scurvy (14).

British troops fighting in North America in 1756 and 1759 suffered losses due to scurvy.

During the Crimean War of 1854–1856, particularly during the siege of the Russian Naval Base at Sebastobol, scurvy was epidemic in the British Army. Dr. Douglas A. Reid, soldier-surgeon of the British Army, credited this to the failure of the army to provide fresh provisions, green vegetables, and lime juice. The French Army and Fleet as well as the Turkish Army also encountered a high incidence of scurvy during the Crimean War (2).

During the Russo-Japanese War of 1904 to 1905, Port Arthur was under siege. The siege lasted for six months. By its end, half of the garrison of 32,000 Russians was afflicated with scurvy (7).

SCURVY AND WAR TIMES

American Revolutionary War

British troops in the New World before the American Revolution observed scurvy during the late winter months. Use of a concoction prepared from spruce or hemlock appeared to have been of benefit in the treatment of scorbutic soldiers.

British forces during the American Revolutionary War period also experienced outbreaks of scurvy during the late winter and early spring months. During the war period of 1775–1783, Sir Gilbert Blane stated that of the 175,990 British men enrolled for war at sea, only 1243 were killed in action (11), but deaths from disease and scurvy claimed 18,545 men. Scurvy was a major cause of these deaths.

During the American Revolution, the Continental Army of General George Washington was supplied with spruce beer and a small amount of lime juice. The United States Navy came into being in 1775 with a fleet of 13 ships. At the end of the American Revolutionary War, the navy was abolished. However, in 1794, the Congress reversed itself and ordered four warships be built. Edwart Cutbush (1772–1843) entered the U.S. Navy as a surgeon in 1799. He was one of the first Americans to employ lemon juice to prevent scurvy. He noted that "a ship furnished plentifully with lemon juice may bid defiance to the scurvy" (24). Dr. William Paul Crillon Barton served as the surgeon on the warship *United States* in 1809. He used lime or lemon juice to prevent scurvy as he was a strong believer in its benefits.

John Boit, an American, commanded the *Columbia* on a four-year trading voyage to the northwest coast of the United States and to China. His diary makes note of the occurrence of scurvy on his voyage. Thus, in 1791, he noted "some of the crew have the scurvy in the gums"; "four seamen laid by the scurvy; their mouths and legs are very bad"; "although there was ten of them in the last stage of the scurvy, still they soon recovered upon the smelling of the turf and eating gress of various kinds" (1).

In subsequent years, the poor provisions supplied the American soldiers resulted in outbreaks of scurvy. For instance, in 1809, United States soldiers stationed on the Mississippi River below New Orleans suffered 600 deaths from scurvy. Fort Atkinson, Nebraska, in 1819–1820, experienced a severe outbreak of scurvy leading to 157 deaths out of 788 troops. Fort McIntosh, Texas, in 1852, and the Ringgold Barracks, Texas, in 1854, both reported that scurvy was a common disease. Both used juice from the American agave to treat the disease with beneficial results (7).

American Civil War

During the American Civil War, more deaths resulted from diarrhea, dysentery, and scurvy than from battle injuries (20). Scurvy was diagnosed in 46,931 Union troops. There was a constant occurrence of cases of scurvy among both the Union and Confederate troops. Several epidemics occurred. One major outbreak occurred in General Sherman's troops during the seige of Atlanta in 1864. Approximately 3000 Union soldiers imprisoned at Andersonville, Georgia, died from scurvy. The physicians of the Civil War (e.g., Drs. Tripler and Letterman) were familiar with scurvy. They were aware of the importance of fresh vegetables and fruits in the prevention and treatment of scurvy. However, wartime conditions prevented their availability and distribution to the troops.

World War I

During World War I, scurvy occurred among civilian populations as a result of rationing. Military personnel were also affected. Military rations were often nutritionally inadequate. Scurvy was extensive in the Indian troops in Mesopotamia in 1915 and 1916 (57,58). During the siege of Kut-el-Amara, 1050 cases of scurvy were reported. All but one case occurred in the Indian troops. The absence of scurvy in the British troops appears to have been related to their use of fresh meat, which provided a small amount of vitamin C. The Indian troops, because of religions scruples, avoided eating meat. Subsequently, with the use of vegetable gardens, scurvy essentially disappeared among the troops.

During World War I, the war, aggravated by the breakups of the government, resulted in the widespread presence of scurvy in Russia. During World War I, scurvy was commonly observed in other European armies, including the French, Serbian, Romanian, Austrian, and German armies. In June 1917 the French Army suffered a serious outbreak of scurvy, due to the lack of fresh vegetables and fruits in the rations.

World War II

During World War II, the United States military avoided scurvy by careful ration planning and concern about the nutritional well-being of the military personnel. As a consequence, the Food and Nutrition Board of the National Academy of Sciences was established to provide guidance for "planning and processing food supplies for national defense." This guidance evolved into the Recommended Dietary Allowances (59). However, scurvy occurred among American prisoners of war in Southeast Asia.

Colonel John E. Olson has written extensively on his experiences during World War II as a Japanese prisoner of war in the O'Donnell Prison Camp, located north of Clark Air Base in the Philippines (60). Colonel Olson fell into the hands of the Japanese on April 9, 1942, on the Bataan peninsula. After participating in the Bataan Death March, he arrived in Camp O'Donnell on April 14, 1942. During the next 70 days, of approximately 9000 American officers and enlisted men, 1253 died (17%). Col. Olson recounted on August 24, 1942, "Scurvy becoming a problem." On September 1942, surveys were made of the hospital patients: "Their results confirmed the generally held opinion that the large morbidity and mortality in the concentration camp were primarily the results of malnutrition and other concomitant conditions" (60).

Subsequently, Maj. General Yoshitaka Kawane and Col. Kurataro Hirano were convicted of war crimes and hanged. They were held responsible for about 10,000 American and Filipino deaths in the infamous Bataan march and 25,000 later deaths in Camp O'Donnell (60).

SEARCH FOR THE NORTHWEST PASSAGE

Voyages from Europe into the Arctic began at the end of the sixteenth century with the hopes of finding a northern passage to the Orient. Expeditions had been made during the summer months to catch fish and whales near Greenland and Spitsbergen. Expeditions that attempted in their explorations to remain over winter in the Arctic often encountered dire consequences. Scurvy was encountered routinely, followed by death. Many of these excursions into the Arctic and Antarctic regions have been summarized vividly, by Ragnar Nicolaysen (10), Kenneth Carpenter (2), Eleanora C. Gordon (61), A. F. Rodgers (62), and H. E. Levis (63).

An example is the voyage of Captain Jens Munk to Hudson Bay in May 1619, on orders from King Christian of Denmark (10,61). His expedition of two ships sailed westward out of Copenhagen in search of the Northwest Passage to China. Forty-eight men were on the frigate *Unicorn* (Enhorningen), and 16 on the sloop *Lambrey* (Lamparanen). In September 1619, after entering Hudson Bay in search of the passage, the expedition encountered heavy snowstorms and decided to winter over in Hudson Bay near the present-day Churchill. Disaster beset the expedition by December 1619. Dysentery complicated with scurvy resulted in a heavy toll of the personnel. Munk states in his journal that by February 16, 1620, only 7 of the crew were healthy and 20 persons had died. By March, 34 were still alive but were sick. He states that their mouths were affected with scurvy (61).

Munk wrote that on May 28, only seven miserable persons were still alive, too weak to do anything. Captain Munk, who stayed on ship (*Enhorningen*), shortly thereafter became ill and immobilized. Two surviving crewman who wintered ashore, themselves debilitated, managed to nurse Captain Munk back to health aided by his eating green shoots that appeared in the Arctic spring. Eventually these three survivors of the 65 who left Denmark in 1619 were able to sail away in their little sloop *Lambrey*. Miraculously the three survivors arrived in Bergen, Norway, on September 21, 1620. Ironically, Munk was arrested and imprisoned for losing the ship *Enhorningen*.

ARCTIC AND ANTARCTIC EXPLORATIONS

During the late 1800s to the early 1900s, a fascination existed for exploration of the Arctic and Antarctic regions. Kenneth Carpenter (2) and Ragnar Nicolaysen (10) have provided a chronological summary of many of these interesting but often tragic expeditions. Most were accompanied by scurvy. Captain R. F. Scott's fatal expedition in 1911–1912 to the South Pole was extensively documented by his own diary (62,63). Scurvy appears to have had a role in this unfortunate venture as Scott's expedition did not take any antiscorbutics with them.

The British expedition to the Arctic in 1847–1859 under McClure on the *Investigator* used real lemon juice from the Mediterranean and was free of scurvy. In a second expedition to the Arctic, Captain George Nares left England in May 1875 with two ships, *Alert* and *Discovery*, in an attempt to reach the North Pole (11,16). The two ships wintered in the ice of the Greenland coast. During this period, Nares sent out sleighing parties. Lime juice was not provided the parties. Soon after traveling on the ice, they suffered scurvy (64). Scurvy weakened one group of 17 men so severely that they could not get back to their ship. Help was provided by a relief party. Fortunately lime juice was available on the ships. Lime juice from West Indian limes, which later proved to have less vitamin C than lemons, was used.

The report of A. H. Smith (64) would indicate that the juice used by the British Navy termed "lime juice" was frequently the juice of lemons and not that of limes. Moreover, lemon juice has approximately four times more vitamin C than lime juice and may account for some of the failures of lime juice to protect sailors against scurvy. These failures placed the use of limes and lemons in the prevention of scurvy in confusion, question, and uncertainty. Nevertheless, the nickname "limey" has been applied to British sailors.

POTATO FAMINE

Although scurvy at sea was largely eliminated by 1800, the disease referred to as "land scurvy" occurred at various times. In many instances the scurvy disappeared when potatoes from the New World were included in the regular meal. Whaling ships spending months at sea relied on potatoes to protect them against scurvy (26).

The potato had long been a staple for the Inca and Aztec populations of Central and South America. In the late sixteenth century, potatoes were introduced into Europe, where they were regarded with suspicion, partly because of the resemblance of the potato flowers to that of the poisonous nightshade. However, during the eighteenth century, the potato began to be generally cultivated and eaten throughout Europe. Its use eliminated scurvy that had occurred in various areas, such as Ireland, Scotland, and Norway. Potatoes as we now know can provide a significant amount of vitamin C. However, dependence on potatoes became a tragedy.

The summer of 1845 was especially cold and wet in Great Britain and elsewhere in Northern Europe. The potato crop was decimated by blight. The crop failed again in 1846. With the potato as a major staple, this resulted in a severe famine in Britain. Along with starvation, scurvy made its appearance. Ireland was particularly hard hit, leading to a major emigration of the population. With a normal crop of potatoes in 1848, scurvy virtually disappeared from the British population.

CALIFORNIA GOLD RUSH

Many of the emigrants to the western United States in the 1840s and 1850s traveled by ship that had traveled around the treacherous Cape Horn. Scurvy outbreaks were common on these long voyages. In 1850, over 36,000 immigrants arrived in San Francisco. Often passengers after arrival developed scurvy from the exertion of unloading and carrying their baggage. Of the miners, it has been estimated that from 1840 to 1855, 1 in 36 had frank scurvy, with a mortality rate of 30% (2,28). During the California gold rush of 1848–1850, it is estimated that at least 10,000 men died of scurvy. Interestingly, the shortages of oranges and limes at that time stimulated the beginning of commercial production of citrus fruits in Southern California.

RUSSIA AND ALASKA

Early contacts of Russia with Alaska were primarily for fur trading. But in 1783, the Russians attempted to establish settlements (29). Three ships with 192 men aboard, under the command of Grigor Ivanovich Shelikof, left Okhotsh, Siberia, in August 1783. One ship became separated in a storm; the other two wintered on Bering Island. In June 1784, the two ships sailed to Kodiak Island. After landing at what is now Karluk, Alaska, many of the Russians developed scurvy and died. Continuing on, the Russians established their first permanent settlement at Three Saints Harbor in 1790. This small settlement of about 50 Russians planted cabbages and potatoes and apparently escaped scurvy. Other settlements by the Russians were not so fortunate and frequently were bothered by scurvy during the winter months. The settlement of Sitka, Alaska, with 200 residents, suffered from starvation and scurvy. It was reported that eight deaths occurred and 60 inhabitants were disabled.

After the purchase of Alaska from Russia in 1867, gold was discovered there but only in small amounts. However, the Klondike gold discovery of 1896–1899, in Canada, resulted in an influx of droves of ill-prepared prospectors. Most of the prospectors entered Canada through Alaskan ports and then by foot, horseback, and dog sled to the gold fields. The numbers of prospectors that arrived far exceeded expectations, resulting in severe food shortages during the winters of 1897–1899. As a result starvation set in as well as scurvy, typhoid, and pneumonia. In some villages, it was estimated that 75% suffered from scurvy, and 10% died. This was the last catastrophic occurrence of scurvy on the North American continent.

WHALING INDUSTRY

Whaling has been conducted for several thousand years. For centuries whales were pursued as a source of oil, meat, and whalebone. An early whaling settlement was established in Greenland around 985 A.D. by the Viking Eric the Red (23). Before the seventeenth century, the Basques from the Bay of Biscay developed a highly profitable whaling enterprise. During the seventeenth and eighteenth centuries, other countries entered the whaling trade. The Dutch, English, German, and Norwegians developed major whaling industries. In the nineteenth century, the United States became the leading whaling country. The American fleet represented about 40,000 men. The average length of a whaling cruise around the year 1850 was 42 months. With such lengthy voyages, scurvy became a curse of whaling. McCord has summarized many of the encounters with scurvy among the whaling expeditions of the nineteenth century (23). In 1925, the last whaling fleet sent out from the United States embarked from New Bedford, Massachusetts. Limited whaling continues in several countries, including Japan and Russia.

EARLY CONCEPT OF VITAMINS

George Budd (1808–1882)

It should be noted that George Budd, a London physician, wrote in 1840 "that scurvy resulted from the lack of an essential factor that would be discovered by organic chemistry or the experiments of physiologists in the near future" (65). He had proposed already in 1842 that accessory food factors were required components of diets and their absence from the diet resulted in recognizable deficiency diseases (66). Budd described three diseases that he considered could be "traced to defective nutrients" (67). He stated, "The first and best known of these is scurvy properly so called; of the second the most distinctive character is a peculiar ulceration of the cornea; the third is chiefly marked by softness of imperfect development of the bones." We now recognize these three conditions as deficiencies of vitamins C, A, and D, respectively. Unfortunately, Budd was more than 50 years ahead of his time. Hence, his nutritional observations and concepts on the existence of accessory food factors received little recognition and thus produced little impact on the nutritional developments of the 1800s.

Casimir Funk (1884–1967)

In 1912, Casimir Funk, a Polish chemist working in the Lister Institute in London, wrote a landmark publication (68,69) (see Fig. 3). In his publication he announced his "vitamine theory," in which he proposed four different vitamins. He chose the term "*vitamine*" because his investigations indicated that the antiberiberi factor was an amine: hence, a "vital amine." Funk proposed four "vitamines," namely, antiberiberi "vitamine," antiscurvy "vitamine," antipellagra "vitamine," and antirickets "vitamine."

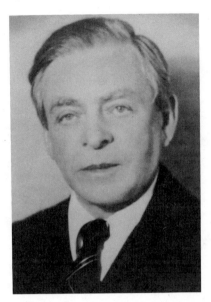

Figure 3   Casimir Funk (1884–1967).

With foresight, Funk wrote: "I must admit that when I chose the name 'vitamine' I was well aware that these substances might later prove not at all to be of an amine nature. However, it was necessary for me to use a name that would sound well and serve as a 'catch-word.'" Although the "vitamine" that Funk isolated proved to have no antiberiberi activity, his theory provided a new concept for interpreting diet-related events.

DISCOVERY OF VITAMIN C

Holst and Frölich

By the end of the 1800s, the cause of scurvy remained uncertain. It was recognized that citrus fruits could cure scurvy, although the concept that the disease was caused by the lack of nutrient in the diet was not accepted. Scurvy was considered to be the result of a specific infection, or ptomaine poisoning, or unsanitary conditions, overwork, and exposure to dampness and cold. The medical community, influenced by Louis Pasteur, was attracted to the germ theory of disease. Hence, at the beginning of the twentieth century, scurvy, beriberi, and rickets, and later pellagra were considered to be caused by a bacterium or bacterial toxin.

At the beginning of the twentieth century, the investigations of Holst and Frölich and the concepts of Funk set the stage for resolving the cause of scurvy. In 1907, Axel Holst (see Fig. 4) with the help of Theodor Frölich, both from Norway, reported that the diseases "ship beriberi" (scurvy) and infantile scurvy could be produced experimentally in the guinea pig (70,71) by feeding a simple diet of oats, barley, rye, and wheat. Feeding the guinea pigs fresh apples, fresh potatoes, fresh cabbage, or fresh lemon juice prevented the disease.

Actually Theobald Smith in 1895 was the first to induce scurvy in guinea pigs fed on an oat and bran diet (14). He noted a disease condition developed that could be prevented with

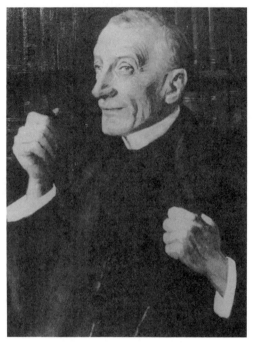

Figure 4   Axel Holst (1860–1931).

supplements of clover, grass, or vegetables such as cabbage (72). Smith was studying a bacillus in swine disease and apparently failed to recognize that he had experimentally induced scurvy in his guinea pigs.

The report of Holst and Frölich stimulated intensive investigations during the next 20 years in an attempt to isolate and characterize the essential nutrient. The first successful attempt to make a highly potent concentrate of vitamin C was that of Harden and Zilva in 1918 (52). During the 1920s, S. S. Zilva, at the Lister Institute in London, was particularly active in vitamin C research and was considered the leader in the field. Of interest, however, in 1927, Albert Szent-Györgyi isolated a reducing agent from adrenal glands, orange juice, and cabbage (73). A sample of the isolates was sent to Zilva, who made the pronouncement that it could not be vitamin C. This error delayed the identification of the vitamin for several years. Extensive investigations were also conducted during the period of 1918–1930 as to the antiscorbutic contents of fruit, fruit juice preparations, and vegetables. These efforts were striking in that the antiscorbutic substance had not yet been isolated or characterized and the analyses were dependent on the use of a guinea pig bioassay. These efforts have been largely summarized in the writings of McCollum and associates (14,15) and of Sherman and Smith (13).

Isolation of Vitamin C: Early Attempts

During the period 1920–1930, several "near misses" occurred in the attempt to isolate and identify vitamin C (38). Among them was that of Karl Paul Link of the University of Wisconsin. He prepared several grams of calcium ascorbate but was unable to demonstrate its antiscorbutic acitivity because the dean at the university refused him a research grant of a few hundred dollars for the bioassay of his of material (65,75). Ironically, years later Link brought millions of dollars to the University of Wisconsin through his research on vitamin K antagonists, such as dicumarol, and patents on rodenticides, such as warfarin (coumadin). Warfarin was named for the Wisconsin Alumni Research Foundation.

Similarly, in 1927 Edward B. Vedder had made a crude preparation of vitamin C. At the time, Col. Vedder was a commissioned pathologist in the Office of the Surgeon General of the U.S. Army. Before he was able to carry out the essential bioassays on his material, he was transferred to another position (76,77). His essay, "A Study of the Antiscorbutic Vitamin," was named the Wellcome Prize Essay in 1932 by the Association of Military Surgeons (77).

Colonel Vedder played an important role also in the discovery of thiamin. While in the Philippines during the period 1909–1912, Vedder tracked down the cause of beriberi; and demonstrated that it was a deficiency disease. He prepared extracts from rice bran that would cure infants dying from beriberi; not being a chemist, he enlisted Dr. Robert Ramapatnam Williams, a chemist, to isolate the lifesaving component in the extract. In 1933, Williams, along with his colleagues Robert E. Waterman and John C. Keresztesy, succeeded in isolating and characterizing the anti-beriberi factor, thiamin.

Isolation, Characterization, Synthesis of Ascorbic Acid

Controversy has existed as to who should be credited with the discovery of vitamin C as the antiscorbutic factor. Two groups were studying the factor:Charles Glen King (see Fig.5) and his associates W. A. Waugh and J. L. Svirbely, at the University of Pittsburgh, in Pennsylvania, and Albert Imre Szent-Györgyi von Nagyrapolt at the University of Szeged, in Hungary. Several reports regarding this controversy have appeared (2,65,78-83). These citations provide interesting reading. Undoubtedly the contributions of the two groups were complementary.

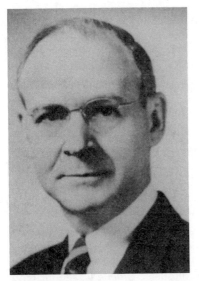

Figure 5   Charles Glen King (1896–1988).

In 1931, Svirbely and King obtained crystalline vitamin C from lemon juice and found it to have the physical and chemical properties associated with hexuronic acid (84). Subsequently, on April 1, 1932, King and Waugh reported that daily feeding of approximately 0.5 mg of the recrystalled vitamin C protected guinea pigs from scurvy and permitted normal growth (84,85). They also reported on the vitamin C activity of hexuronic acid isolated from suprarenal glands by E. C. Kendal at Mayo Clinic in Minnesota. They found the hexuronic acid was identical to their vitamin C in its ability to protect the guinea pig from scurvy (86).

Two weeks later, on April 16, 1932, Svirbely and Szent-Györgyi reported that crystalline hexuronic acid prepared earlier also at the Mayo Clinic from beef adrenal glands had antiscorbutic acitvity (87). Guinea pigs that received 1 mg of the hexuronic acid daily were protected from the development of scurvy. As an interesting background, Svirbely, who was American-born, had moved several months earlier from King's laboratory to that of Szent-Györgyi in Szeged, Hungary. Szent-Györgyi had isolated "hexuronic acid" as a result of his interest in a reducing factor found in adrenal cortex, cabbage, oranges, and other sources (73,87).

When Szent-Györgyi isolated the reducing agent, he knew it was related to sugars, but unsure of which sugar. As he stated, "Ignosco meaning 'don't know' and the ending 'ose' meaning sugar, I called this carbohydrate 'Ignose.' Harden, the editor of the *Biochemical Journal*, did not like jokes and reprimanded me. 'Godnose' was not more successful and so, following Harden's proposition, I called the new substance 'hexuronic acid' since it had 6 C's and was acidic" (73).

Szent-Györgyi had a quantity of hexuronic acid, which he gave to the newly arrived Svirbely to test for vitaminic activity. Szent-Györgyi stated, "I expected he would find it identical to vitamin C. I always had a strong hunch that this was so but never had tested it. I was not acquainted with animal tests in this field and the whole problem was, for me, too glamorous, and vitamins were, to my mind, theoretically uninteresting! Vitamin means that one has to eat it. What one has to eat is the first concern of the chef, not the scientist" (73). Regardless, in 1937 "chef" Albert Szent-Györgyi received the Nobel Prize for physiology and medicine.

The structure of hexuronic acid (vitamin C) was elucidated in 1933 by E. L. Hirst and W. N. Haworth using material isolated by Szent-Györgyi in the chemical laboratory of the Mayo Clinic, Rochester, Minnesota (88). Haworth and Szent-Györgyi adopted the name "L-ascorbic acid" to reflect the antiscorbutic properties of vitamin C. In 1937, Haworth was awarded the Nobel Prize in chemistry for his carbohydrate and vitamin studies. Studies on the chemical properties of vitamin C were greatly facilitated by the discovery of Szent-Györgyi and Svirbely that Hungarian red peppers (paprika) were extraordinarily rich in vitamin C. Thus, they were able shortly to prepare a kilogram of the pure substance from these peppers (73,89). In 1933, ascorbic acid was synthesized by Reichstein, Grussner, and Oppenheimer (90). Patents on the commercial production of vitamin C were arranged with Hoffmann-La Roche. L-Ascorbic acid is now synthesized in large tonnages for human nutrition, animal feeds, pharmaceutical use, and industrial applications.

Albert Szent-Györgyi was born in Hungary in 1893 and died in 1986 at the age of 93. Charles Glen King was born in Entiat, Washington, in 1896 and died in 1988 in Pennsylvania at the age of 92.

Originally the factor that prevented scurvy was designated as the antiscorbutic vitamin. In 1920, Drummond proposed to call the antiscorbutic substance *vitamin C*, and the term was widely adopted (91). In 1933, when hexuronic acid proved to be vitamin C, Haworth and Szent-Györgyi renamed it *ascorbic acid* (73). The term was generally accepted by chemists but raised objections from the American Medical Association because of its therapeutic suggestiveness. The Council on Pharmacy and Chemistry of the American Medical Association introduced the term *cevitamic acid*. This name was not generally accepted and went out of use. Currently vitamin C is commonly used as a generic term by nutritionists and is generally familiar to the public, whereas ascorbic acid, as a specific compound, is usually used by chemists.

CONCLUSION

During the depression years of the 1930s, many cases of scurvy were observed, particularly in the large cities. This was the result of poor housing, insufficient food, and lack of sources of vitamin C in the diet.

Despite our knowledge and the availability of vitamin C, outbreaks of scurvy may still occur, particularly in refugee camps. Two thousand cases of scurvy were reported in 1982 in Somali refugee camps (12); in 1986, over 4000 cases were noted in camps in eastern Sudan (12). Relief provisions are frequently inadequate in vitamin C.

The British Antarctic Survey in 1975 was reported by S. Vallance to have had a basic diet deficient in ascorbic acid (11), reflected in low blood levels of vitamin C in the members. The use of citrus juices and multivitamin tablets resulted in satisfactory blood concentrations of vitamin C.

With the identity of ascorbic acid established and efficient and inexpensive production of the vitamin available, attention could be turned to studies on its role in physiological and biochemical functions. The pathological changes and clinical signs and symptoms associated with a vitamin C deficiency evidenced in the scorbutic patient are not fully explained by our current state of knowledge of the vitamin. Some uncertainty even exists as to the amount of vitamin C required for optimal health (59,92,93). Subsequent chapters of this book may provide definitive answers as to the specific biochemical function(s) of ascorbic acid.

ACKNOWLEDGMENTS

The photographs of the nutrition scientists used in this chapter appeared in Darby, W. J., Jukes, J. H., eds. *Founders of Nutrition Science*, Vols. 1 and 2. Bethesda, MD: American Institute of Nutrition, 1992. The photographs are used with the permission of the American Institute of Nutrition.

The assistance of Ms. Donna Janine Smith in the preparation of the manuscript is deeply appreciated.

REFERENCES

1. Foley GPH. A treatment of dentistry: a causerie on scurvy. J Am Coll Dent 1986; 53:27–30.
2. Carpenter KJ. The History of Scurvy and Vitamin C. Cambridge: Cambridge University Press, 1986.
3. Major RH. Classic Descriptions of Disease. Springfield, IL: Charles C Thomas, 1932:575–578.
4. Mellinkoff SM. History of medicine: James Lind's legacy to clinical medicine. West J Med 1995; 162:367–369.
5. Dickman SR. The search for the specific factor in scurvy. Perspect Biol Med 1981; 24:382–395.

6. Hargreaves R. Seafarer's scourge. Practitioner 1967; 198:292–301.
7. McCord CP. Scurvy as an occupational disease. VII. Scurvy in the world's armies. J Occup Med 1971; 13:586–592.
8. Kinnier Wilson JV. Organic diseases of ancient Mesopotamia. In: Brothwell D, Sandison AT, eds. Diseases in Antiquity. Springfield, IL: Charles C Thomas, 1967.
9. Rosner F. Scurvy in the Talmud. NY State J Med 1972; 72:2818–2819.
10. Nicolaysen R. Arctic nutrition. Perspect Biol Med 1980; 23:295–310.
11. Watt J. Nutrition in adverse environments. I. Forgotten lessons of maritime nutrition. Hum Nutr Appl Nutr 1982; 36A:35–45.
12. Sheehy TW. Scurvy. Ala Med 1990; 60:11–17.
13. Sherman HC, Smith SL. The Vitamins. New York: American Chemical Society Monograph Series, The Chemical Catalog Co., Boston: 1931: 148–200.
14. McCollum EV. A History of Nutrition. Boston: Houghton Mifflin, 1957: 252–265.
15. McCollum EV, Orent-Keiles E, Day HG. The Newer Knowledge of Nutrition. New York: Macmillan, 1939: 398–440.
16. Wilson LG. The clinical definition of scurvy and the discovery of vitamin C. J History Med Allied Sci 1975; 30:40–60.
17. Lee RV. Scurvy: a contemporary historical perspective (Part 2). Conn Med 1983; 47:703–704.
18. Lee RV. Scurvy: a contemporary historical perspective (Part 3). Conn Med 1984; 48:33–35.
19. McBride WM. "Normal" medical science and British treatment of the sea scurvy, 1753–75. J Hist Med Allied Sci 1991; 46:158–177.
20. Bollet AJ. Scurvy and chronic diarrhea in Civil War troops: were they both nutritional deficiency syndromes? J Hist Med Allied Sci 1992; 47:49–67.
21. McCord CP. Scurvy as an occupational disease. I. Introduction. J Occup Med 1971; 13:306–307.
22. McCord CP. Scurvy as an occupational disease. II. Early sea explorations. J Occup Med 1971; 13:348–351.
23. McCord CP. Scurvy as an occupational disease. III. Scurvy during early global circumnavigations. J Occup Med 1971; 13:393–395.
24. McCord CP. Scurvy as an occupational disease. IV. Scurvy and the nations' men-of-war. J Occup Med 1971; 13:441–447.
25. McCord CP. Scurvy as an occupational disease. V. Scurvy and the merchant marines. J Occup Med 1971; 13:484–491.
26. McCord CP. Scurvy as an occupational disease. VI. Scurvy among the whalers. J Occup Med 1971; 13:543–548.
27. McCord CP. Scurvy as an occupational disease. VIII. Scurvy and the slave trade. J Occup Med 1972; 14:45–49.
28. McCord CP. Scurvy as an occupational disease. X. Scurvy among early American western migrants. J Occup Med 1972; 14:321–324.
29. McCord CP. Scurvy as an occupational disease. XI. Scurvy and gold in Alaska. J Occup Med 1972; 14:397–398.
30. McCord CP. Scurvy as an occupational disease. XII. Scurvy in the early American colonies. J Occup Med 1972; 14:556–559.
31. Lind J. A Treatise of the Scurvy in Three Parts. Containing an Inquiry into the Nature, Causes, and Cure of that Disease. Together with a Critical and Chronological View of What Has Been Published on the Subject. 1st ed. Edinburgh: Sands, Murray, and Cochran, printers, 1753.
31a. Krehl WA. James Lind, MD. J Nutr 1953; 50:1–11.
32. Hughs RE. James Lind and the cure of scurvy: an experimental approach. Med Hist 1975; 19:342–351.
33. Editorial: the Cook bicentenary. NZ Med J 1969; 70:257–258.
34. Gluckman LK. Cook's voyages to New Zealand in medical perspective. NZ Med J 1969; 70:219–222.

35. Fite GL. Captain James Cook (1728–1779). JAMA 1969; 209:1217–1218.
36. Wynder EL. James Lind's discovery of the causes of scurvy. Prev Med 1974; 3:300–305.
37. Leach RD. Sir Gilbert Blane, Bart, MD FRS (1749–1832). Ann R Coll Surg Engl 1980; 62: 232–239.
38. Davies MB, Austin J, Partridge DA. Vitamin C: its chemistry and biochemistry. Cambridge: Royal Society of Chemistry, 1991.
39. Claiborne J. Inaugural Essay on Scurvy. University of Pennsylvania, May 22, 1798. Philadelphia: Stephen C. Ustick, printers, 1798.
40. Evans PR. Infantile scurvy: the centenary of Barlow's disease. Br Med J 1983; 287:1862–1863.
41. Still GF. Infantile scurvy: its history. Arch Dis Child 1935; 10:211–218.
42. Vyhmeister IR. The incidence of infantile scurvy: a problem of yesteryear and today. Med Arts Sci 1967; 1:9–22.
43. Barlow T. Infantile scurvy and its relation to rickets. Lancet 1894; ii:1029–1034.
44. Barlow T. On cases described as "acute rickets" which are possibly a combination of rickets and scurvy, the scurvy being essential and the rickets variable. Medico-Chirugical Trans 1883; 66:159–220 (reprinted in Arch Dis Child 1935; 10:223–252).
45. Aspin RK. Illustrations from the Wellcome Institute library: The papers of Sir Thomas Barlow (1845–1945). Med Hist 1993; 37:333–340.
46. Lomax E. Difficulties in diagnosing infantile scurvy before 1878. Med Hist 1986; 30:70–80.
47. Frölich T. Experimentelle untersuchungen uber den infantilen skorbut. Z Hyg Infektionskrankh 1912; 72:155–182.
48. Hess AF, Fish M. Infantile scurvy: the blood, the blood-vessels and the diet. Am J Dis Child 1914; 8:399–405.
49a. Darby WJ, Woodruff CW. Alfred Fabian Hess: a biographical sketch. J Nutr 1960; 71:1–9.
49. Hess AF. Scurvy: Past and Present. Philadelphia: Lippincott, 1920.
50. Hess AF. Scurvy in the world war. Int J Pub Health 1920; I:302–307.
51. Harden A, Zilva SS, Still GF. Infantile scurvy: the antiscorbutic factor of lemon juice in treatment. Lancet 1919; 196:17–18.
52. Harden A, Zilva SS. The antiscorbutic factor in lemon juice. Biochem J 1918; 12:259–269.
53. Parson LG. Scurvy treated with ascorbic acid. Proc R Soc Med 1933; 23:1533.
54. Hughes RW. The rise and fall of the "antiscorbutics": Some notes on the traditional cures for "land scurvy." Med Hist 1990; 34:52–64.
55. Leveille GA, Zabik ME, Morgan KJ. Nutrients in Foods. Cambridge, MA: Nutrition Guild, 1983.
56. Bauernfeind JC. Ascorbic acid technology in agricultural, pharmacentical, food, and industrial applications. In: Seib PA, Tolbert BM, eds. Ascorbic Acid: Chemistry, Metabolism and Uses, Advances in Chemistry Series, 1982, No. 200. Washington, DC: American Chemical Society.
57. Willcox WH. Rations in relation of disease in Mesopotamia. Lancet 1917; II:677.
58. Willcox WH. The treatment and management of diseases due to deficiency of diet: scurvey and beriberi. Br Med J 1920; 3081:73–77.
59. Food and Nutrition Board. Recommended Dietary Allowances. 10th ed. Washington, DC: National Academy Press, 1989.
60. Olson JE. O'Donnell: Andersonville of the Pacific. Kansas City, KS: Published by John E. Olson, Lake Quivira, 1985.
61. Gordon EC. The voyage of Captain Munk to Hudson Bay in 1619: an analysis of a medical catastrophe. Trans Studies Coll Physicians Phila 1989; 11:13–27.
62. Rogers AF. The death of Chief Petty Officer Evans. Practitioner 1974; 212:570–580.
63. Lewis HE. Medical aspects of polar exploration: sixteenth anniversary of Scott's last expedition. Proc R Soc Med 1972; 65:39–42.
64. Smith AH. An historical inquiry into the efficacy of lime juice for the prevention and cure of scurvy. J R Army Med Corps 1919; 32:93–116, 188–208.
65. Stare FJ, Stare IM. Charles Glen King, 1896–1988. J Nutr 1988: 118:1272–1277.

66. Hughes RE. George Budd (1808–1882) and nutritional deficiency diseases. Med Hist 1973; 17:127–135.

67. Budd G. Disorders resulting from defective nutrients. London Med Gaz 1842; 2:632–636.

68. Funk C. The etiology of the deficiency diseases: beri-beri, polyneuritis in birds, epidemic dropsy, scurvy, experimental survy in animals, infantile scurvy, ship beri-beri, pellagra. J State Med 1912; 20:341–368.

69. Griminger P. Casimir Funk. J Nutr 1972; 102:1105–1114.

70. Holst A, Frölich T. Experimental studies relating to ship-beri-beri and scurvy. II. On the etiology of scurvy. J Hyg 1907; 7:634–671.

71. Johnson BC. Axel Holst. J Nutr 1954; 53:1–16.

72. Smith T. Bacilli of Swine Disease. United States Department of Agriculture, Bureau of Animal Industry, Ann Rep, 1895–1896, Washington, D.C.

73. Szent-Györgyi A. Lost in the twentieth century. Annu Rev Biochem 1963; 32:1–14.

74. Fawns HT. Discovery of vitamin C. James Lind and the scurvy. Nurs Times 1975; 872–875.

75. King CG. The discovery and chemistry of vitamin C. Proc Nutr Soc 1953; 12:219–227.

76. Williams RR. Edward Bright Vedder: a biographical sketch. J Nutr 1962; 77:1–6.

77. Vedder EB. Study of antiscorbutic vitamin. Mil Surgeon 1932; 71:505.

78. Moss RW. Free Radical: Albert Szent-Gyorgyi and the Battle over Vitamin C. New York: Paragon House, 1987.

79. Carpenter KJ. Book Review: Free Radical: Albert Szent-Gyorgyi and the Battle over Vitamin C, by Ralph W. Moss. J Nutr 1988; 118:1422–1423.

80. Hurley LS. The identification of vitamin C. J Nutr 1988; 118:1271.

81. Jukes TH. The identification of vitamin C, an historical summary. J Nutr 1988; 118:1290–1293.

82. King CG. The isolation of vitamin C from lemon juice. Fed Proc 1979; 38:2681–2683.

83. Jukes TH. Szent-Györgyi and vitamin C. Nature 1988; 332:390.

84. King CG, Waugh WA. The chemical nature of vitamin C. Science 1932; 75:357–358.

85. Waugh WA, King CG. The isolation and identification of vitamin C. J Biol Chem 1932; 97: 325–331.

86. King CG, Waugh WA. The vitamin C activity of hexuronic acid from suprarenal glands. Science 1932; 76:630.

87. Svirbely JL, Szent-Györgyi A. Hexuronic acid and the antiscorbutic factor. Nature (London) 1932; 129:576.

88. Haworth WN, Hirst EL. Synthesis of ascorbic acid. J Soc Chem Ind (London) 1933; 52: 645–647.

89. Svirbely JL, Szent-Györgyi A. Chemical nature of vitamin C. Biochem J 1933; 27:279–285.

90. Reichstein T, Grussner A, Oppenheimer R. Synthese der d- und l-Ascorbinsaure (C-vitamin). Helv Chim Acta 1933; 16:1019–1033.

91. Drummond JC. The nomenclature of the so-called accessory food factors (vitamins). Biochem J 1920; 14:660.

92. Sauberlich HE. Pharmacology of vitamin C. Annu Rev Nutr 1994; 14:371–391.

93. Sauberlich HE. Vitamin C and cancer. In: Carroll KK, Kritchevsky D, eds. Nutrition and Disease Update: Cancer. Champaign, IL: AOCS Press: 1994: 111–172.

2

An Overview of Ascorbic Acid Chemistry and Biochemistry

CONSTANCE S. TSAO
Linus Pauling Institute, Palo Alto, California

INTRODUCTION

Since the discovery of ascorbic acid (vitamin C), a large number of publications on ascorbic acid have accumulated in the scientific literature (1–18). Many conferences and books have been devoted to ascorbic acid research, in the fields of chemistry, biochemistry, molecular biology, physiology, pharmacology, and analytical methods. Many biochemical changes and clinical and pathological conditions have been reported as associated with vitamin C deficiency and ascorbic acid metabolism disorders. Although the roles of ascorbic acid in a number of enzymatic systems have come to light, still the physiological functions of ascorbic acid have not yet been fully described in a scientifically satisfactory manner.

Ascorbic acid is involved in many physiological functions in living organisms. Its role in the synthesis of collagen in connective tissues is well known. The absence of wound healing and the failure of fractures to repair are classically recognized features of scurvy. These features are attributable to impaired collagen formation due to lack of vitamin C. Ascorbic acid is a strong reducing agent and readily oxidizes reversibly to dehydroascorbic acid. Studies on the interactions of ascorbic acid with various chemicals and metal ions have indicated that ascorbic acid and its oxidation product dehydroascorbic acid, as well as its intermediate monodehydroascorbic acid free radical, may function as cycling redox couples in reactions involving electron transport and membrane electrochemical potentiation. Research on the electron transport and redox coupling reactions has been the subject of numerous biochemical studies. For example, ascorbic acid has been shown to participate in many different neurochemical reactions involving electron transport. Neurons are known to use ascorbic acid for many different chemical and enzymatic reactions, including the synthesis of neurotransmitters and hormones. Studies on the interactions of extracellular ascorbic acid with various plasma membrane proteins suggest that ascorbic acid may function as a neuromodulator. In certain brain regions, ascorbic acid appears to be a signaling molecule, regulating the postsynaptic efficacy of neurotransmitters. Recently, sufficient evidence has accumulated to suggest a role of ascorbic acid in interneuronal communications. It is not known at this time how the information flows through the nervous system by neurochemical processes and how these processes are regulated and controlled. Nevertheless, the participation of ascorbic acid in neuronal communication may explain the fundamental difference between prokaryote and eukaryote organisms, since ascorbic acid is present in all known eukaryotes but in almost none of the prokaryotes.

In a variety of other functions, the role of ascorbic acid in cellular metabolism can be accounted for by its reducing properties to protect cellular components from oxidative damage. It acts as a scavenger for oxidizing free radicals and harmful oxygen-derived species, such as the hydroxyl radical, hydrogen peroxide, and singlet oxygen. Under certain circumstances, however, ascorbic acid may act as a prooxidant to promote the production of reactive free radicals and oxygen-derived species. Certain biochemical reactions are known to be stimulated by the prooxidant activity of ascorbic acid. The ability of the ascorbic acid radical to regulate cell growth has been known for many years. The bactericidal and antiviral activity of ascorbic acid in aqueous solution is presumably attributable to its prooxidant properties. Much research has focused on the antioxidant activity of ascorbic acid, while relatively little has been devoted to the understanding of its functions as a prooxidant. In living organisms, it is desirable to eliminate harmful oxidative species, but it may be equally important to produce a needed amount of oxidative species for biological functions, such as stimulation of biochemical reactions, growth regulation, and defense against bacteria and viruses.

Ascorbic acid is widely used in the food industry as an additive to foods to improve the taste and to restore the vitamin C loss due to processing and storage (4,10). It can prevent oxidation as a preservative or serve as a stabilizer in various food products and beverages. It is used in bread baking, brewing, wine making, and freezing of fruits. In addition, ascorbic acid and some of its derivatives are used in industrial processes, such as polymerization reactions, photographic development and printing, and metal technology. Most of these applications make use of the reducing properties of ascorbic acid.

There have been many articles published with titles similar to the present one. This chapter includes references to some recent publications on the chemical and biochemical aspects of ascorbic acid. Most of them confirm previous research results or extend the research efforts into other biochemical systems. In the near future there certainly will be more such new discoveries, since our current knowledge of ascorbic acid chemical and biochemical processes is still quite incomplete. These new discoveries will be helpful to us in devising new methods and procedures for ascorbic acid to control and prevent diseases as well as to maintain health.

CHEMISTRY

Molecular Structure

L-Ascorbic acid is a dibasic acid with an enediol group built into a five membered heterocyclic lactone ring. The molecule is stabilized by delocalization of the π electrons over the conjugated carbonyl and enediol system. The lactone ring is confirmed to be almost planar. The chemical and physical properties of ascorbic acid are related to its structure (7,9,19–23).

The structure of dehydroascorbic acid, the first oxidation product of ascorbic acid, has been analyzed by x-ray crystallography to be a dimer (23). Nuclear magnetic resonance (NMR) studies have indicated that dehydroascorbic acid in aqueous solution exists as a bicyclic hydrated monomer. Electrochemical studies have indicated that ascorbic acid and dehydroascorbic acid form a reversible redox couple.

The ascorbic acid molecule consists of two asymmetric carbon atoms, C-4 and C-5 (20). Therefore, in addition to L-ascorbic acid itself, there are three other stereoisomers: D-ascorbic acid, D-isoascorbic acid, and L-isoascorbic acid. These three isomers have very little or no antiscorbutic activity.

Synthesis

Ascorbic acid has been synthesized from C-5 sugars, such as L-xylosone, L-lyxose, L-xylose, and L-arabinose (7,19). The reaction involves carboxylation and molecular skeletal rearrangement. Another synthetic approach involves the combination of C-2 and C-4 carbon units. An example of this approach is the condensation between L-threose and ethyl glyoxalate in the presence of sodium cyanide.

The most commonly used starting material for ascorbic acid synthesis is D-glucose. The synthetic process involves the reduction of D-glucose to D-sorbitol, which is oxidized to L-sorbose. Di-O-isopropylidenyl protection of the hydroxyl groups on carbons 2,3 and 4,6 permits the selective oxidation of the C-1 primary alcohol to produce the corresponding 2,3-4,6-di-O-isopropylidene-2-keto-L-gulonic acid. The protected gulonic acid can then be converted directly into ascorbic acid, using nonaqueous conditions. Radioactive labeling studies have indicated that the reaction has undergone a carbon-chain inversion: namely, C-1 of the D-glucose precursor molecule becomes C-6 in the L-ascorbic acid product. In addition to D-glucose, D-galactose and D-galactouronic acid have also been converted into L-ascorbic acid.

Several other synthetic routes of the synthesis of ascorbic acid from glucose do not involve carbon-chain inversion. The C-1 of glucose remains the C-1 of ascorbic acid. Although such syntheses have not proved to be of commercial value, they have found use in the preparation of C-5 deuterated derivatives of L-ascorbic acid.

Chemical Properties

Ascorbic acid in aqueous solution is a strong reducing agent. It can be oxidized to dehydroascorbic acid by a variety of oxidizing agents such as the halogens, quinones, iodate ion, phenolindiphenol, molecular oxygen in the presence of a suitable catalyst metal ion, and activated charcoal. This oxidation process is readily reversible. The reduction back to ascorbic acid may be accomplished by several different reagents, including hydrogen sulfate, hydriodic acid, cysteine, sodium dithionate, and other thiols.

The role of vitamin C in biological systems is related to its oxidation–reduction reactions. Ascorbic acid is oxidized by oxygen to dehydroascorbic acid. The reaction is reversible and both ascorbic and dehydroascorbic acid have antiscorbutic activity and other physiological effects of the vitamin (23). Dehydroascorbic acid still possesses reducing properties, especially in alkaline solutions. It can be further oxidized by oxidative agents such as molecular oxygen, hydrogen peroxide, permanganate, and hypoiodite ion to produce a number of products that are no longer physiologically active. The major products of the process are threonic acid and oxalic acid.

The rate of aerobic oxidation of ascorbic acid depends on the pH, exhibiting maxima at pH 5 and 11.5 (7). In alkaline solutions the reaction is much more rapid and the degradation more extensive. Degradative oxidation occurs slowly under anaerobic conditions. Irradiation of aqueous ascorbic acid with ultraviolet, x-, or γ-radiation causes photochemical oxidation under aerobic or anaerobic conditions. In nonaqueous media, oxidation of ascorbic acid is very slow.

In aqueous solution the oxidation of ascorbic acid to dehydroascorbic acid is a two-electron redox process. Ascorbic acid is a moderately weak acid in the loss of the first hydrogen ion (pKa = 4.25) and a very weak acid in the loss of the second (pKa = 11.79). The intermediate formed from the loss of one electron is the ascorbate radical with a single unpaired electron; it is a strong acid (pKa = −0.45), comparable to mineral acids. The ultraviolet (UV) spectrum of the ascorbate radical measured at a pH range −0.3 to 11 indicates that a single species is present throughout this range of acidity and that the unpaired electron density is spread over all three carbonyl groups.

Ascorbate is a reactive reductant, but its free radical is relatively nonreactive (24). The decay of the ascorbate radical involves the combination of two ascorbate radical ions to form an intermediate with paired electrons, which then disproportionates to form ascorbic acid and dehydroascorbic acid (25). The rate of the reaction depends on the ionic strength and the pH of the solution.

In the absence of a catalyst, the reaction of ascorbic acid with oxygen is slow and the rate is pH-dependent (7,26–28). It is slow in acidic solutions, much faster in alkaline solutions. Electron spin resonance studies have shown that when ascorbate reacts with oxygen in aqueous solution in the pH range of 6.6–9.6, a steady-state concentration of ascorbate radical is produced. Data from the inhibition of the reaction by certain enzymes, such as superoxide dismutase and catalase, suggest that hydrogen peroxide is produced in the process.

The oxidation of ascorbic acid to dehydroascorbic acid, or dehydroascorbic acid to 2,3-diketogulonic acid and other oxidation products, is enhanced by metal ions, of which copper(II) is the most potent (7,29,30). A complex intermediate in the oxidation of ascorbic acid by Cu(II) has been detected spectrophotometrically. A possible mechanism for the reaction is the formation of a ternary complex among ascorbic acid, copper, and oxygen. In general, the reaction rate of ascorbic acid oxidation is first-order in ascorbic acid, in metal ion, and in molecular oxygen. The first oxidation step of ascorbic acid by transition metal ions or their complexes often produces an ascorbate free radical (7,24). This ascorbate radical may react with another metal ion to give the required stoichiometric characteristics. In the process, the transition metal ion frequently is itself reduced.

Oxidation and Degradation Products

The nonenzymatic browning reaction of ascorbic acid leads to the formation of many degradation products (31). The rate of ascorbic acid degradation depends on ascorbic acid concentration, temperature, pH, oxygen, light, and presence of metal ions (28–35). When ascorbic acid is heated in an aqueous solution, the major products are dehydroascorbic acid, 2,3-diketogulonic acid, threonic acid, and oxalic acid. Small amounts of reductones, reductic acids, sugars, and sugar acids have been detected and some have been identified. A group of volatile furan-type compounds and reductones are detected by the gas chromatography method. Some of these browning products have antioxidant activity (35), while others have destructive prooxidant effects, including lipid peroxidation, cytotoxicity, mutagenesis, and adduct formation with proteins and nucleic acids (36).

Synthetic Derivatives and Analogues

Ascorbic acid has several reaction positions that can be used to synthesize a number of derivatives (7,20,37). Many substituted compounds at the C-2, C-3, C-5, and C-6 positions have been synthesized (38,39). Acid-catalyzed esterification of ascorbic acid with an acylating reagent initially produces the O-6-acylated derivative, and under vigorous conditions, a 5,6-diester. The compound ascorbyl 5,6-diacetate is well known. More vigorous conditions still are needed to produce the 2,3,5,6-tetra-acetate. Under basic conditions, electrophilic attack by alkylating and acylating reagents depends on the acidity and steric accessibility of the OH groups in the C-2, C-3, C-5, and C-6 positions. Although the most acidic hydrogen is at the C-2 hydroxyl group, the delocalization of the negative charge in the anion reduces its reactivity and may lead to both C-2 and C-3 alkylations. As a result, selective O-2 derivatization is generally difficult. However, some C-2 inorganic esters, such as 2-O-phosphate and 2-O-sulfate have been synthesized (20,37,38). If both the C-2 and C-3 hydroxyl groups are protected, base-promoted alkylation or acylation takes place at the more sterically accessible primary hydroxyl group on C-6 rather than C-5. Reactions at the C-5 position occur only after derivatizations of C-2, C-3, and C-6 are completed.

The formation of acetals or ketals of ascorbic acid is useful for the protection of the molecule while reactions at the other carbons are carried out. The 5,6-O-derivatives isopropylidene ketal and benzylidene acetal are known. Reactive aldehydes have been used to protect the C-2 and C-3 positions. This process permits the selective modification of the primary and secondary alcohol groups on the side chain to produce a number of side-chain-oxidized derivatives (37,39). Ascorbyl palmitate has been successfully synthesized in nonaqueous medium using an enzyme from a microorganism as a biocatalyst (40).

In addition to the substituted derivatives, compounds with structural features quite different from that of ascorbic acid have been synthesized. For example, a cyclopentenone has been recently synthesized (41). In this molecule, the oxygen of the lactone ring is replaced by a carbon atom. The crystal structure of erythroascorbic acid has been determined (42). This molecule contains a side chain with a methoxy group instead of an ethoxy group. Other examples include a group of bicyclic alkylidene-dimethyloxy butenolides and a series of hydroxylactones, all synthesized using ascorbic acid as a starting material (43–45).

Interaction with Metal Ions

Ascorbic acid is a strong two-electron reducing agent that is readily oxidized in one-electron steps by metal ions and metal complexes (30,46). When ascorbic acid is oxidized, the metal ion, such as Cu(II) or Fe(III), reduces to Cu(I) or Fe(II). However, reaction of Cr(VI) with ascorbic acid produces Cr(V), Cr(IV), and a carbon-based radical (47). Ascorbic acid is a potentially bidentate ligand, presumably forming complexes by coordination with the two oxygen atoms of the 2- and 3-hydroxyl groups (7,30,46). Structures of such complexes in aqueous solutions have been proposed on the basis of electron paramagnetic resonance or NMR data (47,48). However, most of the complexes known are formed with ascorbate monoanion, and very few recorded are with the fully deprotonated dianion. Complexes with the dianion form only in alkaline solutions, and many of the metals also form hydroxyl species in alkaline solutions, which may compete with the ascorbate dianion.

Ascorbic acid forms complexes with many metal ions, including those capable of reducing, such as copper(II) and iron(III). The bonds between the metal and ascorbic acid molecules are weaker than expected when compared with the complexes of similar chelating ligands.

Crystals of a number of complexes of ascorbic acid have been obtained under strictly anaerobic conditions. However, the structures of these complexes are still largely unknown. The x-ray crystal structure of a complex of ascorbic acid and 1,2-diaminocyclohexane platinum(II) does not involve complexation through the 2-OH and 3-OH of the ascorbic acid molecule, but via the direct bonding to C-2 and the deprotonated hydroxyl in C-5. It is already known that platinum(II) at times forms Pt-C bonds where Pt-O bonds might be expected.

The oxidation mechanism of ascorbic acid has been studied for many metal ions and metal complexes capable of oxidizing ascorbic acid. Some of these reactions are catalyzed by copper(II) ions. The kinetics of these reactions seems to involve a pathway in which the copper(II) ion acts as an intermediary for the passage of electrons from ascorbic acid to the reducing metal ion.

Analysis of Ascorbic Acid

Ascorbic acid has strong absorption in the ultraviolet region. This physical property is the basis of spectrophotometric methods for the measurement of ascorbic acid in pharmaceutical preparations, beverages, and fruit and vegetable extracts. Treatment with ascorbic acid oxidase has been used as a blank to correct for interfering substances in biological samples.

Numerous high-performance liquid chromatographic methods have been developed for the analysis of ascorbic acid. The electrochemical detector is suitable for measuring ascorbic acid content in biological fluids and tissues (49–52). It has been developed on the basis of the oxidation–reduction properties of ascorbic acid. Many of the chromatographic systems are designed for the simultaneous measurement of ascorbic and dehydroascorbic acid as well as their isomers and derivatives (52). To measure dehydroascorbic acid, first reduce it to ascorbic acid by a reducing agent such as dithiothreitol before analysis (53). Because of the chromatographic separation, and the selectivity and sensitivity of the electrochemical detector, this method provides greater selectivity and sensitivity than the UV detector. The UV detector may be used for the determination of ascorbic acid in pharmaceutical preparations.

Both the ion exchange and reversed phase chromatographic columns are commonly used. A fused silica capillary column has been used for the measurement of ascorbic acid in fruits and vegetables (53). In certain high-performance liquid chromatography (HPLC) procedures, ascorbic and dehydroascorbic acid are derivatized by treatment with a complexing agent such as borohydride before HPLC analysis (54).

There are several colorimetric methods for the measurement of ascorbic acid. The 2,4-dinitrophenylhydrazine method is commonly used for the determination of total ascorbic acid (ascorbic acid plus dehydroascorbic acid) (55,56). In this method, ascorbic acid is first oxidized to dehydroascorbic acid, which then reacts with 2,4-dinitrophenylhydrazine to form a hydrazone derivative. This derivative can then be measured colorimetrically.

The 2,2′-dipyridyl colorimetric method is based on the reduction of Fe(III) to Fe(II) by ascorbic acid (57). The Fe(II) reacts with 2,2′-dipyridyl to from a complex that can be quantified colorimetrically. This method is based on the reducing properties of ascorbic acid. To measure dehydroascorbic acid, first reduce it to ascorbic acid. A reducing agent, dithiothreitol, has been used satisfactorily for this purpose. The excess of dithiothreitol is removed with N-ethylmaleimide (58). In addition to 2,2′-dipyridyl, ferrozine and Folin phenol reagent have also been used as color-producing agents in this method (59,60).

The fluorometric method is a specific technique for the determination of ascorbic acid by the formation of a fluorescent complex. Fluorescence from the ascorbic acid complex is measured spectrophotometrically (61,62). When interfering substances are separated prior to fluorometric detection, higher precision can be achieved (62).

In addition to the UV, electrochemical, and fluorometric detectors, the mass spectrometer has been used (63). Dehydroascorbic acid has been quantified by measuring the kinetics of a derivatization reaction using mass spectrometry. Another mass spectrometry method is the isotope ratio technique. In this method, a known amount of C^{13} is added to the sample and the amount of ascorbic acid in the sample is calculated by comparing the measured and added amounts of C^{13} (64). New techniques reported using other detectors are the modified spectrophotometric, chemiluminometric, and voltammetric methods (65,66).

Gas chromatographic methods using commercially available silylating agents have been employed in the analysis of ascorbic acid for many years (49). These methods are very convenient but require careful sample preparation to remove water completely before derivatization to the silyl compounds.

Biological methods employing guinea pigs have been used to determine the efficacy of vitamin C for cure or prevention of scurvy (67–70). These methods are still used for establishing biological specificity and antiscorbutic properties of certain chemicals and products.

The enzymatic methods using ascorbate oxidase have the advantage of selectively measuring the biological activity of ascorbic acid. Ascorbic acid reacts with a variety of reagents to produce color products, but the reactions usually are not specific for ascorbic acid. These reactions may be carried out with and without ascorbate oxidase. The amount of interfering substances may be calculated, yielding results with a high degree of selectivity and precision (71,72).

The titration method using 2,6-dichlorophenolindophenol is suitable for a rapid estimation of ascorbic acid concentration when high precision is not required (73).

Interference with Clinical Tests

Ascorbic acid interferes with many urine and blood chemical tests, including the analysis of glucose, uric acid, creatinine, bilirubin, glycohemoglobin, hemoglobin A, cholesterol, triglycerides, urine leukocytes, and inorganic phosphate (74–79). The extent and direction of interference vary, depending on the types of reaction, reagents, and apparatus (74,80,81).

Many clinical tests involve nonspecific color formation by redox reactions. As a strong reducing agent, ascorbic acid in biological samples may interfere with the analytical procedures and give misleading results. It may inhibit color development by causing a time lag or by rereducing oxidized indicators (82). In analyses involving oxidase, peroxidase, or peroxide-generating systems, an interfering action of ascorbic acid is the result of its metal-catalyzed production of hydrogen peroxide (79,80,83).

Nevertheless, many of these undesirable effects can be eliminated by using specific test systems. For example, ascorbic acid destroys vitamin B_{12} in certain test systems, but this can be prevented by using the more specific microbiological or radio assays (84). Furthermore, certain techniques have been developed to minimize the interference of ascorbic acid. A glucose sensor electrode for the detection of hydrogen peroxide has been developed for analytical procedures free of ascorbic acid interference (83).

However, in certain analytical procedures, especially those involving the analysis of multiple constituents in a single sample, the use of a specific method is not possible. For example, in a procedure to analyze urinary amino acids using ninhydrin as an indicator, ascorbic acid and its degradation products form unstable ninhydrin-positive compounds that hamper the analyses (85). Therefore, for nonspecific analytical precedures, experiments must be carried out in the absence of interfering substances. It is necessary for the subject to discontinue supplemental ascorbic acid for a short period prior to the clinical tests.

PHYSIOLOGICAL ASPECTS

Deficiency

The classical vitamin deficiency disease, scurvy, was demonstrated by Lind to be a dietary deficiency resulting from lack of fresh fruit and vegetables (86). Results of a clinical experiment indicated that scorbutic patients recovered from the disease by drinking lemon juice.

The history of vitamin C is associated with the cause, treatment, and prevention of scurvy (13,87,88). The early signs of scurvy include weakness and lassitude. These are followed by swelling of the legs and arms, softening of the gums, hemorrhages from the nose and gums and under the skin, and extensive degeneration of bone and cartilage. Scorbutic patients are highly susceptible to infection. In persons who have marginal vitamin C intake fulminating scurvy is likely to develop if an infection should occur. If the disease is not relieved, death results from exhaustion or acute infections.

This vitamin C deficiency disease affected many people in ancient Egypt, Greece, and Rome. In the Middle Ages, it was endemic in Northern Europe during winters, when fresh fruits and vegetables were unavailable. It affected long sea voyages by outbreaks when vitamin C in rations became depleted.

Intestinal Absorption and Transport

Absorption of ascorbic acid in the intestine occurs through a sodium-dependent active transport system (89–93). The transport of ascorbic acid into the ileum is a carrier-mediated process at low mucosal concentrations of ascorbic acid. At high mucosal concentrations, however, influx of ascorbic acid into the ileum is linearly related to the ascorbic acid concentration, and absorption occurs predominantly by simple diffusion (93). The gastrointestinal absorption is inversely related to the dose (94,95). The amounts absorbed decrease with the age of a person. Ascorbic acid in large doses can cause intestinal discomfort and osmosis diarrhea.

The cellular accumulations of vitamin C in humans and animals are mediated by a variety of specific transporters located at the cell membranes and regulated in a cell-specific manner (96–102). An active transport mechanism for ascorbic acid through the blood–cerebrospinal fluid barrier has also been observed (103).

Transporters for both ascorbic acid and dehydroascorbic acid have been identified, and most of the transport processes are found to be sodium-dependent (98–101). In many biological systems, uptakes of both ascorbic acid and dehydroascorbic acid utilize the glucose transporters (96,104). Certain in vitro studies have indicated that dehydroascorbic acid, not ascorbic acid, is preferentially transported intracellularly (96,105). In the transporting process, extracellular ascorbic acid is first oxidized to dehydroascorbic acid before being transported into cells. The transported dehydroascorbic acid is then reduced back to ascorbic acid, which is nontransportable and remains in the cell. The transport of dehydroascorbic acid via glucose transporters is a sodium-independent process that is kinetically and biologically separable from the reduction of dehydroascorbic acid to ascorbic acid. Kinetic analysis of the uptake of ascorbic acid in human neutrophils has revealed the presence of at least two functional activities of different binding affinities for ascorbic acid, high-affinity and low-affinity activities (105–108). Neutrophils are able to sense an intracellular vitamin C deficiency and make rapid adjustments by absorption of plasma ascorbic acid utilizing the high- and low-affinity membrane transport systems. Both systems show saturation kinetics and are adversely affected by the presence of glucose (107,108).

Tissue Distribution and Body Store

A clue to the metabolic role of ascorbic acid in animals may be deduced by the examination of tissue concentrations. The concentrations of ascorbic acid in tissues are tightly controlled by the body and vary from tissue to tissue (7,109,110). The plasma ascorbic acid concentration of a healthy person is 8–14 mg/L, while adrenal glands, pituitary, thymus, corpus luteum, and retina have concentrations more than 100 times higher. The brain, spleen, lung, testicle, lymph glands, liver, thyroid, small intestinal mucosa, leukocytes, pancreas, kidney, and salivary glands have concentrations 10–50 times that of plasma. The skeletal, smooth and cardiac muscle, and erythrocytes have concentrations about 10 times that of plasma.

In most of these tissues, a common function of vitamin C is the maintenance of structural integrity through collagen synthesis. The high levels in some of the vital organs may protect them against dietary deficiencies and enable them to perform their specialized functions. These functions include synthesizing hormones and neurotransmitters in the adrenals and brain, improving immune response in the spleen and leukocytes, promoting the pentose phosphate metabolic pathway in the liver, and maintaining the transparency of the eye lens and cornea.

Vitamin C is a nutrient for health maintenance (20,109). It exists as an ascorbic acid pool distributed throughout the body (95). In some animals, there is evidence that ascorbic acid may exist in the liver in a bound form that is protected against degradation by liver enzymes. The adult human body accumulates a limited amount (1.5–2 g) of the vitamin. Any intake in excess of the daily rate of metabolism (5–20 mg/day) is absorbed but promptly excreted unchanged in the urine after plasma concentration exceeds the renal threshold of about 14 mg/L. The biological half-life of ascorbic acid is inversely related to the daily intake, 14–40 days in humans with normal intake, and 3–4 days in guinea pigs. In a human on a vitamin-C-free diet scurvy will develop in about 3–4 months; in the guinea pig, 3–4 weeks.

Systemic Conditioning Effect

Humans and animals have several levels of control mechanisms to attain homeostasis of vitamin C. Absorption of ascorbic acid in the intestine is very efficient at low intakes and increasingly poor as ascorbic acid intakes increase (91–94). In the presence of large amounts of ascorbic acid, mechanisms to catabolize and eliminate excess ascorbic acid in animals are activated to remove it more effectively (111,112). When the high dosage is withdrawn, the accelerated catabolic processes probably continue to catabolize ascorbic acid (112,113). In humans and in guinea pigs, prolonged high maternal intake of ascorbic acid during pregnancy increases the metabolism of this vitamin in the neonatal period (114,115). The ingestion of large amounts of ascorbic acid by the mother during pregnancy may condition the newborn babies to require vitamin C in amounts greater than normal intakes.

Guinea pigs fed large amounts of ascorbic acid have a higher rate of catabolism of ascorbic acid to carbon dioxide than do controls (111,112). This effect persists after the ascorbic-acid-treated animals are returned to a normal diet. In comparison with untreated ones, guinea pigs treated previously with large doses of ascorbic acid die earlier of scurvy when put on a scorbutic diet.

The systemic conditioning effect of ascorbic acid in humans has also been reported. In healthy human adults, even moderately increased ascorbic acid intake, 600 mg/day, increases the turnover of plasma ascorbic acid (116). The effect of systemic conditioning after large doses of ascorbic acid is probably not common to all humans. Under certain circumstances, however, some individuals may be more susceptible to this effect than others.

In ascorbic-acid-synthesizing animals, very high dietary ascorbic acid intakes only moderately raise ascorbic acid levels in tissues (110,117,118). In mice and rats, dietary ascorbic acid has unexpectedly caused lower concentrations of ascorbic acid in certain organs, including the adrenal glands, kidney, liver, lung, muscle, and spleen, than the concentrations in such organs of the control animals on ascorbic-acid-free diets (117,118). Tissue ascorbic acid levels in the liver and intestine of sturgeons, an ascorbic-acid-synthesizing fish species, are also not a monotonic increasing function of dietary ascorbic acid intakes (119). These observations suggest that exogenous ascorbic acid intake may interact with the mechanisms for transport, metabolism, elimination, and even biosynthesis of vitamin C in these animals. Indeed, dietary ascorbic acid has caused a decrease in the activities of ascorbic-acid-synthesizing enzymes in mouse liver homogenates, with gulonolactone or glucuronolactone as a substrate (120,121).

Dietary Requirement

There has been much discussion concerning the safety of large doses of ascorbic acid and the amount of vitamin C that needs to be consumed for optimum well-being (84,122–127). Various authorities have recommended amounts varying from 30 to 10,000 mg/day. In humans a daily consumption of 10 mg of ascorbic acid is usually effective to alleviate and cure clinical signs of scurvy, but this does not necessarily provide an acceptable reserve of the vitamin. The 1989 recommended dietary allowance (RDA) for adults in the United States is 60 mg/day, which is designed for the prevention of scurvy with a margin of reserve (127–129). It has been questioned whether the amount of ascorbic acid needed to prevent scurvy is equivalent to the optimal amount for human health (125–127).

There is without doubt a wide margin between the amount of vitamin C needed to prevent scurvy and that required for the maintenance of good health. The guinea pig is an animal species unable to produce vitamin C endogenously and must depend on exogenous intake. About 0.5 mg vitamin C/day will protect young guinea pigs against scurvy, but there are distinct gains in health when the intakes are increased to 10 to 20 times this amount.

Although the optimum amounts of ascorbic acid necessary for the well-being of guinea pigs have been established (110), the optimum amounts for humans are still uncertain.

A quantitative approach to determine human optimal intakes for vitamin C and other vitamins has been proposed (125,126). The vitamin C requirement may be estimated on the basis of its biological activities relating to the biological functions, and on the necessary intakes to maintain the various tissue concentrations needed for these functions in humans. The tissue concentration of ascorbic acid for a specific biochemical reaction is determined experimentally, and the dosage to attain this tissue concentration is determined clinically. The criteria for determining the optimal intakes of vitamin C include its availability in the diet, dose–biological function relationship, plasma and tissue concentration, urinary excretion, toxicity, and epidemiological findings.

In practice, however, there are serious difficulties in establishing optimal individual human needs because these needs are highly variable from person to person (130). The biochemical variations in the human species are of much greater magnitude than those in animals (131). Evidence of differences in the individual need of vitamin C was provided by the outbreak of scurvy in the days of long sea voyages. One member of the crew was observed as suffering from severe scurvy and was about to die of the disease, while many of the crew were quite free of any symptoms. A tolerance test for high doses of ascorbic acid with 60 healthy persons indicated that wide variations exist from individual to individual with respect to the digestive system (132). Three persons ingested a daily dose of 20 g or more of ascorbic acid for more than 5 years without apparent difficulties. In contrast, a daily dose of 500 mg caused diarrhea and discomfort of the intestinal tract in two other persons. On the basis of these observations, a given dose of ascorbic acid may be beneficial to some people but unsuitable for some others, although excess of ascorbic acid is excreted in the urine of most people. Therefore, besides considering information from biochemical and clinical experiments, it is wise also to take into account the health and medical data for each individual.

BIOCHEMISTRY

Biosynthesis

The biosynthesis of ascorbic acid in animals is included in the glucuronic acid metabolic pathway. The metabolic pathway is involved in the metabolism of sugars under normal and disease conditions, and in regulation of physiological functions (5,7,10,133). It is an important pathway for major detoxification processes. The activities of the synthesizing enzymes vary from species to species (134–136).

Most animals can convert D-glucose into L-ascorbic acid (136). Humans and other primates, guinea pigs, Indian fruit bats, some fish and birds, and insects are unable to produce ascorbic acid endogenously. The biosynthesis of ascorbic acid in vertebrates presumably was started in the kidney of amphibians and reptiles, then transferred to the liver of mammals, and eventually lost in primates, fruit bats, and guinea pigs in the process of evolution.

Most of the research on ascorbic acid synthesis in animals have been carried out using the rat (137–139). D-Glucose is converted into L-ascorbic acid via D-glucuronic acid, L-gulonic acid, L-gulonolactone, and 2-keto-L-gulonolactone as intermediates (140). Studies with radioactive labeling technique have indicated that, in the synthetic pathway, inversion of C-1 and C-6 takes place between D-glucuronic acid and L-gulonic acid, while the D-glucose chain remains intact (138).

Animals that cannot synthesize ascorbic acid endogenously lack the oxidizing enzyme L-gulono-γ-lactone oxidase (141). This enzyme is required in the last step of the conversion of L-gulono-γ-lactone to 2-oxo-L-gulono-γ-lactone, which is a tautomer of L-ascorbic acid and, transforms spontaneously into vitamin C. Cloning and chromosomal mapping studies have indicated that the human nonfunctional gene for L-gulono-γ-lactone oxidase has accumulated a large number of mutations without selective pressure since it presumably ceased to function during evolution (142,143).

Certain microorganisms are able to synthesize ascorbic acid or one of its isomers. A bacterial-origin enzyme, L-gulono-γ-lactone dehydrogenase, which catalyzes the oxidation reaction of the synthesis of ascorbic acid, has been isolated and characterized. The physical and chemical properties of this enzyme are entirely different from those of eukaryotic organisms (144).

In vitro and in vivo studies have shown that ascorbic acid biosynthesis is controlled by a direct feedback mechanism, and that the concentration of ascorbic acid in cell culture medium or in the blood regulates the amount of ascorbic acid synthesized in the liver or in hepatocytes of rat or mice (121,136,145). The hepatic ascorbic acid synthesis in mice is stimulated by enhanced glycogenolysis (146). The rate of in vitro ascorbic acid synthesis showed close correlation with the glucose release by hepatocytes (146). The biosynthesis of ascorbic acid is impaired by deficiency of vitamin A, vitamin E, or biotin, but is stimulated by certain drugs, such as barbiturate, chlorobutanol, animopyrine, and antipyrine, and by certain carcinogens, such as 3-methylcholanthrene or 3,4-benzpyrene (147). In mice the injection of glucagon increases ascorbic acid concentrations in the liver and plasma. In hepatocytes, ascorbic acid synthesis is stimulated by glucagon, dibutyryl cyclic adenosine monophosphate (AMP), phenylephrine, vasopressin, and okadaic acid.

The exposure to xenobiotic compounds can induce biosynthesis of enzymes involved in the glucuronic acid pathway, part of the drug detoxification process in the body. In rats, uridine diphosphate (UDP) glucuronosyltransferase gene expression is involved in the stimulation of ascorbic acid biosynthesis by xenobiotics, such as 3-methylcholanthrene and sodium phenobarbital (148).

Metabolism

Ascorbic acid is metabolized in the liver, and to some extent in the kidney, in a series of reactions. The principal pathway of ascorbic acid metabolism involves the loss of two electrons (7,20). The intermediate free radical reversibly forms dehydroascorbic acid, leading to the irreversible formation of the physiologically inactive 2,3-diketogulonic acid (149–151). Diketogulonic acid may be either cleaved to oxalic acid and threonic acid, or decarboxylated to carbon dioxide, xylose, and xylulose, leading eventually to xylonic acid and lyxonic acid. All these metabolites and ascorbic acid itself are excreted in the urine. The amounts of each vary from species to species according to the amounts of ascorbic acid ingested. When the daily ingestion is 60–100 mg, almost the whole amount is absorbed, and urinary oxalate is the major metabolite. When the doses increase to 2–3 g/day, ascorbic acid is excreted largely unchanged in the urine, with very little increase in urinary or plasma oxalic acid.

In rats and guinea pigs, ascorbic acid is metabolized to respiratory carbon dioxide in the breath. Studies with radioactive labeled ascorbic acid indicate that oxalic acid is produced from carbon atoms 1 and 2 while carbon dioxide is produced from the complete metabolism of the entire carbon chain. In contrast to observations in rats, guinea pigs, and monkeys, in humans practically no respiratory carbon dioxide has been detected (152). In humans, carbon dioxide may be formed when ascorbic acid is decomposed prior to ingestion or when the intake is very large (153,154). The formation of carbon dioxide is due to a presystemic effect or the microbiological or chemical degradation of ascorbic acid in the intestines (155). There is no evidence of a catabolic pathway of ascorbic acid to carbon dioxide in humans.

Some other metabolites besides those in the main stream of metabolism have been identified. Ascorbic acid-2-sulfate has been found in humans and 2-O-methyl ascorbic acid in rats (20). 2-O-Methyl ascorbic acid is produced from the enzymatic methylation of ascorbic acid by catechol-O-methyltransferase (156,157). L-Saccharoascorbic acid, an oxidation product of ascorbic acid at the C-6 position, has been found in monkeys. A new metabolite of ascorbic acid, ascorbic-acid-2-O-β-glucuronide, has been identified in human urine and uremic plasma (158). Other identified metabolites of ascorbic acid include glucose, glycogen, and glycine in excreted hippuric acid.

Ascorbate Enzymes

Ascorbic acid is oxidized by two different enzymes, ascorbate oxidase and ascorbate peroxidase. The two oxidized forms of ascorbic acid are reduced by monodehydroascorbate reductase and dehydroascorbate reductase (159).

Ascorbate oxidase belongs to a class of blue multicopper oxidases and catalyzes the oxidation of ascorbate to dehydroascorbate (160). Ascorbate oxidase is associated with the rapidly growing regions in the plant and has been found as protein bound to the cell wall and as soluble protein in the cytosol. It was first discovered in cabbage leaves and later in tissues of squashes, cucumbers, and other plants. It has been the subject of numerous chemical and biological studies (161–165).

Ascorbate peroxidase has been previously reported to be a membrane-bound protein but was also revealed in soluble forms by subsequent studies (159). Ascorbate peroxidase is a hydrogen-peroxide-scavenging enzyme that functions to protect cells from hydrogen peroxide accumulation under normal and stressful conditions. In chloroplast, ascorbate peroxidase catalyzes the reduction of hydrogen peroxide, using ascorbate as an electron donor, to yield water and monodehydroascorbate radical as the primary oxidation product (166). In higher plants and algae, different isoenzymes of ascorbate peroxidase are known and some of their complementary deoxyribonucleic acid (cDNA) crystal structures have been characterized (167–172).

Dehydroascorbate reductase functions as a reducing agent for the regeneration of ascorbate from dehydroascorbate. It has been isolated from various plant and animal tissues (159,173). The ability of cells to recycle ascorbate enzymatically from dehydroascorbate generated by various oxidation pathways depends on the relative activity level of dehydroascorbate reductase and the availability of glutathione (173–176). Recently, a specific glutathione-dependent dehydroascorbate reductase originated from mammalian tissues has been characterized (176). Mammalian thiol-transferases (glutaredoxins) and protein disulfide isomerase have also been reported to have intrinsic dehydroascorbate reductase activity (177,178). These enzymes catalyze the glutathione-dependent two-electron regeneration of ascorbate.

The enzyme monodehydroascorbate radical reductase catalyzes the regeneration of ascorbate from monodehydroascorbate radical using reduced oxidized nicotinamide-adenine dinucleotide phosphate (NADPH) as the electron donor (179,180). It scavenges toxic oxygen-derived species in plant tissues (181,182). The action of this reductase has been detected by pulse radiolysis (183), and its cDNA from cucumber has been cloned and characterized (184,185).

Ascorbic Acid in Plants

Ascorbic acid is found all over the plant world, often in quite large quantities and distributed throughout the plant. The biochemical characteristics of ascorbic acid in plants are still very poorly understood.

Most plants synthesize ascorbic acid from D-glucose, D-galactose, D-glucuronolactone, and D-galacturonic acid and its methyl ester. Galactonolactone, rather than gulonolactone, is the major precursor of ascorbic acid (11,159,186–188). It is synthesized in the cytosol and released to the chloroplast, apoplast, and vacuole, following a concentration gradient. In its function as an antioxidant, ascorbate in the apoplast may be oxidized to dehydroascorbate, which can then be efficiently transported back into the cytosol for regeneration to ascorbate (189).

The metabolism of ascorbic acid in plants is more complex than that observed in animals because of the formation of tartaric acid and two-carbon fragments, in addition to oxalic acid (11,159,188). In some plants, cleavage occurs between C-2 and C-3 to yield threonic acid and oxalic acid, which can be metabolized to carbon dioxide. Ascorbic acid is involved in cellular respiration, carbohydrate biosynthesis, and plant growth. Glutathione is part of the respiration system reversing the ascorbate–dehydroascorbate cycle and helps maintain carbon balance (11,159,187,190). In many metabolic processes, ascorbate oxidase is known to facilitate the transfer of hydrogen from ascorbic acid to molecular oxygen. However, the factors that control ascorbate turnover rate are still unknown.

Dry seeds do not store ascorbic acid but contain dehydroascorbic acid and several dehydroascorbic-acid-reducing proteins. Dehydroascorbic acid reduction plays an important role during the early stage of seed germination (190). Ascorbic acid free radical acts as an electron acceptor for the transplasma membrane redox system to regenerate ascorbate (191–193). The activation of this transplasma membrane redox system is likely involved in the cell growth processes (194–198).

Photosynthesis, which is vitally important to the existence of virtually all life on earth, is a complex process still not fully understood. Although oxygen is essential to the development of all life, high concentrations of oxygen have an adverse effect on a number of important biochemical processes (199,200). In photosynthesis, high concentrations of oxygen inhibit the development of chloroplasts. In the process of illumination of chloroplasts and other photochemical reactions, damaging oxygen-derived species such as hydrogen peroxide, super oxide, singlet oxygen, lipid peroxides, and the hydroxyl radical may be formed. These damaging species are also formed through absorption of environmental chemicals, such as ozone and other pollutants (200–202). Ascorbic acid is part of the antioxidant defense system, which protects plants against photochemical and environmental oxidative stress by destroying these harmful molecules. Spraying with ascorbic acid is effective in protecting plants against environmental chemicals.

Ascorbate has many functions related to plant physiological processes. For example, high concentration of ascorbate increases peroxidase activities. Apoplastic ascorbate affects the activity of cell-wall-associated enzymes in catalyzing lignification (203). During fruit ripening, following the increase in ascorbate concentration, the ascorbate peroxidase activities increase three- to fourfold (204). Ascorbate may play a direct role in delaying senescence in plants (205). However, as senescence progresses, the ascorbate level decreases while chlorophyll is being lost.

BIOCHEMICAL ASPECTS

Oxidation and Hydroxylation

Ascorbic acid is involved in the metabolism of several amino acids, leading to the formation of hydroxyproline, hydroxylysine, norepinephrine, serotonin, homogenistic acid, and carnitine (5,7,20,206,207). Hydroxyproline and hydroxylysine are components of collagens, the fibrous connective tissue in animals. Collagens are principal components of tendons, ligaments, skin, bone, teeth, cartilage, heart valves, intervertebral disks, cornea, eye lens, and the ground substances between cells. When collagen is synthesized, proline and lysine are hydroxylated posttranslationally on the growing polypeptide chain. Hydroxyproline and hydroxylysine are required for the formation of a stable extracellular matrix and cross-links in the fibers. The subsequent triple helix quaternary state of physiologically effective collagen can only be achieved if the requisite proline and lysine residues have been hydroxylated. A deficiency of ascorbic acid reduces the activity of two mixed-function oxidases, prolyl hydroxylase and lysyl hydroxylase, which hydroxylate proline and lysine. The role of ascorbic acid is probably to maintain the iron cofactor in a reduced state at the active sites of the hydroxylases. Some collagen forms in the absence of ascorbic acid, but the fibers are abnormal, resulting in skin lesions and blood vessel fragility, characteristics of scurvy.

Most of the research on collagen biosynthesis related to ascorbic acid has been carried out in cultured cells (208–215). In the collagen synthesizing cells, ascorbic acid is thought to regulate protein synthesis, energy metabolism, and other biological activities. In certain biological systems, the action of ascorbic acid on cells is to promote procollagen secretion and not procollagen synthesis (209,212). In other systems, ascorbic acid stimulates collagen synthesis, independently of hydroxylation, by inducing lipid peroxidation and formation of reactive aldehydes, thereby stimulating collagen gene transcription (213,215).

Another hydroxyproline-containing protein is the plasma complement component C1q, which constitutes an important part of the defense against pathogens. The concentration of C1q is significantly lower in guinea pigs fed a vitamin-C-deficient diet than in those fed a vitamin-C-adequate diet (5,7,216).

Ascorbic acid regulates and participates in enzymatic reactions and transport for neurotransmitters and in hormone biosynthesis (217–221). In the biosynthesis of a variety of neurochemicals, ascorbic acid is involved in many of the hydroxylation and decarboxylation reactions. Tyrosine is normally catabolized to fumaric and acetoacetic acid via homogenistic acid (7,8). Animals deficient in ascorbic acid metabolize tyrosine incompletely. In another metabolic pathway, tyrosine is metabolized in the presence of ascorbic acid to catecholamines by hydroxylation and decarboxylation, forming dopamine, norepinephrine, epinephrine, and adrenocrome. Ascorbic acid is directly involved in the dopamine-β-hydroxylase reaction to produce norepinephrine. The ascorbate free radical may be the primary product of the oxidation. The catecholamine biosynthesis occurs in the adrenal glands and the brain, both with relatively large amounts of ascorbic acid. Ascorbic acid protects catecholamines by direct chemical interactions and by elimination of adrenochrome, a toxic product of catecholamine oxidation, which has been linked to certain mental diseases (7,9). Furthermore, there are complex interactions among catecholamines, their tissue receptors, and ascorbic acid.

The hydroxylation of tyrosine to catecholamines and the hydroxylation of phenylalanine to tyrosine seem to involve the folic acid derivative tetrahydrobiopterin as an electron carrier, and the recycling of ascorbic acid. Ascorbic acid may function to restore this substrate from the oxidized dihydrobiopterin. It has been suggested that dopamine-β-hydroxylase works in conjunction with monodehydroascorbate reductase to recycle tetrahydrobiopterin.

The synthesis of serotonin, a neurotransmitter and vasoconstrictor, involves the hydroxylation and decarboxylation of tryptophan. The initial hydroxylation step, catalyzed by tryptophan hydroxylase, is thought to require ascorbic acid. The cosubstrate for the hydroxylase is tetrahydrobiopterin. Again, it has been suggested that ascorbic acid is able to restore this substrate from its oxidized form, dihydrobiopterin.

Other enzymatic systems responsible for neurotransmitter and hormone synthesis, and dependent on the presence of ascorbic acid and oxygen, are the copper-containing peptidyl glycine amidating monooxygenases, which are found in the atrium, skin, pituitary, and adrenal glands (7,8,218).

Carnitine is a component of heart and skeletal muscles, liver, and other body tissues (7,8). It is essential for the transport of energy-rich activated long-chain fatty acids, from the cytoplasm across the inner mitochondrial membrane to the matrix side, where they are catabolized to acetate. Carnitine is synthesized from lysine and methionine by two hydroxylases through a series of reactions that require ferrous iron and ascorbic acid for full activity (222). A deficiency of vitamin C can decrease the rate of carnitine biosynthesis, decrease the efficiency of renal reabsorption of carnitine, and increase urinary carnitine excretion; these effects may account for the accumulation of triglycerides in the blood and the physical fatigue and lassitude in scurvy (223–225).

Another hydroxylation role for ascorbic acid is the stepwise conversion of cholesterol to bile acid via 7α-hydroxycholesterol (226–229). These reactions require the microsomal enzymatic system containing cytochrome P450-hydroxylases. The activities of these enzymes are depressed in the livers of guinea pigs with marginal vitamin C deficiency. Impaired cholesterol transformation to bile acids causes cholesterol accumulation in the liver and blood, atherosclerotic changes in coronary arteries, and formation of cholesterol gallstone. In hypercholesterolemic humans with low vitamin C status, ascorbic acid administration lowers plasma cholesterol concentration. In lipid metabolism, the oxidation and decarboxylation of fatty acids appear to require ascorbic acid. In an ascorbate-deficient animal, the plasma triglyceride level rises, the postheparin plasma lipolytic activity decreases, and the half-life of plasma triglycerides increases, causing triglyceride accumulation in the liver and arteries.

Detoxification and Bactericidal Activities

One important function of the liver is the metabolism of xenobiotics, such as drugs, poisons, and abnormal metabolites (230,231). Many drugs and lipid-soluble potentially toxic agents produced by the body, such as bilirubin and steroid hormones, are chemically modified by a mixed-function oxidase system in liver microsomes prior to excretion. This oxidase system requires a number of enzymes for hydroxylation and demethylation reactions, cytochrome P450 for electron transport, oxygen, and the presence of a reducing agent such as ascorbic acid. The cytochrome P450 enzymatic system catalyzes the hydrox-

ylation and demethylation of many aromatic chemicals, such as benzene and polychlori-
nated biphenyls, ethanol, various carcinogens, pollutants, and pesticides.

Ascorbic acid participates in the detoxification of a variety of pharmacological and
environmental chemicals (232–240). Several studies have shown that cigarette smokers
who have the same vitamin C intakes as nonsmokers have blood vitamin C levels lower
than those of nonsmokers (234–236). The plasma turnover of ascorbic acid is higher in
smokers than that in nonsmokers (95). Studies from a number of laboratories have indicated
that vitamin C deficiency in guinea pigs results in decreased metabolism of a variety of
pharmacological agents. The administration of toxic chemicals to laboratory animals
increases the rate of ascorbate metabolism and decreases tissue ascorbate content (233,
240). The depletion of vitamin C is associated with a decrease in the activity of many of the
enzymes involved in drug metabolism, and a decrease in the quantity and stability of
cytochrome P450.

Ascorbic acid is known to inhibit the nitrosation of a variety of amines and amides (241–
246). There are many nitrosating agents in the diet capable of reacting with a variety of
amines and amides in the mammalian stomach to produce nitrosamines. Many of these
nitrosamines are highly toxic or carcinogenic. Ascorbic acid inhibits nitrosation reactions
by reacting with nitrosating agents. The reason is that these reactions with ascorbic acid are
generally faster than those between the nitrosating agents and amines or amides.

Phagocytosis, the ingestion and destruction of bacteria by phagocytes, has long been
known to be one of the chief defense mechanisms of the human body against bacterial
attack. The ability of phagocytes to carry out such activities has been shown to be
associated with the presence of ascorbic acid in the white blood cells. Ascorbic acid plays
an important role in aiding phagocytes to function normally and to kill microorganisms
(247–251). It also neutralizes excessive levels of reactive oxidants produced by phagocytes
in cases of chronic infection (251). Ascorbic acid deficiency greatly alters phagocyte
morphological characteristics and mobility and diminishes the level of plasma complement
component C1q and the effectiveness of phagocytes to kill bacteria (216,248,249). A study
of guinea pigs that received various doses of ascorbic acid has indicated that the activities of
phagocytes are positively correlated to serum ascorbic acid levels, and that the number of
bacteria killed per phagocyte increases significantly with increasing doses.

Electron Transport

Ascorbic acid metabolism in animals and plants involves a two-step reversible oxidation
reaction and an irreversible lactone ring opening reaction (5,7). The biochemical and
physiological functions of ascorbic acid primarily depend on its reducing properties and its
role as an electron carrier (164,174,178,179,252,253). By giving up two electrons, ascorbic
acid is converted to dehydroascorbic acid. The loss of one electron, by interaction with
oxygen or metal ions, produces the reactive monodehydroascorbic acid free radical. It is an
important intermediate in a variety of reactions involving the oxidation or reduction of free
radicals present in living cells (24,252,253). These reactions destroy harmful free radicals.
The monodehydroascorbic acid free radical can be reduced back to ascorbic acid by various
enzymes. In certain model systems, however, reactions occur as a result of its redox
potential and not of any enzymatic activity. Dehydroascorbic acid can be reduced back to
ascorbic acid enzymatically, or chemically by a reducing agent, such as glutathione (173).

Ascorbic acid participates in various electron transport reactions and affects the activities of cytochromes, the electron carriers. Several ascorbate oxidoreductases have been

identified (181–185). Some of these are involved in the electron transport reactions with a cytochrome b (179). Monodehydroascorbate oxidoreductase participates in inactivating free radicals and oxidants in living cells. Ascorbic acid is also known as a major electron donor for a transmembrane oxidoreductase of human erythrocytes (254). Cytochrome b561, an electron channel in the membrane secretory vesicles, catalyzes the transmembrane electron transport. It mediates the equilibration of ascorbate-monodehydroascorbate inside the secretory vesicle with the ascorbate redox pair in the cytoplasm. The role for cyto-chrome b561 is to regenerate ascorbate inside the vesicle for use by monooxygenases (255). However, at physiological pH the predominant form of ascorbate monoanion is a poor electron donor because it oxidizes to the stable monodehydroascorbate radical anion. It has been suggested that during the reduction of cytochrome b561, dehydrogenation of the ascorbate monoanion occurs. The reaction mechanism involves a hydrogen atom transfer from the ascorbate monoanion to the cytochrome molecule, rather than an electron transfer (174,256). Another proposed hydrogen atom transfer mechanism of ascorbate is the reac-tion between tocopheroxyl radical and ascorbate (257).

Antioxidant Activity

Molecules containing reactive oxygen are critical to biological systems. There are bio-chemical reactions that result in the formation of oxygen-derived species more reactive than molecular oxygen. Particularly reactive species are the very aggressive oxidants, such as the oxidizing free radicals, singlet oxygen, and the superoxide anion, which attack lipids, proteins, and DNA molecules to cause pathological events.

Since oxygen is required for cell viability it is essential that mechanisms be available to control the reactive oxygen species generated during cellular metabolism and from exog-enous sources, such as radiation and environmental chemicals. For example, the superoxide free radical is capable of forming very aggressive hydroxyl radicals but is normally destroyed by superoxide dismutase, which may depend on ascorbic acid for full activity. Ascorbate and ascorbate radical may function as a cycling redox couple in electron transport and membrane potentiation, or as reducing agents to keep many biochemical substances, including iron- and copper-containing enzymes, in their effective reduced state. Moreover, the reducing properties of ascorbic acid enable it to protect cells and other antioxidants by scavenging oxidizing free radicals. Ascorbic acid reduces stable oxygen, nitrogen, and sulfhydryl radicals and acts as a primary defense against aqueous radicals in the blood and cerebrospinal fluid (258–261). An in vitro study using a spin trapping technique has detected the formation of adducts between the hydroxyl radical and a carbon-centered ascorbate radical (262). These free-radical-scavenging reactions are particularly important in the eye and the extracellular fluid of the lung, where they provide protection against radiation and oxidizing agents, such as ozone and other pollutants (263–265).

Ascorbic acid interacts with certain biological substances to maintain their reducing properties. For example, it is thought to have an essential role in the metabolism of folic acid. Folic acid is involved in many one-carbon transfer reactions in the formation of a wide variety of compounds: purine, thymine, serine, choline, carnitine, creatine, adrenaline, among many others (5,7,127). In these reactions, folic acid must be in its reduced form. The reducing property of ascorbic acid maintains folic acid in its most reduced form.

In vivo experiments have provided strong evidence that ascorbic acid and glutathione, also a water-soluble reducing agent, function together as antioxidants (266,267). On the surface of membrane and in aqueous parts of the cell, ascorbic acid protects glutathione, usually at its own expense, by preventing the oxidation of glutathione. Glutathione deficiency in animals resulted in decreased tissue ascorbic acid concentration and increased tissue dehydroascorbic acid/ascorbic acid ratio. When dehydroascorbic acid is transported into cells, it is presumably reduced to ascorbic acid by glutathione (178,266,267). Administration of ascorbic acid to glutathione-deficient animals decreases the mortality and cell damage that result from oxygen stress.

In vivo and in vitro studies have indicated that ascorbic acid protects tissues, blood components, body fluids, lipids, and lipoproteins against oxidative damage (268–273). Ascorbic acid protects leukocytes and erythrocytes against singlet oxygen and superoxide free radical damage (248,251,271) and destroys nitroxide radicals in the membrane near the membrane surface (249,272). In erythrocytes, the aggressive superoxide free radical may oxidize the heme iron from Fe(II) to Fe(III), to produce nonfunctional methemoglobin (7). This process can be reversed by methemoglobin reductase, which involves cytochrome b5 and ascorbic acid. It has been suggested that ascorbic acid can also directly reduce Fe(III) to Fe(II).

Ascorbic acid prevents metal-ion-dependent initiation and propagation of lipid peroxidation in human low-density lipoproteins (270). Ascorbic acid is reactive enough to intercept oxidants effectively in the aqueous phase before they can cause oxidative damage to lipids (260). Dehydroascorbic acid, the oxidation product of ascorbic acid, also prevents the oxidation of low-density lipoproteins (273).

Although ascorbic acid cannot scavenge lipophilic radicals directly within the lipid compartment, it acts as a synergist with tocopherol for the reduction of lipid peroxide radicals. At the lipid-aqueous interphase, ascorbic acid interacts with the membrane-bound oxidized tocopherol radical to regenerate active tocopherol for more antioxidant functions (257,274,275). The monodehydroascorbic acid radical, a product of this reaction, then disproportionates back to ascorbic acid and dehydroascorbic acid. An in vitro experiment has shown that ascorbic acid prevents the oxidation of vitamin E to tocopherylquinone.

Dietary supplementation with vitamins C and E inhibits in vitro oxidation of lipoproteins in humans (274,275). Guinea pigs fed larger amounts of ascorbic acid have higher concentrations of vitamin E in their tissues than those fed smaller amounts.

Prooxidant Activity

In certain biological systems, ascorbic acid appears to be a prooxidant and functions as such in many biochemical reactions. For example, in vitro studies have indicated that ascorbic acid induces lipid peroxidation and production of reactive aldehydes. These reactions are thought to be required for the stimulation of collagen gene expression in certain collagen-synthesizing cells (213,215). Many in vitro and in vivo studies have demonstrated that the ascorbate free radical is associated with cell growth in various kinds of plants (190–198). Ascorbic acid is toxic to viruses, bacteria, and many types of cultured cells, because of its prooxidant activity (249,276–279). It is particularly toxic to malignant tumor cells but much less toxic to nonmalignant normal cells. The toxic effects of ascorbic acid may be caused by its autooxidation or metal-catalyzed free radical generation and the production of reactive oxidation and degradation products. Furthermore, it has been demonstrated that ascorbic acid in cell culture media generates hydrogen peroxide, and that ascorbic acid inhibits the activity of catalase to decompose hydrogen peroxide (280).

Ascorbic acid has both antioxidant and prooxidant effects on photosensitized peroxidation of lipids in erythrocyte membranes (281,282). It acts as antioxidant and prooxidant in brain tissue homogenates at different concentrations (283). Ascorbate radical has been indirectly detected in experimental brain injury by microdialysis and electron spin resonance spectroscopic technique (284). Because of its reducing properties, ascorbic acid added to the Fenton system increases the rate of hydroxyl radical production (285). In the presence of iron or copper ion, this prooxidant activity derives from the ability of ascorbic acid to reduce Fe(III) and Cu(II) to Fe(II) and Cu(I), respectively, and to generate reactive oxygen-derived species, such as singlet oxygen and hydrogen peroxide. Damage to nucleic acid and proteins results from the binding of either Fe(II) or Cu(I) to metal binding sites on these macromolecules, followed by reaction of the metal complex with hydrogen peroxide. This process leads to the production of active oxygen-derived species that attack functional groups at or near the metal binding sites (286–288), consequently inducing lipid peroxidation, structural change, and cleavage of protein and DNA molecules (289–291). Certain oxidation products of ascorbic acid are also known to be destructive to macromolecules (292). In an enzymatic redox cycling reaction of a naphthoquinone, ascorbic acid appears to be a prooxidant and may increase the potential toxicity of the quinone (293).

In a study with premature infants, high plasma ascorbic acid levels at birth are associated with low antioxidant status (291). However, it is not known whether this phenomenon is the prooxidant effect of ascorbic acid or is related to the systemic conditioning or rebound effect of ascorbic acid as an antioxidant (111,112,116).

Interaction with Mineral Nutrients

Ascorbic acid, as a reducing and chelating agent, interacts with mineral nutrients in diets and tissues. The level of dietary ascorbic acid may have important nutritional consequences through a wide range of inhibitory and enhancing interactions with mineral nutrients (30,294–303). For example, ascorbic acid enhances the intestinal absorption of dietary iron and selenium and reduces the absorption of copper, nickel, and manganese. It apparently has little effect on calcium, zinc, or cobalt and generally has no effect on the toxic minerals cadmium and mercury.

Ascorbic acid has an important role for iron nutrition in humans, and a deficiency interferes with iron metabolism (294–297). For the absorption of dietary nonheme iron, ascorbic acid prevents the formation of insoluble and unabsorbed iron compounds or complexes and reduces the ferric ion to the ferrous ion, which seems to be a requirement for the uptake of iron into the mucosal cells. Ascorbic acid supplementation has been used as a means of reducing iron deficiency in diets low in sources of heme iron. However, the enhancement of iron absorption by ascorbic acid does not occur linearly (84,294). Maximum efficiency of absorption is observed with 25–50 mg ascorbic acid per meal. Therefore, in healthy persons large amounts of dietary ascorbic acid generally do not lead to iron overload.

Ascorbic acid affects the mobilization and distribution of mineral ions throughout the body. For example, ascorbic acid stimulates iron incorporation into ferritin from the iron-bound transferrin, stabilizes ferritin, and enhances iron-induced ferritin translation in human cells (304,305). All these activities are able to increase iron bioavailability. Ascorbic acid also affects the distribution of intracellular iron, favoring its relocation into ferritin while having little effect on the total iron content in the cell (306). On the other hand, in certain experiments, iron overload enhances the oxidative catabolism of ascorbic acid.

Ascorbic acid reacts with certain minerals inside the human body; the products of these reactions may interact with other biochemicals. For example, reaction of chromium(VI) ion with ascorbic acid produces Cr(V) and Cr(IV) ions and carbon-based radicals. Chromium(V) ion and carbon-based radicals are thought to be responsible for Cr-DNA adducts and DNA single-strand breaks (47,307). Another example is the spectroscopic detection of a group of vanadium-diascorbates in human urine (308). These compounds have enzymatic inhibition activities similar to those of ouabain.

ACKNOWLEDGMENT

Appreciation is expressed to Dorothy Munro for her advice and assistance in the preparation of this chapter.

REFERENCES

1. Burns JJ. World Conference on Vitamin C. Vol. 92. New York: New York Academy of Sciences, 1961.
2. King CG, Burns JJ. Second World Conference on Vitamin C. Vol. 258. New York: New York Academy of Sciences, 1975.
3. Burns JJ, Rivers JM, Machlin LJ. Third World Conference on Vitamin C. Vol. 498. New York: New York Academy of Sciences, 1987.
4. Seib PA, Tolbert BM. Ascorbic Acid: Chemistry, Metabolism, and Uses. Advances in Chemistry Series. Washington DC: American Chemical Society, 1982.
5. Basu TK, Schorah CJ. Vitamin C in Health and Disease. London and Canberra: Croom Helm, 1982.
6. Clemetson CAB. Vitamin C. Boca Raton, FL: CRC Press, 1989.
7. Davies MB, Austin J, Partridge DA. Vitamin C: Its Chemistry and Biochemistry. Cambridge: The Royal Society of Chemistry, 1991.
8. Counsell JN, Hornig DH. Vitamin C, Ascorbic Acid. London: Applied Science, 1981.
9. Lewin S. Vitamin C, its Molecular Biology and Medical Potential. London and New York: Academic Press, 1976.
10. Birch GG, Parker KJ. Vitamin C: Recent Aspects of Its Physiological and Technological Importance. New York and Toronto: Wiley, 1974.
11. Chinoy JJ. The Role of Ascorbic Acid in Growth, Differentiation and Metabolism of Plants. The Hague: Kluer Boston, 1987.
12. Nobile S, Woodhill JM. Vitamin C: The Mysterious Redox System, a Trigger of Life. Lancaster: MTP Press, 1981.
13. Carpenter KJ. The History of Vitamin C and Scurvy. Cambridge: Cambridge University Press, 1986.
14. Cheraskin E, Ringsdorf NM Jr, Sisley EL. The Vitamin C Connection. Wellingborough: Thorsons, 1983.
15. Hanck A, Ritzel G. Re-evaluation of Vitamin C. Int J Vitam Nutr Res suppl 16, 1977.
16. Hanck A, Ritzel G. Vitamin C: Recent Advances and Aspects in Virus Diseases, Cancer and in Lipid Metabolism. Int J Vitam Nutr Res suppl 19, 1979.
17. Hanck A. Vitamin C: New Clinical Applications in Immunology, Lipid Metabolism and Cancer. Int J Vitam Nutr Res suppl 23, 1982.
18. Hanck A. Vitamin C in Medicine: Recent Therapeutic Aspects. Int J Vitam Nutr Res suppl 24, 1982.
19. Crawford TC. Synthesis of L-ascorbic acid. In: Seib PA, Tolbert BM, eds. Ascorbic Acid: Chemistry, Metabolism, and Uses. Advances in Chemistry Series. Washington DC: American Chemical Society, 1982:1–36.
20. Tolbert BM, Downing M, Carlson RW, et al. Chemistry and metabolism of ascorbic acid and ascorbate sulfate. Ann NY Acad Sci 1975; 258:48–69.

21. King CG, Waugh WA. The chemical nature of vitamin C. Science 1932; 75:357–358.
22. Svirbely JL, Szent-Györgyi A. The chemical nature of vitamin C. Biochem J 1932; 26:865–870.
23. Tolbert BM, Ward JB. Dehydroascorbic acid. In: Seib PA, Tolbert BM, eds. Ascorbic Acid: Chemistry, Metabolism, and Uses. Advances in Chemistry Series. Washington DC: American Chemical Society, 1982:101–124.
24. Bielski BHJ. Chemistry of ascorbic acid radicals. In: Seib PA, Tolbert BM, eds. Ascorbic Acid: Chemistry, Metabolism, and Uses. Advances in Chemistry Series. Washington DC: American Chemical Society, 1982:81–100.
25. Bielski BHJ, Allen AO, Schwarz HA. Mechanism of disproportionation of ascorbate radicals. J Am Chem Soc 1981; 103:3516–3518.
26. Huelin GE, Coggiola IM, Sidhu GS, Kennett BH. The anaerobic decomposition of ascorbic acid in the pH range of foods and in more acid solutions. J Sci Food Agric 1971; 22:540–542.
27. Velisek J, Davidek J, Janicek G. Behavior of L-dehydroascorbic acid in aqueous solutions. Collect Czech Chem Commun 1972; 37:1465–1470.
28. Niemela K. Oxidative and non-oxidative alkali-catalyzing degradation of L-ascorbic acid. J Chromatogr 1987; 399:235–243.
29. Taqui Kahn MM, Martell AE. Metal ion and metal chelate catalyzed oxidation of ascorbic acid by molecular oxygen. I. Cupric and ferric ion catalyzed oxidation. J Am Chem Soc 1967; 89: 4176–4185.
30. Martell AE. Chelates of ascorbic acid: formation and catalytic properties. In: Seib PA, Tolbert BM, eds. Ascorbic Acid: Chemistry, Metabolism, and Uses. Advances in Chemistry Series. Washington DC: American Chemical Society, 1982:153–178.
31. Tatum JH, Shaw PE, Berry RE. Degradation products from ascorbic acid. J Agric Food Chem 1969; 17:38–40.
32. Reynolds TM. Chemistry of nonenzymatic browning. Adv Food Res 1965; 14:167–283.
33. Kamiya S. Decomposition of L-ascorbic acid: browning reaction of L-ascorbic acid. Nippon Nogeikagaku Kaishi 1960; 34:8–16.
34. Velisek J, Davidek J, Kubelka V, et al. Volatile degradation products of L-dehydroascorbic acid. Z Lebensm Unters Forsch 1976; 162:285–290.
35. Velisek J, Davidek J, El-Zeany BA, et al. Antioxidant activity of some brown pigments in L-ascorbic acid solutions. Z Lebensm Unters Forsch 1974; 154:151–156.
36. Omura H, Tomita Y, Fujiki H, et al. Breaking action of reductones related to ascorbic acid on nucleic acids. J Nutr Sci Vitaminol 1978; 24:263–270.
37. Andrews GC, Grawford TC. Recent advances in the derivatization of L-ascorbic acid. In: Seib PA, Tolbert BM, eds. Ascorbic Acid: Chemistry, Metabolism, and Uses. Advances in Chemistry Series. Washington DC: American Chemical Society, 1982:59–80.
38. Lee CH, Seib PA, Liang YT, et al. Chemical synthesis of several phosphoric esters of L-ascorbic acid. Carbohydr Res 1978; 67:127–138.
39. Bock K, Lundt I, Pedersen C. Preparation of some bromodeoxyaldonic acids. Carbohydr Res 1979; 68:313–319.
40. Humeau C, Girardin M, Coulon D, Miclo A. Synthesis of 6-O-palmityl L-ascorbic acid catalyzed by Candida antartica lipase. Biotech Lett 1995; 17:1091–1094.
41. Schachtner J, Stachel H-D. Synthesis of the (±) carbocyclic analogues of ascorbic and isoascorbic acid. Tetrahedron 1995; 51:9005–9014.
42. Wang XY, Seib PA, Paukstelis JV, et al. Crystal structure of D-erythroascorbic acid. J Carbohydr Chem 1995; 14:1257–1263.
43. Khan MA, Adams H. Simple and efficient stereoselective synthesis of (Z)- and (E)-alkylidene 2,3-dimethoxy-butenolides from L-ascorbic acid and D-isoascorbic acid. J Synthetic Organic Chem 1995; 6:687–692.
44. Saniere M, Charvet I, Le Merrer Y, Depezay J-C. Enantiopure hydroxylactones from L-ascorbic acid and D-isoascorbic acids. Part I. Synthesis of Muricatacin. Tetrahedron 1995; 51:1653–1662.

45. Gravier-Pelletier C, Le Merrer Y, Depezay J-C. Enantiopure hydroxylactones from L-ascorbic acid and D-isoascorbic acids. Part II. Synthesis of (−)-(5R,6S)-6-acetoxy-5-hexadecanolide and its diastereomers. Tetrahedron 1995; 51:1663–1674.

46. Hay RW. Bio-Inorganic Chemistry. Chichester: Ellis Horwood, 1984.

47. Stearns DM, Wetterhahn KE. Reaction of Chromium(VI) with ascorbate produces chromium(V), chromium(IV), and carbon-based radicals. Chem Res Toxicol 1994; 7:219–230.

48. Hayakawa K, Hayashi Y. Detection of a complex intermediate in the oxidation of ascorbic acid by the copper(II) ion. J Nutr Sci Vitaminol 1977; 23:395–401.

49. Sauberlich HE, Green MD, Omaye ST. Determination of ascorbic acid and dehydroascorbic acid. In: Seib PA, Tolbert BM, eds. Ascorbic Acid: Chemistry, Metabolism, and Uses. Advances in Chemistry Series. Washington DC: American Chemical Society, 1982:199–221.

50. Pachla LA, Kissinger PT. Analysis of ascorbic acid by liquid chromatography with amperommetric detection. In: McCormick DB, Wright, eds. Methods in Enzymology. Vol. 62. New York: Academic Press, 1979:15–24.

51. Behrens WA, Madere R. A procedure for the separation and quantitative analysis of ascorbic acid, dehydroascorbic acid, isoascorbic acid, and dehydroisoascorbic acid in food and animal tissue. J Liquid Chromatogr 1994; 17:2445–2455.

52. Tsao CS, Young M. Analysis of ascorbic acid derivatives by high performance liquid chromatography with electrochemical detection. J Chromatogr 1985; 13:855–856.

53. Thompson CO, Trenerry VC. A rapid method for the determination of total L-ascorbic acid in fruits and vegetables by micellar electrokinetic capillary chromatography. Food Chem 1995; 53:43–50.

54. Ito T, Murata H, Yasui Y, et al. Simultaneous determination of ascorbic acid and dehydroascorbic acid in fish tissues by high-performance liquid chromatography. J Chromatogr B 1995; 667:355–357.

55. Roe JH, Keuther CA. The determination of ascorbic acid in whole blood and urine through the 2,4-dinitrophenylhydrazine derivative of dehydroascorbic acid. J Biol Chem 1943; 147:399–407.

56. Schaffert R, Kingsley GR. A rapid, simple method for the determination of reduced, dehydro and total ascorbic acid in biological material. J Biol Chem 1955; 212:59–68.

57. Zannoni V, Lynth M., Goldstein S, Sato P. A rapid micromethod for the determination of ascorbic acid in plasma and tissues. Biochem Med 1974; 11:41–48.

58. Kampfenkel K, Van Montagu M, Inze D. Extraction and determination of ascorbate and dehydroascorbate from plant tissue. Anal Biochem 1995; 225:165–167.

59. Jagota SK, Dani HM. A new colorimetric technique for the estimation of vitamin C using Folin phenol reagent. Anal Biochem 1982; 127:178–182.

60. McGown EL, Rusnak MG, Lewis CM, Tillotson JA. Tissue ascorbic acid analysis using ferrozine compared with the dinitrophenylhydrazine method. Anal Biochem 1982; 119:55–61.

61. Deutsch MJ, Weeks CE. Microfluorometric assay for vitamin C. J Assoc Official Analyt Chem 1965; 48:1248–1256.

62. Moeslinger T, Brunner M, Spieckermann PG. Spectrophotometric determination of dehydroascorbic acid in biological samples. Anal Biochem 1994; 221:290–296.

63. Goldenberg H, Jirovetz L, Krajnik P, et al. Quantitation of dehydroascorbic acid by the kinetic measurement of a derivatization reaction. Anal Chem 1994; 66:1086–1089.

64. Gensler M, Rossmann A, Schmidt H-L. Detection of added L-ascorbic acid in fruit juices by isotope ratio mass spectrometry. J Agric Food Chem 1995; 43:2662–2666.

65. Perez-Rutz T, Martinez-Lozano C, Sanz A. Flow-injection chemiluminometric determination of ascorbic acid based on its sensitized photooxidation. Anal Chim Acta 1995; 308:299–307.

66. Esteve MJ, Farre R, Frigola A, Lopez JC. Comparison of voltammetric and high performance liquid chromatographic methods for ascorbic acid determination in infant formulas. Food Chem 1995; 52:99–102.

67. Machlin LJ, Garcia F, Kuenzig W, et al. Lack of antiscorbutic activity of ascorbate 2-sulfate in the rhesus monkey. Am J Clin Nutr 1976; 29:825–831.

68. Machlin LJ, Garcia JF, Kuenzig W, Brin M. Antiscorbutic activity of ascorbic acid phosphate in the rhesus monkey and the guinea pig. Am J Clin Nutr 1979; 32:325–331.

69. Imai Y, Usui T, Matsuzaki T, Yokotani H, et al. The antiscorbutic activity of L-ascorbic acid phosphate given orally and percutaneously in guinea pigs. Jpn J Pharmacol 1967; 17:317–324.

70. Schulze J, Broz J, Ludwig B. Efficacy of L-ascorbate-2-polyphosphate as a source of ascorbic acid in dogs. Int J Vitam Nutr Res 1992; 63:63–64.

71. Liu TZ, Chin N, Kiser MD, Bigler WN. Specific spectrophotometry of ascorbic acid in serum or plasma by use of ascorbate oxidase. Clin Chem 1982; 28:2225–2228.

72. Moeslinger T, Brunner M, Volf I, Spieckermann PG. Spectrophotometric determination of ascorbic acid and dehydroascorbic acid. Clin Chem 1995; 41:1177–1181.

73. Harris LJ, Olliver M. The reliability of the method for estimating vitamin C by titration against 2,6-dichlorophenol-indophenol. Biochem J 1942; 36:155–182.

74. Koch P, Sidloi M, Tonks DB. Estimation of serum ascorbic acid in patients and the effect of ascorbic acid and its oxidation products on SMA 12/60 parameters. J Biochem 1980; 13: 73–77.

75. Daae LNW, Juell A. Ascorbic acid and test strip reactions for haematuria. Scand J Clin Lab Invest 1983; 43:267–269.

76. Gillenwater JY. Detection of urinary leukocytes by Chemstrip-L. J Urol 1981; 125:383–384.

77. Davie SJ, Gould BJ, Yudkin JS. Effect of vitamin C on glycosylation of proteins. Diabetes 1992; 41:167–173.

78. Weycamp CW, Penders TJ, Muskiet FAJ, van der Slik W. Influence of hemoglobin variants and derivatives on glycohemoglobin determinations, as investigated by 102 laboratories using 16 methods. Clin Chem 1993; 39:1717–1723.

79. Benzie IFF, Strain JJ. The effect of ascorbic acid on the measurement of total cholesterol and triglycerides: possible artefactual lowering in individuals with high plasma concentration of ascorbic acid. Clin Chim Acta 1995; 239:185–190.

80. Siest G, Appel W, Blijenberg GB, et al. Drug interference in clinical chemistry: studies on ascorbic acid. J Clin Chem Clin Biochem 1978; 16:103–110.

81. Freemantle J, Freemantle MJ, Badrick T. Ascorbate interferences in common clinical assays performed on three analyzers. Clin Chem 1994; 40:950–951.

82. White-Stevens RH, Stover LR. Interference by ascorbic acid in test systems involving peroxidase. II. Redox-coupled indicator systems. Clin Chem 1982; 28:589–595.

83. van Os PJHJ, Bult A, van Bennekom WP. A glucose sensor, interference free for ascorbic acid. Anal Chim Acta 1995; 305:18–25.

84. Rivers J. Safety of high-level vitamin C ingestion. Ann NY Acad Sci 1987; 498:445–454.

85. Pollitt RJ, Sandhu B. Ascorbic acid: an unstable ninhydrin-positive urinary constituent running with valine in a commonly used screening system. J Inherited Metab Dis 1980; 3:17–18.

86. Lind J. Treatise on Scurvy. 2nd ed. London: Millar, 1757.

87. Holst A, Frolich T. Experimental studies relating to ship beri-beri and scurvy. II. On the etiology of scurvy. J Hyg 1907; 7:634–671.

88. Chatterjee GC. Effect of ascorbic acid deficiency in animals. In: Sebrell WH, Harris RS. eds. The Vitamins: Chemistry, Physiology, Pathology, Methods. Vol. 1. 2nd ed. New York: Academic Press, 1967:407–457.

89. Spencer RP, Purdy S, Hoeldtke R, et al. Studies on intestinal absorption of L-ascorbic acid-1-C[14]. Gastroenterology 1963; 44:768–773.

90. Spencer RP, Bow TM. In vitro transport of radiolabeled vitamins by the small intestines. J Nucl Med 1964; 5:251–258.

91. Stevenson NR. Active transport of L-ascorbic acid in the human ileum. Gastroenterology 1974; 67:952–956.

92. Stevenson NR, Brush MK. Existence and characteristic of Na^+-dependent active transport of ascorbic acid in guinea pig. Am J Clin Nutr 1969; 22:318–326.

93. Hornig D, Weber F, Wiss O. Site of intestinal absorption of ascorbic acid in guinea pigs and rats. Biochem Biophys Res Comm 1973; 52:168–172.

94. Mellors AJ, Nahrwold DL, Rose RC. Ascorbic acid flux across mucosal border of guinea pig and human ileum. Am J Physiol 1977; 233:E374–E379.

95. Kallner A, Hartmann D, Hornig D. Kinetics of ascorbic acid in humans. In: Seib PA, Tolbert BM, eds. Ascorbic Acid: Chemistry, Metabolism, and Uses. Advances in Chemistry Series. Washington DC: American Chemical Society, 1982:335–348.

96. Vera JC, Rivas CI, Zhang RH, et al. Human HL-60 myeloid leukemia cells transport dehydro-ascorbic acid via the glucose transporters and accumulate reduced ascorbic acid. Blood 1994; 84:1628–1634.

97. Goldenberg H, Schweinzer E. Transport of vitamin C in animal and human cells. J Bioenerg Biomembr 1994; 26:359–367.

98. Siushansian R, Wilson JX. Ascorbate transport and intracellular concentration in cerebral astrocytes. J Neurochem 1995; 65:41–49.

99. Franceschi RT, Wilson JX, Dixon SJ. Requirement for Na-dependent ascorbic acid transport in osteoblast function. Am J Physiol 1995; 268:C1430–C1439.

100. Sharma SK, Johnstone RM, Quastel JH. Active transport of ascorbic acid in adrenal cortex and brain in vitro and the effects of ACTH and steroids. Can J Biochem Physiol 1963; 41:597–604.

101. Toggenburger G, Hausermann M, Mutsch B, et al. Na+-dependent, potential-sensitive L-ascorbate transport across brush border membrane vesicles from kidney cortex. Biochim Biophys Acta 1981; 646:433–443.

102. Morita K, Teraoka K, Oka M, Levine M. Inhibitory action of palytoxin on ascorbic acid transport into cultured bovine adrenal chromaffin cells. J Pharmacol Exp Ther 1966; 276:996–1001.

103. Spector R. Micronutrient homeostasis in mammalian brain and cerebrospinal fluid. J Neurochem 1989; 53:1667–1674.

104. Rybakowski C, Mohar B, Wohlers S, et al. The transport of vitamin C in the isolated human near-term placenta. Eur J Obstet Gynecol Reprod Biol 1995; 62:107–114.

105. Vera JC, Rivas CI, Velasquez FV, et al. Resolution of the facilitated transport of dehydroascorbic acid from its intracellular accumulation as ascorbic acid. J Biol Chem 1995; 270:23706–23712.

106. Bergsten P, Amitai G, Kehr J, et al. Millimolar concentrations of ascorbic acid in purified human mononuclear leukocytes: depletion and reaccumulation. J Biol Chem 1990; 265:2584–2587.

107. Butler JD, Bergsten P, Welch RW, Levine M. Ascorbic acid accumulation in human skin fibroblasts. Am J Clin Nutr 1991; 54:1144S–1146S.

108. Washko P, Rotrosen D, Levine M. Ascorbic acid in human neutrophils. Am J Clin Nutr 1991; 54:1221S–1227S.

109. Hornig D. Distribution of ascorbic acid, metabolites and analogues in man and animals. Ann NY Acad Sci 1975; 258:103–118.

110. Veen-Baigent MJ, Ten Cate AR, Bright-See E, Rao AV. Effects of ascorbic acid on health parameters in guinea pigs. Ann NY Acad Sci 1975; 258:339–354.

111. Angel J, Alfred B, Leichter J, et al. Effect of oral administration of large quantities of ascorbic acid on blood levels and urinary excretion of ascorbic acid in healthy men. Int J Vitam Nutr Res 1975; 45:237–243.

112. Sorensen DI, Devine M, Rivers JM. Catabolism and tissue levels of ascorbic acid following long-term massive doses in the guinea pig. J Nutr 1974; 104:1041–1048.

113. Tsao CS, Leung PY. Urinary ascorbic acid levels following the withdrawal of large doses of ascorbic acid in guinea pigs. J Nutr 1988; 118:895–900.

114. Norkus EP, Rosso P. Effects of maternal intake of ascorbic acid on the postnatal metabolism of this vitamin in the guinea pig. J Nutr 1981; 111:624–628.

115. Cochrane WA. Over nutrition in prenatal and neonatal life, a problem? Can Med Assoc J 1965; 93:893–899.

116. Omaye ST, Skala JH, Jacob RA. Plasma ascorbic acid in adult males: effects of depletion and supplementation. Am J Clin Nutr 1986; 44:257–264.

117. Tsao CS, Leung PY, Young M. Effect of dietary ascorbic acid intake on tissue vitamin C in mice. J Nutr 1987; 117:291–297.

118. Ginter E, Bobeck P. The influence of vitamin C on lipid metabolism. Counsell JN, Hornig DH, eds. In: Vitamin C (Ascorbic Acid). Englewood Cliffs, NJ: Applied Science Publishers, 1982:299–347.

119. Dabrowski K. Primitive actinopterigian fishes can synthesize ascorbic acid. Experientia 1994; 50:745–748.

120. Tsao CS, Young M. Effect of exogenous ascorbic acid intake on biosynthesis of ascorbic acid in mice. Life Sci 1989; 45:1553–1557.

121. Tsao CS, Young M. Enzymatic formation of ascorbic acid in liver homogenate of mice fed dietary ascorbic acid. In Vivo 1990; 4:167–170.

122. Rivers JM. Safety of high level vitamin C ingestion. In: Walter P, Brubacher G, Stähelin H, eds. Elevated Dosages of Vitamins: Benefits and Hazards. Toronto, Lewiston, NY, Bern, and Stuttgart: Hans Haber, 1989:95–102.

123. Prooxidant effects of antioxidant vitamins. Annual Meeting, Experimental Biology 95. Atlanta, GA, April 9–13, 1995.

124. Herbert V. Antioxidants, pro-oxidants, and their effects. JAMA 1994; 272:1659.

125. Levine M, Conry-Cantilena C, Wang Y, et al. Vitamin C pharmacokinetics in healthy volunteers: Evidence for a recommended dietary allowance. Proc Natl Acad Sci USA 1996; 93: 3704–3709.

126. Levine M, Dhariwal KR, Welch RW, et al. Determination of optimal vitamin C requirements in humans. Am J Clin Nutr 1995; 62:1347S–1356S.

127. Gershoff SN. Vitamin C (ascorbic acid): new roles, new requirements? Nutr Rev 1993; 51: 313–326.

128. Harper AE. The recommended dietary allowances for ascorbic acid. Ann NY Acad Sci 1975; 258:491–497.

129. Kallner A. Requirement for vitamin C based on metabolic studies. Ann NY Acad Sci 1987; 498:418–423.

130. Yew MS. Biological variation in ascorbic acid needs. Ann NY Acad Sci 1975; 258:451–457.

131. Williams RJ, Deason G. Individuality in vitamin C needs. Proc Natl Acad Sci USA 1967; 57:1638–1641.

132. Tsao CS. Unpublished data.

133. Knox WE, Goswami MND. Ascorbic acid in man and animals. In: Sobotka H, Stewart CP, eds. Advances in Clinical Chemistry. Vol. 4. New York and London: Academic Press, 1961:121–205.

134. Grollman AP, Lehninger AL. Enzymic synthesis of L-ascorbic acid in different animal species. Arch Biochem Biophys 1957; 69:458–467.

135. Chatterjee IB, Majunder AK, Nandi BK, Subramadian N. Synthesis and some major functions of vitamin C in animals. Ann NY Acad Sci 1975; 258:24–47.

136. Bock KW, Schwarz LR. Formation of L-ascorbic acid in perfused rat liver. Naunyn Schmiedebergs Arch Pharmacol 1974; 284:307–310.

137. Isherwood FA, Chen YT, Mapson LW. Synthesis of L-ascorbic acid in plants and animals. Biochem J 1954; 56:1–15.

138. Horowitz HH, King CG. The conversion of glucose-6-C14 to ascorbic acid by the albino rat. J Biol Chem 1953; 200:125–128.

139. Burns JJ, Mosbach EH. Further observation on the biosynthesis of L-ascorbic acid from D-glucose in the rat. J Biol Chem 1956; 221:107–111.

140. Horowitz HH, King CG. Glucuronic acid as a precursor of ascorbic acid in the albino rat. J Biol Chem 1953; 205:815–821.

141. Burns JJ. Biosynthesis of L-ascorbic acid: basic defect in scurvy. Am J Med 1959; 26:740–748.

142. Nishikimi M, Fukuyama R, Minoshima S, et al. Cloning and chromosomal mapping of the human nonfunctional gene for L-gulonolactone oxidase, the enzyme for L-ascorbic acid biosynthesis missing in man. J Biol Chem 1994; 269:13685–13688.

143. Nishikimi M, Yagi K. Molecular basis for the deficiency in humans of gulonolactone oxidase, a key enzyme for ascorbic acid biosynthesis. Am J Clin Nutr 1991; 54:1203S–1208S.

144. Sugisawa T, Ojima S, Matzinger PK, Hoshino T. Isolation and characterization of a new vitamin C producing enzyme (L-gulono-γ-lactone dehydrogenase) of bacterial origin. Biosci Biotech Biochem 1995; 59:190–196.

145. Bissell DM, Guzelian PS. Ascorbic acid deficiency and cytochrome P-450 in adult rat hepatocytes in primary monolayer culture. Arch Biochem Biophys 1979; 192:569–576.

146. Braun L, Garzo T, Mandl J, Banhegyi G. Ascorbic acid synthesis is stimulated by enhanced glycogenolysis in murine liver. FEBS Lett 1994; 352:4–6.

147. Jaffe GM. Vitamin C. In: Machlin LJ, ed. Handbook of Vitamins. New York and Basel: Marcel Dekker, 1984:199–244.

148. Horio F, Shibata T, Makino S, et al. UDP glucuronosyltransferase gene expression is involved in the stimulation of ascorbic acid biosynthesis by xenobiotics in rats. J Nutr 1993; 123:2075–2084.

149. Ashwell G, Kanfer J, Smiley JD, Burns JJ. Metabolism of ascorbic acid and related uronic acids, aldonic acids and pentoses. Ann NY Acad Sci 1961; 92:105–114.

150. Chan PC, Becker RR, King CG. Metabolic product of L-ascorbic acid. J Biol Chem 1958; 231:231–240.

151. Fituri N, Allawi N, Bentley M, Costello J. Urinary and plasma oxalate during ingestion of pure ascorbic acid: a re-evaluation. Eur Urol 1983; 9:312–315.

152. Baker EM, Levandoski NG, Sauberlich HE. Respiratory catabolism in man of the degradative intermediates of L-ascorbic-1-^{14}C acid. Proc Soc Exp Biol 1963; 113:379–383.

153. Abt AF, von Schuchling SL, Enns T. Vitamin C requirements of man reexamined: new values based on previously unrecognized exhalatory excretory pathway of ascorbic acid. Am J Clin Nutr 1963; 12:21–29.

154. von Schuchling SL, Abt AF. Verification of L-ascorbic-1-^{14}C-acid catabolism to ^{14}C carbon dioxide in the human by liquid scintillation counting. Proc Soc Exp Biol NY 1965; 118:30–37.

155. Kallner A, Hornig D, Pellikka R. Formation of carbon dioxide from ascorbate in man. Am J Clin Nutr 1985; 41:609–613

156. Bowers-Komro DM, McCormick DB, King GA, et al. Confirmation of 2-O-methyl ascorbic acid as the product from the enzymatic methylation of L-ascorbic acid by catechol-O-methyltransferase. Int J Vitam Nutr Res 1982; 52:185–192.

157. Blaschke E, Hertting G. Enzymic methylation of L-ascorbic acid by catechol O-methyltransferase. Biochem Pharm 1971; 20:1363–1370.

158. Gallice P, Sarrazin F, Polverelli M, et al. Ascorbic acid-2-O-β-glucuronide, a new metabolite of vitamin C identified in human urine and uremic plasma. Biochim Biophys Acta 1994; 1199:305–310.

159. Loewus FA, Loewus MW. Biosynthesis and metabolism of ascorbic acid in plants. CRC Crit Rev Plant Sci 1987; 5:101–119.

160. Kroneck PMH, Armstrong FA, Merkle H, Marchesini A. Ascorbate oxidase: molecular properties and catalytic activity. In: Seib PA, Tolbert BM, eds. Ascorbic Acid: Chemistry, Metabolism, and Uses. Advances in Chemistry Series. Washington DC: American Chemical Society, 1982:223–248.

161. Kim Y-R, Yu S-W, Lee S-R, et al. A heme-containing ascorbate oxidase from Pleurotus ostreatus. J Biol Chem 1996; 271:3105–3111.

162. Messerschmidt A, Rossi A, Ladenstein R, et al. X-ray crystal structure of the blue oxidase ascorbate oxidase from zucchini: analysis of the polypeptide fold and a model of the copper sites and ligands. J Med Biol 1989; 206:513–529.

163. Kato N, Esaka M. cDNA cloning and gene expression of ascorbate oxidase in tobacco. Plant Mol Biol 1996; 30:833–837.

164. Farver O, Wherland S, Pecht I. Intramolecular electron transfer in ascorbate oxidase is enhanced in the presence of oxygen. J Biol Chem 1994; 269:22933–22936.

165. bin Saari N, Fujita S, Haraguchi K, Miyazoe R. Neutral and acidic ascorbate oxidases from satsuma mandarin (*Citrus unshiu* marc) isolation and properties. J Sci Food Agric 1995; 68:515–519.

166. Grace S, Pace R, Wydrzynski T. Formation and decay of monodehydroascorbate radicals in illuminated thylakoids as determined by EPR spectroscopy. Biochim Biophys Acta 1995; 1229:155–165.

167. Santos M, Gousseau H, Lister C, et al. Cytosolic ascorbate peroxidase from *Arabidopsis thaliana L* is encoded by a small multigene family. Planta 1996; 198:64–69.

168. Bunkelmann JR, Trelease RN. Ascorbate peroxidase. Plant Physiol 1996; 110:589–598.

169. Ishikawa T, Sakai K, Takeda T, Shigeoka S. Cloning and expression of cDNA encoding a new type of ascorbate peroxidase from spinach. FEBS Lett 1995; 367:28–32.

170. Yamaguchi K, Mori H, Nishimura M. A novel isoenzyme of ascorbate peroxidase localized on glyoxysomal and leaf peroxisomal membranes in pumpkin. Plant Cell Physiol 1995; 36:1157–1162.

171. Patterson WR, Poulos TL. Crystal structure of recombinant pea cytosolic ascorbate peroxidase. Biochemistry 1995; 34:4331–4341.

172. Dalton DA, del Castillo LD, Kahn ML, et al. Heterologous expression and characterization of soybean cytosolic ascorbate peroxidase. Arch Biochem Biophys 1996; 328:1–8.

173. Wells WW, Xu DP, Washburn MP. Glutathione: dehydroascorbate oxidoreductases. Methods Enzymol 1995; 252:30–38.

174. Coassin M, Tomasi A, Vannini V, Unisini F. Enzymatic recycling of oxidized ascorbate in pig heart: one electron vs two-electron pathway. Arch Biochem Biophys 1991; 290:458–462.

175. Washko P, Wang Y, Levine M. Ascorbic acid recycling in human neutrophils. J Biol Chem 1993; 268:15531–15535.

176. Maellaro E, Del Bello B, Sugherini L, et al. Purification and characterization of glutathione-dependent dehydroascorbate reductase from rat liver. Biochem J 1994; 301:471–476.

177. Wells WW, Xu D-P, Yang Y, Rocque PA. Mammalian thioltransferase (glutaredoxin) and protein disulfide isomerase have dehydroascorbate reductase activity. J Biol Chem 1990; 265:15361–15364.

178. Wells WW, Xu DP. Dehydroascorbate reduction. J Bioenerg Biomembr 1994; 26:369–377.

179. Weis W. Ascorbic acid and electron transport. Ann NY Acad Sci 1975; 285:190–200.

180. Stankova L, Rigas DA, Bigley RH. Dehydroascorbate uptake and reduction by human blood neutrophils, erythrocytes, and lymphocytes. Ann NY Acad Sci 1975; 258:238–242.

181. Lumper L, Schneider W, Staudinger HJ. Untersuchungen zur kinetik der mikrosomalen NADH: semidehydroascorbat-oxydoreducktase. Hoppe Seylers Z Physiol Chem 1967; 348:323–328.

182. De Leonardis S, De Lorenzo G, Borraccino G, Dipierro S. A specific ascorbate free radical reductase isozyme participates in the regeneration of ascorbate for scavenging toxic oxygen species in potato tuber mitochondria. Plant Physiol 1995; 109:847–851.

183. Kobayashi K, Tagawa S, Sano S, Asada K. A direct demonstration of the catalytic action of monodehydroascorbate reductase by pulse radiolysis. J Biol Chem 1995; 270:27551–27554.

184. Sano S, Asada K. cDNA cloning of monodehydroascorbate radical reductase from cucumber: a high degree of homology in terms of amino acid sequence between this enzyme and bacterial flavoenzymes. Plant Cell Physiol 1994; 35:425–437.

185. Sano S, Miyake C, Mikami B, Asada K. Molecular characterization of monodehydroascorbate radical reductase from cucumber highly expressed in *Escherichia coli*. J Biol Chem 1995; 270:21354–21361.

186. Saito K. Formation of L-ascorbic acid and oxalic acid from D-glucosone in *Lemna minor*. Phytochem 1996; 41:145–149.

187. Loewus FA, Wagner G, Yang JC. Biosynthesis and metabolism of ascorbic acid in plants. Ann NY Acad Sci 1975; 258:7–23.
188. Loewus FA, Helsper JPFG. Metabolism of L-ascorbic acid in plants. In: Seib PA, Tolbert BM, eds. Ascorbic Acid: Chemistry, Metabolism, and Uses. Advances in Chemistry Series. Washington DC: American Chemical Society, 1982:249–262.
189. Rautenkranz AAF, Li L, Machler F, et al. Transport of ascorbic acid and dehydroascorbic acids across protoplast and vacuole membranes isolated from barley leaves. Plant Physiol 1994; 106:187–193.
190. Arrigoni O. Ascorbate system in plant development. J Bioenerg Biomembr 1994; 26:407–419.
191. Asard H, Horemans N, Caubergs RJ. Involvement of ascorbic acid and b-type cytochrome in plant plasma membrane redox reactions. Protoplasma 1995; 184:36–41.
192. Asard H, Horemans N, Caubergs RJ. Transmembrane electron transport in ascorbate-loaded plasma membrane vesicles from higher plants involves a b-type cytochrome. FEBS Lett 1992; 306:143–146.
193. Horemans N, Asard H, Caubergs RJ. The role of ascorbate free radical as an electron acceptor to cytochrome b-mediated trans-plasma membrane electron transport in higher plants. Plant Physiol 1994; 104:1455–1458.
194. Forti G, Elli G. The function of ascorbic acid in photosynthetic phosphorylation. Plant Physiol 1995; 109:1207–1211.
195. Cordoba F, Gonzalez-Reyes JA. Ascorbate and plant cell growth. J Bioenerg Biomembr 1994; 26:399–405.
196. Navas P, Gomez-Diaz C. Ascorbate free radical and its role in growth control. Protoplasma 1995; 184:8–13.
197. Gonzalez-Reyes JA, Alcain FJ, Caler JA, et al. Stimulation of onion root elongation by ascorbate and ascorbate free radical in Allium cepa L. Protoplasma 1995; 184:31–35.
198. Citterio S, Sgorbati S, Scippa S, Sparvoli E. Ascorbic acid effect on the onset of cell proliferation in pea root. Physiol Plant 1994; 92:601–607.
199. Halliwell B. Ascorbic acid and the illuminated chloroplast. In: Seib PA, Tolbert BM, eds. Ascorbic Acid: Chemistry, Metabolism, and Uses. Advances in Chemistry Series. Washington DC: American Chemical Society, 1982:263–274.
200. Foyer CH, Lelandais M, Kunert KJ. Photooxidative stress in plants. Physiol Plant 1994; 92:696–717.
201. Kubo A, Saji H, Tanaka K, Kondo N. Expression of arabidopsis cytosolic ascorbate peroxidase gene in response to ozone or sulfur dioxide. Plant Mol Biol 1995; 29:479–489.
202. Polle A, Wieser G, Havranek WM. Quantification of ozone influx and apoplastic ascorbate content in needles of Norway spruce trees at high altitude. Plant Cell Environ 1995; 18: 681–688.
203. Otter T, Polle A. The influence of apoplastic ascorbate on the activities of cell wall associated peroxidase and NADH oxidase in needles of Norway spruce. Plant Cell Physiol 1994; 35: 1231–1238.
204. Schantz M-L, Schreiber H, Guillemaut P, Schantz R. Changes is ascorbate peroxidase activities during fruit ripening in Capsicum annuum. FEBS Lett 1995; 358:149–152.
205. Borraccino G, Mastropasqua L, De Leonardis S, Dipierro S. The role of the ascorbic acid system in delaying the senescence of oat leaf segments. Plant Physiol 1994; 144:161–166.
206. Barnes MJ. Function of ascorbic acid in collagen metabolism. Ann NY Acad Sci 1975; 258:264–277.
207. Kipp DE, McElvain M, Kimmel DB, et al. Scurvy results in decreased collagen synthesis and bone density in the guinea pig animal model. Bone 1996; 18:281–288.
208. Shapiro IM, Leboy PS, Tokuoka T, et al. Ascorbic acid regulates multiple metabolic activities of cartilage cells. Am J Clin Nutr 1991; 54:1209S–1213S.
209. Salpeter MM, Liu E, Minor RR, et al. Acetylcholine receptor regulation in L5 muscle cells is independent of increases in collagen secretion induced by ascorbic acid. Am J Clin Nutr 1991; 54:1184S–1187S.

210. Graham MF, Willey A, Adams J, et al. Role of ascorbic acid in procollagen expression and secretion by human intestinal smooth muscle cells. J Cell Physiol 1995; 162:225–233.

211. Geesin JC, Darr D, Kaufman R, Murad S. Ascorbic acid specifically increases type I and type III procollagen messenger RNA levels in human skin fibrobasts. J Invest Dermatol 1988; 90:420–424.

212. Peterkofsky B. Ascorbate requirement for hydroxylation and secretion of procollagen: relationship to inhibition of collagen synthesis in scurvy. Am J Clin Nutr 1991; 54:1135S–1140S.

213. Houglum KP, Brenner DA, Chojkier M. Ascorbic acid stimulation of collagen biosynthesis independent of hydroxylation. Am J Clin Nutr 1991; 54:1141S–1143S.

214. Chan D, Lamande SR, Cole WG, Bateman JF. Regulation of procollagen synthesis and processing during ascorbate-induced extracellular matric accumulation in vitro. Biochem J 1990; 269:175–181.

215. Geesin JC, Hendricks LJ, Gordon JS, Berg RA. Modulation of collagen synthesis by growth factors: the role of ascorbate-stimulated lipid peroxidation. Arch Biochem Biophys 1991; 67: 952–956.

216. Haskell BE, Johnston CS. Complement component C1q activity and ascorbic acid nutriture in guinea pigs. Am J Clin Nutr 1991; 54:1228S–1230S.

217. Diliberto EJ Jr, Daniels AJ, Viveros Multicompartmental secretion of ascorbate and its dual role in dopamine b-hydroxylation. Am J Clin Nutr 1991; 54:1163S–1172S.

218. Eipper BA, Mains RE. The role of ascorbate in the biosynthesis of neuroendocrine peptides. Am J Clin Nutr 1991; 54:1153S–1156S.

219. Rebec GV, Pierce RC. A vitamin as neuromodulator: ascorbate release into the extracellular fluid of the brain regulates dopaminergic and glutamatergic transmission. Progr Neurobiol 1994; 43:537–565.

220. Tolbert LC, Thomas TN, Middaugh LD, Zemp JW. Effect of ascorbic acid on neurochemical, behavioral, and physiological systems mediated by catecholamines. Life Sci 1979; 25:2189–2195.

221. Desole, MS, Anania A, Esposito G, et al. Neurochemical and behavioral changes induced by ascorbic acid and *d*-amphetamine in the rat. Pharmacol Res Comm 1987; 19:441–450.

222. Reboucne CJ. Ascorbic acid and carnitine biosynthesis. Am J Clin Nutr 1991; 54:1147S–1152S.

223. Nelson PJ, Pruitt RE, Henderson LL, et al. Effect of ascorbic acid deficiency on the in vivo synthesis of carnitine. Biochim Biophys Acta 1981; 672:123–127.

224. Ha TY, Otsuka M, Arakawa N. The effect of graded doses of ascorbic acid on the tissue carnitine and plasma lipid concentrations. J Nutr Sci Vitaminol 1990; 36:227–234.

225. Rebouche CJ. Renal handling of carnitine in experimental vitamin C deficiency. Metabolism 1995; 44:1639–1643.

226. Ginter E, Jurcovicova M. Chronic vitamin C deficiency lowers fractional catabolic rate of low-density lipoproteins in guinea pigs. Ann NY Acad Sci 1987; 498:473–475.

227. Ginter E, Bobek P, Jurcovicova M. Role of L-ascorbic acid in lipid metabolism. In: Seib PA, Tolbert BM, eds. Ascorbic Acid: Chemistry, Metabolism, and Uses. Advances in Chemistry Series. Washington DC: American Chemical Society, 1982:381–393.

228. Uchida K, Nomura Y, Takase H. Effect of vitamin depletion on serum cholesterol and lipoprotein levels in ODS (od/od) rats unable to synthesize ascorbic acid. J Nutr 1990; 120:1140–1147.

229. Hallfrisch J, Singh VN, Muller DC, et al. High plasma vitamin C associated with high plasma HDL- and HDL2 cholesterol. Am J Clin Nutr 1994; 60:100–105.

230. Zannoni VG, Holsztynska EJ, Lau SS. Biochemical functions of ascorbic acid in drug metabolism. In: Seib PA, Tolbert BM, eds. Ascorbic Acid: Chemistry, Metabolism, and Uses. Advances in Chemistry Series. Washington DC: American Chemical Society, 1982:349–368.

231. Zannoni VG, Sato PH. Effects of ascorbic acid on microsomal drug metabolism. Ann NY Acad Sci 1975; 258:119–131.

232. Shimpo K, Nagatsu T, Yamada K, et al. Ascorbic acid and adriamycin toxicity. Am J Clin Nutr 1991; 54:1298S–1301S.
233. Ficek W. Vitamin C and DNA content in the thymus and other lymphatic tissues of mice (C57BL) after administration of hydrocortisone. Biochem Arch 1995; 11:21–26.
234. Brown AJ. Acute effects of smoking cessation on antioxidant status. Nutr Biochem 1996; 7:29–39.
235. Schectman G, Byrd JC, Hoffmann R. Ascorbic acid requirements for smokers: analysis of a population survey. Am J Clin Nutr 1991; 53:1466–1470.
236. Pelletier O. Vitamin C and cigarette smokers. Ann NY Acad Sci 1975; 258:156–168.
237. Overman DO, Graham MN, Roy WA. Ascorbate inhibiton of 6-aminonicotinamide teratogenesis in chicken embryos. Teratology 1976; 13:85–94.
238. Kovacikova Z, Ginter E. Effect of ascorbic acid supplementation during the inhalation exposure of guinea pigs to industrial dust on bronchoalveolar lavage and pulmonary enzymes. J Appl Toxicol 1995; 15:321–324.
239. Gonzalez JP, Valdivieso A, Calvo R, et al. Influence of vitamin C on the absorption and first pass metabolism of propranolol. Eur J Clin Pharmacol 1995; 48:295–297.
240. Zannoni VG, Brodfuehrer JI, Smart RC, Susick RL. Ascorbic acid, alcohol, and environmental chemicals. Ann NY Acad Sci 1987; 498:364–388.
241. Tannenbaum SR. Preventive action of vitamin C on nitrosamine formation. In: Walter P, Brubacher G, Stähelin H. Elevated Dosages of Vitamins: Benefits and Hazards. Toronto, Lewiston NY, Bern, and Stuttgart: Hans Haber, 1989:109–113.
242. Cieslik E. The effect of naturally occurring vitamin C in potato tubers on the levels of nitrates and nitrites. Food Chem 1994; 49:233–235.
243. Mirvish SS. Blocking the formation of *N*-nitroso compounds with ascorbic acid in vitro and in vivo. Ann NY Acad Sci 1975; 258:175–180.
244. Kamm JJ, Dashman T, Conney AH, Burns JJ. Effect of ascorbic acid on amine-nitrite toxicity. Ann NY Acad Sci 1975; 258:169–174.
245. Wagner DA, Shuker DEG, Bilmazes C, et al. Effect of vitamins C and E on endogenous synthesis of *N*-nitrosamino acids in humans: precursor–product studies with 15N nitrate. Cancer Res 1985; 45:6519–6522.
246. Ton CCT, Fong LYY. The effects of ascorbic acid deficiency and excess on the metabolism and toxicity of *N*-nitrosodimethylamine and *N*-nitrosodiethylamine in the guinea pig. Carcinogen 1984; 5:533–536.
247. Boxer LA, Vanderbilt B, Bonsib S, et al. Enhancement of chemotactic response and microtubule assembly in human leukocytes by ascorbic acid. J Cell Physiol 1979; 100:119–126.
248. Rawal BD. Bactericidal action of ascorbic acid on *Pseudomonas aeruginosa*: alteration of cell surface as a possible mechanism. Chemotherapy 1978; 24:166–177.
249. Goldschmidt MC. Reduced bactericidal activity in neutrophils from scorbutic animals and the effect of ascorbic acid on these target bacteria in vivo and in vitro. Am J Clin Nutr 1991; 54: 1214S–1220S.
250. Goldschmidt MC, Masin WJ, Brown LR, Wyde PR. The effect of ascorbic acid deficiency on leukocyte phagocytosis and killing of *Actinomyces viscosus*. Int J Vitam Nutr Res 1988; 58: 326–334.
251. Anderson R, Lukey PT. A biological role for ascorbate in the selective neutralization of extracellular phagocyte-derived oxidants. Ann NY Acad Sci 1987; 498:229–247.
252. Sies H. Relationship between free radicals and vitamins: an overview. In: Walter P, Brubacher G, Stähelin H, eds. Elevated Dosages of Vitamins: Benefits and Hazards. Toronto, Lewiston NY, Bern, and Stuttgart: Hans Haber, 1989:215–223.
253. Ghiretti F, Ghiretti-Magaldi A. The effect of vitamin C on the intracellular oxygen transport. In: Hanck A, and Ritzel G, eds. Re-evaluation of Vitamin C. Bern: Verlag Hans Huber, 1977: 41–51.
254. May JM, Qu ZC, Whitesell RR. Ascorbate is the major electron donor for a transmembrane oxidoreductase of human erythrocytes. Biochim Biophys Acta 1995; 1238:127–136.

255. Fleming PJ, Kent UM. Cytochrome b561, ascorbic acid, and transmembrane electron transfer. Am J Clin Nutr 1991; 54:1173S–1178S.

256. Njus D, Jalvkar V, Zu J, Kelley PM. Concerted proton–electron transfer between ascorbic acid and cytochrome b561. Am J Clin Nutr 1991; 54:1179S–1183S

257. Bisby RH, Parker AW. Reaction of ascorbate with the α-tocopheroxyl radical in micellar and bilayer membrane systems. Arch Biochem Biophys 1995; 317:170–178.

258. Barabas J, Nagy E, Degrell I. Ascorbic acid in cerebrospinal fluid: a possible protection against free radicals in the brain. Arch Gerontol Geriat 1995; 21:43–48.

259. Frei B, England L, Ames BN. Ascorbate is an outstanding antixodant in human blood plasma. Proc Natl Acad Sci USA 1989; 86:6377–6381.

260. Frei B. Ascorbic acid protects lipids in human plasma and low-density lipoprotein against oxidative damage. Am J Clin Nutr 1991; 54:1113S–1118S.

261. Niki E. Action of ascorbic acid as a scavenger of active and stable oxygen radicals. Am J Clin Nutr 1991; 54:1119S–1128S.

262. Bernofsky C, Bandara BMR. Spin trapping endogenous radicals in MC-1010 cells: evidence for hydroxyl radical and carbon-centered ascorbyl radical adducts. Mol Cell Biochem 1995; 148:155–164.

263. Ringvold A. The significance of ascorbate in the aqueous humour protection against UV-A and UV-B. Exp Eye Res 1996; 62:261–264.

264. Narra VR, Harapanhalli RS, Howell RW, et al. Vitamins as radioprotectors in vivo. I. Protection by vitamin C against internal radionuclides in mouse testes: implications to the mechanism of damage caused by the Auger effect. Radiat Res 1994; 137:394–399.

265. Garland DL. Ascorbic acid and the eye. Am J Clin Nutr 1991; 54:1198S–1202S.

266. Winkler BS, Orselli SM, Rex TS. The redox couple between glutathione and ascorbic acid: a chemical and physiological perspective. Free Radical Biol Med 1994; 17:333–349.

267. Martensson J, Meister A. Glutathione deficiency decreases tissue ascorbate levels in newborn rats: ascorbate spares glutathione and protects. Proc Natl Acad Sci USA 1991; 88:4656–4660.

268. Chakraborty S, Nandi A, Mukhopadhyay M, et al. Ascorbate protects guinea pig tissues against lipid peroxidation. Free Radical Biol Med 1994; 16:417–426.

269. Rifici VA, Khachadurian AK. Dietary supplementation with vitamins C and E inhibits in vitro oxidation of lipoproteins. J Am Coll Nutr 1993; 12:631–637.

270. Parkkinen J, Vaaranen O, Vahtera E. Plasma ascorbate protects coagulation factors against photooxidation. Thromb Haemost 1996; 75:293–297.

271. Postaire E, Regnault C, Simonet L, et al. Increase of singlet oxygen protection of erythrocytes by vitamin E, vitamin C, and β-carotene intakes. Biochem Mol Biol Int 1995; 35:371–374.

272. Zhang Y, Fung LWM. The role of ascorbic acid and other antioxidants in the erythrocyte in reducing membrane nitroxide radicals. Free Radical Biol Med 1994; 16:215–222.

273. Retsky KL, Freeman MW, Frei B. Ascorbic acid oxidation product(s) protect human low density lipoprotein against atherogenic modification. J Biol Chem 1993; 268:1304–1309.

274. Niki E, Noguchi N, Tsuchihashi H, Gotoh N. Interaction among vitamin C, vitamin E, and β-carotene. Am J Clin Nutr 1995; 62:1322S–1326S.

275. Chan AC. Partners in defense, vitamin E and vitamin C. Can J Physiol Pharmacol 1993; 71: 725–731.

276. Hovi T, Hirvimies A, Stenvik M, et al. Topical treatment of recurrent mucocutaneous herpes with ascorbic acid-containing solution. Antiviral Res 1995; 27:263–270.

277. Peterkofsky B, Prather W. Cytotoxicity of ascorbate and other reducing agents toward cultured fibroblasts as a result of hydrogen peroxide formation. J Cell Physiol 1977; 90:61–70.

278. Leung PY, Miyashita K, Young M, Tsao CS. Cytotoxic effect of ascorbate and its derivatives on cultured malignant and nonmalignant cell lines. Anticancer Res 1993; 13:475–480.

279. Andersson M, Grankvist K. Ascorbate-induced free radical toxicity to isolated islet cells. Int J Biol 1995; 27:493–498.

280. Orr CWM. The inhibition of catalase (hydrogen-peroxide: hydrogen peroxide oxidoreductase, EC 1.11.1.6) by ascorbate. Methods Enzymol 1970; 18:59–62.

281. Girotti AW, Thomas JP, Jordan JE. Prooxidant and antioxidant effects of ascorbate on photosensitized peroxidation of lipids in erythrocyte membranes. Photochem Photobiol 1985; 41: 267–276.

282. Heikkila RE, Manzino L. Ascorbic acid, redox cycling, lipid peroxidation, and the binding of dopamine receptor antagonists. Ann NY Acad Sci 1987; 498:63–76.

283. Li CL, Werner P, Cohen G. Lipid peroxidation in brain: interactions of L-DOPA/dopamine with ascorbate and iron. Neurodegeneration 1995; 4:147–153.

284. Kihara T, Sakata S, Ikeda M. Direct detection of ascorbyl radical in experimental brain injury: microdialysis and an electron spin resonance spectroscopic study. J Neurochem 1995; 65: 282–286.

285. Zhao MJ, Jung L. Kinetics of the competitive degradation of deoxyribose and other molecules by hydroxyl radicals produced by the Fenton reaction in the presence of ascorbic acid. Free Radical Res 1995; 23:229–243.

286. Stadtman ER. Ascorbic acid and oxidative inactivation of proteins. Am J Clin Nutr 1991; 54: 1125S–1128S.

287. Chou W-Y, Tsai W-P, Lin C-C, Chang G-G. Selective oxidative modification and affinity cleavage of pigeon liver malic enzyme by the Cu^{2+}-ascorbate system. J Biol Chem 1995; 270: 25935–25941.

288. Reinheckel T, Wiswedel I, Noack H, Augustin W. Electrophoretic evidence for the impairment of complexes of the respiratory chain during iron/ascorbate induced peroxidation in isolated rat liver mitochondria. Biochim Biophys Acta 1995; 1239:45–50.

289. Littlefield NA, Hass BS. Damage in DNA by cadmium or nickel in the presence of ascorbate. Ann Clin Lab Sci 1995; 25:485–492.

290. Garland D, Zigler JS, Kinoshita J. Structural changes in bovine lens crystallins induced by ascorbate, metal, and oxygen. Arch Biochem Biophysics 1986; 251:771–776.

291. Silver KM, Gibson AT, Powers HJ. High plasma vitamin C concentrations at birth associated with low antioxidant status and poor outcome in premature infants. Arch Dis Child 1994; 71: F40–F44.

292. Nagaraj RH, Monnier VM. Protein modification by the degradation products of ascorbate: formation of a novel pyrrole from the Maillard reaction of L-threose with proteins. Biochim Biophys Acta 1995; 1253:75–84.

293. Jarabak R, Jarabak J. Effect of ascorbate on the DT-diaphorase-mediated redox cycling of 2-methyl-1,4-naphthoquinone. Arch Biochem Biophys 1995; 318:418–423.

294. Solomons NW. Biological interaction of ascorbic acid and mineral nutrients. In: Seib PA, Tolbert BM, eds. Ascorbic Acid: Chemistry, Metabolism, and Uses. Advances in Chemistry Series. Washington DC: American Chemical Society, 1982:550–569.

295. Hallberg L, Brune M, Rossander L. The role of vitamin C in iron absorption. In: Walter P, Brubacher G, Stähelin H, eds. Elevated Dosages of Vitamins: Benefits and Hazards. Toronto, Lewiston NY, Bern, and Stuttgart: Hans Haber, 1989:103–108.

296. Baader SL, Bill E, Trautwein AX, et al. Mobilization of iron from cellular ferritin by ascorbic acid in neuroblastoma SK-N-SH cells: an EPR study. FEBS Lett 1996; 381:131–134.

297. Hunt JR, Gallagher SK, Johnson LK. Effect of ascorbic acid on apparent iron absorption by women with low iron stores. Am J Clin Nutr 1994; 59:1381–1385.

298. Sandstrom B, Cederblad A. Effect of ascorbic acid on the absorption of zinc and calcium in man. Int J Vitam Nutr Res 1987; 57:87–90.

299. Davidsson L, Almgren A, Juillerat M-A, Hurrell RF. Manganese absorption in humans: the effect of phytic acid and ascorbic acid in soy formula. Am J Clin Nutr 1995; 62:984–987.

300. Morcos SR, El-Shobaki FA, El-Hawary Z, Saleh N. Effect of vitamin C and carotene on the absorption of calcium from the intestine. Ernaehrungswiss 1976; 15:387–390.

301. Milne DB, Omaye ST. Effect of vitamin C on copper and iron metabolism in the guinea pig. Int J Vitam Nutr Res 1980; 50:301–308.

302. Johnson MA, Murphy CL. Adverse effects of high dietary iron and ascorbic acid on copper status in copper-deficient and copper-adequate rats. Am J Clin Nutr 1988; 47:96–101.

303. Calabrese EJ, Stoddard A, Leonard DA, Dinardi SR. The effects of vitamin C supplementation on blood and hair levels of cadmium. Ann NY Acad Sci 1987; 498:347–353.

304. Bridges KR, Cudkowicz A. Effect of iron chelators on the transferrin receptor in K562 cells. J Biol Chem 1984; 259:12970–12977.

305. Toth I, Rogers JT, McPhee JA, et al. Ascorbic acid enhances iron-induced ferritin translation in human leukemia and hepatoma cells. J Biol Chem 1995; 270:2846–2852.

306. Bridge KR, Hoffman KE. The effects of acorbic acid on the intracellular metabolism of iron and ferritin. J Biol Chem 1986; 261:14273–14277.

307. Stearns DM, Kennedy LJ, Courtney KD, et al. Reduction of chromium(VI) by ascorbate leads to chromium-DNA binding and DNA strand breaks in vitro. Biochemistry 1995; 34:910–919.

308. Kramer HJ, Krampitz G, Backer A, et al. Vanadium-diascorbates are strong candidates for endogenous ouabain-like factors in human urine: effect on Na-K-ATPase enzyme kinetics. Biochem Biophys Res Comm 1995; 213:289–294.

3

Antioxidant and Prooxidant Properties of Vitamin C

BARRY HALLIWELL and MATTHEW WHITEMAN
King's College, University of London, London, England

INTRODUCTION

Ascorbic acid is widely regarded as an essential antioxidant in the human body and has even been called "the most important antioxidant in human plasma" (1). Although vitamin C is known to be essential in the human diet for the action of several hydroxylase enzymes—lysine, proline, and dopamine β-hydroxylase are examples (2)—hard evidence to support the widespread belief in the antioxidant powers of ascorbate is surprisingly limited. For example, little evidence has yet been obtained to substantiate the common view that ascorbate regenerates α-tocopherol from the α-tocopheryl radical (3). In addition, vitamin C can exert prooxidant effects in vitro, but no one is sure yet whether this is relevant in vivo. The purpose of the present chapter is to review what we do (and do not!) know and to suggest how our state of ignorance might be remedied.

BASIC DEFINITIONS: WHAT IS AN ANTIOXIDANT?

Antioxidant is a term frequently used but rarely defined. Often the term is implicitly restricted to chain-breaking antioxidant inhibitors of lipid peroxidation, such as α-tocopherol. However, free radicals generated in vivo frequently damage proteins and deoxyribonucleic acid (DNA) as well as lipids, and so the author has introduced a broader definition: an *antioxidant* is any substance that, when present at low concentrations compared to those of an oxidizable substrate, significantly delays or prevents oxidation of that substrate (4,5). The term *oxidizable substrate* covers almost everything found in living cells, including proteins, lipids, carbohydrates and DNA.

When reactive oxygen species (ROS) and reactive nitrogen species (RNS) (see Table 1) are generated in living systems, a wide variety of antioxidants comes into play. Their relative importance as protective agents depends on which ROS or RNS is generated, how

59

Table 1   Reactive Oxygen and Reactive
Nitrogen Species[a]

Reactive oyxgen species (ROS)	
Radicals	Nonradicals
Superoxide, $O_2^{\cdot-}$	Hydrogen peroxide, H_2O_2
Hydroxyl, $OH^\cdot$	Hypochlorous acid, HOCl
Peroxyl, $RO_2^\cdot$	Ozone, O_3
Alkoxyl, $RO^\cdot$	Singlet oxygen $^1\Delta g$
Hydroperoxyl, $HO_2^\cdot$	
Reactive nitrogen species (RNS)	
Radicals	Nonradicals
Nitric oxide, $NO^\cdot$	Nitrous acid, HNO_2
Nitrogen dioxide, $NO_2^\cdot$	Dinitrogen tetroxide, N_2O_4
	Dinitrogen trioxide, N_2O_3
	Peroxynitrite, $ONOO^-$
	Peroxynitrous acid, ONOOH
	Nitryl cation, NO_2^+
	Alkyl peroxynitrites, ROONO

[a]*ROS* is a collective term that includes both oxygen radicals and certain nonradicals that are oxidizing agents and/or are easily converted into radicals (HOCl, O_3, $ONOO^-$, $^1O_2$, H_2O_2). *RNS* is also a collective term including nitric oxide and nitrogen dioxide radicals, as well as such nonradicals as HNO_2 and N_2O_4. $ONOO^-$ is often included in both categories, and HOCl could equally well be called a "reactive chlorine species." "Reactive" is not always an appropriate characterization; H_2O_2, $NO^\cdot$, and $O_2^{\cdot-}$ react quickly with very few molecules, whereas $OH^\cdot$ reacts quickly with almost everything. $RO_2^\cdot$, $RO^\cdot$, HOCl, $NO_2^\cdot$, $ONOO^-$, and O_3 have intermediate reactivities.

it is generated, where it is generated, and which target of damage is measured. For example, if human blood plasma is tested for its ability to inhibit iron ion-dependent lipid peroxidation, the proteins transferrin and caeruloplasmin are found to be the most important protective agents (6,7). When plasma is exposed to nitrogen dioxide, uric acid appears to exert some protective effect against damage to biomolecules by this toxic oxidizing gas (8). By contrast, when hypochlorous acid (HOCl) is added to plasma, uric acid appears to have little protective role (9).

Similarly, if the oxidative stress remains constant but a different target of oxidative damage is measured, different answers can result. For example, when plasma is exposed to gas-phase cigarette smoke, lipid peroxidation occurs, an event which can be inhibited by both endogenous and added ascorbic acid (10). By contrast, ascorbic acid has no effect on oxidative damage to plasma proteins by cigarette smoke as measured by the carbonyl assay (11). Some known carcinogens (such as diethylstilbestrol) are powerful inhibitors of in vitro lipid peroxidation (12) but can accelerate oxidative DNA damage in vivo (13). This is a stark illustration of how careful one has to be in equating "antioxidant" with "safe molecule."

The preceding definition emphasizes the importance of the source of stress and the target ("oxidizable substrate") measured when defining antioxidants. Change either of these, and the relative protective effectiveness of different antioxidants will change. Hence there is no universal "best" biological antioxidant.

ANTIOXIDANT PROPERTIES OF ASCORBATE IN VITRO

Ascorbate readily undergoes oxidation, forming an intermediate radical of low reactivity (for further details see Chaps. 2 and 4). The poor reactivity of this radical may account for many of ascorbate's antioxidant effects: a fairly reactive radical combines with ascorbate and a much less reactive radical (ascorbate radical) is formed (14). Buettner (15) has summarized the one-electron reduction potentials of various biologically relevant systems: Table 2 is a selection from the data he presents. Of course, these are standard potentials and the redox behavior of substances is much affected by such factors as temperature, concentration, and pH. Nevertheless, Table 2 illustrates the important point that ascorbate is thermodynamically close to the bottom of the pecking order for oxidizing radicals; i.e., it will tend to quench more-reactive species such as $OH^{.}$, $O_2^{.-}$ and urate radical. The ascorbate radical is relatively unreactive, being neither strongly oxidizing nor strongly reducing (14,15). In particular, it is thermodynamically unlikely that ascorbate radical reduces O_2 to $O_2^{.-}$ (15), a conclusion consistent with experimental data (14–16).

As predicted, ascorbate has a multiplicity of antioxidant properties in vitro, summarized in Table 3. It may also be an important protective agent against damage by reactive nitrogen

Table 2 Some Standard Reduction Potentials

	Couple	Standard reduction potential (mV)
Highly oxidizing	$OH^{.}$, H^+/H_2O	2310
	$RO^{.}$, H^+/ROH (aliphatic alkoxyl)	1600
	$HO_2^{.}$, H^+/H_2O_2	1060
	$O_2^{.-}$, $2H^+/H_2O_2$	940
	$RS^{.}/RS^-$ (cysteine)	920
	$HU^{.-}$, H^+/UH_2^- (urate)	590
	$\alpha T^{.}$, $H^+/\alpha TH$ (α-tocopherol)	500
	Trolox C ($TO^{.}$, H^+/TOH)	480
	H_2O_2, H^+/H_2O, $OH^{.}$	320
	Ascorbate$^{.-}$, H^+/ascorbate$^-$	282
	Ferricytochrome c/ferrocytochrome c	260
	Ubisemiquinone H^+/ubiquinol	200
	Fe^{3+}-EDTA/Fe^{2+}-EDTA	120
	Fe^{3+}-citrate/Fe^{2+}-citrate	~100
	Fe^{3+}-ADP/Fe^{2+}-ADP	~100
	Ubiquinone, H^+/ubisemiquinone	−36
	Dehydroascorbate/ascorbate$^{.-}$	−174
	Fe^{3+}-ferritin/ferritin + Fe^{2+}	−190
	$O_2/O_2^{.-}$	−330
	Fe^{3+}-transferrin/Fe^{2+}-transferrin	−400 (pH 7.3)
	Paraquat/paraquat$^{.-}$	−448
	O_2/H^+, $HO_2^{.}$	−460
	$CO_2/CO_2^{.-}$	−1800
Highly reducing	H_2O/e^-_{aq}	−2840

EDTA, ethylenediaminetetraacetic acid; ADP, adenosine diphosphate.
Data selected from the extensive compilation in Ref. 15.

Table 3   Ascorbic Acid as an Antioxidant In Vitro[a]

Scavenges O_2^- and $HO_2^{\cdot}$ (overall rate constant $> 10^5/M^{-1}s^{-1}$ at pH 7.4).

Scavenges water-soluble peroxyl ($RO_2^{\cdot}$) radicals (lipophilic ascorbate esters can also scavenge lipid-soluble $RO_2^{\cdot}$ radicals).

Scavenges thiyl and sulphenyl radicals.

"Repairs," and so prevents damage by, radicals arising by attack of $OH^{\cdot}$ or $RO_2^{\cdot}$ on uric acid.

Can reduce carcinogenic nitrosamines to inactive products.

Powerful scavenger of hypochlorous acid and a substrate for the enzyme myeloperoxidase (possibly slowing HOCl formation, although its effects on the enzyme are complex).

Inhibits lipid peroxidation by hemoglobin- or myoglobin-H_2O_2 mixtures and prevents peroxide-dependent heme breakdown to release iron ions, by being preferentially oxidized.

Powerful scavenger and quencher of singlet O_2 in aqueous solution.

May regenerate α-tocopherol from α-tocopheryl radicals in membranes and lipoproteins.

Scavenges nitroxide radicals.

Scavenges $OH^{\cdot}$ radicals (rate constant $> 10^9/M^{-1}s^{-1}$).

Protects plasma lipids against peroxidation induced by activated neutrophils.

May protect membranes and lipoproteins against lipid peroxidation induced by species present in cigarette smoke.

Powerful scavenger of O_3 and $NO_2^{\cdot}$ in human body fluids, probably protects lung lining fluids against inhaled oxidizing air pollutants.

Can react with damaging radicals generated from certain therapeutic agents (e.g., phenylbutazone), preventing the damaging effects of these radicals.

[a]For discussions see Refs. 5, 15, 18–34.

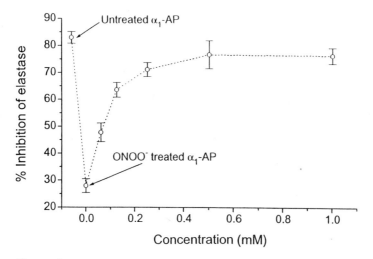

Figure 1   Protection by ascorbate against inactivation of α_1-antiproteinase by peroxynitrite. For details of experimental conditions see Ref. 17. Ascorbate was present at the final concentrations stated; peroxynitrite was 0.5 mM.

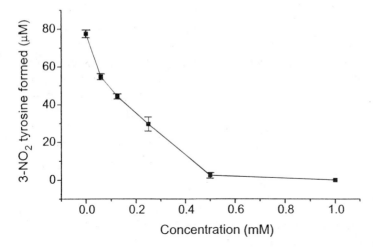

Figure 2 Protection by ascorbate against nitration of tyrosine by peroxynitrite. For details of experimental conditions see Ref. 17. Peroxynitrite and tyrosine were 1.0 mM and ascorbate was present at the final concentrations stated.

species, such as peroxynitrite: Figures 1 and 2 show that ascorbate protects against nitration of tyrosine and inactivation of α_1-antiproteinase by $ONOO^-$ (17). Ascorbate in respiratory tract lining fluids may be especially important in protecting against damage by inhaled oxidizing air pollutants, such as O_3 and $NO_2^{\cdot}$ (23).

PROOXIDANT PROPERTIES OF ASCORBATE

In vitro, however, vitamin C can also exert prooxidant properties. The classic system of Udenfriend (35) for making hydroxyl radicals consists of an iron chelate, H_2O_2, and ascorbate. The ascorbate acts as reductant to the iron, easily permitted by the relative reduction potentials (Table 2).

$$Fe^{3+} + ascorbate \rightarrow Fe^{2+} + ascorbate^{\cdot} \tag{1}$$
$$Fe^{2+} + H_2O_2 \rightarrow Fe^{3+} + OH^{\cdot} + OH^- \tag{2}$$

Iron–ascorbate mixtures are frequently used to stimulate lipid peroxidation in vitro (36); again, the ascorbate functions mainly by reducing iron ions. Instillation of ascorbate and iron or copper ions into the stomach of animals led to $OH^{\cdot}$ generation (37,38), and the mixture of metal ions and ascorbate in some vitamin pills has been claimed to generate $OH^{\cdot}$ once the pills dissolve (39). A mixture of ascorbate and copper ions (which will also generate $OH^{\cdot}$) inactivates the enzyme catalase (40). Several authors have described cytotoxic and mutagenic effects of ascorbate on isolated cells (41), which probably involve interaction of ascorbate with transition metal ions added to (or contaminating) the cell growth media (5). Prooxidant effects of ascorbate are also well known to food scientists. For example, Porter (42) referred to the actions of ascorbate in foods as follows: "Of all the paradoxical compounds, ascorbic acid probably tops the list. It is truly a two-headed Janus, a Dr. Jekyll–Mr. Hyde, an oxymoron of antioxidants."

Hence, when metal ions are present, ascorbate can often stimulate free radical damage in vitro. For example, a copper ion–ascorbate–H_2O_2 mixture causes severe oxidative damage to the bases of DNA by generating OH· (43). An interesting apparent exception is low-density lipoprotein (LDL): even in the presence of copper ions, ascorbate delays oxidation of LDL, both by recycling of vitamin E and by other mechanisms (44,45). However, once LDL oxidation is well under way, and presumably all the α-tocopherol has been oxidized, vitamin C can accelerate LDL oxidation; i.e., it can become prooxidant (46).

It should be noted that these in vitro prooxidant effects are not unique to ascorbate; they can be demonstrated with many reducing agents. For example, there is considerable current interest in the antioxidant effects of plant phenolics (e.g., in wine), such as the flavonoids (47–49). However, several plant phenolics can be made to exert prooxidant effects in vitro (47,50). Often, they inhibit lipid peroxidation, but, when mixed with iron or copper ions, they can damage other biological molecules, including DNA and proteins, in vitro.

PHYSIOLOGICAL RELEVANCE OF THE ANTIOXIDANT EFFECTS OF ASCORBATE: WHAT IN VIVO DATA DO WE HAVE?

We know that vitamin C is essential in the human diet; insufficient intake causes disease (scurvy) and the role of ascorbate as a cofactor for several enzymes is well established (2). Ascorbate is also often said to aid the absorption of inorganic iron from the gut by reducing Fe(III) to the more easily absorbable Fe^{2+}. Ascorbate is present in gastric juice and may aid in eliminating nitrosamine carcinogens originating from the diet or formed in the stomach, hence helping to protect against one cause of stomach cancer (51). The recommended daily allowance (RDA) for vitamin C (40 mg/day in the United Kingdom, 60 mg/day in the United States, higher for smokers) may be sufficient to do all these things (51,52). However, the strong epidemiological evidence for the protective effect of ascorbate against certain forms of cancer (51–53) is not evidence that this anticancer action is exerted by an antioxidant mechanism. A similar comment may be made about the reported effect of ascorbate on hemostatic factors (54).

Nevertheless, it seems chemically very likely that ascorbate does exert some antioxidant properties in vivo. It scavenges many ROS and RNS (Table 3) and it is widely distributed in cells and extracellular fluids at concentrations that should scavenge ROS and RNS (Figs. 1 and 2) (15,55). But how can this be proved?

In some cases involving naturally occurring putative antioxidants, it has been possible to remove the compound in question and look for evidence of increased oxidative damage. For example, mutants of *Escherichia coli* genetically engineered to lack both manganese superoxide dismutase (MnSOD) and iron superoxide dismutase (FeSOD) show severe damage when grown aerobically (56) and damage can be minimized by introducing a gene coding for SOD, even mammalian CuZnSOD (57). These experiments illustrate the physiological role of SOD. For ascorbate, the effect of removing it from the diet can be studied in experimental animals unable to synthesize ascorbate such as the guinea pig or a mutant rat strain (58,59). Surprisingly little work has been reported that measures accurately parameters of oxidative damage in these animals in relation to ascorbate intake, although studies of ascorbate–vitamin E interactions have been carried out in guinea pigs (3). An early study on guinea pigs showed that a vitamin C–deficient diet led to increased exhalation of pentane and ethane, suggestive of increased lipid peroxidation in vivo (60). However, the validity of such hydrocarbon measurements as an index of lipid peroxidation has repeatedly been questioned (61,62).

If ascorbate is really acting as an antioxidant in vivo is it depleted under conditions of oxidative stress? The answer seems to be yes. Thus it becomes oxidized to dehydroascorbate in synovial fluid in the knee joints of patients with active rheumatoid arthritis (63,64). Presumably ascorbate is acting to scavenge ROS or RNS derived from the many activated phagocytes present. Ascorbate is also oxidized in the plasma of patients with adult respiratory distress syndrome, in which there is often massive infiltration of neutrophils into the lung, where they become activated (65). This loss of ascorbate would at first sight seem unexpected, since enzymic systems exist in vivo to reduce ascorbate radical back to ascorbate at the expense of reduced oxidized nicotinamide-adenine dinucleotide (NADH) (the NADH-semidehydroascorbate reductase enzyme) or of GSH (the dehydroascorbate reductase enzyme) (2,66). However, these enzymes seem to be largely intracellular, and so ascorbic acid is rapidly depleted in human extracellular fluids under conditions of oxidative stress, presumably by the reactions

$$\text{ascorbate} \xrightarrow{\text{radical attack}} \text{ascorbate radical} \tag{3}$$

$$2 \text{ ascorbate radical} \rightarrow \text{ascorbate} + \text{dehydroascorbate} \tag{4}$$

$$\text{dehydroascorbate} \xrightarrow{\text{rapid nonenzymic breakdown}} \text{oxalate, threonate, other oxidation products} \tag{5}$$

Glutathione deficiency in newborn rats and in guinea pigs is lethal, but death can be prevented by high doses of ascorbate. The onset of scurvy in guinea pigs fed a diet low in ascorbate is delayed substantially by GSH precursors. Hence there is evidence for interactions between GSH and ascorbate in vivo (67).

Can breakdown products of ascorbate be measured under conditions of oxidative stress? Direct electron paramagnetic resonance (EPR) measurement of ascorbate radical has given promising results which are, in general, consistent with oxidation of ascorbate at sites of oxidative stress (15,68,69).

RELEVANCE OF PROOXIDANT EFFECTS: IS ASCORBATE TOXIC TO HUMANS?

Medical and lay interest in "optimal" ascorbate intakes was raised by claims that that megadoses (10 g/day or more) can protect against the common cold and can be used to treat cancer (70). The alleged anticancer effect has never been independently confirmed (71). Indeed, perusal of one of the original papers (72) reveals the worrying observation that four cancer patients died of hemorrhagic tumor necrosis soon after vitamin C treatment had been started. Vitamin C does not cure the common cold or prevent its occurrence; debate continues as to whether there is a small effect on disease severity (73,74).

Several reports have appeared about alleged toxic effects of high vitamin C intake (Table 4). In general, data are limited and documentation is often inadequate. For example, it is often said at meetings that increased vitamin C intake predisposes to kidney stones, and that people who stop taking large doses of ascorbate become scorbutic, but I have been unable to find convincing literature documentations of either of these phenomena (hence note c in Table 4).

However, the possibility of prooxidant effects should not be dismissed lightly. There is good evidence for an ongoing background level of oxidative damage to DNA, lipids, and

Table 4   Reported Toxic Effects of Vitamin C[a]

Stomach cramps, nausea, diarrhea (with multigram doses)[b]
Sodium overload (if sodium salt taken),[c] acidosis (if free acid taken)[c]
Increased risk of oxalosis, perhaps leading to kidney stones[c]
"Rebound effect," cessation of megadoses leading to very low ascorbate levels[c]
Serious cardiovascular disturbances when excess ascorbic acid given to iron-overloaded patients[d]
Hemolysis in patients with glucose-6-phosphate dehydrogenase deficiency[d]
Glycation of lens proteins[e]
Hemolysis in paroxysmal nocturnal hemoglobinuria[d]

[a]For further discussions see Refs. 75–91.
[b]Effects reported from several centers.
[c]Effects not well established; variable or poorly documented literature reports.
[d]Literature reports consistent with in vitro data, but few in number.
[e]In vitro effect only (75); bulk of epidemiological evidence is consistent with a protective effect of vitamin C against cataract (76,77).

proteins in the human body (92), and the pattern of damage to DNA bears the "chemical fingerprint" of attack by OH· (93). Stadtman et al. (94,95) have argued that oxidative protein damage involving metal ion-dependent OH· generation occurs in vivo; this can be accelerated by ascorbate in vitro. Ames et al. (96) and Totter (97) propose that oxidative damage to DNA is a major contributor to the age-related increase in the development of human cancer. If they are right, even a small rise in OH· generation over a lifetime could increase the incidence of cancer. So we must be very sure that ascorbic acid is really safe before proposing large intakes on a regular basis.

What data relating ascorbate to levels of oxidative DNA damage are available? Very few. Fraga et al. (98) showed that very severe dietary ascorbate restriction (5 mg/day) increased baseline levels of oxidative DNA damage (measured as 8-hydroxydeoxyguanosine) in human spermatozoa.

Relevance of Prooxidant Effects

Are the prooxidant effects of ascorbate (and of plant phenolics) relevant in vivo? A major factor would presumably be the availability of "catalytic" transition metal ions. This relates to another important nutritional question: What is the optimal intake of iron? Iron is essential for human health, especially in children and pregnant women, but could too much iron intake cause harm? In the healthy human body, iron and copper ions are largely sequestered in forms unable to catalyze free radical reactions (6,99). Hence the antioxidant properties of ascorbate (and any dietary plant phenolics that are absorbed through the gut) probably predominate over prooxidant effects. Nothing can ever be completely sequestered, however: metals are always in transit within and between cells. Hence it is possible that interactions of metal ions with ascorbate contribute to basal oxidative damage. The author believes that the antioxidant properties of ascorbate greatly predominate over prooxidant damaging reactions in most healthy people.

However, some apparently healthy people are not. It has been stated that twice as many adult men in the United States have hemochromatosis as have real iron-deficiency anemia (85,87) and the prevalence of iron overload due to homozygous hemochromatosis in apparently healthy Australians was about 1 in 300 (78). Giving vitamin C to iron-overloaded patients without administering an iron chelating agent (such as desferal) has been reported to produce deleterious clinical effects (Table 4). A simple solution to the problem of hemochromatosis would be including screening for the hemochromatosis gene (or checking of blood iron status, e.g., by measurement of serum ferritin levels or percentage transferrin saturation) in routine medical examinations. Such screening may be justified by the devastating consequences of prolonged iron overload (e.g., hepatoma) and the ease with which it can be prevented or treated if diagnosed at an early stage (88). Iron-overloaded patients have subnormal plasma ascorbate levels (89,90): one should probably not try to "correct" this without bringing the iron overload under control.

A second caveat is that injury to human tissues, probably by any cause, leads to release of "catalytic" transition metal ions (99,100). This effect has been widely demonstrated, e.g., in humans suffering from brain injury (100), those subjected to cardiopulmonary bypass (101), patients in liver failure (102), individuals with rheumatoid arthritis (103), and cancer patients given chemotherapy (104,105). The first clinical trial claiming to rebut Pauling's early work on anticancer effects of megadose vitamin C involved patients who had received chemotherapy; it is not impossible that iron overload could have negated any benefits of the administered ascorbate. However, a later trial avoided this problem (71) and the result was still negative.

As we get older, we get sicker. In advanced human atherosclerotic lesions, metal ions catalytic for free radical reactions can be measured (106,107): indeed, the lesion contents will stimulate $OH^.$ formation in the presence of H_2O_2 and ascorbate in vitro (106,107). There are repeated (but controversial) suggestions (108–112) that high body iron and/or copper (113) stores are associated with increased risk of cancer and cardiovascular disease. Could this be because the more iron or copper is in a tissue, the more is potentially mobilizable to catalyze free radical reactions after an injury (114)? If this is the case, then ascorbate could be harmful, not helpful. Indeed, it has been argued that the decline in ascorbate at the onset of many oxidative stresses is beneficial (6,99,100), first because the ascorbate is helping to scavenge radicals and recycle α-tocopherol, and second because ascorbate removal minimizes its potential prooxidant interactions with metal ions released by tissue damage. Thus it is possible that giving lots of ascorbate to sick people may not be a good thing.

Another question is whether ascorbate could promote excessive uptake of iron into the human body, since the reduction of ferric ions to Fe^{2+} by ascorbate is believed to facilitate iron uptake in the gut. There is no clear evidence for this in healthy subjects (115–117), but the issue needs to be addressed in relation to hemochromatosis.

CONCLUSION

Ascorbate is essential in the human diet, but many unanswered questions remain about its properties. In healthy subjects, the RDA for ascorbate probably helps protect against various diseases, including stomach cancer, probably by reducing nitrosamines. Gey et al. (52,118) reviewed several epidemiological studies and concluded that ~50 μM ascorbate plasma concentrations are associated with decreased risk of cardiovascular disease. Such levels are easily achievable by diet alone. The studies of Fraga et al. (98,119) showed that 60 mg/day of ascorbate seemed to be enough to normalize levels of oxidative DNA damage in sperm. In sperm collected from human volunteers, only very low seminal fluid ascorbate levels were associated with elevated DNA damage. A high intake of vitamin C appears not to be protective against breast cancer (120), and, apart from those related to stomach cancer, many other studies are equivocal about the protective effects of ascorbate (121).

In the Linxian study (122), supplementation of a Chinese population with molybdenum plus vitamin C at doses about twice the U.S. RDA (120 mg, 30 μg) showed no evidence of a reduction in cancer incidence or mortality.

Hence there is no clear evidence for any great benefit to be obtained by megadose vitamin C, and we cannot yet prove that it is not harmful over a lifetime. The authors favor a diet with plenty of fruits and vegetables and avoidance of smoking. In their view, supplementation with ascorbate (if any) should use only amounts close to the RDA.

REFERENCES

1. Frei B, England L, Ames BN. Ascorbate is an outstanding antioxidant in human blood plasma. Proc Natl Acad Sci USA 1989; 86:6377–6381.
2. Sauberlich HE. Pharmacology of vitamin C. Annu Rev Nutr 1994; 14:371–391.
3. Burton GW, Wronska U, Stone L, et al. Biokinetics of dietary RRR-α-tocopherol in the male guinea pig at three dietary levels of vitamin C and two levels of vitamin E: evidence that vitamin C does not "spare" vitamin E in vivo. Lipids 1990; 25:199–210.
4. Halliwell B, Gutteridge JMC. Free Radicals in Biology and Medicine. 2nd ed. Oxford: Clarendon Press, 1989.
5. Halliwell B. How to characterize a biological antioxidant. Free Radical Res Commun 1990; 9:1–32.
6. Halliwell B, Gutteridge JMC. The antioxidants of human extracellular fluids. Arch Biochem Biophys 1990; 280:1–8.
7. Gutteridge JMC, Quinlan GJ. Antioxidant protection against organic and inorganic oxygen radicals by normal human plasma: the important primary role for iron-binding and iron-oxidising proteins. Biochim Biophys Acta 1992; 1159:248–254.
8. Halliwell B, Hu ML, Louie S, et al. Interaction of nitrogen dioxide with human plasma: antioxidant depletion and oxidative damage. FEBS Lett 1992; 313:62–66.
9. Hu ML, Louie S, Cross CE, et al. Antioxidant protection against hypochlorous acid in human plasma. J Lab Clin Med 1992; 121:257–262.
10. Frei B, Forte TM, Ames BN, Cross CE. Gas phase oxidants of cigarette smoke induce lipid peroxidation and changes in lipoprotein properties in human blood plasma. Biochem J 1991; 247:133–138.
11. Reznick AZ, Cross CE, Hu M, et al. Modification of plasma proteins by cigarette smoke as measured by protein carbonyl formation. Biochem J 1992; 286:607–611.
12. Wiseman H, Halliwell B. Carcinogenic antioxidants: diethylstilboestrol, hexoestrol and 17 α-ethynyl-oestradiol. FEBS Lett 1993; 322:159–163.
13. Roy D, Liehr JG. Elevated 8-hydroxydeoxyguanosine levels in DNA of diethylstilboestrol-treated syrian hamsters: covalent DNA damage by free radicals generated by redox cycling of diethylstilboestrol. Cancer Res 1991; 51:3882–3885.
14. Bielski BHJ, Richter HW. Some properties of the ascorbate free radical. Ann NY Acad Sci 1975; 258:231–237.
15. Buettner GR. The pecking order of free radicals and antioxidants: lipid peroxidation, α-tocopherol and ascorbate. Arch Biochem Biophys 1993; 300:535–543.
16. Halliwell B, Foyer CH. Ascorbic acid, metal ions and the superoxide radical. Biochem J 1976; 155:697–700.
17. Whiteman M, Halliwell B. Protection against peroxynitrite-dependent tyrosine nitration and α₁-antiproteinase inactivation by ascorbic acid. Free Rad Res 1996; 25:275–283.
18. Bendich A, Machlin LJ, Scandurra O, et al. The antioxidant role of vitamin C. Adv Free Radical Biol Med 1986; 2:419–444.
19. Chow CK, Thacker RR, Changchit C, et al. Lower levels of vitamin C and carotenes in plasma of cigarette smokers. J Am Coll Nutr 1986; 5:305–312.

20. Wayner DDM, Burton GW, Ingold KU, et al. The relative contributions of vitamin E, urate, ascorbate and proteins to the total peroxyl radical-trapping antioxidant activity of human blood plasma. Biochim Biophys Acta 1987; 924:408–419.

21. Halliwell B, Wasil M, Grootveld M. Biologically-significant scavenging of the myeloperoxidase-derived oxidant hypochlorous acid by ascorbic acid: implications for antioxidant protection in the inflamed rheumatoid joint. FEBS Lett 1987; 213:15–18.

22. Chou PT, Khan AU. L-ascorbic acid quenching of singlet delta molecular oxygen in aqueous media: generalized antioxidant property of vitamin C. Biochem Biophys Res Commun 1983; 115:932–937.

23. Cross CE, van der Vliet A, O'Neill CA, et al. Oxidants, antioxidants and respiratory tract lining fluids. Environ Health Perspect 1994; 102 (suppl 10):185–191.

24. Rice-Evans C, Okunade G, Khan R. The suppression of iron release from activated myoglobin by physiological electron donors and by desferrioxamine. Free Radical Res Commun 1989; 7:45–54.

25. Aruoma OI, Halliwell B. Inactivation of α_1-antiproteinase by hydroxyl radicals: the effect of uric acid. FEBS Lett 1989; 244:76–80.

26. Asmus KD. Sulfur-centered free radicals. In: Slater TF, ed. Radioprotectors and Anticarcinogens. London: Academic Press, 1987:23–42.

27. Sevilla MD, Yan M, Becker D, Gillich S. ESR investigations of the reactions of radiation-produced thiyl and DNA peroxyl radicals: formation of sulfoxyl radicals. Free Radical Res Commun 1989; 6:21–24.

28. Cabelli DE, Bielski BHJ. Kinetics and mechanism for the oxidation of ascorbic acid/ascorbate by HO_2/O_2^- radicals: a pulse radiolysis and stopped-flow photolysis study. J Phys Chem 1983 87:1809–1812.

29. Wayner DDM, Burton GW, Ingold KU. The antioxidant efficiency of vitamin C is concentration-dependent. Biochim Biophys Acta 1986; 884:119–123.

30. Evans PJ, Cecchini R, Halliwell B. Oxidative damage to lipids and α_1-antiproteinase by phenylbutazone in the presence of haem proteins: protection by ascorbic acid. Biochem Pharmacol 1992; 44:981–984.

31. Evans PJ, Akanmu D, Halliwell B. Promotion of oxidative damage to arachidonic acid and α_1-antiproteinase by anti-inflammatory drugs in the presence of the haem proteins myoglobin and cytochrome c. Biochem Pharmacol 1994; 48:2173–2179.

32. Nishikimi M. Oxidation of ascorbic acid with superoxide anion generated by the xanthine-xanthine oxidase system. Biochem Biophys Res Commun 1975; 63:463–468.

33. Nandi A, Chatterjee IB. Scavenging of superoxide radical by ascorbic acid. J Biosci 1987; 11:435–441.

34. Nihro Y, Miyataka H, Sudo T, et al. 3-O-Alkylascorbic acids as free radical quenchers: synthesis and inhibitory effect on lipid peroxidation. J Med Chem 1991; 34:2152–2157.

35. Udenfriend S, Clark CT, Axelrod J, Brodie BB. Ascorbic acid in aromatic hydroxylation. J Biol Chem 1954; 208:731–739.

36. Wills ED. Lipid peroxide formation in microsomes: the role of non-haem iron. Biochem J 1969; 113:325–332.

37. Slivka A, Kang J, Cohen G. Hydroxyl radicals and the toxicity of oral iron. Biochem Pharmacol 1986; 35:553–556.

38. Kadiiska MB, Hanna PM, Hernandez L, Mason RP. In vivo evidence of hydroxyl radical formation after acute copper and ascorbic acid intake: electron spin resonance evidence. Mol Pharmacol 1992; 42:723–729.

39. Maskos Z, Koppenol WH. Oxyradicals and multi-vitamin tablets. Free Radical Biol Med 1991; 11:609–610.

40. Orr CWM. Studies on ascorbic acid. I. Factors influencing the ascorbate-mediated inhibition of catalase. Biochemistry 1967; 6:295–300.

41. Shamberger RJ. Genetic toxicology of ascorbic acid. Mutat Res 1984; 133:135–159.

42. Porter WL. Paradoxical behaviour of antioxidants in food and biological systems. Toxicol Ind Health 1993; 9:93–122.

43. Aruoma OI, Halliwell B, Gajewski E, Dizdaroglu M. Copper ion-dependent damage to the bases in DNA in the presence of hydrogen peroxide. Biochem J 1991; 273:601–604.

44. Esterbauer H, Striegl G, Puhl H, Rotheneder M. Continuous monitoring of in vitro oxidation of human low density lipoprotein. Free Radical Res Commun 1989; 6:67–75.

45. Retsky KL, Freeman MW, Frei B. Ascorbic acid oxidation product(s) protect human low density lipoprotein against atherogenic modification. J Biol Chem 1993; 268:1304–1309.

46. Stait SE, Leake DS. Ascorbic acid: can either increase or decrease low density lipoprotein modification. FEBS Lett 1994; 341:263–267.

47. Laughton MJ, Halliwell B, Evans PJ, Hoult JRS. Antioxidant and pro-oxidant actions of the plant phenolics quercetin, gossypol and myricetin. Biochem Pharmacol 1989; 38:2859–2865.

48. Kanner J, Frankel E, Granit R, et al. Natural antioxidants in grapes and wines. J Agric Food Chem 1994; 42:64–69.

49. Hertog MGL, Feskens EJM, Hollman PCH, et al. Dietary antioxidant flavonoids and risk of coronary heart disease: the Zutphen elderly study. Lancet 1993; 342:1007–1011.

50. Hodnick WF, Kung FS, Roettger WJ, et al. Inhibition of mitochondrial respiration and production of toxic oxygen radicals by flavonoids. Biochem Pharmacol 1986; 35:2345–2357.

51. Block G. Vitamin C and cancer prevention: the epidemiologic evidence. Am J Clin Nutr 1991; 53:270S–282S.

52. Gey F. Ten year retrospective on the antioxidant hypothesis of arteriosclerosis: threshold plasma levels of antioxidant micronutrients related to minimum cardiovascular risk. J Nutr Biochem 1995; 6:206–236.

53. Ocké MC, et al. Average intake of anti-oxidant (pro) vitamins and subsequent cancer mortality in the 16 cohorts of the seven countries study. Int J Cancer 1995; 61:480–484.

54. Khaw KT, Woodhouse P. Interrelation of vitamin C, infection, haemostatic factors, and cardiovascular disease. Br Med J 1995; 310:1559–1563.

55. Bergsten P, et al. Millimolar concentrations of ascorbic acid in purified human mononuclear leukocytes. J Biol Chem 1990; 265:2584–2587.

56. Touati D. The molecular genetics of superoxide dismutase in E. coli. An approach to understanding the biological role and regulation of SODs in relation to other elements of the defence system against oxygen toxicity. Free Radical Res Commun 1989; 8:1–9.

57. Natvig DO, Imlay K, Touati D, Hallewell RA. Human copper-zinc superoxide dismutase complements superoxide dismutase-deficient Escherichia coli mutants. J Biol Chem 1989; 262:14697–14701.

58. Kuwai T, Nishikimi M, Ozawa T, Yagi K. A missense mutation of L-gulono-γ-lactone oxidase causes the inability of scurvy-prone osteogenic disorder rats to synthesise L-ascorbic acid. J Biol Chem 1992; 267:21973–21976.

59. Kimura H, Yamada Y, Morita Y, et al. Dietary ascorbic acid depresses plasma and low density lipoprotein peroxidation in genetically scorbutic rats. J Nutr 1992; 122:1904–1909.

60. Kunert KJ, Tappel AL. The effect of vitamin C on in vivo lipid peroxidation in guinea pigs as measured by pentane and ethane production. Lipids 1983; 18:271–274.

61. Cailleux A, Allain P. Is pentane a normal constituent of human breath? Free Radical Res Commun 1993; 18:323–327.

62. Mendis S, Sobotka PA, Euler DE. Expired hydrocarbons in patients with acute myocardial infarction. Free Radical Res 1995; 23:117–122.

63. Lunec J, Blake DR. The determination of dehydroascorbic acid and ascorbic acid in the serum and synovial fluid of patients with rheumatoid arthritis. Free Radical Res Commun 1985; 1:31–39.

64. Blake DR, Hall ND, Treby DA, et al. Protection against superoxide and hydrogen peroxide in synovial fluid from rheumatoid patients. Clin Sci 1981; 61:483–486.

65. Cross CE, Forté T, Stocker R, et al. Oxidative stress and abnormal cholesterol metabolism in patients with adult respiratory distress syndrome. J Lab Clin Med 1990; 115:396–404.
66. Wells WW, Xu DP. Dehydroascorbate reduction. J Bioenerg Biomembr 1994; 26:369–377.
67. Meister A. On the antioxidant effects of ascorbic acid and glutathione. Biochem Pharmacol 1992; 44:1905–1915.
68. Buettner GR, Jurkiewicz BA. Ascorbate free radical as a marker of oxidative stress: an EPR study. Free Radical Biol Med 1993; 14:49–55.
69. Kunitano R, Miyauchi Y, Inoue M. Synthesis of a cytochrome c derivative with prolonged in vivo half-life and determination of ascorbyl radicals in the circulation of the rat. J Biol Chem 1992; 267:8732–8738.
70. Serafini A. Linus Pauling: A Man and His Science. New York: Paragon House, 1991.
71. Moertel CG. Megadoses of vitamin C are valuable in the treatment of cancer: negative. Nutr Rev 1986; 44:28–32.
72. Cameron E, Campbell A. The orthomolecular treatment of cancer. II. Clinical trial of high dose ascorbic acid supplements in advanced human cancer. Chem Biol Interact 1974; 9:285–315.
73. Hemila H. Vitamin C and the common cold. Br J Nutr 1992; 67:3–16.
74. Seshli MA. Possible adverse health effects of vitamin C and ascorbic acid. Semin Oncol 1983; X:299–304.
75. Ortwerth BJ, Slight SH, Prabhakaram M, et al. Site-specific glycation of lens crystallins by ascorbic acid. Biochim Biophys Acta 1992; 1117:207–215.
76. Taylor A. Cataract: relationships between nutrition and oxidation. J Am Coll Nutr 1993; 12:138–146.
77. Bendich A, Langseth L. The health effects of vitamin C supplementation: a review. J Am Coll Nutr 1995; 14:124–136.
78. Leggett BA, Halliday JW, Brown NN, et al. Prevalence of haemochromatosis amongst asymptomatic Australians. Br J Haematol 1990; 74:525–530.
79. McLaran CJ, Bett JHN, Nye JA, Halliday JW. Congestive cardiomyopathy and haemochromatosis—rapid progression possibly accelerated by excessive ingestion of ascorbic acid. Aust NZ J Med 1982; 12:187–188.
80. Rowbotham B, Roeser HP. Iron overload associated with congenital pyruvate kinase deficiency and high dose ascorbic acid ingestion. Aust NZ J Med 1984; 14:667–669.
81. Nienhuis AW. Vitamin C and iron. N Engl J Med 1981; 304:170–171.
82. Tsao CS, Leung PY. Urinary ascorbic acid levels following the withdrawal of large doses of ascorbic acid in guinea pigs. J Nutr 1988; 118:895–900.
83. Mehta JB, Singhal SB, Mehta BC. Ascorbic-acid-induced haemolysis in G-6-PD deficiency. Lancet 1990; ii:944.
84. Campbell GD, Steinberg MH, Bower JD. Ascorbic acid-induced hemolysis in G-6-PD deficiency. Ann Intern Med 1975; 82:810.
85. Cook JD, Skikne BS, Lynch SR, Reusser ME. Estimates of iron sufficiency in the US population. Blood 1986; 68:726–731.
86. Iwamato N, et al. Haemolysis induced by ascorbic acid in paroxysmal nocturnal haemoglobinuria. Lancet 1994; 343:357.
87. Edwards CQ, Griffen LM, Goldgar D, et al. Prevalence of hemochromatosis among 11,065 presumably healthy blood donors. N Engl J Med 1988; 318:1355–1362.
88. Stremmel W, Riedel HD, Niederau C, Strohmeyer G. Pathogenesis of genetic haemochromatosis. Eur J Clin Invest 1993; 23:321–329.
89. Young IS, Trouton TG, Torney JJ, et al. Antioxidant status and lipid peroxidation in hereditary haemochromatosis. Free Radical Biol Med 1994; 16:393–397.
90. Cohen A, Cohen IJ, Schwartz E. Scurvy and altered iron stores in thalassemia major. N Engl J Med 1981; 304:158–160.
91. Moser U, Hornig D. High intakes of vitamin C: a contributor to oxalate formation in man? Trends Pharmacol Sci 1982: 480–483.

92. Halliwell B. Free radicals and antioxidants: a personal view. Nutr Rev 1994; 52:253–265.
93. Halliwell B, Dizdaroglu M. The measurement of oxidative damage to DNA by HPLC and GC/MS techniques. Free Radical Res Commun 1992; 16:75–87.
94. Fucci L, Oliver CN, Coon MJ, Stadtman ER. Inactivation of key metabolic enzymes by mixed-function oxidation reactions: possible implication in protein turnover and ageing. Proc Natl Acad Sci USA 1983; 80:1521–1525.
95. Stadtman ER. Oxidation of free amino acids and amino acid residues in proteins by radiolysis and by metal-catalyzed reactions. Annu Rev Biochem 1983; 62:797–821.
96. Ames BN, Shigenaga MK, Hagen TM. Oxidants, antioxidants and the degenerative diseases of aging. Proc Natl Acad Sci USA 1993; 90:7915–7922.
97. Totter JR. Spontaneous cancer and its possible relationship to oxygen metabolism. Proc Natl Acad Sci USA 1980; 77:1763–1767.
98. Fraga CG, Motchnik PA, Shigenaga MK, et al. Ascorbic acid protects against endogenous oxidative DMA damage in human sperm. Proc Natl Acad Sci USA 1991; 88:11003–11006.
99. Halliwell B, Gutteridge JMC. Oxygen free radicals and iron in relation to biology and medicine: some problems and concepts. Arch Biochem Biophys 1986; 246:501–514.
100. Halliwell B, Cross CE, Gutteridge JMC. Free radicals, antioxidants and human disease: where are we now? J Lab Clin Med 1992; 119:598–620.
101. Moat NE, Evans TE, Quinlan GJ, Gutteridge JMC. Chelatable iron and copper can be released from extracorporeally circulated blood during cardiopulmonary bypass. FEBS Lett 1993; 328:103–106.
102. Evans PJ, Evans RW, Bomford A, et al. Metal ions catalytic for free radical reactions in the plasma of patients with fulminant hepatic failure. Free Radical Res 1994; 20:139–144.
103. Rowley DA, Gutteridge JMC, Blake D, et al. Lipid peroxidation in rheumatoid arthritis: thiobarbituric-acid-reactive material and catalytic iron salts in synovial fluid from rheumatoid patients. Clin Sci 1984; 66:691–695.
104. Halliwell B, Aruoma OI, Mufti G, Bomford A. Bleomycin-detectable iron in serum from leukaemic patients before and after chemotherapy: therapeutic implications for treatment with oxidant-generating drugs. FEBS Lett 1988; 241:202–204.
105. Carmine TC, Evans P, Bruchelt G, et al. Presence of iron catalytic for free radical reactions in patients undergoing chemotherapy: implications for therapeutic management. Cancer Lett 1995; 94:219–226.
106. Smith C, Mitchinson MJ, Aruoma OI, Halliwell B. Stimulation of lipid peroxidation and hydroxyl radical generation by the contents of human atherosclerotic lesions. Biochem J 1992; 286:901–905.
107. Swain J, Gutteridge JMC. Prooxidant iron and copper, with ferroxidase and xanthine oxidase activities in human atherosclerotic material. FEBS Lett 1995; 368:513–515.
108. Burt MJ, Halliday JW, Powell LW. Iron and coronary heart disease. Br Med J 1993; 307:575–576.
109. Knekt P, et al. Body iron stores and risk of cancer. Int J Cancer 1994; 56:379–382.
110. Sempos CT, Looker AC, Gillum RF, Makuo DM. Body iron stores and risk of coronary heart disease. N Engl J Med 1994; 330:1119–1124.
111. Magnusson MK, Sigfusson N, Sigvaldason H, et al. Low iron binding capacity as a risk factor for myocardial infarction. Circulation 1994; 89:102–108.
112. Salonen JT, Nyysönen K, Korpela H. High stored iron levels are associated with excess risk of myocardial infarction in Eastern Finnish men. Circulation 1992; 86:803–811.
113. Salonen JT, Salonen R, Korpela H, et al. Serum copper and the risk of acute myocardial infarction; a prospective population study in men in Eastern Finland. Am J Epidemiol 1991; 134:268–276.
114. Chevion M, Jiang Y, Har-El R, et al. Copper and iron are mobilized following myocardial ischemia: possible predictive criteria for tissue injury. Proc Natl Acad Sci USA 1993; 90:1102–1106.

115. Bendich A, Cohen M. Ascorbic acid safety: analysis of factors affecting iron absorption. Toxicol Lett 1991; 51:189–201.

116. Cook JD, Watson SS, Simpson KM, et al. The effect of high ascorbic acid supplementation on body iron stores. Blood 1984; 64:721–726.

117. Hunt JR, Gallagher SK, Johnson LA. Effect of ascorbic acid on apparent iron absorption by women with low iron stores. Am J Clin Nutr 1994; 59:1381–1385.

118. Gey KF, Moser UK, Jordan P, et al. Increased risk of cardiovascular disease at suboptimal plasma concentrations of essential antioxidants: an epidemiological update with special attention to carotene and vitamin C. Am J Clin Nutr 1993; 57(suppl):787S–797S.

119. Jacob RA, et al. Immunocompetence and oxidant defense during ascorbate depletion of healthy men. Am J Clin Nutr 1991; 54:1302S–1309S.

120. Hunter DJ, et al. A prospective study of the intake of vitamins C, E and A and the risk of breast cancer. N Engl J Med 1993; 329:234–240.

121. Byers T, Perry G. Dietary carotenes, vitamin C, and vitamin E as protective agents in human cancers. Annu Rev Nutr 1992; 12:139–159.

122. Blot, WJ, et al. Nutrition intervention trials in Linxian, China: supplementation with specific vitamin/mineral combinations, cancer incidence, and disease-specific mortality in the general population. J Natl Cancer Inst 1993; 85:1483–1492.

4

The Vitamin C Radical and Its Reactions

WOLF BORS

Institut für Strahlenbiologie, GSF Research Center Neuherberg, Oberschleissheim, Germany

GARRY R. BUETTNER

Free Radical Research Institute, The University of Iowa, Iowa City, Iowa

PROPERTIES OF THE ASCORBATE RADICAL

The ascorbate radical is an important intermediate in reactions involving the antioxidant function of ascorbate. However, its generation by and reaction with enzymes are also known. In this chapter, we discuss: (1) the physicochemical properties and reactions of the ascorbate radical, (2) its formation during antioxidant interactions, and (3) the in vivo detection of ascorbate radical by electron paramagnetic resonance (EPR) spectroscopy as a promising tool for noninvasive monitoring of oxidative stress. But first, we wish to clear up confusion and offer some suggestions for order to the multitude of descriptions and abbreviations used in the literature for the compounds involved.

Nomenclature

In the literature there exist many different names and abbreviations for the various species involved in the chemistry of vitamin C. For example, SDA, MDAA, AR, AFR, plus others, have been used for the ascorbate radical alone. In this review we use $AscH_2$, $AscH^-$, and Asc^{2-} to denote the undissociated form of ascorbic acid, the physiologically dominant ascorbate monoanion ($pK_1 = 4.1$) (1), and the ascorbate dianion ($pK_2 = 11.79$) (1), respectively; $AscH^{\cdot}$ and $Asc^{\cdot-}$ for the neutral ascorbyl and the anionic ascorbate radicals (with a pK value of -0.86 (2) only $Asc^{\cdot-}$ is relevant in biology); DHA for dehydroascorbic and DHAA for its hydrolyzed form, both products of the two-electron oxidation of vitamin C (3) (see Fig. 1 for the structures of each of these species.). Although there is no International Union of Pure and Applied Chemistry (IUPAC) convention for these abbreviations, we suggest that researchers use them because they are simple, yet they convey accurately the chemical aspects of the species being discussed.

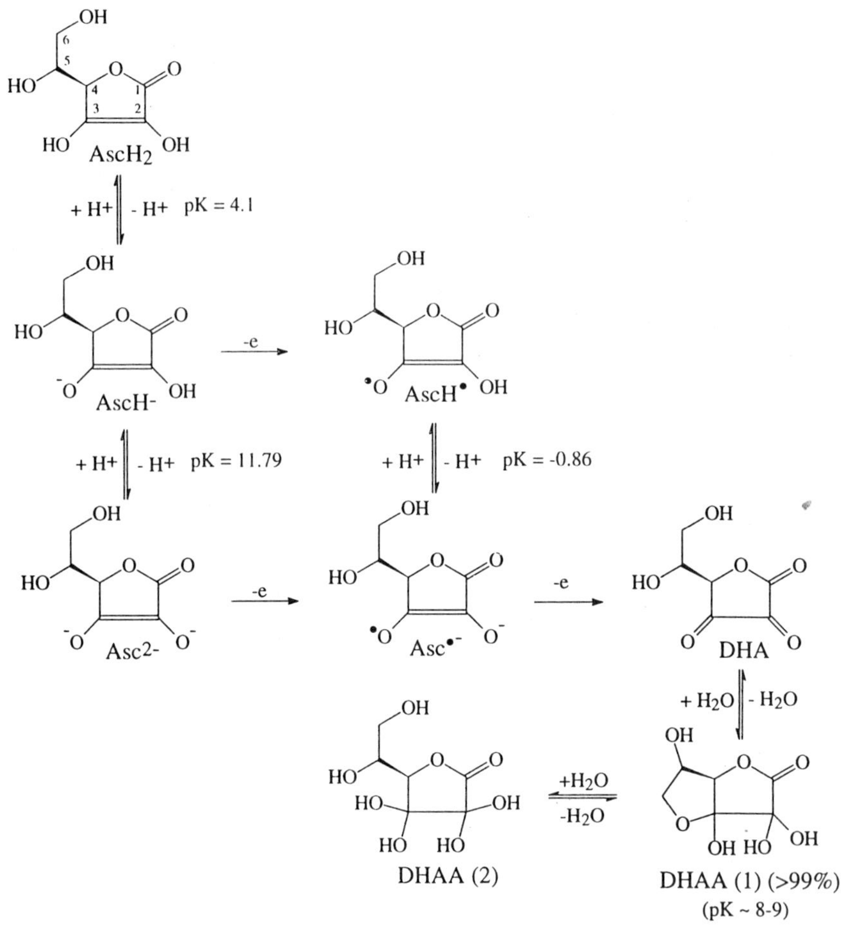

Figure 1 The equilibrium and redox species in the ascorbic acid–dehydroascorbic acid system.

Physicochemical Properties

The most detailed studies on the kinetics of ascorbate and ascorbate radical reactions have been carried out using pulse radiolysis (4–12). Photosensitized generation of Asc$^{\bullet-}$ is less suitable for these types of kinetics studies as it is prone to side reactions diminishing the yield of Asc$^{\bullet-}$ (13,14). The reaction of ascorbate with HO$^{\bullet}$ is quite complex as a result of formation of intermediates (4,7,12); thus generation of Asc$^{\bullet-}$ for kinetic studies is preferably done with other electrophilic species such as halogen radical (4,7) or especially azidyl radicals (15–17).

The National Institute of Standards and Technology (NIST) Solution Kinetics Database (18) contains quite a number of rate constants for the generation of Asc$^{\bullet-}$, almost two-thirds of them reactions of AscH$^-$ with peroxyl radicals (19–21), most others with inorganic radicals. However, the NIST Database has only a limited number of the reactions of AscH$^-$ with phenoxyl radicals (15,17,22–26); these are included in Table 1. Table 1 also contains four rate constants for reductive reactions of DHA with flavonoid aroxyl radicals, leading to

Table 1   Rate Constants for Ascorbate Radical (Asc$^{\cdot-}$) Formation

Radical	Substrate	pH	$k/M^{-1}s^{-1}$	Comment	Ref.
		Substrate: ascorbic acid (AscH$_2$)			
HO$^{\cdot}$	AscH$_2$	1.5	8.25×10^9	See text	4
Br$_2^{\cdot-}$	AscH$_2$	1.5	1.1×10^8		4
I$_2^{\cdot-}$	AscH$_2$	1.5	5.0×10^6		4
(SCN)$_2^{\cdot-}$	AscH$_2$	1.5	1.0×10^7		4
HO$_2^{\cdot}$	AscH$_2$	0.3–1	1.6×10^4		9
SO$_3^{\cdot}$	AscH$_2$	3.6	2.3×10^6		27
SO$_5^{\cdot-}$	AscH$_2$	3.6	1.3×10^7		27
CCl$_3$OO$^{\cdot}$	AscH$_2$	1.0	1.4×10^7	H$_2$O/iPOH (8:1)	28
CH$_3$OO$^{\cdot}$	AscH$_2$	3.1	4.0×10^5	10% DMSO	21
		Substrate: ascorbate monoanion (AscH$^-$)			
HO$^{\cdot}$	AscH$^-$	7.0	1.28×10^{10}	See text	4
Br$_2^{\cdot-}$	AscH$^-$	7.0	1.1×10^9		4
I$_2^{\cdot}$	AscH$^-$	7.0	1.4×10^8		4
(SCN)$_2^{\cdot-}$	AscH$^-$	7.0	6.0×10^8		4
O$_2^{\cdot-}$	AscH$^-$	≥8.0	5.0×10^4	pH-dep. 0.1–11	9
SO$_3^{\cdot-}$	AscH$^-$	6.8	9.2×10^6	pH 2–12	27
SO$_5^{\cdot-}$	AscH$^-$	6.7	1.4×10^8		27
CCl$_3$OO$^{\cdot}$	AscH$^-$	7.0	5.3×10^8	H$_2$O/iPOH (8:1)	28
CH$_3$OO$^{\cdot}$	AscH$^-$	7.0	1.8×10^6	40% DMSO	21
α-Tocopheroxyl	AscH$^-$	?	1.55×10^6	H$_2$O/iPOH/acetone	23
α-Tocopheroxyl	AscH$^-$	?	9.0×10^5	CTAB micelles-EPR	22
α-Tocopheroxyl	AscH$^-$	≥7.0	3.0×10^{5a}	DMPC bilayer; LFP	24
Trolox-O$^{\cdot}$	AscH$^-$	7.0	1.45×10^7	Also thermodynamic data	24
Trolox-O$^{\cdot}$	AscH$^-$	8.5	1.12×10^7	Kinetic modeling	17
Hydroxyaceto- phenone-O$^{\cdot}$	AscH$^-$	9.5	1.7×10^9	Also iso-AscH$^-$	25
Trp-O$^{\cdot}$	AscH$^-$	7.0	9.3×10^7	Phosphate buffer	15
VP-16-O$^{\cdot}$	AscH$^-$	8.5	3.5×10^7	Kinetic modeling	Unpublished
Fisetin-O$^{\cdot}$	AscH$^-$	8.5	8.65×10^4	Kinetic modeling	17
Dihydroquer-O$^{\cdot}$	AscH$^-$	8.5	1.6×10^5	Kinetic modeling	17
Rutin-O$^{\cdot}$	AscH$^-$	8.5	1.25×10^6		17
Quercetin-O$^{\cdot}$	AscH$^-$	8.5	4.75×10^6		17
Kaempferol-O$^{\cdot}$	AscH$^-$	8.5	5.2×10^6		17
Luteolin-O$^{\cdot}$	AscH$^-$	8.5	9.9×10^6		17
		Substrate: dehydroascorbic			
Fisetin-O$^{\cdot}$	DHA	8.5	6.9×10^4	Kinetic modeling	17
Rutin-O$^{\cdot}$	DHA	8.5	1.7×10^5	Kinetic modeling	17
Luteolin-O$^{\cdot}$	DHA	8.5	1.65×10^6	Kinetic modeling	17
Quercetin-O$^{\cdot}$	DHA	8.5	1.2×10^7	Kinetic modeling	17

[a]This is the best estimate for the rate constant of ascorbate with the tocopheroxyl radical in a biological membrane.

Table 2   Rate Constants for Formation of Derivatives of Ascorbate Radical from Derivatives of Ascorbate

Radical	Substrate	pH	$k/M^{-1}s^{-1}$	Comment	Ref.
		Substrates: O-methylated derivatives			
HO˙	1-O-methyl	6.8	2.5×10^{10}		10
HO˙	2-O-methyl	3.5–6.8	2.7×10^{9}		10
HO˙	3-O-methyl	6.4–7.9	3.0×10^{10}		10
HO˙	2,3-O-dimethyl	6.8	4.3×10^{9}		10
$Br_2^{˙-}$	1-O-methyl	6.8	3.7×10^{8}		10
$Br_2^{˙-}$	2-O-methyl	3.5–6.8	6.1×10^{8}		10
$Br_2^{˙-}$	3-O-methyl	6.4–7.9	7.5×10^{7}		10
		Substrates: 6-O-galactosyl derivatives			
HO˙	6-O-α-gal.	6.5	6.1×10^{9}	Also decay rates	12
HO˙	6-O-β-gal.	6.8	5.8×10^{9}	Also decay rates	12
$N_3^{˙}$	6-O-α-gal.	7.9	3.3×10^{9}	Also decay rates	12
$N_3^{˙}$	6-O-β-gal.	7.8	2.7×10^{9}	Also decay rates	12
		Substrates: 6-O-fatty acid derivatives			
α-Tocopheroxyl	6-Caprylate (8)	?	3.0×10^{5}	CTAB micelles; stop-flow EPR	22
α-Tocopheroxyl	6-Laurate (12)	?	7.0×10^{4}	CTAB micelles; stop-flow EPR	22
α-Tocopheroxyl	6-Palmitate (16)	?	3.0×10^{3}	CTAB micelles; stop-flow EPR	22

Asc˙⁻. Listed in Table 2 are the rate constants for radical formation of various ascorbate derivatives (10,12,22). When comparing the reactivity of AscH$_2$ with that of AscH⁻, we see that in nearly every case ascorbate monoanion demonstrates much greater reactivity for electron (hydrogen atom) transfer than the diacid (4,9,21,27,28).

Once formed, Asc˙⁻ decays relatively slowly. In simple buffered solutions, the nearly exclusive mode of decay is disproportionation. This somewhat "slow" decay of Asc˙⁻ may seem rather unusual, for example, slow compared to decay of HO˙ or RO˙. According to the most detailed study by Bielski et al. (7), the stability of Asc˙⁻ is proposed to be due to obligatory dimer formation as an intermediate during the disproportionation reaction.

$$2\ Asc^{˙-} \overset{k_1}{\underset{k_{-1}}{\rightleftharpoons}} (Asc)_2^{2-} \tag{1}$$

$$(Asc)_2^{2-} + H^+ \overset{k_2}{\rightarrow} AscH^- + DHA \tag{2}$$

$$(Asc)_2^{2-} + H_2O \overset{k_3}{\rightarrow} Asc^- + DHA + OH^- \tag{3}$$

$$\text{Net Reaction:}\quad 2\ Asc^{˙-} + H^+ \overset{k_{obs}}{\rightarrow} AscH^- + DHA \tag{4}$$

Thus, in the absence of phosphate (discussed later) we have

$$-d\frac{[\text{Asc}^{\cdot-}]}{dt} = -2k_{\text{obs}}[\text{Asc}^{\cdot-}]^2$$

where

$$k_{\text{obs}} = \frac{k_1}{[1 + (k_1/k_2\,[\text{H}^+] + k_3)]}$$

An increase in ionic strength has been observed both to increase and to decrease the rate of dismutation of $\text{Asc}^{\cdot-}$ (7,29). However, a most important observation is that phosphate buffer accelerates the dismutation (7). This acceleration is attributed to the ability of various protonated forms of phosphate to donate a proton efficiently to the radical dimer, reaction 2. It is quite possible that other buffers may similarly act as proton donors, thereby accelerating $\text{Asc}^{\cdot-}$ dismutation. Figure 2 shows the pH dependence of the rate of $\text{Asc}^{\cdot-}$ dimutation. At neutral pH, i.e., pH approximately 7.4, changes in ionic strength have an insignificant effect on this rate. However, the presence of 45 mM phosphate buffer shifts this curve up; at pH 7.4 the rate constant increases by a factor of approximately 10.3, from 1.41×10^5 to 1.45×10^6 ($\text{M}^{-1}\text{s}^{-1}$). As anticipated, derivatization of ascorbate alters the rate of der-$\text{Asc}^{\cdot-}$ decay. Considerable prolongation of the der-$\text{Asc}^{\cdot-}$ lifetime was observed when the 6-position was elongated by saturated fatty acids (22)—with a concomitant decrease for the scavenging of the α-tocopheroxyl radical by the respective parent compounds. In contrast, 6-substitution with α- or β-galactosyl residues caused a doubling of the decay rate (12).

Pulse-radiolytic studies of ascorbate radical reactions have been mainly concerned with the reactivity toward redox-active substrates (6,9,11,17). As shown in Table 3, the reaction

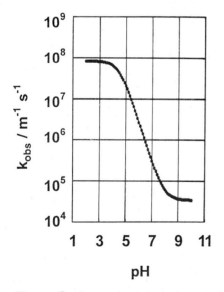

Figure 2 The calculated observed rate constants for the disproportionation of ascorbate radical as a function of pH. These observed rate constants were determined from data presented in Ref. 7.

Table 3   Rate Constants for Ascorbate Radical (Asc⁻) Reactions

Reactant	pH	$k/M^{-1}s^{-1}$	$E°'/mV^a$	Ref.
$HO_2^·$	0.3–1	5×10^9	1060	9
$O_2^{·-}$	≥8.0	2.6×10^8	950	9
O_2	8.6	$<5 \times 10^2$	−330	6
Asc⁻	7.4	1.4×10^5	282	7[b,c]
Asc⁻ in 45 mM phosphate	7.4	1.2×10^6	282	7
Ferric/ferrous iron complexes				
$[Fe(N)_6]^{3-}$	7.0	4.0×10^6	425	11
Fe(III)-EDTA	7.0	4.0×10^6	117	11
Cytochrome c (Fe^{3+})	7.4	6.6×10^3	262	6
Cytochrome b_5 (Fe^{2+})	7.0	$<10^4$	0	11
Phenolates				
Dopamine	8.4	3.6×10^2	?	6
Quercetin-O⁻	8.5	1.55×10^3	398	17
Fisetin-O⁻	8.5	3.85×10^4	214	17
Rutin-O⁻	8.5	5.2×10^4	275	17
Luteolin-O⁻	8.5	1.55×10^5	299	17
Kaempferol-O⁻	8.5	2.8×10^6	209	17
Dihydroquer-O⁻	8.5	1.2×10^7	83	17
Cytochrome b_5 reductase: E-FADH⁻	7.0	4.3×10^6	−147	11
Aroxyl radicals/semiquinones				
Luteolin-O·	8.5	1.95×10^6	299	17
Quercetin-O·	8.5	1.45×10^7	398	17
Rutin-O·	8.5	3.5×10^7	275	17
Dihydroquercetin-O·	8.5	4.65×10^7	83	17
Fisetin-O·	8.5	7.1×10^7	214	17
Kaempferol-O·	8.5	3.4×10^8	209	17
Cytochrome b_5 reductase: E-FAD·⁻	7.0	3.7×10^5	−88	11
Quinoid structures				
Fisetin(=O)	8.5	3.75×10^3	−249	17
Rutin(=O)	8.5	4.1×10^4	−211	17
Quercetin(=O)	8.5	1.15×10^6	−233	17
Luteolin(=O)	8.5	1.65×10^7	−115	17

[a]$E°'$ is the standard one-electron reduction potential of the reactant at neutral pH.
[b]This rate constant holds over a range of ionic strengths, e.g., 1–200 mM, but in the absence of proton donors such as phosphate.
[c]See Fig. 1.

rates are under strong control of the respective one-electron reduction potentials. The standard reduction potential of the ascorbate radical–ascorbate couple at pH 7 is $+ 282$ mV and for the dehydroascorbic acid–ascorbate radical couple is -174 mV (pH-independent) (30–32). Most of the data in Table 3 were obtained by kinetic modeling of pulse-radiolytic data, i.e., calculations of the changes in the kinetics of the formation and decay of the flavonoid aroxyl radical (the only species that could be observed) by changing the concentrations of ascorbate. The iterative optimization program is based on a set of differential equations that is derived from all the pertinent reactions in the system (17). We have also investigated this system by observing either the flavonoid aroxyl or the ascorbate radical by EPR spectroscopy. Using these approaches we could verify that some of the fast radical–radical electron-exchange reactions are reversible on the slower time scale of EPR spectroscopy (Bors W, Michel C, and Stettmaier K, manuscript submitted).

Both $AscH^-$ and $Asc^{\cdot-}$ are considered to be strong reductants (vis-à-vis cytochrome b_5 and NADH-cytochrome b_5 reductase; $Asc^{\cdot-}$ can also be an oxidant) (31). However, ascorbate seems to be unable to reduce disulfides (33); that inability at first may seem inconsistent with its reducing ability. However, the first step of disulfide reduction (a one-electron transfer) would produce the disulfide radical anion. This is a very strong reducing species; the reduction potential ($E^{\circ\prime}$) for the $GSSG/GSSG^{\cdot-}$ couple is -1500 mV; Thus, its formation is thermodynamically difficult (32).

The weak (UV-visible) absorption spectrum of the ascorbate radical (at pH 6.4 $\lambda_{max} = 360$ nm, $\varepsilon_{360} = 3,300$ M^{-1} cm^{-1}) (7,34) makes it impossible to observe it directly in steady-state experiments, especially in complex biological material. Consequently, EPR spectroscopy of $Asc^{\cdot-}$ is the preferred method for observing it (35). Detailed EPR studies of $Asc^{\cdot-}$ in 1972 (36) and 1973 (37) have accurately established the g-factor (2.00518) and coupling constants (1.76 G, 0.07 G, 0.19 G for a^{H4}, a^{H5}, and a^{H6}, respectively, in aqueous solution) (36) as well as the effect of different solvents (37). Although proton nuclear magnetic resonance (NMR) experiments have suggested a bicyclic structure for the ascorbate radical (38), analogous to that of DHAA (1) of Fig. 1 the EPR parameters are consistent with the structure of the ascorbate radical presented in Fig. 1. Corroborating the pulse-radiolytic and EPR data are quantum mechanical calculations on the optimized geometries of the various radical and ionic intermediates (39) and reaction pathways with hydroxyl radical (40). Both the quasi aromaticity of the radical and the lower pK values as compared to those of the model compound triose reductone are likely explanations of the stability of the ascorbate radical.

In most biological experiments the actual steady-state concentrations of $Asc^{\cdot-}$ observed are $\sim 10^{-7}$ M, often 10^{-8}–10^{-10} M (41). These low concentrations dictate that for successful detection care must be taken to use the optimal EPR instrument settings, especially for the time resolution needed for kinetic for $EPR/Asc^{\cdot-}$ experiments. We have found that a modulation amplitude of 0.6–0.7 G produces the greatest EPR signal height for $Asc^{\cdot-}$ (42). When using a TM cavity we also have observed that a nominal microwave power of ≈ 40 mW also maximizes the signal height for $Asc^{\cdot-}$ in room temperature aqueous solutions (42). However, saturation effects begin at ≈ 16 mW nominal power. Thus, if absolute concentrations of $Asc^{\cdot-}$ are needed, then standardization and quantitation calculations must take into account these possible saturation effects.

The extreme sensitivity of EPR detection of $Asc^{\cdot-}$ coupled with the efficiency of metal catalysis of ascorbate oxidation have been used to estimate iron concentrations in reagents in the range of 1–1000 nM (41). Thus, the $Asc^{\cdot-}$ can provide investigators with information on several aspects of a system. But one must always keep in mind that what is being monitored is $[Asc^{•-}]_{ss}$. A kinetic argument has been made that the dominant route of $Asc^{•-}$ decay will usually be via disproportionation (43). However, the relative stability of $Asc^{•-}$, compared to that of radicals such as $HO^{•}$ and $RO^{•}$, gives a time resolution suitable for kinetic EPR spectroscopy (14,22,44,45,46).

Enzymology

The unusual stability of the ascorbate radical has apparently dictated that enzymatic systems are required to reduce the potential transient accumulation of $Asc^{•-}$. An enzyme, NADH:monodehydroascorbate reductase (EC 1.6.5.4), has apparently evolved for that purpose. It is quite common in plants (47–51), where it plays a major role in stress-related responses. In animal organs it exists predominantly in the retina (52,53). Other sources indicate that the enzyme functions as a transmembrane electron-carrier system (54,55); e.g., in mitochondria and chromaffin granules, its activity depends on the thiol–disulfide redox balance (56). Recently, the presence of a soluble ascorbate radical reductase, which differs from the known membrane-bound enzyme, has been reported (57). In addition, a mitochondrial enzyme has been described, which has distinct properties such as molecular weight and catalytic parameters (58). In a timely report Kobayashi et al. (59) have determined the absolute rate constant of the cucumber ascorbate radical reductase at pH 7.4 to be $2.6 \times 10^8 \ M^{-1}s^{-1}$. The fact that in animal tissues this enzyme is far less ubiquitous than in plant tissues has been explained by the predominant role of the glutathione-dependent dehydroascorbate reductase enzyme (EC 1.8.5.1) in controlling the ascorbate–dehydroascorbic redox balance (60). Furthermore, L-DHAA appears to be the major transport form of this vitamin across membranes (61). Thus, these enzymes play a major role in reducing DHAA to $AscH^-$, thereby keeping the antioxidant function of vitamin C operating at maximum efficiency.

The fact that several enzymes aside from ascorbate oxidase (47,62) also take advantage of the univalent redox cycling of ascorbate, i.e., generate ascorbate radicals during their turnover, for example, ascorbate peroxidase (EC 1.11.1.11) (48,63,64), dopamine-β-hydroxylase (EC 1.14.17.1) (62,65), and ascorbate-cytochrome b_5 reductase (EC 1.10.2.1) (66) indicates that "nature" considers this cycle as somewhat innocuous and not prone to severely toxic side reactions.

GENERATION AND REACTIVITY OF Asc$^{•-}$ IN ANTIOXIDANT INTERACTIONS

Despite the fact that the original proposal of Szent-Györgyi and colleagues of certain flavonoids protecting the antiscorbutic effects of ascorbic acid (67–69) did not mention the involvement of ascorbate radicals, a recent study on flavonoid–ascorbate interactions by pulse radiolysis and kinetic modeling confirmed this intermediate as an essential link (17). This study, incidentally, was instigated by another observation of Szent-Györgyi and colleagues (70), where they showed a prooxidant and cytotoxic effect of ascorbate involving univalent reduction of quinones and a concomitant formation of $Asc^{•-}$ by EPR spectroscopy. Because these reactions are evidently controlled by the respective redox potentials, the cytotoxicity of most biologically relevant quinones (e.g., antibiotics) may be partially explained by such reactions, in addition to potential futile redox cycling generating superoxide anion (71–73).

Quite recently, a report on the formation of $Asc^{•-}$ by the reaction of ascorbate with peroxynitrite, the presumed cytotoxic product of $\cdot$NO reacting with $O_2{}^{\cdot-}$, provided a potential link between these biologically relevant radicals and the vitamin C antioxidant systems (74–76).

$$AscH^- + O=NOOH \rightarrow Asc^{\cdot-} + \cdot NO_2 + H_2O \tag{5}$$

$$AscH^- + \cdot NO_2 \rightarrow Asc^{\cdot-} + NO_2{}^- \tag{6}$$

where

k_{obs} for reaction 5 at pH 7.4 is 47 $M^{-1}s^{-1}$ (7)

Phenols

One of the most important and intensely investigated reactions with ascorbate is the reduction of tocopheroxyl radicals forming $Asc^{\cdot-}$

$$AscH^- + \alpha\text{-}TO^{\cdot} \rightarrow Asc^{\cdot-} + \alpha\text{-}TOH \tag{7}$$

First observed in a pulse-radiolytic study (23) and since confirmed (22,24,77–80), rate constants for this reaction under various conditions (22–24) as well as EPR evidence of this redox cycling (22,77,79,80) have been reported; see Table 1. Even though superior analogues of α-tocopherol have been chemically synthesized (81–83) and lipophilic derivatives of ascorbate can be nearly as effective (with only a minor decrease in the rate constant with α-tocopheroxyl radical with lengthening of the C6-side chain) (22), the potential biological importance of reaction 7 must not be underestimated.

Because the tocopheroxyl radical is a good reactant for ascorbate, it is easily hypothesized that other phenoxyl radicals could also be reduced with the concomitant formation of $Asc^{\cdot-}$. This was first demonstrated by Schuler (34) and since corroborated for a number of pharmacologically relevant phenols (84–89), such as probucol (86,87) and etoposide (VP-16) (88,89). Yet the fact that certain p- (70) and o-semiquinones (25) are not reduced by ascorbate again points to the importance of the respective redox potentials of the radical species involved in controlling the reaction.

Thiols

A recurrent problem in the understanding of the interrelationships of biological antioxidative systems is the question of the extent to which the glutathione and the ascorbate redox cycling system may act synergistically in direct chemical reactions (90), in addition to the known interaction in their respective enzyme systems (56,63). Despite evidence to the contrary (89), it seems to be reasonable to expect such interaction, yet it may be difficult to prove as the primary link: the thiyl radical is hard to observe directly and has an altogether too short lifetime. Furthermore, with dihydrolipoic acid (DHLA) as a recently popular alternative thiol reductant (88,89), the thiyl radical, as a free radical, never actually occurs as cyclization to the radical disulfide anion is an extremely rapid intramolecular process ($\geq 1 \times 10^7$ s^{-1} (unpublished data from our laboratory). Whether this distinction between dihydrolipoic acid (DHLA) and reduced glutathione (GSH) is also the basis of the additive reducing effect of AscH$^-$ and GSH toward the etoposide phenoxyl radical (33)—whereas DHLA and AscH$^-$ do show a synergistic effect with both etoposide (88) and probucol phenoxyl radicals (86)—is the basis of ongoing kinetic studies in our laboratory. Since the thiols are capable of reducing the etoposide (88) but not the probucol phenoxyl radical (86), we are interested in whether this reactivity is kinetically or thermodynamically controlled.

ASCORBATE RADICALS IN PLANTS

The ascorbate radical was first observed by EPR spectroscopy over three decades ago. Since then interest in $Asc^{\cdot-}$ has grown. In plants and plant tissue the first reports of altered $Asc^{\cdot-}$ levels from environmental stress appeared in the early 1990s (91,92). Plants have an extensive system to handle ascorbate radicals (93,94) in addition to the redox cycling system mentioned (47–51). In addition to $Asc^{\cdot-}$ formation in response to oxidative stress (47,92,94), or during wounding (50), they may actually use $Asc^{\cdot-}$ formation as a signaling event in development (95). Because both the univalent and bivalent redox cycles of ascorbate are highly intertwined in plants, it augurs well to further explore the EPR technique for such studies.

ASCORBATE RADICAL EPR INTENSITY AS A MEASURE OF OXIDATIVE STRESS

The details of the EPR spectrum of $Asc^{\cdot-}$ in aqueous solutions were understood in 1972/73 (36,37) and soon thereafter studies of $Asc^{\cdot-}$ in cell cultures and animal organs were initiated (96,97). However, almost two decades passed before EPR spectroscopy of $Asc^{\cdot-}$ became an established method in cell and animal studies. It is now recognized that the monitoring of $Asc^{\cdot-}$ formation by EPR is an excellent marker of oxidative stress (98–102). Buettner and Jurkiewicz have provided thermodynamic and kinetic arguments for the use of $[Asc^{\cdot-}]_{ss}$ as a marker of oxidative stress (99). They have detailed some of the experimental considerations needed to allow a reasonable interpretation of the EPR data (41,99,102). In brief, an increase in $[Asc^{\cdot-}]_{ss}$ correlates with an increase in oxidative stress. However, to be able to make such an inference one must control pH and ascorbate concentration in the system. In addition, changes in oxygen levels as well as in catalytic metal activity must be considered. Examples of using the EPR $Asc^{\cdot-}$ signal to gain information on various biological systems follow.*

Cell Cultures

The study of $Asc^{\cdot-}$ in conjunction with cell cultures is proceeding on two fronts: (1) use of changes in $[Asc^{\cdot-}]_{ss}$ to reflect oxidative stress and (2) the possible involvement of $Asc^{\cdot-}$ in cell signaling and cell development.

Oxidative Stress

These investigations have used EPR to monitor $[Asc^{\cdot-}]_{ss}$ when the cell cultures are exposed to different stresses. The cells have ranged from isolated rat hepatocytes (98), to Ehrlich ascites tumor cells (103), L1210 murine leukemia cells (44), and even simple thyroid microsomes (104). Following the change in $[Asc^{\cdot-}]_{ss}$ with time via kinetic EPR spectroscopy can provide very useful information. Figure 3 provides an example of the change in $[Asc^{\cdot-}]_{ss}$ observed in a whole cell incubation of L1210 murine leukemia cells (44). Edelsfosine, an ether lipid anticancer drug that is membrane-active, is introduced at the arrow. Within a minute we observe a dramatic increase in oxidative flux as reflected by a rapid rise in $[Asc^{\cdot-}]_{ss}$. These results demonstrate the rapid response of the cells to this

---

*A recent study suggests that conjugated cytochrome c, which is not a substrate for either cytochrome c reductase or cytochrome c oxidase and also is not reduced by $O_2^{\cdot-}$, can be used indirectly to monitor $Asc^{\cdot-}$ levels in the circulation of rats (133).

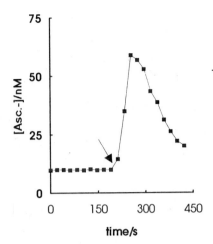

Figure 3 Edelfosine increases oxidative stress in L1210 murine leukemia cell suspensions as reflected by changes in $(Asc^{.-})_{ss}$ (44). Docosahexaenonic acid enriched L1210 cells (5×10^6 cells/ml) were incubated in room temperature 0.9% NaCl solution that contained 20 μM Fe^{2+} and 100 μM ascorbate. Edelfosine 40 μM, a membrane-active ether lipid anticancer drug, was added at the arrow. Vehicle alone produced no significant change in $(Asc^{.-})_{ss}$. EPR spectra were collected with a Bruker ESP 300 electron spin resonance spectrometer.

oxidative stress. The fall of $[Asc^{.-}]_{ss}$ indicates a depletion of some necessary component: oxidizable substrate, ascorbate, or perhaps oxygen. Supporting experiments suggest oxidizable membrane lipids are being depleted (44).

Asc·– and Cell Signaling

Ascorbate radical has been proposed to activate transplasma membrane electron transport systems (95,105–109). Cell-impermeable oxidants that can accept electrons from this electron transport system appear to stimulate cell growth (105). $Asc^{.-}$ is poorly taken up by cells compared to $AscH^-$. Thus, $Asc^{.-}$ appears to serve as an oxidant that can act as an external electron acceptor. $AscH^-$ is regenerated, but cell "signaling" can also occur, resulting in stimulated growth. Data that have been presented suggest this to be the case for HL-60 cells (105,109) and onion root meristems (107,108), two quite different eukaryotic cells.

Body Fluids

It would be ideal to learn something about free radical oxidations from body fluids. When freshly extracted fluids are examined by EPR, $Asc^{.-}$ is quite likely observed. Fresh whole blood gives a very weak $Asc^{.-}$ EPR signal (110). However, when plasma from this same blood is examined, a much stronger, easily detectable signal is observed (79,101,111–116). Fresh serum also yields detectable $Asc^{.-}$ (111,117–119). The much lower $[Asc^{.-}]_{ss}$ seen in whole blood compared to plasma or serum undoubtedly results from the ability of red cells to reduce $Asc^{.-}$. There have been successes in gaining information on the "oxidative state" of plasma. However, careful attention to controls and most importantly the level of ascorbate present must be known (99,102). Other fluids also have $Asc^{.-}$ present that may provide information. $Asc^{\cdot-}$ in synovial fluid has been used to indicate the presence of catalytic metals (120). $Asc^{\cdot-}$ has been observed in semen and may provide an indication of sperm robustness (121). $Asc^{\cdot-}$ in cow's milk has potential to indicate the state of "freshness" (122,123). In a related application, $Asc^{\cdot-}$ has been used to study potential antioxidant components of infant formulas (123).

In all these examples, it is clear that to gain information from $Asc^{\cdot-}$, the mechanisms by which it may be formed must be understood.

Perfused Tissue/Organs

Changes in ascorbate radical EPR intensity have been observed when rabbit aorta or iliac artery has been subjected to changes in flow (115). These results implied that the endothelium was the principal source of flow-related free radical production. This radical production appears to be another example of the beneficial effects of physiological free radical production.

When isolated rat hearts were subjected to ischemic reperfusion episodes, an increased level of $Asc^{\cdot-}$ was observed in the perfusion buffer (112). The transient increase commenced on reperfusion and was dissipated usually within 30 min. These data were interpreted to indicate that at reperfusion ascorbate, probably mostly as DHAA, was released from the tissue, resulting in an increase in radical production. In similar experiments with isolated rat liver, an increase in $Asc^{\cdot-}$ has also been observed on reperfusion after ischemia (124). Thus, $Asc^{\cdot-}$ has potential to provide information about oxidative events during ischemia–reperfusion episodes.

Care must be exercised in designing and interpreting all experiments where perfusion buffers are used as it has been clearly shown that the heart can extract the adventitious metals present in the buffer. These metals, particularly copper, will alter the experimental results (125). It is best to remove these metals from all buffers used so that the best interpretation of the data is possible (126).

Whole Animals

Two approaches have been used to gain information from $Asc^{\cdot-}$ about oxidative events in whole animals. Both are ex vivo approaches in which fluid is routed from the body via tubing to the EPR for examination.

Mori et al. (127,128) have devised a method to route blood from a femoral artery of a rat through the EPR spectrometer and return it to the animal. This approach monitors $Asc^{\cdot-}$ in whole blood. The researchers observed that $[Asc^{\cdot-}]_{ss}$ increases, as predicted, when ascorbate or iron-citrate is infused into the animal.

At this same time, Sharma et al. (129) developed a similar system to circulate coronary venous blood from dogs through a flat cell in an EPR cavity and return it to the animal. An intravenous infusion pump is used to control the flow rate so that the transit time from heart to EPR is constant. These investigators have observed that $[Asc^{\cdot-}]_{ss}$ is increased on infusion of ascorbate or when metal-mediated oxidative stress is induced by infusion of iron or copper salts.

Of special interest is the observation that infusion of sodium nitroprusside, an antihypertensive drug, produced a dramatic rise in $[Asc^{\cdot-}]$ consistent with the initiation of oxidative stress by this compound. Myocardial ischemia reperfusion experiments demonstrated that on reperfusion after a 20 min ischemic episode the $[Asc^{\cdot-}]_{ss}$ in the blood from the coronary vein increased. This increase was blunted by superoxide dismutase–catalase and by metal chelators, all consistent with radical formation on reoxygenation of the ischemic myocardium.

Still another approach uses microdialysis to produce an EPR sample for detection of $Asc^{\cdot-}$ (130–132). Microdialysis tubing is placed in the region of interest. The low-molecular-weight ascorbate-system species diffuse into the solution in the tubing and can then be examined by EPR. This approach has been used to monitor oxidative stress in the brain of rats. As predicted, the presence of iron salts or H_2O_2 increased the $Asc^{\cdot-}$ concentration in the dialysate. Other stresses such as cold injury also produced increases in $Asc^{\cdot-}$, indicating the potential of this system to prove oxidative events.

Humans

Investigations on the use of ascorbate radical to probe for human health status are exceedingly limited. Early work used lyphilized tissue samples for EPR examination (96,97). In these preparations, the EPR signals observed were those of the immobilized $Asc^{\cdot-}$. Most interesting was the observation of a very strong $Asc^{\cdot-}$ EPR signal from lyphilized erythrocytes of patients with acute lymphatic leukemia. A completely different EPR spectrum was obtained from erythrocytes of patients with acute myeloid leukemia. The unique spectrum obtained from acute lymphatic leukemia patients was never observed in erythrocytes from patients with other types of leukemia or other diseases of the hematopoietic or lymphatic system.

Recent work with human plasma ascorbate radical has as a goal probing for oxidative stress (112,116). In cardiac ischemia–reperfusion the depletion of plasma ascorbate was monitored via $Asc^{\cdot-}$ using EPR (112). This study suggests that transient changes in plasma ascorbate status induced during cardiac arrest and reperfusion may be a useful clinical marker for oxidative stress This change in ascorbate is reflected in the plasma $[Asc^{\cdot-}]_{ss}$.

Another study of $Asc^{\cdot-}$ in human plasma was directed toward monitoring intensive care patients with sepsis (116). The study found that sepsis patients have significantly more catalytic iron in serum than healthy control persons, while ascorbate in sepsis patients was less than in control patients. Yet $[Asc^{\cdot-}]_{ss}$ was nearly the same. However, a 1 g bolus injection of ascorbate to sepsis patients resulted in only a minor increase in $[Asc^{\cdot-}]_{ss}$ and plasma ascorbate, as compared to those of control patients. These results suggest that quite different ascorbate metabolism occurs in the sepsis patient. How to interpret this with respect to improvement of patient health is not yet known, but it suggests that quite a difference in ascorbate metabolism exists between healthy control and sepsis patients.

Skin

One of the most informative uses of $Asc^{\cdot-}$ has been in studies of skin. The first investigation of $Asc^{\cdot-}$ in this organ (SKH-1 hairless mouse) demonstrated that UV light increased endogenous $[Asc^{\cdot-}]_{ss}$ and that in skin treated with chlorpromazine, a photoactive drug, UV light produced an even greater increase in $[Asc^{\cdot-}]_{ss}$ (133). In complementary experiments using the EPR spin trapping agent α-(4-pyridyl 1-oxide)-N-tert-butylnitrone (POBN) applied to the skin, a carbon-centered radical presumably from lipid peroxidation products was detected. This radical signal was blunted when an iron chelating agent (Desferal) was applied prior to UV exposure (134). These results demonstrate that UV light does indeed produce free radicals in skin and that iron present in the skin may exacerbate the free radical oxidative stress.

If membrane-derived free radicals are involved in the deleterious effects of UV light on skin, then tocopherol-based antioxidants may reduce this damage. Indeed, Jurkiewicz et al. (135) in the SKH-1 mouse model have used EPR detection of Asc$^{\cdot-}$ as well as POBN spin trapping to demonstrate that topical application of tocopherol sorbate reduces UV light-mediated free radical formation. But most exciting is that they have also demonstrated that tocopherol sorbate protects against photoaging and UV light–induced skin tumor formation. This study is the first actually to correlate photoaging and UV light–induced tumor formation with free radical production. Thus, the development of effective antioxidants and the methods to deliver them to the skin for protection against UV light is well justified.

Timmons and Davies (136) have used these techniques to demonstrate that application of organic peroxides to murine skin results in an increase in the endogenous Asc$^{\cdot-}$ EPR signal. This radical formation requires that the peroxide penetrates the skin stratum corneum. These observations are the first steps needed to correlate peroxide-induced free radical formation with its deleterious effects in skin tissue.

SUMMARY

Asc$^{\cdot-}$ is both thermodynamically and kinetically a very domesticated free radical. It is a pi radical with low reactivity. Thus, it is an ideal radical to be formed as a product when ascorbate, a donor antioxidant, reacts to repair dangerously oxidizing radicals, such as peroxyl and alkoxyl radicals, and less dangerous, but potentially bothersome, phenolic radicals, such as those from flavonoids and tocopherol. Its low reactivity results in a "relatively" long lifetime, making it an ideal marker for ongoing free radical oxidations in solutions, cells, tissues, and even whole organisms. Perhaps one of the most powerful aspects of its use as a marker of oxidative stress is that it can provide information on the system in real time (99,102).

REFERENCES

1. Weast RC. Handbook of Chemistry and Physics, 67th ed. Boca Raton, FL: CRC Press, 1986:D161.
2. Davis HF, McManus HJ, Fessenden RW. An ESR study of free-radical protonation equilibria in strongly acid media. J Phys Chem 1986; 90:6400–6404.
3. Lewin S. Vitamin C: its molecular biology and medical potential. New York: Academic Press, 1976.
4. Schöneshöfer M. Pulsradiolytische Untersuchung zur Oxidation der Ascorbinsäure durch OH-Radikale and Halogen-Radikalkomplexe in wäßriger Lösung. Z Naturforsch 1972; 27b: 649–659.
5. Bansal KM, Schöneshöfer M, Grätzel M. Polarographic studies on the pulse-radiolytic oxidation of ascorbic acid in aqueous solution. Z Naturforsch 1973; 28b:528–529.
6. Bielski BHJ, Richter HW, Chan PC. Some properties of the ascorbate free radical. Ann NY Acad Sci 1975; 258:231–237.
7. Bielski BHJ, Allen AO, Schwarz HA. Mechanism of disproportionation of ascorbate radicals. J Am Chem Soc 1981; 103:3516–3518.
8. Bielski BHJ. Chemistry of ascorbic acid radicals. Adv Chem Ser 1982; 200:81–100.
9. Cabelli DE, Bielski BHJ. Kinetics and mechanism for the oxidation of ascorbic acid/ascorbate by HO$_2$/(O$_2^-$) radicals: a pulse radiolysis and stopped-flow photolysis study. J Phys Chem 1983; 87:1809–1812.
10. Cabelli DE, Bielski BHJ, Seib PA. A pulse radiolysis study of the oxidation of methyl-substituted ascorbates. Radiat Phys Chem 1984; 23:419–429.

11. Kobayashi K, Harada Y, Hayashi K. Kinetic behavior of the monodehydroascorbate radical studied by pulse radiolysis. Biochemistry 1991; 30:8310–8315.

12. Nakata K, Morita N, Taniguchi R, Horii H. Oxidized intermediates formed from α- and β-galactosyl ascorbic acid by pulse radiolysis. Bioelectrochem Bioenerg 1995; 38:85–89.

13. Kim H, Rosenthal I, Kirschenbaum LJ, Riesz P. Photosensitized formation of ascorbate radicals by chloroaluminum phthalocyanine tetrasulfonate: an electron spin resonance study. Free Radical Biol Med 1992; 13:231–238.

14. Kim H, Kirschenbaum LJ, Rosenthal I, Riesz P. Photosensitized formation of ascorbate radicals by riboflavin: an ESR study. Photochem Photobiol 1993; 57:777–784.

15. Hoey BM, Butler J. The repair of oxidized amino acids by antioxidants. Biochim Biophys Acta 1984; 791:212–218.

16. Alfassi ZB, Huie RE, Neta P, Shoute LCT. Temperature dependence of the rate constants for reactions of inorganic radicals with organic reductants. J Phys Chem 1990; 94:8800–8805.

17. Bors W, Michel C, Schikora S. Interaction of flavonoids with ascorbate and determination of their univalent redox potentials: a pulse radiolysis study. Free Radical Biol Med 1995; 19: 45–52.

18. Ross AB, Mallard WG, Helman WP, et al. NDRL-NIST Solution Kinetics Database, Version 2. Gaithersburgh, MD: NIST Standard Reference Data, 1994.

19. O'Neill P, Davies S. Interaction of peroxyl radical adducts of DNA bases with reductants. In: Rotilio G, ed. Superoxide and Superoxide Dismutase in Chemistry, Biology and Medicine. Amsterdam: Elsevier, 1986:44–45.

20. Lal M, Schöneich C, Mönig J, Asmus KD. Rate constants for the reactions of halogenated organic radicals. Int J Radiat Biol 1988; 54:773–785.

21. Neta P, Huie RE, Mosseri S, et al. Rate constants for reduction of substituted methylperoxyl radicals by ascorbate ions and N,N,N',N'-tetramethyl-p-phenylenediamine. J Phys Chem 1989; 93:4099–4104.

22. Liu ZL, Han ZX, Yu KC, et al. Kinetic ESR study on the reaction of vitamin E radical with vitamin C and its lipophilic derivatives in cetyltrimethylammonium bromide micelles. J Phys Org Chem 1992; 5:33–38.

23. Packer JE, Slater TF, Willson RL. Direct observation of a free radical interaction between vitamin E and vitamin C. Nature 1979; 278:737–738.

24. Bisby RH, Parker AW. Reaction of ascorbate with the α-tocopheroxyl radical in micellar and bilayer membrane systems. Arch Biochem Biophys 1995; 317:170–178.

25. Bors W. Semiquinone and phenoxyl radicals of phenolic antioxidants and model compounds: generation, spectral and kinetic properties. Life Chem Rep 1985; 3:16–21.

26. Bors W, Michel C, Saran M. Unpublished data.

27. Huie RE, Neta P. Oxidation of ascorbate and a tocopherol analogue by the sulfite-derived radicals SO_3^- and SO_5^-. Chem Biol Interact 1985; 53:233–238.

28. Neta P, Huie RE, Maruthamuthu P, Steenken S. Solvent effects in the reactions of peroxyl radicals with organic reductants. Evidence for proton-transfer-mediated electron transfer. J Phys Chem 1989; 93:7654–7659.

29. Wieczorek P, Ogonski T, Machoy Z. Interaction of Na, Li, Cs, K ions with ascorbyl radicals. Z Naturforsch 1987; 42c:215–216.

30. Williams NH, Yandell JK. Outer-sphere electron transfer reactions of ascorbate anions. Aust J Chem 1982; 35:1133–1144.

31. Iyanagi T, Yamazaki I, Anan KF. One-electron oxidation–reduction properties of ascorbic acid. Biochim Biophys Acta 1985; 806:255–261.

32. Buettner GR. The pecking order of free radicals and antioxidants: lipid peroxidation, α-tocopherol, and ascorbate. Arch Biochem Biophys 1993; 300:535–543.

33. Fleming JE, Bensch KG, Schreiber J, Lohmann W. Interaction of ascorbic acid with disulfides. Z Naturforsch 1983; 38c:859–861.

34. Schuler RH. Oxidation of ascorbate anion by electron transfer to phenoxyl radicals. Radiat Res 1977; 69:417–433.

35. Buettner GR, Jurkiewicz BA. Chemistry and biochemistry of ascorbic acid. In: Cadenas E, Packer L, eds. Handbook of Antioxidants. New York: Marcel Dekker, 1996.

36. Laroff GP, Fessenden RW, Schuler RH. The ESR spectra of radical intermediates in the oxidation of ascorbic acid and related substances. J Am Chem Soc 1972; 94:9062–9073.

37. Steenken S, Olbrich G. EPR investigations concerning the structure of the ascorbic acid radical in water, alcohol, and DMSO. Photochem Photobiol 1973; 18:43–48.

38. Sapper H, Pleyer-Weber A, Lohmann W. ^{1}H-NMR- und ESR-Messungen zur Struktur der Dehydroascorbinsäure und des Semidehydroascorbatradikals. Z Naturforsch 1982; 37c: 129–131.

39. Abe Y, Okada S, Horii H, et al. A theoretical study on the mechanism of oxidation of L-ascorbic acid. J Chem Soc [Perkin Trans II] 1987; 715–720.

40. Abe Y, Okada S, Nakao R, et al. A molecular orbital study on the reactivity of L-ascorbic acid towards OH radical. J Chem Soc [Perkin Trans II] 1992; 2221–2227.

41. Buettner GR. Ascorbate oxidation: UV absorbance of ascorbate and ESR spectroscopy of the ascorbyl radical as assays for iron. Free Radical Res Comm 1990; 10:5–9.

42. Buettner GR, Kiminyo KP. Optimal EPR detection of weak nitroxide spin adduct and ascorbyl free radical signals. J Biochem Biophys Method 1992; 24:147–151.

43. Roginsky VA, Stegmann HB. Ascorbyl radical as natural indicator of oxidative stress: quantitative regularities. Free Radical Biol Med 1994; 17:93–103.

44. Wagner BA, Buettner GR, Burns CP. Increased generation of lipid-derived and ascorbate free radicals by L1210 cells exposed to the ether lipid edelfosine. Cancer Res 1993; 53:711–713.

45. Buettner GR, Need MJ. Hydrogen peroxide and hydroxyl free radical production by hematoporphyrin derivative, ascorbate and light. Cancer Lett 1985; 25:297–304.

46. Buettner GR, Doherty TP, Bannister TD. Hydrogen peroxide and hydroxyl radical formation by methylene blue in the presence of ascorbic acid. Radiat Environ Biophys 1984; 23: 235–243.

47. Arrigoni O, Dipierro S, Borraccino G. Ascorbate free radical reductase, a key enzyme of the ascorbic acid system. FEBS Lett 1981; 125:242–244.

48. Hossain MA, Nakano Y, Asada K. Monodehydroascorbate reductase in spinach chloroplasts and its participation in regeneration of ascorbate for scavenging H_2O_2. Plant Cell Physiol 1984; 25:385–395.

49. Hausladen A, Kunert KJ. Effects of artificially enhanced levels of ascorbate and GSH on the enzymes monodehydroascorbate reductase, dehydroascorbate reductase and GSH reductase in spinach (Spinacia oleracea). Physiol Plant 1990; 79:384–388.

50. Grantz A, Brummell DA, Bennett AB. Ascorbate free radical reductase RNA levels are induced by wounding. Plant Physiol 1995; 108:411–418.

51. Polle A, Morawe B. Seasonal changes of the antioxidative systems in foliar buds and leaves of field-grown beech trees (Fagus sylvatica, L.) in a stressful climate. Bot Acta 1995; 108:314–320.

52. Bando M, Obazawa H. Ascorbate free radical reductase and ascorbate redox cycle in the human lens. Jpn J Ophthalmol 1988; 32:176–186.

53. Bando M, Obazawa H. Activities of ascorbate free radical reductase and H_2O_2-dependent NADH oxidase in senile cataractous human lenses. Exp Eye Res 1990; 50:779–784.

54. Sun I, Morre DJ, Crane FL, et al. Monodehydroascorbate as an electron acceptor for NADH reduction by coated vesicle and Golgi apparatus fractions of rat liver. Biochim Biophys Acta 1984; 797:266–275.

55. Wakefield LM, Cass AEG, Radda GK. Electron transfer across the chromaffin granule membrane: use of EPR to demonstrate reduction of intravesicular ascorbate radical by the extravesicular mitochondrial NADH:ascorbate radical oxidoreductase. J Biol Chem 1986; 261: 9746–9752.

56. Villalba JM, Canalejo A, Burón MI, et al. Thiol groups are involved in NADH-ascorbate free radical reductase activity of rat liver plasma membrane. Biochem Biophys Res Comm 1993; 192:707–713.

57. Rose RC. Ascorbic acid metabolism in protection against free radicals: a radiation model. Biochem Biophys Res Comm 1990; 169:430–436.
58. Deleonardis S, Delorenzo G, Borraccino G, Dipierro S. A specific ascorbate free radical reductase isozyme participates in the regeneration of ascorbate for scavenging toxic oxygen species in potato tuber mitochondria. Plant Physiol 1995; 109:847–851.
59. Kobayashi K, Tagawa S, Sano S, Asada K. A direct demonstration of the catalytic action of monodehydroascorbate reductase by pulse radiolysis. J Biol Chem 1995; 270:27551–27554.
60. Rose RC. The ascorbate redox potential of tissues: a determinant or indicator of disease? News Physiol Sci 1989; 4:190–195.
61. Bigley R, Stankova L, Roos D, Loos J. Glutathione-dependent dehydroascorbate reduction: a determinant of dehydroascorbate uptake by human polymorphonuclear leukocytes. Enzyme 1980; 25:200–204.
62. Skotland T, Ljones T. Direct spectrophotometric detection of ascorbate free radical formed by dopamine β-monooxygenase and by ascorbate oxidase. Biochim Biophys Acta 1980; 630: 30–35.
63. Asada K. Ascorbate peroxidase - a hydrogen peroxide-scavenging enzyme in plants. Physiol Plant 1992; 85:235–241.
64. Grace S, Pace R, Wydrzynski T. Formation and decay of monodehydroascorbate radicals in illuminated thylakoids as determined by EPR spectroscopy. Biochim Biophys Acta 1995; 1229:155–165.
65. DiLiberto EJ, Allen PL. Mechanism of dopamine-β-hydroxylation: semidehydroascorbate as the enzymic oxidation product of ascorbate. J Biol Chem 1981; 256:3385–3393.
66. Everling FB, Weis W, Staudinger H. Kinetische Studien an einer Ascorbat: ferricytochrom b₅-Oxidoreduktase (EC 1.1.2.?). Hoppe Seylers Z Physiol Chem 1969; 350:1485–1492.
67. Rusznyak S, Szent-Györgyi A. Vitamin P: flavonols as vitamins. Nature 1936; 138:27
68. Bentsath A, Rusznyak S, Szent-Györgyi A. Vitamin nature of flavones. Nature 1936; 138:798.
69. Bentsath A, Rusznyak S, Szent-Györgyi A. Vitamin P. Nature 1937; 139:326–327.
70. Pethig R, Gascoyne PRC, McLaughlin JA, Szent-Györgyi A. Ascorbate-quinone interactions: electrochemical, free radical, and cytotoxic properties. Proc Natl Acad Sci USA 1983; 80: 129–132.
71. Sies H. Quinone redox cycling and the protective effect of DT diaphorase. In: Crastes de Paulet A, Dousté-Blazy L, Paoletti R, eds. Free Radicals, Lipoproteins and Membrane Lipids. New York: Plenum Press, NATO ASI Ser 1990, A189:381–388.
72. O'Brien PJ. Molecular mechanisms of quinone cytotoxicity. Chem Biol Interact 1991; 80: 1–41.
73. Mason RP. Free radical metabolites of toxic chemicals and drugs as sources of oxidative stress. In: Spatz L, Bloom AD, eds. Biological Consequences of Oxidative Stress. New York: Oxford University Press, 1992:23–49.
74. Shi XL, Rojanasakul Y, Gannett P, et al. Generation of thiyl and ascorbyl radicals in the reaction of peroxynitrite with thiols and ascorbate at physiological pH. J Inorg Biochem 1994; 56:77–86.
75. Bartlett D, Church D, Bounds P, Koppenol WH. The kinetics of the oxidation of L-ascorbic acid by peroxynitrite. Free Radical Biol Med 1995; 18:85–92.
76. Squadrito GL, Jin X, Pryor WA. Stopped-flow kinetic study of the reaction of ascorbic acid with peroxynitrite. Arch Biochem Biophys 1995; 322:53–59.
77. Scarpa M, Rigo A, Maiorino M, et al. Formation of α-tocopherol radical and recycling of α-tocopherol by ascorbate during peroxidation of phosphatidylcholine liposomes: an EPR study. Biochim Biophys Acta 1984; 801:215–219.
78. Tomasi A, Bini A, Botti B, et al. Glutathione, vitamin C, and vitamin E interaction in model systems of biological interest. Med Biol Environ 1992; 20:63–66.
79. Sharma MK, Buettner GR. Interaction of vitamin C and vitamin E during free radical stress in plasma: an ESR study. Free Radical Biol Med 1993; 14:649–653.

80. Roginsky VA, Stegmann HB. Kinetics of the reaction between ascorbate and free radical from vitamin E as studied by ESR steady-state method. Chem Phys Lipids 1993; 65: 103–122.

81. Burton GW, Ingold KU. Vitamin E: application of the principles of physical organic chemistry to the exploration of its structure and function. Accounts Chem Res 1986; 19:194–201.

82. Hughes L, Burton GW, Ingold KU, et al. Custom design of better in vivo antioxidants structurally related to vitamin E. In: Phenolic Compounds in Food and their Effects on Health II. Washington, DC, ACS Sympos Ser, 1992, 507:184–199.

83. Barclay LRC, Vinqvist MR, Mukai K, et al. Chain-breaking phenolic antioxidants—steric and electronic effects in polyalkylchromanols, tocopherol analogs, hydroquinones, and superior antioxidants of the polyalkylbenzochromanol and naphthofuran class. J Org Chem 1993; 58: 7416–7420.

84. Pelizzetti E, Meisel D, Mulac WA, Neta P. On the electron transfer from ascorbic acid to various phenothiazine radicals. J Am Chem Soc 1979; 101:6954–6959.

85. Rao DNR, Fischer V, Mason RP. GSH and ascorbate reduction of the acetaminophen radical formed by peroxidase: detection of the GSH disulfide radical anion and the ascorbyl radical. J Biol Chem 1990; 265:844–847.

86. Kagan VE, Freisleben HJ, Tsuchiya M, et al. Generation of probucol radicals and their reduction by ascorbate and dihydrolipoic acid in human low density lipoprotein. Free Radical Res Comm 1991; 15:265–276.

87. Kalyanaraman B, Darley-Usmar VM, Wood J, et al. Synergistic interaction between the probucol phenoxyl radical and ascorbic acid in inhibiting the oxidation of low density lipoprotein. J Biol Chem 1992; 267:6789–6795.

88. Stoyanovsky D, Yalowich J, Gantchev T, Kagan VE. Tyrosinase-induced phenoxyl radicals of etoposide (VP-16): interaction with reductants in model systems, K562 leukemic cell and nuclear homogenates. Free Radical Res Comm 1993; 19:371–386.

89. Kagan VE, Yalowich JC, Day BW, et al. Ascorbate is the primary reductant of the phenoxyl radical of etoposide in the presence of thiols both in cell homogenates and in model systems. Biochemistry 1994; 33:9651–9660.

90. Winkler BS, Orselli SM, Rex TS. The redox couple between glutathione and ascorbic acid: a chemical and physiological perspective. Free Radical Biol Med 1994; 17:333–349.

91. Stegmann HB, Schuler P. Ascorbic acid as indicator of damage to forest: a correlation with air quality. Z Naturforsch 1991; 46c:67–70.

92. Westphal S, Wagner E, Knollmüller M, et al. Impact of aminotriazole and paraquat on the oxidative defence system of spruce monitored by monodehydroascorbic acid. A test for oxidative stress causing agents in forest decline. Z Naturforsch 1992; 47c:567–572.

93. Miyake C, Asada K. Ferredoxin-dependent photoreduction of the monodehydroascorbate radical in spinach thylakoids. Plant Cell Physiol 1994; 35:539–549.

94. Foyer CH, Lelandais M, Kunert KJ. Photooxidative stress in plants. Physiol Plant 1994; 92: 696–717.

95. Gonzalez-Reyes JA, Alcain FJ, Caler JA, et al. Stimulation of onion root elongation by ascorbate and ascorbate free radical in Allium cepa L. Protoplasma 1995; 184:31–35.

96. Lohmann W, Bensch KG, Schreiber J, Mueller E. Paramagnetic changes in pulmonary tumors. Z Naturforsch 1981; 36c:5–8.

97. Lohmann W. Ascorbic acid and cancer. Ann NY Acad Sci 1987; 498:402–417.

98. Tomasi A, Albano E, Bini A, et al. Ascorbyl radical is detected in rat isolated hepatocytes suspensions undergoing oxidative stress: an early index of oxidative damage in cells. In: Poli G, Cheeseman KH, Dianzani MU, Slater TF, eds. Free Radicals in the Pathogenesis of Liver Injury. Oxford: Pergamon Press, Adv Biosci 1988; 76:325–334.

99. Buettner GR, Jurkiewicz BA. Ascorbate free radical as a marker of oxidative stress: an EPR study. Free Radical Biol Med 1993; 14:49–55.

100. Koyama K, Takatsuki K, Inoue M. Determination of superoxide and ascorbyl radicals in the circulation of animals under oxidative stress. Arch Biochem Biophys 1994; 309:323–328.

101. Pietri S, Seguin JR, d'Arbigny P, Culcasi M. Ascorbyl free radical—a noninvasive marker of oxidative stress in human open-heart surgery. Free Radical Biol Med 1994; 16:523–528.

102. Buettner GR, Jurkiewicz BA. Ascorbate radical: a valuable marker of oxidative stress. In: Favier AE, Cadet J, Kalyanaraman B, et al., eds. Analysis of Free Radicals in Biological Systems. Basel: Birkhäuser, 1995:145–164.

103. Pethig R, Gascoyne PRC, McLaughlin JA, Szent-Györgyi A. Enzyme-controlled scavenging of ascorbyl and 2,6-dimethoxy-semiquinone free radicals in Ehrlich ascites tumor cells. Proc Natl Acad Sci USA 1985; 82:1439–1442.

104. Nakamura M, Ohtaki S. Formation and reduction of ascorbate radicals by hog thyroid microsomes. Arch Biochem Biophys 1993; 305:84–90.

105. Alcain FJ, Burón MI, Rodriguez-Aguilera JC, et al. Ascorbate free radical stimulates the growth of a human promyelocytic leukemia cell line. Cancer Res 1990; 50:5887–5891.

106. Navas P, Gomez-Diaz C. Ascorbate free radical and its role in growth control. Protoplasma 1995; 184:8–13.

107. Hidalgo A, Gonzalez-Reyes JA, Navis P. Ascorbate free radical enhances vacuolization in onion root meristems. Plant Cell Environ 1989; 12:455–460.

108. Hidalgo A, Gonzalez-Reyes JA, Navis P. Cell Biol Intern Rep 1990; 14:133–141.

109. Navas P, Alcain FJ, Buron I, et al. Growth factor-stimulated trans plasma membrane electron transport in HL-60 cells. FEBS Lett 1992; 299:223–226.

110. Buettner GR. Unpublished obervations.

111. Minakata K, Suzuki O, Saito SI, Harada N. Ascorbate radical levels in human sera and rat plasma intoxicated with paraquat and diquat. Arch Toxicol 1993; 67:126–130.

112. Pietri S, Culcasi M, Stella L, Cozzone PJ. Ascorbyl free radical as a reliable indicator of free radical mediated myocardial ischemic and post-ischemic injury: a real time continuous flow ESR study. Eur J Biochem 1990; 193:845–854.

113. Pedro MA, Gatty RM, Augusto O. *In vivo* free radical formation monitored by the ascorbyl radical. Quimica Nova 1993; 16:370–372.

114. Minetti M, Forte T, Soriani M, et al. Iron-induced ascorbate oxidation in plasma as monitored by ascorbate free radical formation. Biochem J 1992; 282:459–465.

115. Laurindo FRM, Pedro MA, Barbeiro HV, et al. Vascular free radical release: ex vivo and in vivo evidence for a flow-dependent endothelial mechanism. Circ Res 1994; 74:700–709.

116. Galley HF, Davies MJ, Webster NR. Ascorbyl radical formation in patients with sepsis: effect of ascorbate loading. Free Radical Biol Med 1996; 20:139–143.

117. Sasaki R, Kurokawa T, Tero-Kubota S. Nature of serum ascorbate radical and its quantitative estimation. Tohoku J Exp Med 1982; 136:113–119.

118. Sasaki R, Kobayasi T, Kurokawa T, Shibuya D, Tero-Kubota S. Significance of the equilibrium constant between serum ascorbate radical and ascorbate acids in man. Tohoku J Exp Med 1984; 144:203–210.

119. Sasaki R, Kurokawa T, Shibuya D, et al. Use of K value of ascorbic acid as a clinical index of attack by oxygen radicals. J Clin Biochem Nutr 1989; 6:57–63.

120. Buettner GR, Chamulitrat W. The catalytic activity of iron in synovial fluid as monitored by the ascorbate free radical. Free Radical Biol Med 1990; 8:55–56.

121. Kiminyo KP, Buettner GR. Unpublished observations.

122. Nakamura M. Ascorbate radicals in fresh cow's milk. J Biochem 1994; 116:621–624.

123. Champagne ET, Hinojosa O, Clemetson CAB. Production of ascorbate free radicals in infant formulas and other media. J Food Sci 1990; 55:113–116.

124. Togashi H, Shinzawa H, Yong H, et al. Ascorbic acid radical, superoxide, and hydroxyl radical are detected in reperfusion injury of rat liver using ESR spectroscopy. Arch Biochem Biophys 1994; 308:1–7.

125. Powell SR, Wapnir RA. Adventitious redox-active metals in Krebs-Henseleit buffer can contribute to Langendorff heart experimental results. J Mol Cell Cardiol 1992; 26:749–778.

126. Buettner GR. In the absence of catalytic metals ascorbate does not autoxidize at pH7: ascorbate as a test for catalytic metals. J Biochem Biophys Method 1988; 16:27–40.

127. Wang X, Liu J, Mori A, et al. Direct detection of circulating free radicals in the rat using electron spin resonance spectrometry. Free Radical Biol Med 1992; 12:121–126.

128. Mori A, Wang XY, Liu JK. Electron spin resonance assay of ascorbate free radicals in vivo. Methods Enzymol 1994; 233:149–154.

129. Sharma MK, Buettner GR, Spencer KT, Kerber RE. Ascorbyl free radical as a real-time marker of free radical generation in briefly ischemic and reperfused hearts: an EPR study. Circ Res 1994; 74:650–658.

130. Kihara T, Sakata S, Ikeda M. Direct detection of ascorbyl radical in experimental brain injury: microdialysis and an electron spin resonance spectroscopic study. J Neurochem 1995; 65: 282–286.

131. Isoda H, Akagi K, Hasegawa T, et al. Detection of an increase in ascorbate radical in an irradiated experimental tumour system using ESR. Int J Radiat Biol 1995; 68:467–473.

132. Matsuo Y, Kihara T, Keda M, et al. Role of neutrophils in radical production during ischemia and reperfusion of the rat brain: effect of neutrophil depletion on extracellular ascorbyl radical formation. J Cereb Blood Flow Metab 1995; 15:941–947.

133. Buettner GR, Motten AG, Hall RD, Chignell CF. ESR detection of endogenous ascorbate free radical in mouse skin: enhancement of radical production during UV irradiation following topical application of chlorpromazine. Photochem Photobiol 1987; 46:161–164.

134. Jurkiewicz BA, Buettner GR. Ultraviolet light-inducted free radical formation in skin: an electron paramagnetic resonance study. Photochem Photobiol 1994; 59:1–4.

135. Jurkiewicz BA, Bissett DL, Buettner GR. Effect of topically applied tocopherol on ultraviolet radiation-mediated free radical damage in skin. J Invest Dermatol 1995; 104:484–488.

136. Timmins GS, Davies MJ. Free radical formation in murine skin treated with tumour promoting organic peroxides. Carcinogenesis 1993; 14:1499–1503.

5

Vitamin C and Redox Cycling Antioxidants

LESTER PACKER
University of California, Berkeley, California

Vitamin C sits squarely in the middle of the body's antioxidant network. On one side, it can restore the major lipophilic antioxidant, vitamin E, as well as itself scavenging water-soluble radicals. On the other side, it can itself be restored by thiols such as glutathione, ultimately utilizing reduced nicotinamide-adenine dinucleotide phosphate (NADPH) or reduced nicotinamide-adenine dinucleotide (NADH) as a source of reducing equivalents (Fig. 1). The evidence for regeneration of vitamin C and its ability, in turn, to regenerate vitamin E, is quite strong in vitro and in cellular systems. There are also suggestive reports from in vivo work which indicate that both types of regeneration may be important in the whole animal, as well.

VITAMIN C REDOX CYCLING IN VITRO

Regeneration of Vitamin E by Vitamin C

As long ago as 1941, it was observed that vitamin C increased the antioxidant potency of vitamin E in lard and cottonseed oil (1), and in 1968 Tappel suggested that vitamin C could regenerate vitamin E from the vitamin E radical, formed when vitamin E quenches a lipid peroxyl radical (2). In 1978, Packer et al. (3) confirmed this suggestion. This group found that pulse radiolysis of a solution containing vitamin E resulted in the formation of a transient species whose absorption spectrum matched that of phenoxyl radicals, which they identified as the vitamin E radical. If vitamin C was also present, the absorption spectrum after the pulse was initially that of vitamin E, but rapidly converted to that of the vitamin C radical. This is consistent with vitamin C–mediated regeneration of vitamin E, at the expense of formation of the vitamin C radical. Packer et al. further suggested that vitamin C could be regenerated from its radical form by NADH-dependent processes.

Niki et al. also found that vitamin C regenerated the vitamin E radical formed by

95

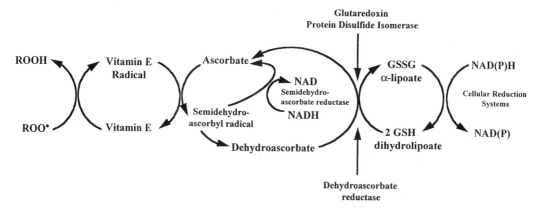

Figure 1 Ascorbate and redox cycling antioxidants. Ascorbate regenerates vitamin E from its radical form, generating the semidehydroascorbyl radical. This radical can be reduced to ascorbate by semidehydroascorbate reductase or disproportionate to dehydroascorbate and ascorbate. Dehydroascorbate can also be reduced to ascorbate by using thiols such as glutathione or dihydrolipoate as a source of reducing equivalents, whose oxidized forms are then reduced by cellular reduction systems utilizing NADPH or NADH. NADPH, reduced nicotinamide-adenine dinucleotide phosphate; NADH, reduced nicotinamide-adenine dinucleotide.

quenching peroxyl radicals generated by oxidation of methyl linoleate in solution (4). In this study the authors note that these results are for vitamin E and vitamin C in homogeneous solution, whereas in biological systems vitamin E is found in lipid environments (membranes and lipoproteins) and vitamin C is found in the aqueous compartment. (5) The same results have since been observed in membrane systems. In phosphatidyl choline liposomes in which lipid peroxidation was initiated by lipid-soluble peroxyl radical generators, vitamin C in solution was ineffective in retarding peroxidation whereas vitamin E in the membrane phase caused an inhibition period before peroxidation; however, if vitamin C was added to the aqueous phase in the presence of vitamin E in the membrane phase, it lengthened the inhibition period considerably (6). Similar results were seen in dilinoleoyl phosphatidyl choline liposomes (5). This suggests that vitamin C cannot scavenge peroxyl radicals directly, but can regenerate tocopherol from the tocopheroxyl radical, whose chromanoxyl head is near the surface of the membrane.

Regeneration of Vitamin C

In regenerating vitamin E from its radical form, as well as in scavenging radicals, vitamin C forms the semidehydroascorbyl radical, a relatively long-lived radical. It has long been known that plant and animal tissues contain a NADH-dependent semidehydroascorbate reductase enzyme (EC 1.6.5.4), which can reduce the radical back to vitamin C using NADH as a source of reducing equivalents (7) (Fig. 1). This enzyme has been found in microsomal membranes from rat liver (8), as well as in the outer mitochondrial membrane (9) and plasma membrane (10). Tissue distribution in rat and guinea pig appears to parallel distribution of ascorbate, suggesting that this pathway may be a significant source of ascorbate regeneration (9).

The semidehydroascorbyl radical decays almost entirely via disproportionation, to ascorbate and dehydroascorbate (the two-electron oxidation product of ascorbate). Dehydroascorbate can have several fates, and the relative contributions of each to ascorbate metabolism is a matter of active research. It can irreversibly decompose to diketogluconic acid, or it can be converted to ascorbate in a glutathione-dependent reaction. The latter occurs both enzymatically and nonenzymatically.

Dehydroascorbate is chemically converted back to ascorbate by glutathione in a coupled reaction (11). This reaction is highly pH-dependent and is quite rapid at pH 7.5 but virtually nonexistent at pH 6.0 (12). The chemical reaction is rapid enough that it must be taken into account when investigating enzymatic mechanisms of reduction, and pH must be carefully controlled. Dihydrolipoic acid, which is the reduced form of α-lipoate, can also directly reduce dehydroascorbate at an even more rapid rate than glutathione (12); unlike glutathione, which is not absorbed in usable form when given as a dietary supplement, α-lipoate is absorbed, transported to tissues, and reduced to dihydrolipoate (13–15). Hence it represents a thiol reductant of vitamin C that may be useful as a dietary supplement.

The existence of a dehydroascorbate reductase (E.C. 1.8.5.1), which utilizes gluathione as a reducing substrate, is well known in plant cells, and the enzyme has been purified from spinach (16) and peas (17). Though early attempts to detect such an enzyme in mammalian tissues were unsuccessful (18), more recent investigations indicate that various tissues contain dehydroascorbate reductase activity, including erythrocytes (19), kidney (20), corneal epithelium (20), colonic mucosa (21), and liver (22). The enzyme has recently been purified from rat liver and characterized (22). It is a protein of approximately 31,000 molecular weight (MW) with a K_m for dehydroascorbate of 245 μM and for reduced glutathione (GSH) of 2.8 mM. The extent to which it may be responsible for conversion of dehydroascorbate to ascorbate in vivo is not known.

Wells et al. suggest that enzymatic reduction of dehydroascorbate may also be catalyzed by glutaredoxin (thioltransferase) or by protein disulfide isomerase (23). Protein disulfide isomerase is a 57 kD protein found on the lumen side of the endoplasmic reticulum, where it is thought to catalyze rearrangements of disulfide bonds required in native protein folding (23,24). Mammalian glutaredoxin is a cytosolic enzyme of MW 12 kD that catalyzes the reduction of ribonucleotide (25). Both enzymes have been shown to have significant dehydroascorbate reductase activity (23), and this group has suggested that the dehydroascorbate reductase activity reported in many tissues may actually be at least partially the result of the activity of these two enzymes.

The exact contributions of semidehydroascorbate reductase, chemical reduction of dehydroascorbate by glutathione, and enzyme-catalyzed reduction of dehydroascorbate by glutathione (whether by dehydroascorbate reductase, protein disulfide isomerase, or glutaredoxin) to regeneration of vitamin C in various tissues and in the whole animal have yet to be elucidated.

Low-Density Lipoprotein

Human low-density lipoprotein (LDL) and its surrounding plasma serve as an example of both vitamin E recycling by ascorbate and ascorbate recycling by thiols.

In studies of nonspecific plasma lipid peroxidation induced by the water-soluble peroxyl radical generator AAPH, activated polymorphonuclear leukocytes, or the lipid-soluble peroxyl radical generator 2, 2'-azo-bis(2,4-dimethyl-valeronitrile) (AMVN), Frei et al. found that antioxidants were depleted by peroxyl radical exposure, with ascorbate depleted first in all cases (26). For AAPH- and polymorphonuclear neutrophil leukocyte– (PMN)-induced peroxidation, ascorbate was completely protective against lipid peroxidation until it was depleted, at which point lipid peroxidation commenced (27). In the case of the lipid-soluble AMVN generation of radicals, ascorbate was not completely protective, but was still the first antioxidant depleted, followed by α-tocopherol (26). After ascorbate was depleted in the AMVN system, lipid peroxidation greatly accelerated. These results suggest that ascorbate acts directly to quench peroxyl radicals generated in the aqueous phase (by AAPH or PMN) but acts perhaps indirectly when radicals are generated in the lipid phase (AMVN), by recycling vitamin E. In these studies plasma lipid peroxidation was measured, but direct measurements of LDL oxidation were not made; however, the major lipids in plasma are from lipoproteins, and these results probably mainly reflect events in the lipoproteins.

Because LDL is separated from plasma during its isolation, it is difficult to study directly the effects of aqueous or hydrophilic plasma antioxidants or supplementation of these antioxidants (e.g., vitamin C or thiols such as dihydrolipoic acid) on LDL oxidation. However, such antioxidants can be added to isolated LDL preparations and their effects examined. This has been done in a number of studies.

Sato et al. (28) found that oxidation of human LDL induced by either AAPH or AMVN, as assessed by formation of lipid hydroperoxides, was suppressed by addition of exogenous ascorbate. In the AMVN system, if ascorbate was added before α-tocopherol was consumed, it retarded α-tocopherol consumption as well as lipid peroxidation. However, if ascorbate was added after all α-tocopherol had been consumed, it had no suppressive effect on LDL oxidation. This strongly suggests that ascorbate is acting indirectly in this system, by recycling vitamin E. Jialal and Grundy studied the oxidative modification of human LDL and its prevention by ascorbate compared with probucol (29). Probucol is a lipid-lowering drug with antioxidant properties that has been shown to retard the progression of atherosclerosis. Isolated human LDL was oxidized either by human monocyte-derived macrophages or in a cell-free system by Cu^{2+}. Both ascorbate and probucol inhibited oxidation of LDL in both systems, as assessed by TBARS content and by increase in electrophoretic mobility. However, the effects of the two substances on LDL antioxidants were quite different. In LDL oxidized by copper, α-tocopherol, γ-tocopherol, and β-carotene were virtually completely destroyed, and addition of probucol had no effect on this destruction. In contrast, addition of ascorbate preserved 69% of α-tocopherol, 88% of γ-tocopherol, and 95% of β-carotene. The two compounds, though both preventing LDL oxidation, clearly work by different mechanisms. The preservation of LDL antioxidants by ascorbate is consistent with its ability to recycle tocopherol; since β-carotene is not depleted until α-tocopherol is gone, its preservation could be an indirect effect of the ascorbate-mediated recycling of tocopherol. Interestingly, probucol can, itself, be recycled by vitamin C in a manner similar to the recycling of vitamin E, as shown by Kagan et al. (30). The probucol radical was generated by incubation of LDL with peroxyl radical generators such as 2,2'-azo-bis(2,4-dimethyl-valeronitrile) (AMVN); the appearance of the probucol radical was delayed if ascorbate was included in the reaction mix.

In our laboratory we took the approach of detecting tocopheroxyl radicals (produced when vitamin E quenches a lipid peroxyl radical) and ascorbyl radicals (produced when vitamin C regenerates vitamin E from the tocopheroxyl radical) in human LDL. We detected these radicals by electron spin resonance (ESR) spectroscopy (31). Both the tocopheroxyl and ascorbyl radicals produce characteristic ESR spectra (Fig. 2). The concentration of α-tocopherol in human LDL is high enough that its signal can be detected without the use of supplementation to bolster its levels; ascorbate concentrations in the aqueous medium can be manipulated to produce a concentration sufficiently great as to allow detection of the ascorbyl radical. Low-density lipoprotein oxidation was induced by

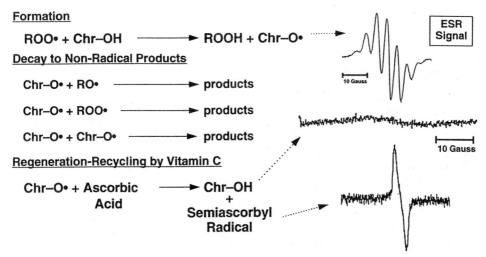

Formation

$$ROO\bullet + Chr–OH \longrightarrow ROOH + Chr–O\bullet$$

Decay to Non-Radical Products

$$Chr–O\bullet + RO\bullet \longrightarrow products$$

$$Chr–O\bullet + ROO\bullet \longrightarrow products$$

$$Chr–O\bullet + Chr–O\bullet \longrightarrow products$$

Regeneration-Recycling by Vitamin C

$$Chr–O\bullet + Ascorbic\ Acid \longrightarrow Chr–OH + Semiascorbyl\ Radical$$

ESR Signal

10 Gauss

10 Gauss

Figure 2 Some reactions of vitamin E radicals formed in the course of lipid peroxidation and vitamin E recycling by ascorbate. When vitamin E (Chr–OH) reduces a lipid peroxyl radical to a lipid hydroperoxide, the one-electron oxidation product, the vitamin E radical (Chr–O•), is produced, with a characteristic ESR signal. In the presence of ascorbate the ESR signal for the E radical disappears (middle ESR spectrum) as the vitamin E radical is reduced to vitamin E. The ESR signal for the semiascorbyl radical then appears (bottom ESR spectrum). In the absence of reductants, vitamin E radicals react to form nonradical products. ESR, electron spin resonance.

lipoxygenase + soybean oil or by AMVN. In some cases tocopheroxyl radicals were produced in LDL directly by irradiation with ultraviolet (UV) light (at λ 290 nm, at which tocopherol has a strong absorbence peak). When the LDL suspension was irradiated in the ESR cavity with UV light or exposed to peroxyl radical-generating systems, the tocopheroxyl (vitamin E) radical signal appeared immediately. The magnitude of the vitamin E radical signal was a function of the LDL concentration in the suspensions and the LDL vitamin E content. The LDL suspensions were irradiated in the presence or the absence of ascorbate. When ascorbate was added to the LDL suspension, tocopheroxyl radical ESR signals from endogenous vitamin E could not be observed. Instead, the characteristic ESR signal of the ascorbyl radical was detected (Fig. 2). This signal decreased in time and was substituted by the progressive appearance of the tocopheroxyl radical signal. The ascorbate-induced delay in the reappearance of the vitamin E chromanoxyl radical signal was concentration-dependent (Fig. 3). The UV irradiation did not induce ascorbyl radical ESR signal in the absence of LDL. This indicates that ascorbate was sparing tocopherol via recycling of its radical (whose signal remained undetectable as long as ascorbate was present).

To test whether thiols can affect the reduction of vitamin E radicals in LDL by regeneration of vitamin C, we studied the time course of UV irradiation–induced tocopheroxyl radicals in the presence of dihydrolipoic acid. Dihydrolipoic acid alone decreased the vitamin E radical ESR signal by about 30–35% but did not cause its transient disappearance as in the presence of ascorbate. However, when dihydrolipoic acid was added to the LDL suspension in combination with ascorbate, again only ascorbyl radical

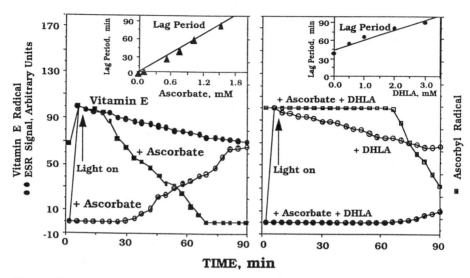

Figure 3 Ultraviolet B–induced vitamin E radicals in human LDL suspensions. LDL was irradiated with UVB light, in the absence or presence of ascorbate (left graph) or ascorbate + dihydrolipoate (DHLA) (right graph), and ESR spectra were obtained for vitamin E and semidehydroascorbyl radicals. Circles represent the vitamin E radical signal; squares represent the semidehydroascorbyl radical signal. Insets: Left, Lag period for reappearance of tocopheroxyl radical signal correlates with the ascorbate concentration. Right, Lag period for reappearance of tocopheroxyl radical signal correlates with the DHLA concentration. DHLA, dihydrolipoic acid; LDL, low-density lipoprotein; UVB, ultraviolet B; ESR, electron spin resonance.

signals could be found in the ESR spectrum, which decayed over time and was substituted by the appearing vitamin E radical signal (Fig. 3). However, the delay in the appearance of the vitamin E chromanoxyl radical signal was much longer than in the presence of ascorbate alone. At a given concentration of ascorbate, the duration of the delay was dependent on the concentration of DHLA added. Essentially the same results were obtained in systems in which oxidation of LDL was induced by generation of peroxyl radicals. Hence, a powerful reducing thiol such as dihydrolipoic acid can preserve ascorbate and, indirectly, vitamin E in LDL through recycling mechanisms such as those outlined in Figure 1.

One aspect in which ascorbate regeneration of vitamin E may be important is in tocopherol-mediated peroxidation (TMP) of LDL. At low peroxyl radical fluxes, formation of the tocopheroxyl radical may result in initiation and propagation of free radical chain reactions in LDL and the formation of lipid hydroperoxides (32). This occurs only at low radical fluxes because higher fluxes would tend to produce more than one tocopheroxyl radical in an LDL particle, and the tocopheroxyl radicals would be more likely to react with each other in a termination reaction. It has been shown that, in the absence of other antioxidants in the aqueous or lipid phase, peroxidation of LDL exposed to a low flux of peroxyl radicals decreases as tocopherol is consumed (33), and supplementation of LDL with tocopherol increases the rate at which the LDL is oxidized (34,35). The LDL can be protected from TMP by other antioxidants which recycle the tocopherol radical. In the lipid phase, the most important of these is ubiquinol, while in the aqueous phase, the most important is ascorbate (32). Thus, adequate levels of ascorbate in plasma may be crucial to protection of LDL from TMP.

VITAMIN C REDOX CYCLING IN CELLULAR SYSTEMS

It has been shown in a variety of cells and tissues that both ascorbate and dehydroascorbate are transported across the cell membrane. Although simple diffusion may account for some movement across the membrane, the major transport is carrier-mediated. For ascorbate, there appears to be a Na^+ cotransporter which can actively transport ascorbate into cells (36). Dehydroascorbate is transported into cells by the glucose transporter-1 (GLUT1) (37).

One strategy for cell accumulation of ascorbate is transport of dehydroascorbate across the cell membrane, followed by its reduction. Erythrocytes and neutrophils represent two examples of this process.

In erythrocytes May et al. (38) demonstrated, using ^{14}C-labeled ascorbate and dehydroascorbate, that dehydroascorbate is taken up by erythrocytes via the glucose transporter at a rate 10 times greater than that for ascorbate, and that the dehydroascorbate is reduced to ascorbate within the erythrocyte. These authors calculated that the erythrocyte dehydroascorbate reduction system was capable of regenerating the ascorbic acid present in whole blood every 3 min. Hence, recycling of dehydroascorbate by erythrocytes may play a major role in maintaining the antioxidant reserve of the blood.

An excellent example of ascorbate recycling comes from neutrophils. Activated neutrophils kill bacteria though a "respiratory burst" during which transient high concentrations of oxidants are developed. The neutrophils must be themselves protected from these oxidants, and it appears that ascorbate plays a major role in such protection. Activated neutrophils accumulate ascorbate, with intracellular ascorbate levels rising from about 2 mM to about 10 mM. Evidence indicates that when neutrophils are activated, some oxidants are released to the extracellular environment. These oxidants are neutralized by ascorbate, which is converted to dehydroascorbate in the process. The neutrophil membrane contains a carrier for dehydroascorbate (but not ascorbate), so when the extracellular concentration of dehydroascorbate increases, it diffuses into the neutrophil down its concentration gradient (39). Inside the neutrophil, the dehydroascorbate is converted back to ascorbate, presumably by a dehydroascorbic acid reductase that utilizes glutathione as a substrate, although the exact mechanism in neutrophils has not been elucidated (40,41). This simultaneously raises the intracellular ascorbate concentration at a time when the cell needs maximum antioxidant protection against its own oxidative burst and keeps the intracellular dehydroascorbate concentration low, maintaining a gradient for continued entry from the extracellular space (Fig. 4). This is unique example of a cellular use of ascorbate recycling mechanisms to maximize antioxidant protection at the precise time that it is most needed.

Evidence for this scheme has been presented by Washko et al. (41). These researchers observed a 10-fold increase in intracellular ascorbate concentration in activated neutrophils. They also observed an accumulation of ascorbate in unactivated neutrophils incubated in a solution containing ascorbate and a superoxide-generating system (xanthine/xanthine oxidase). When oxidation of the extracellular ascorbate to dehydroascorbate was prevented in this system (by superoxide dismutase and catalase), accumulation of intracellular ascorbate did not occur. If neutrophils were incubated in solutions containing dehydroascorbic acid, but not ascorbic acid, intracellular ascorbic acid concentrations increased over 10-fold in a period of 30 min, while intracellular dehydroascorbate concentrations were unchanged.

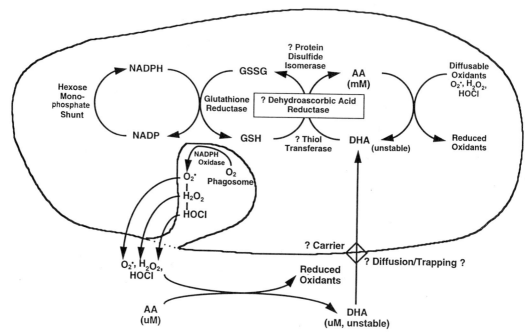

Figure 4 Model for vitamin C recycling in neutrophils. Extracellular ascorbate is oxidized to dehydroascorbate by oxidants that leak from the cell during the respiratory burst. The dehydroascorbate crosses the cell membrane and is reduced to ascorbate in the interior of the cell, keeping intracellular dehydroascorbate concentrations low and maintaining a concentration gradient from outside to inside, while increasing intracellular ascorbate concentrations. In this way the cell can increase intracellular ascorbate concentrations into the millimolar range. AA, ascorbic acid; DHA, dehydroascorbic acid; GSH, reduced gluathione; GSSG, glutathione disulfide. (From Washko et al., 1993.)

Neutrophils from patients with chronic granulomatous disease cannot produce superoxide, and when activated are not able to initiate an oxidative burst. When these neutrophils were exposed to an activator in the presence of ascorbate, no intracellular ascorbate accumulation was seen, consistent with the necessity for conversion of ascorbate to dehydroascorbate before it can cross the membrane. All of these observations support the recycling scheme for ascorbate accumulation in activated neutrophils.

In addition, in several cell membrane systems synergistic protection from oxidation by vitamins E and C has been observed. These include platelets (42), erythrocytes (43), microsomes (44), retinal tissue (45), and polymorphonuclear leukocytes (46). Human low-density lipoprotein (LDL) is the lipid system in which vitamin E and vitamin C interactions are perhaps most well studied, and will be discussed in a separate section.

VITAMIN C REDOX CYCLING IN VIVO

The in vitro and cellular evidence is quite strong for both regeneration of vitamin E by vitamin C and regeneration of vitamin C by enzymatic and nonenzymatic mechanisms.

There is also in vivo evidence for both types of regeneration, though the evidence is largely indirect. Most studies involve the induction of a deficiency state along with supplementation of a putative recycling antioxidant.

In 1959, Rosenberg and Culik reported that symptoms of vitamin E deficiency in rats and vitamin C deficiency in guinea pigs could be prevented by the administration of α-lipoic acid (47). This in vivo work is in agreement with vitamin C redox recycling demonstrated in vitro. It has since been shown that α-lipoate is taken up and reduced to dihydrolipoate in various cells and tissues (13,14,47,48). Hence, it is possible that stores of vitamin C were maintained by regeneration by dihydrolipoate of vitamin C, which in turn can regenerate vitamin E. Since vitamin E is lipid-soluble and vitamin C is water-soluble, it seems unlikely that α-lipoate simply replaced both vitamins. However, at the time of this study, no measurements of vitamins C or E were made.

Podda et al. showed, in hairless mice, a similar ability of α-lipoate to prevent symptoms of vitamin E deficiency (13). Adult hairless mice fed a vitamin E–deficient diet high in polyunsaturated fatty acids start to lose weight after 3 weeks and show clear symptoms of vitamin E deficiency, more obvious as a result of the lack of fur, with muscular dystrophy and neurological changes after 6 weeks (Fig. 5). Histological analysis of symptomatic animals showed muscular changes typical of vitamin E deficiency. These symptoms were prevented if the vitamin E–deficient animals were given dietary α-lipoic acid. Vitamin E levels had decreased greatly in liver, kidney, heart, brain, and skin in both E-deficient and E-deficient α-lipoate-supplemented animals, compared to controls. Vitamin C concentrations were also decreased in all these tissues except brain, but in heart, liver, and kidney, animals were E-deficient and α-lipoate-supplemented exhibited protection of ascorbate levels ($p < 0.01$). Although sparing of vitamin C by α-lipoate through a separate antioxidant function of α-lipoate cannot be ruled out, it appears more likely that recycling of C by dihydrolipoate is the cause of the sparing of vitamin C, as this has been demonstrated in vitro. Hence, recycling of vitamin C by thiols, and subsequent recycling of vitamin E, may play a significant role in vivo.

Other work supports this conclusion. The development of scurvy can be prevented by the administration of dehydroascorbate, indicating that in vivo mechanisms of conversion have a significant effect. Guinea pigs (which cannot synthesize their own vitamin C) can be rescued from development of scurvy on a vitamin C–deficient diet if they are fed glutathione monoester, which bolsters tissue levels of glutathione (49). Meister et al. have used the inhibitor of γ-glutamylcysteine synthetase, buthionine sulfoximine (BSO), to decrease cellular glutathione levels in vivo (50). When animals are made glutathione-deficient with BSO, they are found to have greatly decreased tissue levels of ascorbic acid, consistent with a role for glutathione in regeneration of ascorbic acid. Furthermore, mortality induced by BSO administration can be prevented by large doses of ascorbic acid, but not by dehydroascorbic acid (51). Thus, when glutathione supplies are limited, dehydroascorbate apparently cannot be converted to ascorbate.

We investigated the effect of BSO on lens antioxidants and cataract development in newborn rats (52). Its administration resulted in cataract formation in 100% of the animals treated. If α-lipoic acid was also given, cataract formation decreased, affecting 40% of the animals. Administration of BSO also caused loss of α-tocopherol, ascorbate, and glutathione from lens tissue. α-Lipoate was protective against all of these losses (Table 1). This is consistent with a role for dihydrolipoate in regeneration of ascorbate, in turn regenerating vitamin E and maintaining cellular antioxidant levels, thus preventing oxidative damage that leads to cataract formation.

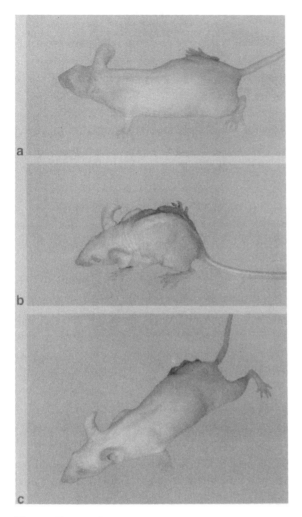

Figure 5 Adult 12-week-old hairless mice after 6 weeks of a, normal control diet; b, vitamin E–deficient diet; c, vitamin E–deficient, α-lipoic-supplemented diet. The animal on the vitamin E–deficient diet shows symptoms of vitamin E deficiency, with muscular dystrophy and weight loss.

Table 1

Treatment[a]	Vitamin E (nmol/g lens)	Glutathione (μmol/g lens)	Vitamin C (nmol/g lens)
Control	5.8 ± 1.3	3.05 ± 1.2	477 ± 31
+ BSO	1.6 ± 0.6	1.79 ± 0.16	263 ± 33
+ BSO + LA	5.2 ± 0.9	2.56 ± 0.08	423 ± 61
LA	5.5 ± 0.5	—	580 ± 50

[a]BSO, buthionine sulfoximine; LA, α-lipoic acid.

CONCLUSION

Vitamin C is a major aqueous antioxidant which also appears to regenerate vitamin E in the lipid phase in both membranes and lipoproteins. The regeneration of vitamin C, ultimately dependent on NADH or NADPH, may be a significant contributor to its antioxidant potency and may also contribute to the potency of vitamin E. The exact role of such regeneration in vivo has not been elucidated and offers a fruitful area of future research.

REFERENCES

1. Golumbic C, Mattill HA. Antioxidants and the autoxidation of fats. XIII. The antioxygenic action of ascorbic acid in association with tocopherols, hydroquinones and related compounds. J Am Chem Soc 1941; 63:1279–1280.
2. Tappel AL. Will antioxidant nutrients slow aging processes? Geriatrics 1968; 23:97–105.
3. Packer JE, Slater TF, Willson RL. Direct observation of a free radical interaction between vitamin E and vitamin C. Nature 1979; 278:737–738.
4. Niki E, Saito T, Kawakami A, Kamiya Y. Inhibition of oxidation of methyl linoleate in solution by vitamin E and vitamin C. J Biol Chem 1984; 259:4177–4182.
5. Doba TG, Burton W, Ingold KU. Antioxidant and co-antioxidant activity of vitamin C: the effect of vitamin C, either alone or in the presence of vitamin E or a water-soluble vitamin E analogue, upon the peroxidation of aqueous multilamellar phospholipid liposomes. Biochim Biophys Acta 1985; 835:298–303.
6. Niki E, Kawakami A, Yamamoto Y, Kamiya Y. Synergistic inhibition of oxidation of soybean phosphatidylcholine liposomes in aqueous dispersion by vitamin E and vitamin C. Bull Chem Soc Jpn 1982; 58:1971–1975.
7. Schneider W, Staudinger H. Reduced nicotinamide-adenine dinucleotide-dependent reduction of semidehydroascorbic acid. Biochim Biophys Acta 1965; 96:157–159.
8. Hara T, Minakami S. On functional role of cytochrome b5. II. NADH-linked ascorbate radical reductase activity in microsomes. J Biochem 1971; 69:325–330.
9. Dilberto EJ, Dean G, Carter C, Allen PL. Tissue, subcellular, and submitochondrial distributions of semidehydroascorbate reductase: possible role of semidehydroascorbate reductase in cofactor regeneration. J Neurochem 1982; 39:563–568.
10. Goldenberg H. Insulin inhibits NADH-semidehydroascorbate reductase in rat liver plasma membrane. Biochem Biophys Res Comm 1980; 94:721–726.
11. Hopkins FG, Morgan JMC. Some relations between ascorbic acid and glutathione. Biochem J 1936; 30:1446–1462.
12. Winkler BS, Orselli SM, Rex TS. The redox couple between glutathione and ascorbic acid: a chemical and physiological perspective. Free Radical Biol Med 1994; 17:333–349.
13. Podda M, Tritschler HJ, Ulrich H, Packer L. α-Lipoic acid supplementation prevents symptoms of vitamin E deficiency. Biochem Biophys Res Commun 1994; 204:98–104.
14. Podda M, Han D, Koh B, et al. Conversion of lipoic acid to dihydrolipoic acid in human keratinocytes. Clin Res 1994; 42:41a.
15. Handelman GJ, Han D, Tritschler H, Packer L. Alpha-lipoic acid reduction by mammalian cells to the dithiol form, and release into the culture medium. Biochem Pharmacol 1994; 47:1725–1730.
16. Foyer CH, Halliwell B. Purification and properties of dehydroascorbate reductase from spinach leaves. Phytochemistry 1977; 16:1347–1350.
17. Yamaguchi M, Joslyn MA. Purification and properties of dehydroascorbic acid reductase of peas. Arch Biochem Biophys 1952; 38:451–465.
18. Borsook H, Davenport HW, Jeffreys CEP, Warner RC. The oxidation of ascorbic acid and its reduction in vitro and in vivo. J Biol Chem 1937; 117:237–279.
19. Hughes RE. Reduction of dehydroascorbic acid by animal tissues. Nature 1964; 203:1068–1069.

20. Rose RC. Renal metabolism of the oxidized form of ascorbic acid (dehydro-L-ascorbic acid). Am J Physiol 1989; 256:F52–F56.

21. Choi J-L, Rose RC. Regeneration of ascorbic acid by rat colon. Proc Soc Exp Biol Med 1989; 190:369–378.

22. Maellaro E, Del Bello B, Sugherini L, et al. Purification and characterization of glutathione-dependent dehydroascorbate reductase from rat liver. Biochem J 1994; 301:471–476.

23. Wells WW, Xu DP, Yang Y, Rocque PA. Mammalian thioltransferase (glutaredoxin) and protein disulfide isomerase have dehydroascorbate reductase activity. J Biol Chem 1990; 265:15361–15364.

24. Carmichael DF, Morin JE, Dixon JE. Purification and characterization of a thiol:protein disulfide oxidoreductase from bovine liver. J Biol Chem 1977; 252:7163–7167.

25. Luthman M, Ericksson S, Holmgren A, Thelander L. Glutathione-dependent hydrogen donor system for calf thymus ribonucleotide diphosphate reductase. Proc Natl Acad Sci USA 1979; 76:2158–2162.

26. Frei B, Stocker R, England L, Ames BN. Ascorbate: the most effective antioxidant in human blood plasma. In: Emerit I, ed. Antioxidants in Therapy and Preventive Medicine. New York: Plenum Press, 1990.

27. Frei B, Stocker R, Ames BN. Antioxidant defenses and lipid peroxidation in human blood plasma. Proc Natl Acad Sci USA 1988; 85:9748–9752.

28. Sato K, Niki E, Shimasaki H. Free radical-mediated chain oxidation of low density lipoprotein and its synergistic inhibition by vitamin E and vitamin C. Arch Biochem Biophys 1990; 279:402–405.

29. Jialal I, Grundy SM. Preservation of the endogenous antioxidants in low density lipoprotein by ascorbate but not by probucol during oxidative modification. J Clin Invest 1991; 87:597–601.

30. Kagan VE, Freisleben HJ, Tsuchiya M, et al. Generation of probucol radicals and their reduction by ascorbate and dihydrolipoic acid in human low density lipoproteins. Free Radical Res Commun 1991; 15:265–276.

31. Kagan VE, Serbinova EA, Forte T, et al. Recycling of vitamin E in human low density lipoproteins. J Lipid Res 1992; 33:385–397.

32. Thomas SR, Neuzil J, Mohr D, and Stocker R. Coantioxidants make α-tocopherol an efficient antioxidant for low-density lipoprotein. Am J Clin Nutr 1995; 62 (suppl):1357S–1364S.

33. Stocker R, Bowry VW, Frei B. Ubiquinol-10 protects human low density lipoprotein more efficiently against lipid peroxidation than does alpha-tocopherol. Proc Natl Acad Sci USA 1991; 88:1646–1650.

34. Bowry VW, Stocker R. Tocopherol-mediated peroxidation: the prooxidant effect of vitamin E on the radical initiated oxidation of human low-density lipoprotein. J Am Chem Soc 1993; 115:6029–6044.

35. Bowry VW, Ingold KU, Stocker R. Vitamin E in human low-density lipoprotein: when and how this antioxidant becomes a pro-oxidant. Biochem J 1992; 288:341–342.

36. Rose RC. Transport of ascorbic acid and other water-soluble vitamins. Biochim Biophys Acta 1988; 947:335–366.

37. Vera JC, Rivas CI, Fischbarg J, Golde DW. Mammalian facilitative hexose transporters mediate the transport of dehydroascorbic acid. Nature 1993; 364:79–82.

38. May JM, Qu Z, Whitesell RR. Ascorbic acid recycling enhances the antioxidant reserve of human erythrocytes. Biochemistry 1995; 34:12721–12728.

39. Washko P, Rotrosen D, Levine M. Ascorbic acid transport and accumulation in human neutrophils. J Biol Chem 1989; 264:18996–19002.

40. Meister A. On the antioxidant effects of ascorbic acid and glutathione. Biochem Pharmacol 1992; 44:1905–1915.

41. Washko PW, Wang Y, Levine M. Ascorbic acid recycling in human neutrophils. J Biol Chem 1993; 268:15531–15535.

42. Chan AC. Partners in defense, vitamin E and vitamin C. Can J Physiol Pharmacol 1993; 71: 725–731.

43. Constantinescu A, Han D, Packer L. Vitamin E recycling in human erythrocyte membranes. J Biol Chem 1993; 268:10906–10913.

44. Leung HW, Vang MJ, Mavis RD. The cooperative interaction between vitamin E and vitamin C in suppression of peroxidation of membrane phospholipids. Biochim Biophys Acta 1981; 664:266–272.

45. Stoyanovsky DA, Goldman R, Darrow RM, et al. Endogenous ascorbate regenerates vitamin E in the retina directly and in combination with exogenous dihydrolipoic acid. Curr Eye Res 1995; 14:181–189.

46. Ho CT, Chan AC. Regeneration of vitamin E in rat polymorphonuclear leukocytes. FEBS Lett 1992; 306:269–272.

47. Rosenberg HR, Culik R. Effect of α-lipoic acid on vitamin C and vitamin E deficiencies. Arch Biochem Biophys 1959; 80:86–93.

48. Handelman GJ, Han D, Tritschler H, Packer L. α-lipoic acid reduction by mammalian cells to the ditiol form, and released into the culture medium. Biochem Pharmacol 1994; 47:1725–1730.

49. Martensson J, Han J, Griffith OW, Meister A. Glutathione ester delays the onset of scurvy in ascorbate-deficient guinea pigs. Proc Natl Acad Sci USA 1993; 90:317–321.

50. Martensson J, Jain A, Stole E, et al. Inhibition of glutathione synthesis in the newborn rat: a model for endogenously produced oxidative stress. Proc Natl Acad Sci USA 1991; 88:9360–9364.

51. Martensson J, Meister A, Martensson J. Glutathione deficiency decreases tissue ascorbate levels in newborn rats: ascorbate spares glutathione and protects. Proc Natl Acad Sci USA 1991; 88:4656–4660.

52. Maitra I, Serbinova E, Tritschler H, Packer L. Alpha-lipoic acid prevents buthionine sulfoximine-induced catract formation in newborn rats. Free Radical Biol Med 1995; 18:823–829.

6

Regeneration of Vitamin C

WILLIAM W. WELLS and CHE-HUN JUNG
Michigan State University, East Lansing, Michigan

INTRODUCTION

Ascorbic acid (AA) is an essential nutrient for higher animal and plant cell functions. Since human cells lack the complete biosynthetic pathway—i.e., they have lost the gene coding for L-gulonolactone oxidase—a dietary AA deficiency leads to the disease scurvy. Despite this well-known fact, when one cultures human cells in the absence of AA, in a strict sense, the cells are scorbutic. Even when AA is added to culture media, the loss of AA through oxidation and degradation has been reported to have a half-life of 0.9 h (1). Moreover, we have observed that fetal calf serum typically has no AA detected by using very sensitive high-performance liquid chromatography (HPLC)–electrochemical detection measurements. When AA is oxidized in the presence of trace amounts of transition metals such as iron or copper, it is often prooxidative, promoting the formation of cytotoxic reactive oxygen species (ROS) such as $O_2^{\cdot-}$, H_2O_2, and $^{\cdot}OH$ (2). A more desirable source of AA, sometimes used in culture media, is L-ascorbic acid 2-phosphate (3). This derivative is stable to oxidation–reduction reactions, yet is convertible to low levels of AA through the action of cellular plasma membrane alkaline phosphatase (4).

Ascorbic acid participates in many cellular oxidation–reduction reactions including hydroxylation of polypeptide proline residues, dopamine, and those reactions accompanying oxidation of AA. The first oxidation product of AA via a single electron step is ascorbic acid free radical (AA$^{\cdot}$), which may rapidly (10^5 $M^{-1}s^{-1}$) disproportionate to AA and dehydroascorbate (DHA) (5). Alternatively, AA$^{\cdot}$ can be directly reduced to AA by reduced nicotinamide-adenine dinucleotide (NADH) catalyzed by membrane-bound AA$^{\cdot}$ reductase (6,7). Dehydroascorbate must be recycled to AA by a two-electron reaction involving either cellular thiols such as glutathione (GSH), cysteine, or cysteamine, or reduction products of pharmacological agents such as α-lipoic acid (8,9). The recycling of DHA to AA by GSH, the most abundant nonprotein thiol (10), was estimated to have a $T_{0.5}$ of 15 min at pH 7.0 and

25°C (11), whereas the degradation of DHA at the same pH and temperature, in vitro, to nonrecyclable products, e.g., 2,3-diketogulonic acid, was reported to have a $T_{0.5}$ of 2 min (12). Thus, in order for cells to maintain a high AA/DHA ratio under normal conditions, they must promote a vigorous catalytic regeneration capability. In this chapter, we will focus primarily on the ability of cells to accomplish the regeneration of AA from DHA chemically or enzymatically under normal conditions or in the diseased state.

ASCORBIC ACID FREE RADICAL REDUCTASE

In most AA oxidation reactions AA· is a common intermediate (5). The direct recycling of AA· to AA is catalyzed by the NADH-dependent AA· reductase activity largely associated with cellular organelles (6,7). The apparent K_m for AA· in the recycling to AA is 4×10^{-6} M (13). Alternatively, AA· is generated by a reversal of the disproportionation reaction. However, the equilibrium constant for this reaction at pH 6.4 and 25°C is 5×10^{-9} (14). Coassin et al. (15) have analyzed the relative involvement of the single-electron AA· reductase on the basis of enzyme content of tissues and the enzyme turnover measured in vitro. When compared with the two-electron pathway, the former was estimated indirectly to be more prominent.

In contrast, the contribution of the GSH-dependent pathway was tested, in vivo, by the recent studies from Meister's laboratory (16). These workers reasoned that newborn rat pups, given buthionine sulfoximine (BSO), the specific inhibitor of γ-glutamylcysteine synthetase, would have depressed tissue levels of GSH. If the GSH-dependent AA regeneration pathway was significant, in vivo, they anticipated seeing deleterious effects on AA recycling. The results of these studies showed that GSH deficiency caused depletion of AA levels in rat pup tissues and that the DHA/AA ratio increased significantly. Rat pups that showed 90% mortality as a result of the BSO administration were spared (11% mortality) when simultaneously given AA intraperitoneally. Administration of an equal level of DHA to that of AA provided no beneficial action. Indeed, DHA was especially toxic, producing 100% rat mortality, confirming the known toxicity of DHA when given to normal rats (17,18). These studies demonstrated that the regeneration of AA from AA· is not sufficient to protect GSH-deficient animals from the tissue damage generated by reactive oxygen species. Accordingly, we turn our attention to the vital interdependence of AA regeneration and normal GSH metabolism.

REDUCED GLUTATHIONE–LINKED RECYCLING OF ASCORBIC ACID

Chemical Recycling

In 1928, Szent-Györgyi showed the recovery of the "reducing substance" from its oxidized state using glutathione as the reducing agent (19). Pfankuch described reduction of DHA by cysteine (20), and Borsook et al. (21) and Schultze et al. (22) extended the studies of the reduction of DHA to AA by GSH. Borsook et al. found no evidence for enzymatic reduction of DHA by GSH using the technology available in 1937. Several investigators (23,24) still argue that only the chemical reduction of DHA by cellular monothiols, chiefly GSH, is necessary to maintain optimal cellular AA/DHA. The argument in favor of this position is typically based on the failure to detect significant catalytic activity in specific tissues (24–26). For example, Winkler (26) has maintained that DHA reductase activity could not be detected in retinal pigment epithelium when assayed at pH 7.5, in vitro. However, in collaboration with Winkler (unpublished results), we have shown that DHA reductase activity could be detected when extracts of retinal pigment epithelium were concentrated and assayed at the cytoplasm pH 6.9 (28). In a later section of this chapter, we will point out that the regeneration of AA from DHA by reduction with GSH in the mitochondria is probably chemical-based. This is because the pH of the mitochondrial matrix is reported to be 7.5 under conditions of state 4 respiration (succinate) (29). At this pH, the difference between catalyzed and uncatalyzed reduction of DHA by GSH is difficult to measure. Furthermore, there is no published evidence for DHA reductase activity in purified mitochondria.

Enzyme-Linked Recycling

In 1941, Crook characterized plant AA oxidase activity and showed that plants have detectable DHA reductase activity dependent on GSH (30). Studies on the GSH-dependent DHA reductase activity in plants progressed more rapidly than in mammals. The DHA reductases were purified and characterized from various plant sources by several laboratories (31–33). The first report of a mammalian DHA reductase came from the study of human erythrocytes by Christine et al. (34), although the enzyme activity was not purified. Hughes (35) and Grimble and Hughes (36) provided evidence for catalytic activity in guinea pig tissues other than blood cells. Extracts from various tissues contained GSH-dependent DHA reductase activity with properties such as relative thermostability and sensitivity to proteolysis and sulfhydryl modifying agents. These properties are universal for the known DHA reductases, particularly of the thioltransferase-like class. Subsequently DHA reductase activity from carp hepatopancreas and kidney and from rat liver were studied (37).

In 1990, it was shown that two purified mammalian proteins, thioltransferase (also known as glutaredoxin) and protein disulfide isomerase (PDI), had DHA reductase activity (38). By following DHA reductase activity of crude rat liver cytosol fractions, Maellaro et al. (39) discovered a 31 kDa protein with DHA reductase activity, but without thiol-disulfide oxidoreductase activity. No other intrinsic activity was reported for this new DHA reductase. A similar enzyme of 32 kDa was recently purified and characterized from human erythrocytes (40). These findings increased the number of human erythrocyte DHA reductases to two, the first being thioltransferase (38). In a study of the recycling of ascorbate in erythrocytes subjected to extracellular ferricyanide, May et al. (41) argued for a role for ascorbate in reducing ferricyanide via a transmembrane oxidoreductase (42,43). Their model included either GSH or NADH for regeneration of the AA from DHA, yet they proposed no known enzymatic pathway for the reduction by either reductant. In a recent extension of these studies, the authors conclude that in human erythrocytes, ascorbate regeneration from DHA is largely GSH-dependent and does not involve the semi-DHA free radical (44). Finally, DelBello et al. (45) noted that a NADPH-dependent DHA reductase activity in rat liver cytosol was associated with the well-known 3α-hydroxy-steroid dehydrogenase.

The kinetic properties of the known GSH-dependent DHA reductases, taken from the original publications, have been compared in a recent report (40) and are shown in Table 1. Thioltransferase has the highest turnover number, 374 min^{-1}, and the highest efficiency, k_{cat}/K_m, 2.4×10^4 M^{-1} s^{-1} for DHA, among the known enzymes. The relative abundance of the two major mammalian DHA reductases, thioltransferase and the 32 kDa protein in, for

Table 1 Kinetic Parameters for Mammalian Dehydroascorbate Reductases[a]

Parameter	Human RBC DHA reductase[b]	Rat liver DHA reductase[c]	Pig liver thioltransferase[d]	Bovine protein disulfide isomerase[e]
k_{cat} (min^{-1})[e]	316 ± 1	140 ± 4	374 ± 20	16 ± 1
K_m(app) (mM)[f] DHA	0.21 ± 0.06	0.25 ± 0.62	0.26 ± 0.09	2.8 ± 0.4
GSH	3.5 ± 0.3	2.8 ± 0.6	3.5 ± 0.3	2.9 ± 0.4
k_{cat}/K_m $(M^{-1}s^{-1})$				
DHA	$2.47 ± 0.64 × 10^4$	$9.52 ± 3.64 × 10^3$	$2.43 ± 0.85 × 10^4$	93 ± 14
GSH	$1.51 ± 0.11 × 10^3$	$0.83 ± 0.30 × 10^3$	$1.81 ± 0.2 × 10^3$	91 ± 14

[a]RBC, red blood cell; DHA, dehydroascorbate; GSH, glutathione.
[b]Human erythrocyte DHA reductase, pH 7.2 (Ref. 40).
[c]pH 7.2 (Ref. 39).
[d]pH 6.9 (Ref. 84).
[e]k_{cat} Values were calculated by dividing V_{max}(app) by the molar concentration of the enzymes.
[f]K_m(app) Values were calculated by nonlinear least-squares fit to the velocity versus substrate concentration data using the PSI-Plot 3.5 software.

example, human tissues, is not completely known. However, a recent analysis of thioltransferase expression in various human tissues allows some speculation about the relative contribution of thioltransferase to the catalytic regeneration of AA from DHA (46). The complete comparison of the two major cytosolic DHA reductases and their contribution to the total cellular activity remains for the cloning of the human 32 kDa DHA reductase and an analysis of its distribution and expression in human tissues. Stomach was reported by Grimble and Hughes to be abundant in DHA reductase activity (36), consistent with its being the highest immunologically detectable pig thioltransferase (47). The AA concentration in gastric secretions of various species including humans is several times higher than that of plasma (48). Accumulated data demonstrate that a considerable amount of ascorbate is secreted in the reduced form into the digestive tract and absorbed predominantly in its oxidized form, DHA. A quantity of AA, equivalent to the daily requirement, is secreted into the digestive tract of scurvy-prone animals including humans. This suggests an important function for the vitamin in the stomach, especially with respect to its antioxidant properties in the prevention of nitrosation. Nitrite can react with dietary amines and amides to create N-nitroso compounds implicated in gastric carcinogenesis. Abscorbic acid reacts with nitrite, converting it to nitric oxide, and generating DHA in the process. In other studies, it was reported that patients with chronic gastritis have significantly lower stomach AA content. These data suggest the disruption of the stomach AA recycling process in these patients. Ascorbic acid may play another vital role nutritionally by enhancing the reduction of ferric ions to ferrous ions, the preferred redox state of iron for absorption. Thus, stomach tissue has a special requirement for DHA transport followed by AA regeneration. These functions are consistent with the relatively high levels of thioltransferase in the stomach. Human heart tissue is rich in thioltransferase messenger ribonucleic acid (mRNA) (46) and this may be related to the necessity to regenerate particularly high levels of DHA resulting from the mitochondrial respiration–derived $O_2^{·-}$ and H_2O_2. Choi and Rose (49) investigated the regeneration of AA by rat colon. They obtained a crude ammonium sulfate precipitate fraction that, after dialysis, catalyzed the reduction of DHA in a NADPH-dependent manner. It is possible that this activity was fortuitous and due to 3α-hydroxysteroid dehydrogenase (44) although this has not been confirmed. The k_{cat} and k_{cat}/K_m for this enzyme suggest that 3α-hydroxysteroid dehydrogenase plays no significant physiological role in AA regeneration.

PARTICIPATION OF MITOCHONDRIA IN DIHYDROLIPOIC ACID–LINKED ASCORBIC ACID RECYCLING

The regeneration of AA from DHA within mitochondria has received less attention than the same process elsewhere in cells. However, mitochondria generate abundant superoxide free radicals as a product of oxidative reactions with molecular oxygen (50). Ascorbic acid may scavenge these reactive radicals or participate in the reduction of α-tocopheryl radicals. Therefore, it is important to evaluate to what extent mitochondria may potentially regenerate AA from DHA by GSH, by NADH (AA⁺ reductase), or pharmacologically by dihydrolipoic acid. Mitochondria contain a pool of GSH and GSSG that represents between 10% and 20% of the total cellular content (51–54).

In addition to nonenzymatic regeneration of AA from DHA by GSH in mitochondria (see the section, Chemical Recycling), dihydrolipoic acid, a more powerful reductant than GSH, $E^{o\prime} = -0.32$ V (55) and $E^{o\prime} = -0.24$ V (56), respectively, is present in extremely low concentrations conjugated to α-keto acid dehydrogenases (57). However, recent studies of the efficacy of α-lipoic acid in alleviation of oxygen-linked cytotoxicity (58) or in disease states such as diabetic polyneuropathy (59) raised the possibility that under these conditions, sufficient dihydrolipoic acid may be generated in tissues to influence significantly the level and redox status of AA, especially in cells under severe oxygen stress. In mitochondria, the reduction of pharmacological doses of α-lipoic acid would likely be mediated by the lipoamide dehydrogenase activity of the α-keto acid dehydrogenases and electrons derived from substrate oxidation (60,61). To explore this possibility, rat liver mitochondria were analyzed for their ability to reduce DHA to AA in an α-lipoic acid–dependent or –independent manner (9). The α-lipoic acid–dependent reduction was stimulated by factors that increased the NADH-dependent reduction of α-lipoic acid to dihydrolipoic acid in coupled reactions. Optimal conditions for DHA reduction to AA were achieved in the presence of pyruvate, α-lipoic acid, and adenosine triphosphate (ATP). Electron transport inhibitors, rotenone, and antimycin A further enhanced the DHA reduction. The reactions were strongly inhibited by 1 mM iodoacetamide or sodium arsenite. Mitoplasts were qualitatively similar to intact mitochondria in DHA reduction activity. Pyruvate dehydrogenase and α-ketoglutarate dehydrogenase reduced DHA to AA in an α-lipoic acid, coenzyme A, and pyruvate or α-ketoglutarate–dependent fashion. The DHA was also catalytically reduced to AA by purified lipoamide dehydrogenase in an α-lipoic acid ($K_{0.5} = 1.4 \pm 0.8$ mM) and lipoamide ($K_{0.5} = 0.9 \pm 0.3$ mM)-dependent manner.

Earlier studies had shown the dihydrolipoate-dependent reduction of DHA to AA in vitro (8). In addition, Kagan et al. (61) suggested that mitochondrial reduction of α-lipoic acid to dihydrolipoic acid by α-keto acid dehydrogenases may largely account for the cellular α-lipoic acid reduction process. This hypothesis was discussed in a recent review by Packer et al. (59). The present author's studies demonstrated that α-keto acid dehydrogenase complexes of mitochondria and mitoplasts and isolated lipoamide dehydrogenase have α-lipoic acid–dependent dehydroascorbic acid reducing activity mediated by the catalytic formation of dihydrolipoic acid (Scheme A). The rate of dihydrolipoic acid or lipoamide reduction of DHA to AA (Scheme A, reaction 2) is believed to be more rapid than reaction 1.

$$(1) \quad \alpha\text{-Lipoic Acid} + \text{HADH} + \text{H}^+ \overset{\text{LDH}}{\rightleftharpoons} \text{Dihydrolipoic Acid} + \text{HAD}^+$$
$$\quad\quad (\text{Lipoamide}) \quad\quad\quad\quad\quad\quad\quad\quad\quad\quad (\text{Dihydrolipoamide})$$

$$(2) \quad \text{Dihydrolipoic Acid} + \text{DHA} \rightarrow \text{AA} + \alpha\text{-Lipoic Acid}$$
$$\quad\quad (\text{Dihydrolipoamide}) \quad\quad\quad\quad\quad\quad (\text{Lipoamide})$$

Scheme A

A similar reaction was demonstrated in a study by Bunik and Follmann (60) in which α-lipoic acid, reduced to dihydrolipoate, promoted the reduction of oxidized thioredoxin from *Escherichia coli*. The k_{cat} for DHA reduction by α-lipoic acid or lipoamide dependent in the presence of lipoamide dehydrogenase was estimated to be 16 and 661 s^{-1}, respectively. The apparent $K_{0.5}$ values for α-lipoic acid and lipoamide, 1.4 and 0.9 mM, respectively, were used to calculate $k_{cat}/K_{0.5}$ of 1.2×10^4 and 7.3×10^5 M^{-1} s^{-1}. In the α-keto acid dehydrogenase systems, a model for exogenous α-lipoic acid was drawn (Fig. 1) to illustrate the satellite reactions observed from these studies. Figure 2 illustrates a proposed reaction among α-lipoic acid, lipoamide, NADH, and DHA catalyzed by purified lipoamide dehydrogenase in vitro. If the preceding process is actively engaged, in vivo, when α-lipoic acid is administered therapeutically, a significant contribution to cellular AA regeneration from DHA would be likely. These present findings offer an explanation for the ability of α-lipoic acid to relieve the symptoms of scurvy in guinea pigs fed an AA-deficient diet (62).

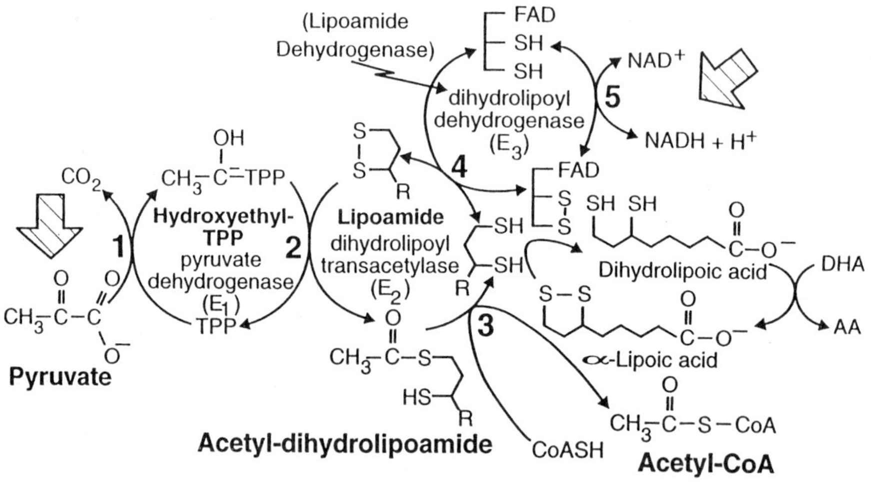

Figure 1 A model illustrating the proposed interaction among α-lipoic acid, DHA, and the pyruvate dehydrogenase complex (E$_1$–E$_3$). Reducing equivalents may enter the system from substrates, pyruvate, or NADH (large arrows) to stimulate dihydrolipoate-mediated reduction of DHA to AA. DHA, dehydroascorbate; NADH, reduced nicotinamide-adenine dinucleotide; AA, ascorbic acid. (From Ref. 9.)

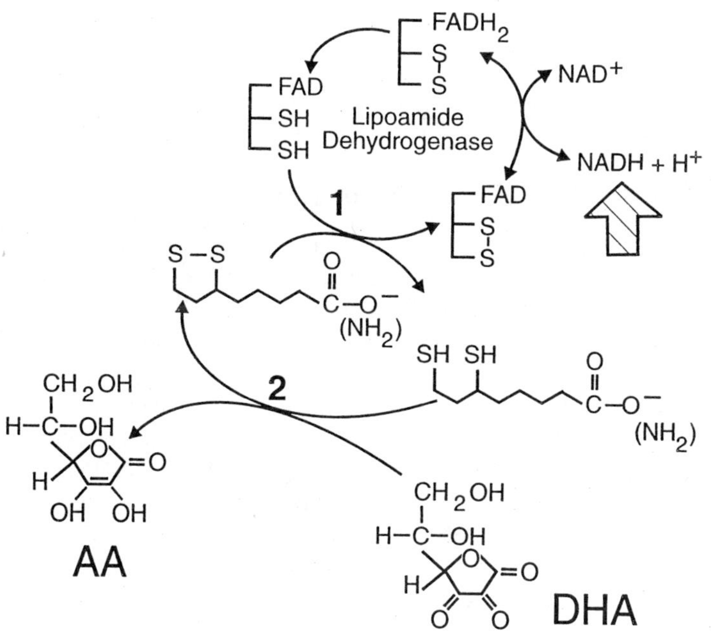

Figure 2 A model illustrating the α-lipoate- or lipoamide-mediated reduction of DHA to AA catalyzed by lipoamide dehydrogenase. Reducing equivalents are derived from NADH (large arrow). DHA, dehydroascorbate; AA, ascorbic acid; NADH, reduced nicotinamide-adenine dinucleotide. (From Ref. 9.)

THE ESSENTIAL ROLE OF ASCORBIC ACID IN INSULIN RELEASE

As a result of the detectable DHA reductase activity of PDI and the known ability of DHA to oxidize protein thiols to disulfides (63–65), the authors proposed the interaction of DHA and AA in the formation of insulin as a model protein disulfide (66). We reasoned that animals deficient in AA should be unable to synthesize insulin normally. This seemed feasible, since Sigal and King (67) had reported that scorbutic guinea pigs had abnormal glucose tolerance test results. These observations were confirmed by Banerjee (68,69), who used a crude hypoglycemia bioassay in rabbits to quantitate the insulin content of pancreases from scorbutic and normal guinea pigs. Banerjee concluded that the insulin content of the scorbutic guinea pig was diminished to about one-eighth that of the normal guinea pig. In a recent study (70), we found that the insulin content of the pancreas of scorbutic guinea pigs was not diminished, but was actually increased about twofold. Moreover, analysis of the insulin from the pancreas of scorbutic guinea pigs revealed only normal insulin; i.e., no evidence appeared for the presence of insulin precursors such as reduced proinsulin. This suggested that AA (and DHA) might not be essential for protein disulfide formation. We did confirm that pancreatic islets from scorbutic guinea pigs failed to release insulin immediately after elevation of D-glucose from 1.7 to 20 mM. When 5 mM L-ascorbic acid 2-phosphate was added to the perfusion medium concurrently with elevation of D-glucose, islets from scorbutic guinea pigs released insulin as rapidly as control guinea pig islets and to a greater extent. L-Ascorbic acid 2-phosphate without elevated D-glucose did not stimulate insulin release by islets from normal or scorbutic guinea pigs. These findings identified a new function of vitamin C in the induction of glucose competence leading to insulin release from pancreatic islets. The precise mechanism for this effect of AA is unknown and under current investigation.

PROTEIN-LINKED ASCORBIC ACID REGENERATION

We proposed a catalytic mechanism for thioltransferase (TT) in which a thiohemiketal between TT and DHA was formed as an intermediate (Fig. 3) (71). The chemical reduction of DHA to AA by GSH may follow a similar path. During the studies of thioltransferase as a thiol-disulfide oxidoreductase, Gravina and Mieyal (72) found that thioltransferase had a specificity for GSH-containing substrates and consequently proposed that a chemical reaction to form GSH-containing mixed disulfides may be prerequisite for enzyme catalysis (73). These authors proposed that DHA reduction catalyzed by thioltransferase may proceed similarly; i.e., DHA would form a thiohemiketal with GSH by a chemical reaction, and then the thiohemiketal would serve as a preferable substrate of thioltransferase (the first reaction of Scheme B). In a recent study of DHA reduction by GSH, we tried to isolate the

Scheme B

thiohemiketal (DHA-SG) by reacting GSH with a molar excess of DHA. The amount of AA produced by GSH, detected by a HPLC-electrochemical method (9), and the amount of GSH consumed by the reduction as measured by 5,5'-dithiobis-(2-nitrobenzoic acid) (DTNB) (74) were analyzed (unpublished results). The decrease of thiol was virtually stoichiometric with the production of AA (2:1), indicating that no significant amount of the thiohemiketal accumulated. This observation suggested that the second reaction in Scheme B is much faster than the first, and that the first reaction is the rate-limiting step. This also suggested that TT, with an exceptionally low active site thiolate pK_a (3.8), may react with DHA much faster than GSH and therefore enhance DHA reduction rate, in keeping with our previously proposed mechanism (Fig. 3) (71).

It is well known that GSH is the most abundant nonprotein thiol in most cells. However,

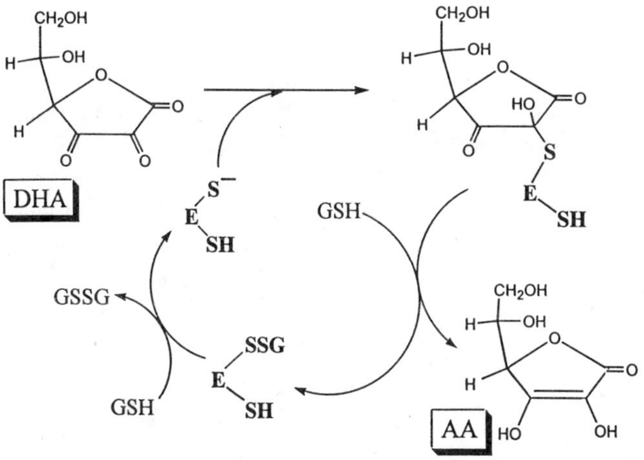

Figure 3 Proposed scheme for the DHA reductase mechanism of thioltransferase. Reaction of the nucleophilic C22 leads to the thiohemiketal intermediate. Glutathione continues the reduction process, releasing AA and the GS mixed disulfide of TT. A second mole of GSH regenerates the enzyme to its S⁻ form and produces GSSG. GSSG is converted to 2GSH by NADPH catalyzed by GSSG reductase. DHA, dehydro-ascorbate; AA, ascorbic acid; GS, glutathionyl; TT, thioltransferase; GSH, glutathione; GSSG, glutathione disulfide; NADPH, reduced nicotinamide-adenine dinucleotide phosphate.

the concentration of reactive thiols on cellular proteins is as high as that of glutathione (75), although the contribution by protein thiols as antioxidants or in DHA reduction has been chiefly disregarded. In preliminary experiments, when rat cytosolic proteins were exposed to DHA, the thiol concentration of proteins decreased. Concurrently, DHA covalently attached to proteins was subsequently released as AA by monothiols such as GSH (unpublished data). During site-directed mutagenesis studies, TT showed a higher activity when one of the active site cysteines, C25, was converted to serine (76). This suggested that the dithiol nature of the TT active site might not be an essential feature for DHA reductase catalysis. Therefore, protein thiols which are accessible to free GSH may also facilitate DHA interaction. Dehydroascorbate not only reacts rapidly with monothiols such as GSH and cysteine (77), but also reacts with protein thiols reversibly (78). The contribution of protein thiols to DHA recycling to AA is under close investigation in the authors' laboratory. While DHA can react with amide nitrogens of, e.g., glutamine (79), or amino groups on lysine residues (80) to form Schiff bases, these reactions produce more stable derivatives, leading in some cases to Maillard-type fucsin products with cytotoxic consequences.

Since cellular DHA reduction is closely tied with GSH (66), it is essential to consider the cellular glutathione/glutathione disulfide (GSH/GSSG) ratios (81). Preliminary observations in guinea pigs, pair-fed a scorbutigenic diet but given drinking water containing 0.1% sodium ascorbate, indicated the presence of significant levels of altered plasma proteins associated with elevated plasma protein bound DHA (unpublished results). The elevated plasma DHA levels corresponded with the restriction of nutrients by paired feeding, suggesting that the enhanced DHA production is associated with an inadequate regeneration of GSH via diminished hexose phosphate shunt activities predominantly in the liver.

Dhariwal et al. (82) have reported that the DHA content of plasma extracts is extremely low if not nonexistent. The analysis of plasma DHA usually depends on the initial stabilization of plasma extracts from AA oxidation and DHA degradation followed by reduction of DHA to AA, and finally analysis of the total AA by electrochemical detection and quantification of HPLC peaks (83). We investigated the possibility of the presence of DHA in plasma of nutritionally restricted guinea pigs in comparison with that of well-nourished animals. We found that the level of unbound plasma DHA was infinitely small in scorbutic guinea pig plasma, whereas a substantial pool of DHA was bound to plasma proteins presumably as thiohemiketals. The results showed that an aliquot of plasma, initially treated with β-mercaptoethanol before extraction of the sample with 10% metaphosphoric acid, revealed an increase in the AA of up to 25% of the total pool. A similar fraction of DHA was not seen in plasma from control well-fed animals (unpublished results). These observations prompted us to ask whether the phenomenon of dehydroascorbylation of proteins might not be more universal in vivo. Currently, we have no information regarding the consequences of protein dehydroascorbylation on protein functions nor on the fate of the modified proteins although it is evident the process occurs. Dehydroascorbylation and dedehydroascorbylation of cellular proteins such as enzymes might represent a novel mechanism of protein function modification worthy of future investigation.

ACKNOWLEDGMENTS

This work was supported by NIH Grants DK-44456 and CA-51972. We thank Carol McCutcheon for typing the manuscript.

REFERENCES

1. Feng J, Melcher AH, Brunette DM, Moe DK. Determination of L-ascorbic acid levels in culture medium: concentration in commercial media and maintenance of levels under conditions of organ culture. In Vitro 1977; 13:91–99.
2. Miller DM, Aust SD. Studies of ascorbate-dependent, iron-catalyzed lipid peroxidation. Arch Biochem Biophys 1989; 271:113–119.
3. Kurata S, Hata R. Epidermal growth factor inhibits transcription of type I collagen genes and production of type I collagen in cultured human skin fibroblasts in the presence and absence of L-ascorbic acid 2-phosphate a long-acting vitamin C derivative. J Biol Chem 1991; 266:9997–10003.
4. Hitomi K, Torii Y, Tsukagoshi N. Increase in the activity of alkaline phosphatase by L-ascorbic acid 2-phosphate in a human osteoblast cell line, HuO-3N1. J Nutr Sci Vitaminol 1992; 38: 535–544.
5. Bielski BHJ. Chemistry of ascorbic acid radicals. In: Seib PA, Tolbert BM, eds. Ascorbic Acid: Chemistry, Metabolism, and Uses. American Chemical Society, Advances in Chemistry Series 200, 1982:81–100.
6. Kersten H, Kersten W, Staudinger H. Zum wirkungsmechanismus der ascorbinsäure. I. Isolierung einer ascorbinsäureabhängigen DPNH-oxidase aus nebennierenmikrosomen. Biochim Biophys Acta 1958; 27:598–608.
7. Schulze H-U, Gallenkamp H, Staudinger H. Untersuchungen zum mikrosomalen NADH-abhängigen electronentransport. Hoppe Seylers Z Physiol Chem 1970; 351:809–817.
8. Bast A, Haenen GRMM. Regulation of lipid peroxidation by glutathione and lipoic acid: involvement of liver microsomal vitamin E free radical reductase. In: Emerit I, Packer L, Auclair C, eds. Advances in experimental medicine and biology. New York: Plenum Press, 1990:111–116.

9. Xu D-P, Wells WW. α-Lipoic acid dependent regeneration of ascorbic acid from dehydroascorbic acid in the rat liver mitochondria. J Bioenerg Biomem 1996; 28:77–85.

10. Jocelyn PC. Biochemistry of the SH Group. New York: Academic Press, 1972:10.

11. Mapson LW. IV. Biochemical systems A. synthesis of ascorbic acid. In: Sebrell WH Jr, Harris RS, eds. The Vitamins. New York: Academic Press, 1954:232.

12. Ball EG. Studies on oxidation-reduction XXIII: ascorbic acid. J Biol Chem 1937; 118:219–239.

13. von Lumper L, Schneider W, Staudinger H. Untersuchungen zur kinetik der mikrosomalen NADH: semidehydroascorbat-oxydoreduktase reductase. Hoppe Seylers Z Physiol Chem 1967; 348:323–328.

14. Foerster G von, Weiss W, Staudinger H. Messung der elektronenspinresonanz an semidehydroascorbinsaure. Justus von Liebigs Ann Chem 1965; 690:155–169.

15. Coassin M, Tomasi A, Vannini V, Ursini F. Enzymatic recycling of oxidized ascorbate in pig heart: one-electron vs two-electron pathway. Arch Biochem Biophys 1991; 290:456–462.

16. Meister A. On the antioxidant effects of ascorbic acid and glutathione. Biochem Pharmacol 1992; 44:1905–1915.

17. Patterson JW. The diabetogenic effect of dehydroascorbic and dehydroisoascorbic acids. J Biol Chem 1950; 183:81–88.

18. Patterson JW. Some effects of dehydroascorbic acid on the central nervous system. Am J Physiol 1951; 165:61–65.

19. Szent-Györgyi A. CLXXIII. Observations on the function of peroxidase systems and the chemistry of the adrenal cortex: description of a new carbohydrate derivative. Biochem J 1928; 22:1387–1409.

20. Pfankuch E. Enzyme reduction of dehydroascorbic acid. Naturwissenschaften 1934; 22:821.

21. Borsook H, Davenport HW, Jeffreys CEP, Warner RC. The oxidation of ascorbic acid and its reduction in vitro and in vivo. J Biol Chem 1937; 117:237–279.

22. Schultze MO, Stotz E, King CG. Studies on the reduction of dehydroascorbic acid by guinea pig tissues. J Biol Chem 1938; 122:395–406.

23. Winkler BS, Orselli SM, Rex TS. The redox couple between glutathione and ascorbic acid: a chemical and physiological perspective. Free Radical Biol Med 1994; 17:333–349.

24. Pietronigro DD, Hovespian M, Demopoulos HB, Flamm ES. Reductive metabolism of ascorbic acid in the central nervous system. Brain Res 1985; 333:161–164.

25. Stahl RL, Liebes LF, Silber R. A reappraisal of leukocyte dehydroascorbate reductase. Biochim Biophys Acta 1985; 839:119–121.

26. Winkler BS. Unequivocal evidence in support of the nonenzymatic redox coupling between glutathione/glutathione disulfide and ascorbic acid/dehydroascorbic acid. Biochim Biophys Acta 1992; 1117:287–290.

27. Meister A. Glutathione-ascorbic acid antioxidant system in animals. J Biol Chem 1994; 269:9397–9400.

28. Roos A, Boron WF. Intracellular pH. Physiol Rev 1981; 61:296–434.

29. Addanki S, Cahill FD, Sotos JF. Determination of intramitochondrial pH and intramitochondrial-extramitochondrial pH gradient of isolated heart mitochondria by the use of 5,5-Dimethyl-2,4-oxazolidinedione. J Biol Chem 1968; 243:2337–2348.

30. Crook EM. The system dehydroascorbic acid-glutathione. Biochem J 1941; 35:226–236.

31. Foyer CH, Halliwell B. Purification and properties of dehydroascorbate reductase from spinach leaves. Phytochem 1977; 16:1347–1350.

32. Hossain MA, Asada K. Purification of dehydroascorbate reductase from spinach and its characterization as a thiol enzyme. Plant Cell Physiol 1984; 25:85–92.

33. Yamaguchi M, Joslyn MA. Purification and properties of dehydroascorbic acid reductase of peas (Pisum sativum). Arch Biochem Biophys 1952; 38:451–465.

34. Christine L, Thomas G, Iggo B, et al. The reduction of dehydroascorbic acid by human erythrocytes. Clin Chim Acta 1956; 1:557–569.

35. Hughes RE. Reduction of dehydroascorbic acid by animal tissues. Nature (London) 1964; 203:1068–1069.

36. Grimble RF, Hughes RE. A dehydroascorbic acid reductase factor in guinea pig tissues. Experientia (Basel) 1967; 23/5:362.

37. Yamamoto Y, Sato M, Ikeda S. Biochemical studies on L-ascorbic acid in aquatic animals. VIII. Purification and properties of dehydro-L-ascorbic acid reductase in carp hepato pancreas. Bull Jpn Soc Sci Fish 1977; 43:53–57.

38. Wells WW, Xu DP, Yang Y, Rocque PA. Mammalian thioltransfease (glutaredoxin) and protein disulfide isomerase have dehydroascorbate reductase activity. J Biol Chem 1990; 265:15361–15364.

39. Maellaro E, Del Bello B, Sugherini L, et al. Purification and characterization of glutathione-dependent dehydroascorbate reductase from rat liver. Biochem J 1994; 301:471–476.

40. Xu DP, Washburn MP, Sun GP, Wells WW. Purification and characterization of a glutathione dependent dehydroascorbate reductase from human erythrocytes. Biochem Biophys Res Commun 1996; 221:117–121.

41. May JM, Qu Z-C, Whitesell RR. Ascorbic acid recycling enhances the antioxidant reserve of human erythrocytes. Biochemistry 1995; 34:12721–12728.

42. Zamudio I, Cellino M, Canessa-Fischer M. The relation between membrane structure and NADH: (acceptor) oxidoreductase activity of erythrocyte ghosts. Arch Biochem Biophys 1969; 129:336–345.

43. Zamudio I, Canessa M. Nicotinamide-adenine dinucleotide dehydrogenase activity of human erythrocyte membranes. Biochim Biophys Acta 1966; 120:165–169.

44. May JM, Qu Z-C, Whitesell RR, Cobb SE. Ascorbate recycling in human erythrocytes: role of GSH in reducing dehydroascorbate. Free Radical Biol Med 1996; 20:543–551.

45. DelBello B, Maellaro E, Sugherini L, et al. Purification of NADPH-dependent dehydroascorbate reductase from rat liver and its identification with 3α-hydroxysteroid dehydrogenase. Biochem J 1994; 304:385–390.

46. Meyer EB, Wells WW. Cloning, sequencing and expression of human placental thioltransferase. FASEB J 1995; 9:A1463.

47. Gan ZR, Wells WW. Immunological characterization of thioltransferase from pig liver. J Biol Chem 1988; 263:9050–9054.

48. Dabrowski K. Gastro-intestinal circulation of ascorbic acid. Comp Biochem Physiol 1990; 95A:481–486.

49. Choi J-L, Rose RC. Regeneration of ascorbic acid by rat colon. Proc Soc Exp Biol Med 1989; 190:369–374.

50. Chance B, Sies H, Boveris A. Hydroperoxide metabolism in mammalian organs. Physiol Rev 1979; 59:527–604.

51. Jocelyn PC, Kamminga A. The non-protein thiol of rat liver mitochondria. Biochim Biophys Acta 1974; 343:356–362.

52. Meredith MJ, Reed DJ. Status of the mitochondrial pool of glutathione in the isolated hepatocyte. J Biol Chem 1982; 257:3747–3753.

53. Wahlländer A, Soboll S, Sies H. Hepatic mitochondrial and cytosolic glutathione content and the subcellular distribution of GSH S-transferases. FEBS Lett 1979; 97:138–140.

54. Griffith OW, Meister A. Origin and turnover of mitochondrial glutathione. Proc Natl Acad Sci USA 1985; 82:4668–4672.

55. Searles RL, Sanadi DR. α-Ketoglutaric dehydrogenase. VIII. Isolation and some properties of flavoprotein component. J Biol Chem 1960; 235:2485–2491.

56. Scott EM, Duncan IW, Ekstrand V. Purification and properties of glutathione reductase of human erythrocytes. J Biol Chem 1963; 238:3928–3933.

57. Stockstad ELR, Seaman GR, Davis RJ, Hunter SH. Assay of thioctic acid. In: Glick D, ed. Methods of Biochemical Analysis. New York: Wiley Interscience, 1956:23–47.

58. Burkart B, Koike T, Brenner H-H, et al. Dihydrolipoic acid protects pancreatic islet cells from inflammatory attack. Agents Actions 1993; 38:60–65.

59. Packer L, Witt EH, Tritschler HJ. α-Lipoic acid as a biological antioxidant. Free Radical Biol Med 1995; 19:227–250.

60. Bunik V, Follman H. Thioredoxin reductase dependent on α-ketoacid oxidation by α-ketoacid dehydrogenase complexes. FEBS Lett 1993; 336:197–200.

61. Kagan VE, Shvedova A, Serbinova E, et al. Dihydrolipoic acid: a universal antioxidant both in membrane and in the aqueous phase: reduction of peroxyl, ascorbyl, and chromanoxyl radicals. Biochem Pharmacol 1992; 44:1637–1649.

62. Rosenberg HR, Culik R. Effect of α-lipoic acid on vitamin C and vitamin E deficiency. Arch Biochem Biophys 1959; 80:86–93.

63. Venetianer P, Straub FB. The mechanism of action of the ribonuclease-reactivating enzyme. Biochim Biophys Acta 1964; 89:189–190.

64. Venetianer P, Straub FB. Studies on the mechanism of action of the ribonuclease-reactivating enzyme. Acta Physiol Acad Sci Hung 1965; 27:303–315.

65. Cameron E. Protocol for the use of vitamin C in the treatment of cancer. Med Hypotheses 1991; 36:190–194.

66. Wells WW, Xu DP. Dehydroascorbate reduction. J Bioenerg Biomembr 1994; 26:369–371.

67. Sigal A, King CG. The relationship of vitamin C to glucose tolerance in the guinea pig. J Biol Chem 1936; 116:489–492.

68. Banerjee S. Vitamin C and carbohydrate metabolism, Part I. The effect of vitamin C on the glucose tolerance test in guinea pigs. Ann Biochem Exp Med 1943; 3:157–164.

69. Banerjee S. Vitamin C and carbohydrate metabolism. Part IV. The effect of vitamin C on the insulin content of the pancreas of guinea pigs. Ann Biochem Exp Med 1944; 4:33–36.

70. Wells WW, Dou C-Z, Dybas LN, et al. Ascorbic acid is essential for release of insulin from scorbutic guinea pig pancreatic islets. Proc Natl Acad Sci USA 1995; 92:11869–11873.

71. Wells WW, Yang Y, Deits TL, Gan Z-R. Thioltransferases. In: Meister A, ed. Advances in Enzymology and Related Areas of Molecular Biology. New York: John Wiley, 1993:149–201.

72. Garavina SA, Mieyal JJ. Thioltransferase is a specific glutathionyl mixed disulfide oxidoreductase. Biochemistry 1993; 32:3368–3376.

73. Mieyal JJ, Garavina S, Mieyal PA, et al. Glutathionyl specificity of thioltransferases: mechanistic and physiological implications. Packer L, Cadenas E, eds. Biothiols in Health and Disease. New York: Marcel Dekker, 1995:305–372.

74. Ellman GL. Tissue sulfhydryl groups. Arch Biochem Biophys 1959; 82:70–77.

75. Jocelyn PC. The effect of glutathione on protein sulfhydryl groups in rat liver homogenates. Biochem J 1962; 85:480–485.

76. Yang Y, Wells WW. Identification and characterization of the functional amino-acids at the active center of pig liver thioltransferase by site-directed mutagenesis. J Biol Chem 1991; 266:12759–12765.

77. Drake BB, Smythe CV, King CG. Complexes of dehydroascorbic acid with three sulfhydryl compounds. J Biol Chem 1942; 143:89–98.

78. Meacham J. Ascorbic acid oxidizes thiol groups of plasma proteins. Eperientia 1968; 24:125.

79. Yin D. Lipofuscin-like fluorophores can result from reactions between oxidized ascorbic acid glutamine, carbonyl-protein cross-linking may represent a common reaction in oxygen radical and glycosylation-related aging processes. Mech Age Dev 1992; 62:35–46.

80. Ortwerth BJ, Slight SH, Prabhakaram M, et al. Site-specific glycation of lens crystallins by ascorbic acid. Biochim Biophys Acta 1992; 1117:207–215.

81. Gilbert HF. Molecular and cellular aspects of thiol-disulfide exchange. In: Meister A, ed. Advances in Enzymology. New York: Academic Press, 1990:59–172.

82. Dhariwal K, Hartzell WO, Levine M. Ascorbic acid and dehydroascorbic acid measurement in human plasma and serum. Am J Clin Nutr 1991; 54:712–716.

83. Bode AM, Yavarow CR, Fry DA, Vargas T. Enzymatic basis for altered ascorbic acid and dehydroascorbic acid levels in diabetes. Biophys Res Commun 1993; 191:1347–1353.

84. Wells WW, Xu DP, Washburn MP. Glutathione: dehydroascorbate oxidoreductases. Methods Enzymol 1995; 252:30–38.

7

Protein Glycation by the Oxidation Products of Ascorbic Acid

BERYL J. ORTWERTH
Mason Eye Institute, University of Missouri, Columbia, Missouri

VINCENT M. MONNIER
Institute of Pathology, Case Western Reserve University, Cleveland, Ohio

INTRODUCTION

Protein glycation has increasingly been implicated in the etiology of diabetes. This is in large part due to the results of the Diabetes Control and Complications Study (1), which showed that decreasing the blood glucose levels in diabetic patients resulted in a corresponding decrease in the development of diabetic complications. Consistent with this finding is the observation that 2-aminoguanidine, an inhibitor of glycation-initiated protein modification, delays the onset of diabetic disorders in retina (2), kidney (3), and nervous tissue (4), as well as the membrane thickening of blood vessels (5). While glycated hemoglobin (Hb_{Alc}) has for many years been used as a diagnostic tool for average blood glucose levels (6), it is now clear that other serum proteins (7,8), enzymes (9,10), and likely all proteins are subject to glycation.

In addition to diabetes, glycated proteins also increase with age; this is likely a significant modification reaction in proteins with a long systemic half-life such as collagen, matrix proteins, and lens crystallins (11,12). A strong case is being made for involvement of glycation in the accumulation of amyloid proteins in Alzheimer's disease (13–15) and in renal failure (16). In spite of glucose's sluggish reactivity, most investigators logically conclude that it is the major sugar responsible for the protein modifications associated with diabetic complications. However, all sugars are reactive in this regard, including fructose (17,18), metabolic intermediates (19), and fructose-3-phosphate (20). Of these sugars, fructose-3-phosphate accumulates to significant levels in diabetes and degrades to 3-deoxyglucosone (21). This is important because osones have been proposed as the proximate initiators of the advanced protein modifications seen in diabetes (22).

Ascorbic acid (AA), or more precisely the oxidation products of AA, also glycate proteins and rapidly produce protein-bound adducts and protein cross-links (23,24). This evidence comes largely from in vitro studies, but compounds synthesized by reacting AA with proteins have also been isolated from aged tissues and from cataract proteins (25,26). The rate of protein glycation by AA, therefore, depends upon its oxidation rate in tissues. Significant in this regard are the observations that AA is increasingly oxidized in cataracts (27,28) and that AA is markedly depleted in the serum of diabetics (29,30). The involvement of AA in glycation reactions is a relatively new concept for both glycation researchers and scientists interested in AA metabolism and nutrition. While the antioxidative properties of AA protect against glycation-associated oxidation, the resulting AA oxidation products are likely more effective agents for long-term protein damage. This chapter seeks to correlate the available evidence supporting AA glycation with some comparisons to similar reactions with glucose.

GLYCATION REACTIONS

In strictest terms, glycation refers to the nonenzymatic covalent attachment of sugars to protein molecules. This modification reaction was previously termed nonenzymatic glycosylation or, broadly, the Maillard reaction (31). In the early stage of this reaction the carbonyl group of the open chain sugars reacts with either the N-terminal α-amino group of proteins or lysine ε-amino groups to form an initial Schiff base, which is readily reversible and in equilibrium with a glycoamine structure (32). The initial Schiff base can spontaneously undergo an internal rearrangement to produce the Amadori compound, a 1-deoxy, 2-keto sugar adduct on the lysine amino group (33). This structure exhibits a greater degree of stability and is capable of reforming a hemiacetal ring structure (34). The glucose Amadori compound can then slowly degrade to yield several compounds, including 3-deoxyglucosone (35). Reduction of either the Schiff base by $NaCNBH_3$ (36) or the Amadori compound by $NaBH_4$ (37) produces a stable alditol-lysine adduct, which is resistant to acid hydrolysis and cannot undergo further reactions.

The incubation of sugars with proteins for extended periods leads to the formation of browning products. A portion of these are protein-bound and are collectively referred to as advanced glycation end products (AGEs). This term includes the protein-bound adducts of nonsugar structure which are responsible for the visible light chromophores, fluorophores, protein cross-links, and antigenic determinants typically seen in these reactions (38,39).

ASCORBIC ACID AS A GLYCATING AGENT

When proteins are incubated with millimolar (mM) levels of AA in the presence of air, extensive browning products, fluorophores, and protein cross-links form after only several days of incubation (23,40,41). Further, the dialyzed proteins display the same properties as glycated proteins, including (1) binding to a boronate affinity column due to bound carbohydrates (50–60% binding after 1 week incubation) (42); (2) covalent incorporation of radioactivity from [1-^{14}C]AA into protein, which is markedly stimulated by $NaCNBH_3$ (41), to as much as 1.0 mole/mole protein (42); (3) increased incorporation of radioactivity from NaB^3H_4 into the dialyzed protein product, again as much as 1.0 mole of [^{3}H] incorporated mole protein; (4) formation of protein–protein cross-links detectable by sodium dodecyl sulfate-polyacrylamide gel electrophoresis (SDS-PAGE), which can be prevented by either $NaBH_3$ (41) or 2-aminoguanidine; (5) amino acid analysis of AA-glycated proteins with $NaCNBH_3$ that shows a decrease in lysine residues only, with the initial formation of adducts which elute near sugar glycation adducts in a standard amino acid profile (41); (6) formation of protein-bound fluorophores with 350/420 excitation/

emission maxima, which are typical of AGEs; and (8) formation of many volatile compounds with AA and amino acids which are the same as those obtained with sugars under the same conditions (43,44).

Incorporation into Protein

The incorporation of AA into protein has been reported to be equivalent to 30 nmoles of AA/mg protein after 2 weeks of aerobic incubation with 5–20 mM levels of AA (41,45), and 2 nmoles of AA/mg protein with tracer levels of AA (25 μM) (40). The rate of incorporation with AA is roughly sevenfold higher than with glucose when $NaCNBH_3$ is present to stabilize the Schiff base. This is a minimum value, however, since only [1-^{14}C]AA was available for these experiments and carbon 1 of AA is rapidly lost by decarboxylation during the incubation, producing unlabeled glycating species. The binding of AA to ovarian proteins, which may represent glycation, has also been reported (46). Simple measurements of AA binding to protein, however, must be viewed with caution. Since AA exists in ionized form, it can readily form ionic bonds with macromolecules (47). Also model building suggests that AA can form adducts with Schiff bases involving lysine amino groups (48). However, this represents reversible binding only, because no incorporation of AA can be detected after trichloroacetic acid precipitation of AA-reacted proteins under anaerobic conditions.

Reactions with millimolar (mM) levels of AA show increasing browning and protein cross-linking for several weeks (42), even though the original AA is usually completely oxidized in approximately 3 days even in the presence of transition metal chelating agents (24). Incubations without the addition of chelating agents display a very rapid oxidation of AA with extensive protein fragmentation (23). This is likely due to the AA-mediated formation of hydroxyl radicals (49). This prooxidant activity of AA, however, is not responsible for either the glycation or cross-linking reactions as these reactions proceed readily in the presence of chelating agents, and with the addition of quenchers for each oxygen free radical species and various free radical destroying enzymes (50).

Conditions for Ascorbic Acid Glycation

Ascorbic acid itself is not capable of glycating or cross-linking lens proteins, but first must undergo oxidation. Reactions carried out for as long as 12 weeks in the absence of oxygen showed no protein modification. The addition of glutathione prevented AA incorporation as well as AA-induced protein cross-linking even in the presence of air (51), because of its ability to reduce dehydroascorbic acid (DHA) back to AA rapidly (52). Oxygen was shown to be required only for the oxidation of AA, because equimolar quantities of DHA produced the same extent of protein cross-linking in the absence of oxygen as AA did in the presence of air (51). Ascorbic acid glycation reactions in vitro are routinely carried out in 0.1 M phosphate buffer and 1.0 mM transition metal chelating agents to prevent the formation of oxygen free radicals. This radical formation stems from the presence of 3.0 μM Fe and 7.0 μM Cu (53) in the reagent grade phosphate salts used to prepare the buffer. However, AA can still be oxidized in the presence of chelators and rapidly form AGEs.

This is in marked contrast to glycation reactions with glucose. While glucose readily forms stable Amadori compounds, it is unable to form AGEs or protein cross-links in the presence of either chelating agents or hydroxyl radical quenchers (54,55). This argues for a necessary hydroxyl radical cleavage of glucose to form more reactive compounds. There is ample evidence for free radical generation by sugars (56,57), and more specifically by

Amadori compounds (58) in the presence of trace metal ions, but the concentration of free radicals produced is very low in vitro (58). The extent to which these reactions occur and form AGEs from glucose in vivo is not known. Oxidation measurements in vitro show that while AA is oxidized slowly in the absence of transition metal ions or in the presence of proteins (which can bind these metal ions), no oxidation of even tracer levels of glucose was observed (59). When oxygen free radicals were generated by the ultraviolet (UV) light irradiation of human lens sensitizers, AA was oxidized at a rate at least three orders of magnitude more rapidly than glucose (59). These facts may explain why extremely high concentrations of glucose (0.25–1.0 M) are required for AGE formation under in vitro conditions (60,61), whereas physiological levels of AA (2.0 mM) are sufficient to produce protein cross-links (23), albeit after 12 weeks of incubation.

Protein Cross-Linking

The incubation of 14 mg/ml protein solutions with 20 mM AA caused the loss of about 50% of the total lysine content in the presence of NaCNBH$_3$ after 6 days. In the absence of NaCNBH$_3$ only 20% of the lysine was modified, but an additional loss of arginine and histidine was observed as cross-linking was allowed to occur. These data argue for the formation of Lys–Arg and Lys–His in addition to Lys–Lys cross-links (24). This was confirmed in a protein cross-linking assay, which measured the sugar-dependent incorporation of [^{14}C]lysine into protein (62). The DHA caused the incorporation of lysine into homopolymers of lysine, arginine, and histidine, but not into polymers of alanine, serine, or aspartic acid. The relative cross-linking ability of various sugars measured in this assay corresponded to the formation of polymeric proteins by the same sugars as detected by SDS-PAGE. The relative cross-linking activity of various AA oxidation products in the absence of air is shown in Figure 1. Glucose exhibited no cross-linking in the presence of DTPA, but shorter chain sugars such as ribose and threose are reactive under these conditions. The cross-linking activity, like sugar incorporation, was inversely proportional

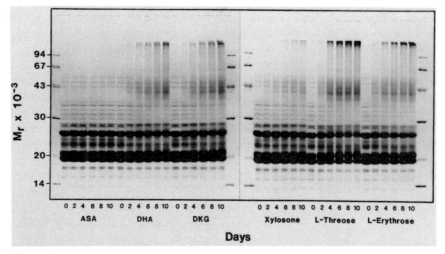

Figure 1   Relative cross-linking activity of ascorbic acid oxidation products with lens proteins in the absence of air. ASA, ascorbic acid; DHA, dehydroascorbic acid; DKG, diketogulonic acid.

to the chain length of the sugar (62), which correlated with the extent of open chain sugar present (63). Similarly short-chain sugars were more active in the synthesis of the specific cross-link pentosidine (64,65). Ascorbic acid cross-linking favored the formation of internal protein cross-links and cross-links between adjacent subunits in a multisubunit protein (42). The crosslinking of monomeric proteins such as lysozyme, ribonuclease, or γ-crystallin into protein dimers or trimers could be demonstrated, but proceeded much more slowly (42).

REACTING SPECIES AND PRODUCTS FORMED

Oxidation Products

The exact oxidation products which are responsible for glycation and AGE formation are not known. The formation of DHA, diketogulonic acid (66), and L-threose (67), as well as decarboxylation reactions leading to xylosone and 3-deoxyxylosone formation (68), has been demonstrated under glycation reaction conditions (see Fig. 2 for structures of AA degradation products). The reaction of DHA with proteins was initially studied by food chemists (69,70) under the elevated temperatures and conditions used in the processing of foodstuffs. The principal product observed was a soluble red compound (2,2'-nitrilo di-2(2)-deoxy-L-ascorbic acid) (71) with an absorption maximum in the visible range at 512–513 nm (72). This product resulted from a Strecker degradation (72) of a DHA–lysine Schiff base adduct releasing scorbamic acid, which reacts with an additional DHA molecule (72). This deamination reaction produces a hydroxylysine residue in the attached protein. Upon further reaction, a yellow compound, which represents a DHA trimer held together by two nitrogens (73), was formed.

Products with Cyanoborohydride

During in vitro reactions of lens proteins with [1-^{14}C]AA in the presence of NaCNBH$_3$, the incorporation of radioactivity correlated directly with the levels of DHA and diketogulonic acid present (24). This analysis, however, was limited by the fact that only the incorporation of compounds containing carbon 1 of AA could be measured. During this assay a rapid loss

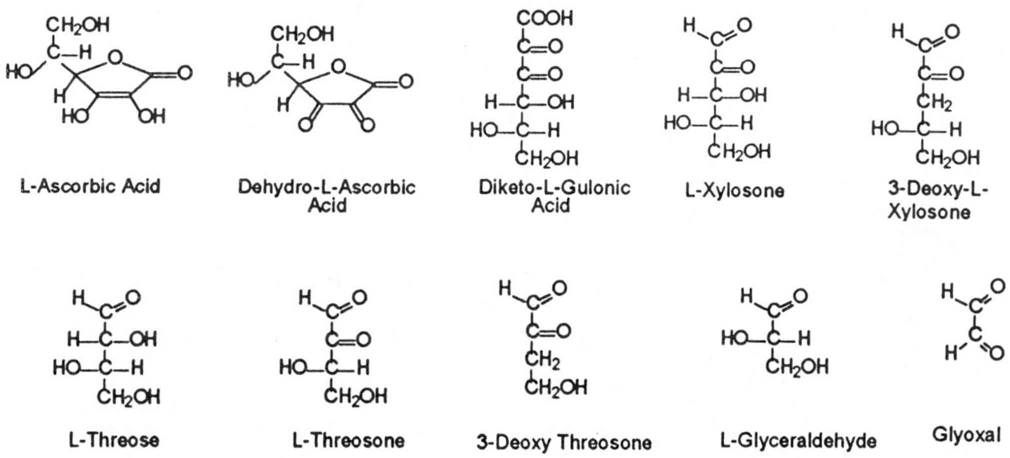

Figure 2 Glycation-reactive degradation products of ascorbic acid.

of 35% of the total radioactivity, which likely reflected decarboxylation (66), was observed (24). All of the initial oxidation products of AA cause AGE formation. The activity of individual compounds could not be assessed, because all degrade along a common pathway. Reductic acid, however, is an ascorbate analogue, which can be oxidized to dehydroreductic acid, but cannot degrade further. This compound was capable of forming glycation adducts and protein cross-links (24), arguing for a possible role of DHA in AGE formation. Other data, however, show that [1-^{14}C]DHA must be decarboxylated to yield browning pigments (74). This was concluded because isolated browning pigments contained no radioactivity. With time, numerous oxidation products of AA are formed; however, the majority of these are not glycation-active (75).

Carboxymethyllysine Formation

To identify the initial reacting species in AA glycation, 2.0 mg/ml solutions of either N-α-acetyllysine or polylysine were incubated with 20 mM AA and NaCNBH$_3$. Amino acid analysis of the hydrolyzed material showed that half of the lysine residues were converted to a single product (Fig. 3). This compound was identified as N^ε-(carboxymethyl)-L-lysine (CML) by comparison to an authentic standard using thin layer chromatography, gas chromatography, and amino acid analysis (76). The CML was as readily formed from polylysine with either AA or DHA, but at a 5- to 10-fold slower rate with diketogulonic acid. [1-^{14}C]Ascorbic acid formed [^{14}C]CML, presumably labeled in the carboxyl group. The data argue for a reaction of the ε-amino group of lysine at the C-2 position in DHA, stabilized by NaCNBH$_3$, with an ensuing cleavage between carbons 2 and 3 of DHA. In the absence of NaCNBH$_3$ the rate of synthesis was similar (10-fold lower) with every AA

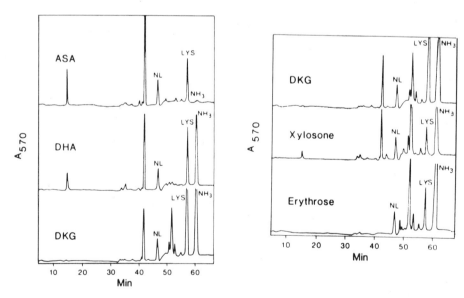

Figure 3 Products of reactions of ascorbic acid oxidation products with polylysine in the presence of NaCNBH$_3$ analyzed by acid hydrolysis and amino acid analysis. N^ε-(carboxymethyl)-L-lysine is the peak at 42 min. ASA, ascorbic acid; DHA, dehydroascorbic acid; DKG, diketogulonic acid.

oxidation product. This could represent either oxidation of an Amadori compound or a reductive reaction of the lysine with glyoxal (77). While glucose also produces CML (78), the reaction proceeds more rapidly with AA. In long-lived tissue proteins, CML is present, increases with age (79,80), and may represent the major antigenic determinant in AGE-modified proteins (81).

The reaction of α-crystallin with DHA and $NaCNBH_3$, followed by proteolytic cleavage, produced peptides with varying levels of modification (82). Only lysine-containing peptides were modified, and in every case fast atom bombardment mass spectrometry showed a mass increase of 58, corresponding to CML formation. The extent of modification varied from 5% to 40% in various peptides, likely reflecting the extent of exposure of the lysine residues in the protein.

Incubation of polylysine with diketogulonic acid (DKG) produced an array of products different from DHA (Fig. 3). This was likely due to the instability of DKG, which released L-threose as the main product, as well as xylosone and 3-deoxyxylosone, by decarboxylation. Incubation of these compounds with polylysine produced adducts similar to those seen with DKG. These compounds were all very effective cross-linking agents as shown by SDS-PAGE, and by the incorporation of [^{14}C]lysine in the cross-linking assay (62). This occurs in the presence of DTPA, and, except for AA, in the absence of oxygen. This is in marked contrast to hexoses, which are inactive under these conditions in both cross-linking assays.

Of all the oxidation products of AA, L-threose is most associated with AGE formation and protein cross-linking due to its high reactivity in the Maillard reaction. Measurements of threose formation during AA degradation (66) show rapid formation, reaching steady-state levels after 12 h. These levels differ with AA, DHA, and DKG, likely reflecting the relative rates of degradation of these compounds compared to the degradation rate of threose. Threose degrades with a half-life of several days at neutral pH, but is markedly accelerated by the presence of lysine (83). The degradation products of threose include low levels of glyceraldehyde and 3-deoxythreosone (84), both of which may be more active than threose in AGE formation. Also, osones can react directly with arginine residues in protein, providing an alternate route to cross-link formation (85).

Fluorophore Formation

Incubating AA alone causes fluorophore formation, but a marked stimulation is seen when amino acids are included in the incubation mixture (86). This is assumed to be due to a glycation-initiated reaction at the α-amino group. The extent of fluorophore formation can be increased 10- to 40-fold with aromatic amino acids, suggesting that glycation adducts are further reacting with the amino acid side chains. These data may support an interaction between glycated lysines in proteins with the side chains of neighboring amino acids. The fluorescence spectrum of AA and amino acids has been reported to resemble the spectrum of the age pigment, lipofuscin (87). The fluorescence spectrum of proteins reacted with AA in air is almost identical to that of proteins isolated from cataract lenses (40,41,88) and aged collagen (89). After prolonged incubation in vitro, longer wavelength fluorophores are formed (28). These fluorophores may remain protein-bound throughout their formation or may be produced in solution and only later form adducts with protein (28). A similar increase of long wavelength fluorophores is also seen in cataract lenses (90,91), extending into the visible light spectrum (92). The spectra obtained with AA and most amino acids or with protein exhibit λ_{max} values of 320–350 nm for excitation and 400–430 nm for emission, which are the same as those seen with sugars (93).

PROTECTIVE MECHANISMS

The presence of millimolar levels of AA in tissues and the observation that AA is the principal soluble antioxidant protecting against oxidative stress (94) both argue that extensive oxidation of AA occurs continuously in vivo. To guard against the potential of these oxidation products to modify protein by a glycation mechanism, the organism has developed several protective mechanisms.

Glutathione and Dehydroascorbate Reductase

While AA is readily oxidized by oxygen in the presence of metal ions and by all oxygen free radicals (59), the DHA produced is readily reduced back to AA by a chemical reaction with glutathione (52). The resulting oxidized glutathione can in turn be reduced by glutathione reductase with the formation of NADPH, which is reoxidized by the pentose phosphate pathway (95). In several tissues it has been shown that DHA is the species transported into cells (96,97), which is then immediately reduced to AA by glutathione. This reaction can also be catalyzed enzymatically by dehydroascorbate reductase (98). Even the formation of ascorbyl free radical leads to dismutation to produce AA and DHA, which is reduced by glutathione (99). At any given time, however, an equilibrium level of DHA is present, usually 5% or less of the total AA (100,101). This opening of the lactone ring of DHA occurs spontaneously, giving rise to DKG and other degradation products which cannot be reduced back to AA. Levels of DKG have been measured in lens tissue (101) and shown to be equivalent to DHA levels, as they are during the degradation of AA in vitro (24).

Aldose Reductase

The principal cross-linking agent produced by AA oxidation may be L-threose. This sugar can be rapidly reduced to the polyol threitol by aldose reductase in spite of its L configuration (82). This enzyme can also reduce osones, producing 3-deoxyfructose from 3-deoxyglucosone (102). Therefore, this enzyme reduces the glycation potential of all aldose sugars and their derivatives. The incubation of rat lenses with [1-^{13}C]threose produced solely [1-^{13}C]threitol within the lens as detected by nuclear magnetic resonance (NMR) spectrometry (82). This was due to the high levels of aldose reductase in these lenses. Similarly, sorbitol accumulation in tissues with high glucose levels during diabetes is due to the activity of aldose reductase (103).

Aldehyde Dehydrogenase

In several mammalian species, and especially in humans, aldose reductase is present at lower levels. The incubation of [1-^{13}C] xylose with bovine lens extracts produced high levels of xylitol, but an equal amount of xylonic acid (104). Similar experiments with L-threose produced threitol and two compounds with carboxylic acid resonances at carbon 1. Bovine and human lenses contain an aldehyde dehydrogenase activity that rapidly converts aldehydes and sugars to carboxylic acids with a corresponding reduction of nicotinamide-adenine dinucleotide (NAD) (105). This activity is also capable of oxidizing L-threose to L-threonic acid, which, like threitol, is incapable of initiating glycation reactions.

Assays of human lenses show the presence of threitol (21,82,106), arguing for the oxidation of AA to threose in this tissue. Also crude bovine lens homogenates produced threitol and threonic acid when incubated with [1-^{14}C]L-threose in vitro. In spite of these protective enzymes, however, as much as 20% of the radioactivity was incorporated into protein, presumably as a result of the rapid glycating ability of L-threose (82). The addition of increasing NADH stimulated threitol formation in the total bovine lens homogenate system (107). Maximum stimulation, however, did not prevent incorporation of [1-^{14}C] threose into protein (107). Inhibition of aldose reductase with Sorbinil increased protein incorporation. The extent of threose glycation at the physiological rate of AA oxidation in vivo, however, is not known.

FREE RADICALS AND ULTRAVIOLET LIGHT SENSITIZERS

Free Radical Generation During Glycation

Incubations containing reducing sugars and protein in phosphate buffer generate oxygen free radicals. Superoxide anion (59,108,109) and H_2O_2 (110) have been demonstrated in reactions containing proteins and glucose. Assays for these reactive oxygen species, however, show the formation of micromolar or smaller (μM) quantities. This is thought to be mediated by the formation of dicarbonyl sugars (osones) (111,112); however, Amadori compounds are likely a richer source (113). In the presence of metal ions, hydroxyl radical formation has been demonstrated during glycation reactions as determined by the hydroxylation of benzoate (21,114). This radical has also been shown to cause protein fragmentation, but it can readily be prevented by the inclusion of chelating agents (115).

Similarly, incubations of dehydroascorbic acid with proteins generated free radicals. Electron spin resonance (EPR) detected several free radical compounds, likely due to scorbamic acid and derivatives, but signals for superoxide anion were also seen (116). The ability of AA to quench superoxide with a 10^5 rate constant (117), however, would prevent superoxide or H_2O_2 damage to protein until the AA was totally oxidized in vitro. Also DHA is capable of detoxifying oxygen free radicals (118). The presence of AA and other reducing agents, along with the absence of free metal ions, would argue that the production of oxygen free radicals by glycation mechanisms may not be the cause of significant protein damage in vivo.

Protein Photolysis by Ultraviolet Light

The irradiation of proteins from aged human lenses with ultraviolet A (UVA) light caused the photolysis of Cys, Met, His, and Trp residues (119). This activity is due to the protein-bound chromophores, which are capable of acting as UVA sensitizers. The incubation of lens proteins with AA produces protein-bound AGEs which have identical absorption and fluorescent spectra and cause an equivalent amount of protein photolysis when irradiated with UVA light in vitro (88). These properties increase with time of glycation, and after 4 weeks the dialyzed lens proteins exhibited the loss of 50 nmol/ml of Trp, and 90 nmole/ml of His, as well as the synthesis of 50 nmol/ml of H_2O_2 after a 1 h irradiation with UVA light. Similar results were obtained with DHA under nitrogen and with L-threose, but not with either glucose or fructose as the glycating agent. The proteins reacted with AA in air or AA oxidation products showed extensive protein cross-linking, which correlated with the loss of Lys, Arg, and His residues only. The sensitizer activity was not due to the oxidation of Trp residues, because ribonuclease (RNase) A, which is devoid of Trp, exhibited the same activity.

Reactive Oxygen Species Generated by Ultraviolet Light

The preceding protein photolysis was mediated by oxygen free radicals. Ascorbic acid–glycated proteins produced 23 μM superoxide anion as measured by cytochrome C reduction in vitro (88). This was in addition to the 140 μM superoxide anion, which dismutated to H_2O_2 under the conditions of the assay. Superoxide anion was responsible for almost no protein oxidation because the bulk of the Cys and Met oxidation was probably due to H_2O_2. The His and Trp photolysis was mediated exclusively by singlet oxygen. As much as 1.0 mM singlet oxygen was generated after 1 h of irradiation, as detected by the oxidation of increasing levels of added His (120). Little or no evidence could be found for the formation of hydroxyl radical during irradiation. Both superoxide radical and singlet oxygen were readily quenched by the addition of AA during the irradiation. Up to 1.4 mM AA was oxidized in the presence of 5.0 mM AA. This demonstrates the ability of AA to compete effectively with the radicals quenched by proteins and water molecules present in the solvent (120). This oxidation of AA is likely important in vivo because the increased AA oxidation products generated can further react with proteins, forming more AGE products, which in turn will display increased sensitizer activity.

ADVANCED GLYCATION END PRODUCTS

Because of the multiplicity of the stochastic processes affecting proteins in aging and age-related diseases, specific probes to assess and understand the mechanism of damage by glycating agents are necessary. Ideally, these chemical probes would be such that they would allow separation of modifications due to ascorbate vs. glucose or other sugars, as well as those resulting from oxidative vs. nonoxidative pathways. The structure of advanced glycation end products (AGEs)/Maillard reaction products that can be synthesized from ascorbate and detected in biological tissues as of today is shown in Figure 4.

CARBOXYMETHYLLYSINE

The mechanistic relationship between ascorbate and carboxymethyllysine (CML) formation was discussed earlier. Both in vitro and in vivo CML is the major known AGE (also called glycoxidation product) (89). It is a nonspecific marker of protein modification by

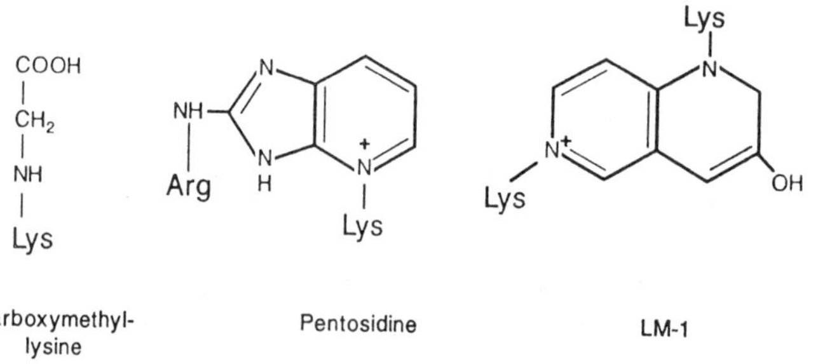

Figure 4 Structure of advanced glycation end products that can be synthesized from ascorbate and detected in tissues.

ascorbate since it can be formed by all sugars tested so far (76,78), including lipid peroxidation, which leads to formation of glyoxal (121), a known precursor of CML (77,60). In human skin collagen and lens crystallins CML increases with age to reach 1.7 and 7 mmol/mol Lys at 80 years, respectively (79,80). The higher levels in lens compared to skin suggest but do not prove that CML is formed from ascorbate. Interestingly, there is a close relationship between H_2O_2 and CML formation in vitro, since catalase prevents CML formation from Amadori products of glucose (123). Thus, extent of CML formation in the lens may reflect intracellular H_2O_2 levels.

Pentosidine

Pentosidine is a fluorescent protein cross-link involving lysine and arginine residues crosslinked by a pentose sugar. It is assayed in protein hydrolysates by reverse-phase high-performance liquid chromatography (HPLC) using a fluorescence detector at 335/385 nm. Like CML, it is a ubiquitous glycoxidation product. Its levels increase curvilinearly in skin to reach approximately 75 pmol/mg collagen at 80 years (124), but less than 5 pmol/mg protein in lens (26). Pentosidine levels in lens increase with the degree of pigmentation of crystallins in cataractous lens and are highest in so-called brunescent lenses, in which extensive oxidative modifications of crystallins have been reported (26). Overall, pentosidine levels are too low to account for the extensive cross-linking and insolubilization of proteins in lens and other tissues (65), and pentosidine should therefore be regarded as marker for glycoxidation.

Pentosidine formation from ascorbate or dehydroascorbate requires oxidative conditions, but it will also form under anaerobic conditions from 2,3-diketogulonic acid (DKG) (68). Its precise mechanism of formation remains to be established. One possible intermediate is xylosone, a degradation product of DKG (68). However, xylose and threose among the various degradation products of ascorbate can act as pentosidine precursors (65,125). Thus, like CML, pentosidine is a nonspecific AGE which can be formed in vitro from most reducing sugars under appropriate conditions. However, it is now clearly established that, in contrast to CML, it cannot form via lipid peroxidation (65,125). In that sense it is a specific marker for glycoxidation, whether initiated by sugars or ascorbate.

Fluorophore LM-1

Fluorophore LM-1 was originally discovered in enzymatically digested human lens protein hydrolysate (25). It is fluorescent at 440 nm upon excitation at 366 nm, i.e., at longer wavelengths than pentosidine. Fluorophore LM-1 was also isolated from an acid hydrolysate of albumin that was incubated with ascorbate or ribose. With age LM-1 levels increase fivefold in water-insoluble human lens crystallins and levels are associated with degree of lens pigmentation, except for brunescent lenses, in which levels are not different from those of age-matched controls (25).

In contrast to pentosidine, the formation of which requires oxidative conditions when ascorbate or dehydroascorbate are precursors, LM-1 can also form from DHA or DKG without oxygen (25). This suggests that LM-1 could form directly from DHA or DKG *prior to* decarboxylation. Furthermore, neither glucose nor fructose could form LM-1 over a period of 22 days at 37°C under conditions in which sugar autoxidation would be sufficient to generate arabinose (60), itself a possible precursor of LM-1. Thus, LM-1 has the potential of being a specific marker for ascorbate-mediated modifications.

The structure of LM-1 has been recently elucidated (125). It is a lysine dimer crosslinked by a pentose and three-carbon chain fused into a heterocyclic naphthyridium ring similar to that of crosslines A and B (126). Levels in cataractous lens from individuals in their seventies vary from 7 to 20 pmol/mg protein (125).

Advanced Glycation End Product Formation During Diabetes and Experimental Galactosemia

Considerable data are now available on the relationship between AGE formation and hyperglycemia in experimental animals and humans. Skin levels of pentosidine, carboxymethyllysine, fluorescence at 360/440 nm accumulate with age at a higher rate in diabetic than normal skin (127,128). Levels correlate with severity of complications, and their formation rate is decreased by tight control of glycemia over many years (127–130). In all these studies, there is a close correlation among the various AGEs, suggesting that they originate from glycoxidation of glucose-derived Amadori products rather than from ascorbate.

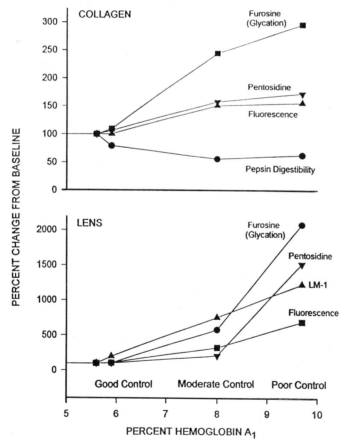

Figure 5 Differential effects of hyperglycemia on collagen glycation, fluorescence, and solubility compared to glycation, pentosidine, fluorescence levels in lens crystallins from diabetic dogs as a function of mean glycemia over a period of 5 years.

The data, however, are different in lenses from hyperglycemic animals and individuals. First, whereas pentosidine level was found elevated in lenses from diabetic individuals, CML level was not elevated (12). Second, in a study involving diabetic dogs with good, moderate, and poor control of glycemia, lenticular levels of pentosidine were normal whereas those of LM-1 were elevated in dogs with moderate hyperglycemia (131). Interestingly, there was a sharp increase in glycated crystallin and pentosidine levels in lenses from poorly controlled dogs (Fig. 5). Third, treatment of galactosemic rats with an aldose reductase inhibitor normalized pentosidine and fluorescence levels in lens (132) without significantly affecting levels in collagen (133). Thus, these studies suggest that the mechanism of formation of AGEs in the hyperglycemic lens is different from that of collagen.

The differential effects of diabetes on lens levels of pentosidine and LM-1 strongly argue against a common precursor for both AGEs. The data are compatible with a mechanism whereby moderate hyperglycemia would be sufficient for ascorbate to become oxidized to form LM-1 and crystallin-linked fluorescence. In contrast, impaired lens membrane permeability in poorly controlled dogs would lead to glucose influx, increased crystallin glycation, and glycoxidation, thereby explaining the concomitant increase in both. However, the recent finding that the galactosemic rat lens becomes permeable to diketogulonic acid, a pentosidine precursor, suggests an alternative or perhaps additional mechanism by which oxidation of ascorbate into DKG would occur in the aqueous humor, followed by passive uptake into lens cells (134).

AREAS FOR FUTURE INVESTIGATION

The oxidation of AA produces L-threose, 3-deoxyxylosone, threosone, glyceraldehyde, glyoxal, and possibly methyl glyoxal, all of which are capable of producing AGEs and protein cross-links. The relative amounts of each produced under glycation reaction conditions and the relative ability of each to form AGEs need to be determined. Also, if reactions are carried out in the absence of chelating agents, an evaluation must be made of the levels of reactive oxygen species produced, and whether the oxidation products of AA by these reactive oxygen species are different from those obtained by molecular oxygen. This is especially important because AA represents the major detoxifying compound for oxygen free radicals in cells. Very little is known about the Amadori compounds produced by AA oxidation products, much less the structure of AA-specific AGEs. In many cases, however, the Amadori products may be too reactive to isolate, and the AGEs produced by these products may resemble those produced by glucose degradation products.

Carboxymethyllysine is produced by the oxidative degradation of fructosyl-lysine, by the reaction of DHA with proteins, as well as by lipid peroxidation. Which of these reactions is responsible for the increased levels of CML seen in vivo with aging is not known. Similarly, both reactions give rise to pentosidine. These compounds cannot be readily used to distinguish the relative contributions of AA and glucose to AGE formation. Compounds unique to AA glycation need to be isolated, their structure determined, and their levels quantified in aged and diabetic tissues. In this way the contribution of AA glycation can be estimated. The myriad AGE compounds produced as in all glycation reactions make the isolation of specific compounds most difficult. Since many of the structures known have multiple aromatic rings attached to a multiply charged lysine residue, present HPLC columns function poorly to separate these molecules. Antibodies can be used in quantitative enzyme-linked immunosorbent assay (ELISA) with tissue extracts or with tissue sections. It is essential, however, that these antibodies be raised against known AGE haptens, rather than crude glycated proteins, because the latter antibodies mainly recognize CML (81).

The major factors controlling the rate of protein glycation with AA in vivo should be the relative rates of AA oxidation and DHA reduction. While these processes are occurring continuously, there is a steady-state level of DHA, which can delactonize irreversibly to form DKG and ensuing glycation active compounds. The rate of this reaction in tissues needs to be established. The single factor hampering the establishment of AA metabolism is the lack of a commercial source for uniformly labeled AA. Because all of the glycation compounds discussed would be unlabeled, [1-^{14}C]Ascorbic acid simply cannot provide information about decomposition products. Metabolic studies are needed to determine not only the rates of oxidation, but also the ability of protective mechanisms to function in aged and diabetic tissues. Such studies are necessary to evaluate the importance of AA glycation in tissue abnormalities.

Ascorbic acid glycation has received little attention because of the logical correlation between glucose levels and tissue damage in diabetes. The requirements established for AGE formation in vitro argue that glucose may not be a significant route for protein damage in vivo. This will require valid data on the ability of glucose to be degraded by protein-bound metal ions, and whether this oxygen free radical process can proceed without being preempted by AA quenching.

ACKNOWLEDGMENTS

Research support is from the National Eye Institute EY02035 and EY07070 (to BJO), EY07099 (to VMM); the National Institute on Aging (AG05601) (to VMM); from Research to Prevent Blindness, Inc., and from the Howard Hughes and Flo Dickey Funk summer fellowship programs.

REFERENCES

1. The Diabetes Control and Complications Trial Research Group. The effect of intensive treatment of diabetes on the development and progression of long-term complications in insulin-dependent diabetes mellitus. N Engl J Med 1993; 329:977–986.
2. Hammes H-P, Martin S, Federlin K, et al. Aminoguanidine treatment inhibits the development of experimental diabetic retinopathy. Proc Natl Acad Sci USA 1991; 88:11555–11558.
3. Vlassara H, Striker LJ, Teichberg S, et al. Advanced glycation end products induce glomerular sclerosis and albunimuria in normal rats. Proc Natl Acad Sci USA 1994; 91:11704–11708.
4. Camerson NE, Cotter MA, Dines K, Love A. Effects of aminoguanidine on peripheral nerve function and polyol pathway metabolites in streptozotocin-diabetic rats. Diabetologia 1992; 35:946–950.
5. Brownlee M, Vlassara H, Kooney A, et al. Aminoguanidine prevents diabetes-induced arterial wall protein cross-linking. Science 1986; 232:1629–1632.
6. Koenig RJ, Peterson CM, Jones RL, et al. Correlation of glucose regulation and hemoglobin A$_{1c}$ in diabetes mellitus. N Engl J Med 1976;417–420.
7. Guthrow EC, Morris MA, Day JF, et al. Enhanced nonenzymatic glucosylation of human serum albumin in diabetes mellitus. Proc Natl Acad Sci USA 1979; 76:4258–4261.
8. Miyata T, Inagi R, Wada Y, et al. Glycation of human β$_2$-microglobulin in patients with hemodialysis-associated amyloidosis: identification of the glycated sites. Biochemistry 1994; 33:12215–12221.

9. Blakytny R, Harding JJ. Glycation (non-enzymatic glycosylation) inactivates glutathione reductase. Biochem J 1992; 288:303–307.

10. Yamaoka T, Oda A, Bannai C, et al. The effect of nonenzymatic glycation on recombinant human aldose reductase. Diabetes Res Clin Pract 1995; 27:165–169.

11. Monnier VM, Kohn RR, Cerami A. Accelerated age-related browning of human collagen in diabetes mellitus. Proc Natl Acad Sci USA 1984; 81:583–587.

12. Lyons TJ, Silvestri G, Dunn JA, et al. Role of glycation in modification of lens crystallins in diabetic and nondiabetic senile cataracts. Diabetes 1991; 40:1010–1015.

13. Vitek MP, Bhattacharya K, Glendening JM, et al. Advanced glycation end products contribute to amyloidosis in Alzheimer disease. Proc Natl Acad Sci USA 1994; 91:4766–4770.

14. Smith MA, Taneda S, Richey PL, et al. Advanced Maillard reaction end products are associated with Alzheimer disease pathology. Proc Natl Acad Sci USA 1994; 91:5710–5714.

15. Yan S-D, Chen X, Schmidt A-M, et al. Glycated tau protein in Alzheimer disease: a mechanism for induction of oxidant stress. Proc Natl Acad Sci USA 1994; 91:7787–7791.

16. Garlick RL, Bunn HF, Spiro RG. Nonenzymatic glycation of basement membranes from human glomeruli and bovine sources. Diabetes 1988; 37:1144–1150.

17. McPherson JD, Shilton BH, Walton DJ. Role of fructose in glycation and cross-linking of proteins. Biochemistry 1988; 27:1901–1907.

18. Dills WL. Protein fructosylation: fructose and the Maillard reaction (review). Am J Clin Nutr 1993; 58:779S–787S.

19. Swamy MS, Tsai C, Abraham A, Abraham EC. Glycation mediated lens crystallin aggregation and cross-linking by various sugars and sugar phosphates in vitro. Exp Eye Res 1993; 56: 177–185.

20. Szwergold, BS, Kappler F, Brown TR. Identification of fructose 3-phosphate in the lens of diabetic rats. Science 1990; 247:451–454.

21. Lal S, Szwergold BS, Taylor AH, et al. Metabolism of fructose-3-phosphate in the diabetic rat lens. Arch Biochem Biophys 1995; 318:191–199.

22. Kato H, Cho RK, Okitani A, Hayase F. Responsibility of 3-deoxyglucosone for the glucose-induced polymerization of proteins. Agric Biol Chem 1987:51:683–689.

23. Ortwerth BJ, Feather MS, Olesen PR. The precipitation and cross-linking of lens crystallins by ascorbic acid. Exp Eye Res 1988; 47:155–168.

24. Slight SH, Feather MS, Ortwerth BJ. Glycation of lens proteins by the oxidation products of ascorbic acid. Biochem Biophys Acta 1990; 1038:367–374.

25. Nagaraj RH, Monnier VM. Isolation and characterization of a blue fluorophore from human eye lens crystallins: in vitro formation from Maillard reaction with ascorbate and ribose. Biochim Biophys Acta 1992; 1116:34–42.

26. Nagaraj RH, Sell DR, Prabhakaram M, et al. High correlation between pentosidine protein crosslinks and pigmentation implicates ascorbate oxidation in human lens senescence and cataractogenesis. Proc Natl Acad Sci USA 1991; 88:10257–10261.

27. Rawal UM, Patel US, Desai RJ. Biochemical studies on cataractous human lenses. Indian J Med Res 1978; 67:161–164.

28. Lohmann W, Schmehl W, Strobel J. Nuclear cataract: oxidative damage to the lens. Exp Eye Res 1988, 43:859–862.

29. Som S, Basu S, Mukherjee D, et al. Ascorbic acid metabolism in diabetes mellitus. Metabolism 1981; 30:572–577.

30. McLennan S, Yue DK, Fisher E, et al. Deficiency of ascorbic acid in experimental diabetes. Diabetes 1988; 37:359–361.

31. Ledl F, Schleicher E. New aspects of the Maillard reaction in foods and in the human body. Angew Chem 1990; 29:565–706.

32. Higgins PJ, Bunn F. Kinetic analysis of the nonezymatic glycation of hemoglobin. J Biol Chem 1981; 256:5204–5208.

33. Yaylayan VA, Huyghues-Despointes A. Chemistry of Amadori rearrangement products: analysis, synthesis, kinetics, reactions, and spectroscopic properties (review). Crit Rev Food Sci Nutr 1994; 34:321–369.

34. Mossine VV, Glinsky GV, Feather MS. The preparation and characterization of some Amadori compounds (1-amino-1-deoxy-D-fructose derivatives) derived from a series of aliphatic ω-amino-acids. Carbohydr Res 1994, 262:257–270.

35. Baker JR, Zyzak DV, Thorpe SR, Baynes JW. Chemistry of the fructosamine assay: D-glucosone is the product of oxidation of amadori compounds. Clin Chem 1994, 40:1950–1955.

36. Friedman M, Williams DL, Masri MS. Reductive alkylation of proteins with aromatic aldehydes and sodium cyanoborohydride. J Peptide Protein Res 1974; 6:183–185.

37. Bunn FH, Haney DN, Gabbay KE, Gallop PM. Further identification of the nature and linkage of the carbohydrate in hemoglobin A_{1c}. Biochem Biophys Res Commun 1975; 67:103–109.

38. Bucala R, Cerami A. Advanced glycosylation: chemistry, biology and implications for diabetes and aging. Adv Pharmacol 1992; 23:1–34.

39. Brownlee M. The pathological implications of protein glycation. Clin Invest Med 1995; 18: 275–281.

40. Bensch KG, Fleming JE, Lohmann W. The role of ascorbic acid in senile cataract. Proc Natl Acad Sci USA 1985; 82:7193–7196.

41. Ortwerth BJ, Olesen PR, Ascorbic acid-induced crosslinking of lens proteins: evidence supporting a Maillard reaction. Biochim Biophys Acta 1988; 956:10–22.

42. Prabhakaram M, Ortwerth BJ. The glycation and cross-linking of isolated lens crystallins by ascorbic acid. Exp Eye Res 1992; 55:451–459.

43. Niemela K. Oxidative and non-oxidative alkali-catalysed degradation of L-ascorbic acid. J Chromatogr 1987; 399:235–243.

44. Seck S, Crouzet J. Formation of volatile compounds in sugar–phenylalanine and ascorbic acid–phenylalanine model systems during heat treatment. J Food Sci 1981; 46:790–793.

45. Dickerson JE Jr, Lou MF, Gracey RW. Ascorbic acid mediated alteration of α-crystallin secondary structure. Curr Eye Res 1994; 14:163–166.

46. Sharma SC, Wilson CWM. Study of binding of L-ascorbic acid to ovarian tissue proteins. Indian J Med Res 1978; 67:598–603.

47. Bensch KG, Koerner O, Lohmann W. On a possible mechanism of action of ascorbic acid: formation of ionic bonds with biological molecules. Biochem Biophys Res Comm 1981; 101: 312–316.

48. Otto P, Ladik J, Szent-Gyorgy A. Quantum chemical calculations of model systems for ascorbic acid adducts with Schiff bases of lysine side chains: possibility of internal charge transfer in proteins. Proc Natl Acad Sci USA 1979; 76:3849–3851.

49. Stadtman ER. Ascorbic acid and oxidative inactivation of proteins. Am J Clin Nutr 1991; 54: 1125S–1128S.

50. Prabhakaram M, Ortwerth BJ. The glycation-associated crosslinking of lens proteins by ascorbic acid is not mediated by oxygen free radicals. Exp Eye Res 1991; 53:261–268.

51. Ortwerth BJ, Olesen PR. Glutathione inhibits the glycation and crosslinking of lens proteins by ascorbic acid. Exp Eye Res 1988; 47:737–750.

52. Winkler BS. Unequivocal evidence in support of the nonenzymatic redox coupling between glutathione/glutathione disulfide and ascorbic acid/dehydroascorbic acid. Biochim Biophys Acta 1992; 1117:287–290.

53. Buettner GR. In the absence of catalytic metals ascorbate does not autoxidize at pH 7: ascorbate as a test for catalytic metals. J Biochem Biophys Methods 1988; 16:27–40.

54. Watkins NG, Neglia-Fisher CI, Dyer DG, et al. Effect of phosphate on the kinetics and specificity of glycation of protein. J Biol Chem 1987; 262:7207–7212.

55. Fu MX, Knecht KJ, Thorpe SR, Baynes JW. Role of oxygen in cross-linking and chemical modification of collagen by glucose. Diabetes 1992; 41:42–48.

56. Thornalley PJ. Monosaccharide autoxidation in health and disease. Environ Health Perspect 1985; 64:297–307.
57. Wolff SP, Jiang ZY, Hunt JV. Protein glycation and oxidative stress in diabetes mellitus and ageing. Free Radical Biol Med 1991; 10:339–352.
58. Mullarkey CJ, Edelstein D, Brownlee M. Free radical generation by early glycation products: a mechanism for accelerated atherogenesis in diabetes. Biochem Biophys Res Commun 1990; 173:932–939.
59. Giangiacomo A, Olesen PR, Ortwerth BJ. Ascorbic acid and glucose oxidation by UVA-generated oxygen free radicals. Invest Ophthalmol Vis Sci 1996; 37:1549–1556.
60. Wells-Knecht KJ, Zyzak DV, Litchfield JE, et al. Mechanism of autoxidative glycosylation: identification of glyoxal and arabinose as intermediates in the autoxidative modification of proteins by glucose. Biochemistry 1995; 34:3702–3709.
61. Shaw SM, Crabbe MJC. Monitoring the progress of non-enzymatic glycation in vitro. Int J Peptide Protein Res 1994; 44:594–602.
62. Prabhakaram M, Ortwerth BJ. Determination of glycation crosslinking by the sugar-dependent incorporation of [^{14}C]lysine into protein. Anal Biochem 1994; 216:305–312.
63. Bunn HF, Higgins PJ. Reaction of monosaccharides with proteins: possible evolutionary significance. Science 1981; 213:222–224.
64. Grandhee SK, Monnier VM. Mechanism of formation of the Maillard protein cross-link pentosidine. J Biol Chem 1991; 266:11649–11653.
65. Dyer DG, Blackledge JA, Thorpe SR, Baynes JW. Formation of pentosidine during non-enzymatic browning of proteins by glucose. J Biol Chem 1991; 266:11654–11660.
66. Shin DB, Feather, MS. The degradation of L-ascorbic acid in neutral solutions containing oxygen. J Carbohydr Chem 1990; 9:461–469.
67. Lopez MG, Feather MS. The production of threose as a degradation product from L-ascorbic acid. J Carbohydr Chem 1992; 11:799–806.
68. Shin DB, Feather MS. 3-Deoxy-L-glycero-pentos-2-ulose (3-deoxy-L-xylosone) and L-threo-pentos-2-ulose (L-xylosone) as intermediates in the degradation of L-ascorbic acid. Carbohydr Res 1990; 208:246–250.
69. Ziderman II, Gregorski KS, Lopez SV, Friedman M. Thermal interaction of ascorbic acid and sodium ascorbate with proteins in relation to nonenzymatic browning and Maillard reactions. J Agric Food Chem 1989; 37:1480–1486.
70. Nishimura K, Ohtsuru M, Nigota K. Effect of dehydroascorbic acid on ovalbumin. J Agric Food Chem 1989; 37:1539–1543.
71. Kurata T, Fujimaki M, Sakurai Y. Red pigment produced by the reaction of dehydro-L-ascorbic acid with amino acids. Agric Biol Chem 1973; 37:1471–1477.
72. Hayaski T, Namiki M. Tri (2-deoxy-L-ascorbyl) amine: a novel compound related to a fairly stable free radical. Tetrahedron Lett 1979; 46:4467–4470.
73. Hayashi T, Hoshii Y, Namiki M. On the yellow product and browning of the reaction of dehydroascorbic acid with amino acids. Agric Biol Chem 1983; 47:1003–1009.
74. Sawamura M, Takemoto K, Li Z-F. ^{14}C studies on browning of dehydroascorbic acid in an aqueous solution. J Agric Food Chem 1991; 39:1735–1737.
75. Tatum JH, Shaw PE, Berry RE. Degradation products from ascorbic acid. J Agr Food Chem 1969; 17:38–40.
76. Slight SH, Prabhakaram M, Shin DB, et al. The extent of N^{ε}-(carboxymethyl) lysine formation in lens proteins and polylysine by the autoxidation products of ascorbic acid. Biochim Biophys Acta 1992; 1117:199–206.
77. Glomb MA, Monnier VM. Mechanism of protein modification by glyoxal and glycolaldehyde, reactive intermediates of the Maillard reaction. J Biol Chem 1995; 270:10017–10026.
78. Dunn JA, Ahmed MU, Murtiashaw MH, et al. Reaction of ascorbate with lysine and protein under autoxidizing conditions formation of N^{ε}-(carboxymethyl) lysine by reaction between

lysine and products of autoxidation of ascorbate. Biochemistry 1990; 29:10964–10970.

79. Dunn JA, McCance DR, Thorpe SR, et al. Age dependent accumulation of N^ε-(carboxymethyl) lysine and N^ε-(carboxymethyl) hydroxylysine in human skin collagen. Biochemistry 1991; 30:1205–1210.

80. Dunn JA, Patrick JS, Thorpe SR, Baynes JW. Oxidation of glycated proteins: age-dependent accumulation of N^ε-(carboxymethyl)lysine in lens proteins. Biochemistry 1989; 28:9464–9468.

81. Reddy S, Bichler J, Wells-Knecht KJ, et al. N^ε-(Carboxymethyl)lysine is a dominant advanced glycation end product (AGE) antigen in tissue proteins. Biochemistry 1995; 34:10872–10878.

82. Ortwerth BJ, Slight SH, Prabhakaram M, et al. Site-specific glycation of lens crystallins by ascorbic acid. Biochim Biophys Acta 1992; 1117:207–215.

83. Ortwerth BJ, Speaker JA, Prabhakaram M, et al. Ascorbic acid glycation: the reactions of L-threose in lens tissue. Exp Eye Res 1994; 58:665–674.

84. Li EY, Feather MS. The degradation of L-threose at Maillard reaction conditions. Carbohydr Res 1994; 256:41–47.

85. Shin DB, Hayase F, Kato H. Polymerization of proteins caused by reaction with sugars and the formation of 3-deoxyglucosone under physiological conditions. Agric Biol Chem 1988; 52:1451–1458.

86. Yin D. Lipofuscin-like fluorophores can result from reactions between oxidized ascorbic acid and glutamine. Carbonyl-protein cross-linking may represent a common reacting in oxygen radical and glycosylation-related ageing processes. Mech Ageing Dev 1992; 62:35–46.

87. Yin D, Brunk UT. Oxidized ascorbic acid and reaction products between ascorbic and amino acids might consitute part of age pigments. Mech Ageing Dev 1991; 61:99–112.

88. Ortwerth BJ, Linetsky MK, Olesen PR. Ascorbic acid glycation of lens proteins produces UVA sensitizers similar to those in human lens. Photochem Photobiol 1995; 62:454–462.

89. Baynes JW. Role of oxidative stress in development of complications in diabetes. Diabetes 1991; 40:405–412.

90. Lohmann W, Wunderling M, Schmehl W. Nuclear cataract and ascorbic acid. Naturwissenschaften 1986; 73:266–267.

91. Kurzel RB, Wolbarsh ML. Spectral studies on normal and cataractous intact human lenses. Exp Eye Res 1973; 17:65–71.

92. Yu N-T, Cai M-Z, Ho DJ-Y, Kuck JFR. Automated laser-scanning-microbeam fluorescence/Raman image analysis of human lens with multichannel detection: evidence for metabolic production of a green fluorophor. Proc Natl Acad Sci USA 1988; 85:103–106.

93. Ghiggeri GM, Candiano G, Delfino G, Queirolo C. Reaction of human serum albumin with aldoses. Carbohydr Res 1985; 145:113–122.

94. Niki E. Action of ascorbic acid as a scavenger of active and stable oxygen radicals. Am J Clin Nutr 1991; 54:1119S–1124S.

95. Sasaki H, Giblin FJ, Winkler BS, et al. A protective role for glutathione-dependent reduction of dehydroascorbic acid in lens epithelium. Invest Ophthalmol Vis Sci 1995; 36:1804–1817.

96. Welch RW, Wang Y, Crossman A Jr, et al. Accumulation of vitamin C (ascorbate) and its oxidized metabolite dehydroascorbic acid occurs by separate mechanisms. J Biol Chem 1995; 270:12584–12592.

97. May JM, Qu Z-C, Whitesell RR. Ascorbic acid recycling enhances the antioxidant reserve of human erythrocytes. Biochemistry 1995; 34:12721–12728.

98. Bigley R, Riddle M, Layman D, Stankova L. Human cell dehydroascorbate reductase. Kinetic and functional properties. Biochim Biophys Acta 1981; 659:15–22.

99. Roginsky VA, Stegmann HB. Ascorbyl radical as natural indicator of oxidative stress: quantitative regularities. Free Radical Biol Med 1994; 17:93–103.

100. Iheanacho EN, Stocker R, Hunt NH. Redox metabolism of vitamin C in blood of normal and malaria-infected mice. Biochim Biophys Acta 1993; 1182:15–21.

101. Kern HL, Zolot SL. Transport of vitamin C in the lens. Curr Eye Res 1987; 6:885–896.

102. Feather MS, Flynn TG, Munro KA, et al. Catalysis of reduction of carbohydrate 2-oxoaldehydes (osones) by mammalian aldose reductase. Biochim Biophys Acta 1995; 1244:10–16.

103. Narayanan S. Aldose reductase and its inhibition in the control of diabetic complications. Ann Clin Lab Sci 1993; 23:148–158.

104. Li EY, Feather MS. The conversion of D-xylose to xylitol and D-xylonic acid by a bovine lens preparation. J Carbohydr Chem 1994; 13:499–505.

105. Crabbe MJC, Hoe ST. Aldehyde dehydrogenase, aldose reductase, and free radical scavengers in cataract. Enzyme 1991; 45:188–193.

106. Tomana M, Prchal JT, Garner LC, et al. Gas chromatographic analysis of lens monosaccharides. J Lab Clin Med 1984; 103:137–142.

107. Ortwerth BJ, Speaker JA, Prabhakaram M. Aldose reductase protects, but does not prevent, the glycation of lens proteins by L-threose. In: Labuza TP, Reineccius GA, eds. Maillard Reactions in Chemistry, Food and Health. Cambridge: The Royal Society of Chemistry, 1994: 292–299.

108. Azevedo M, Falcao J, Raposo J, Manso CM. Superoxide radical generation by Amadori compounds. Free Rad Res Commun 1988; 4:331–335.

109. Sakurai T, Sugioka K, Nakano M. $O_2{}^-$ generation and lipid peroxidation during the oxidation of a glycated polypeptide, glycated polylysine, in the presence of iron-ADP. Biochim Biophys Acta 1990; 1043:27–33.

110. Jiang ZY, Wollard ACS, Wolff SP. Hydrogen peroxide production during experimental protein glycation. FEBS Lett 1990; 268:69–71.

111. Wolff SP, Crabbe MJC, Thornalley PJ. The autoxidation of glyceraldehyde and other simple monosaccharides. Experientia 1984; 40:244–246.

112. Yim H-S, Kang S-O, Hah Y-C, et al. Free radicals generated during the glycation reaction of amino acids by methylglyoxal. J Biol Chem 1995; 270:28228–28233.

113. Smith PR, Thornalley PJ. Mechanism of the degradation of non-enzymatically glycated proteins under physiological conditions. Eur J Biochem 1992; 210:729–739.

114. Hunt JV, Dean RT, Wolff SP. Hydroxyl radical production and autoxidative glycosylation. Biochem J 1988; 256:205–212.

115. Hunt JV, Wolff SP. Oxidative glycation and free radical production: a causal mechanism of diabetic complications. Free Rad Res Commun 1991; 12–13:115–123.

116. Yano M, Hayashi T, Namiki M. Formation of free-radical products by the reaction of dehydroascorbic acid with amino acids. J Agric Food Chem 1976; 24:815–819.

117. Butler J, Koppenol WH, Margoliash E. Kinetics and mechanism of the reduction of ferricytochrome C by the superoxide anion. J Biol Chem 1982; 257:10747–10750.

118. Frimer AA, Gilinsky-Sharon P. Reaction of superoxide with ascorbic acid derivatives: insight into the superoxide-mediated oxidation of dehydroascorbic acid. J Org Chem 1995; 60:2796–2801.

119. Ortwerth BJ, Olesen PR. UVA photolysis using the protein-bound sensitizers present in human lens. Photochem Photobiol 1994; 60:53–60.

120. Linetsky M, Ortwerth BJ. Quantitation of the reactive oxygen species generated by the UVA irradiation of ascorbic acid-glycated lens proteins. Photochem Photobiol 1996; 63:649–655.

121. Loidl-Stahlhofen A, Spiteller G. α-Hydroxyaldehydes, products of lipid peroxidation. Biochim Biophys Acta 1994; 1211:156–160.

122. Fu MX, Requena JR, Jenkins AJ, et al. The advanced glycation end product, N^ε-(carboxymethyl)lysine is a product of both lipid peroxidation and glycoxidation reactions. J Biol Chem 1996; 271:9982–9986.

123. Ahmed MU, Thorpe SR, Baynes JW. Identification of N-ε-carboxymethyllysine as a degradation product of fructoselysine in glycated protein. J Biol Chem 1986; 261:4889–4894.

124. Sell DR, Carlson EC, Monnier VM. Differential effects of Type 2 (non-insulin-dependent) diabetes mellitus on pentosidine formation in skin and glomerular basement membrane. Diabetologia 1993; 36:936–941.

125. Graham L, Monnier VM, Nagaraj RH. Structure elucidation of an ascorbate/ribose derived

lys–lys crosslink present in the human lens. Invest Ophthalmol Suppl 1996; 37:5886.

126. Nakamura K, Hosegawa T, Fukunaga Y, Ienaga K. Crosslines A and B as candidates for the fluorophores in age- and diabetes-related crosslinked proteins, and their diacetates produced by the late products of the Maillard reaction of N-α-acetyl-L-lysine with D-glucose. J Chem Soc Chem Commun 1992; 114:992–994.

127. Sell DR, Lapolla A, Odetti P, et al. Pentosidine formation in skin correlates with severity of complications in individuals with long-standing IDDM. Diabetes 1992; 41:1286–1292.

128. McCance DR, Dyer DG, Dunn JA, et al. Maillard reaction products and their relation to complications in insulin-dependent diabetes mellitus. J Clin Invest 1993; 91:2470–2478.

129. Beisswenger PJ, Moore LL, Brinck-Johnson T, Curphey TJ. Increased collagen-linked pentosidine levels and advanced glycosylation end products in early diabetic nephropathy. J Clin Invest 1993; 92:212–217.

130. Monnier VM, Sell DR, Fogarty J, et al. Diabetes 1995; 44:112A.

131. Nagaraj RH, Kern TS, Sell DR, et al. Evidence of a glycemic threshold in diabetic dog lens but not in collagen. Diabetes. In press.

132. Nagaraj RH, Prabhakaram M, Ortwerth BJ, Monnier VM. Suppression of pentosidine formation in galactosemic rat lens by an inhibitor of aldose reductase. Diabetes 1994; 43:580–586.

133. Richard S, Tamas C, Sell DR, Monnier VM. Tissue-specific effects of aldose reductase inhibition on fluorescence and cross-linking of extracellular matrix in chronic galactosemia. Diabetes 1991; 40:1049–1056.

134. Saxena P, Saxena A, Monnier VM. High galactose levels in vitro and in vivo impair ascorbate regeneration and increase ascorbate-mediated glycation in cultured rat lens (submitted).

8

Ascorbate Membrane Transport Properties

RICHARD C. ROSE
Finch University of Health Sciences, Chicago Medical School, North Chicago, Illinois

JOHN X. WILSON
University of Western Ontario, London, Ontario, Canada

This chapter focuses on the cellular properties by which ascorbic acid (AA) is directed to its sites of action in the body. Although most vertebrate species synthesize AA from glucose, humans and other primates must acquire food that contains vitamin C. We must also protect the vitamin as it passes through the harsh environment of the stomach, bring about its absorption in the intestine, and deliver it into cells of the various tissues that will use it in functions discussed elsewhere in this text. Even in vertebrate species which can synthesize vitamin C, this capability is limited to few cell types (e.g., hepatocytes) and other cells must take up the vitamin from the blood. In essence, AA needs to be distributed among a large number of body compartments and it must be at the appropriate concentration in each one.

THE ROLE OF AA COMPARTMENTATION AND MECHANISMS BY WHICH IT IS ACHIEVED

Some Physicochemical Properties of AA and Cell Membranes

Ascorbic acid has several chemical properties that allow it to be selectively moved throughout the body (1). It is a lactone ($C_6H_8O_6$) with a molecular weight of 176 (Fig. 1). In an aqueous environment, the hydroxyl groups at positions 2 and 3 ionize with pK values of 4.17 and 11.57. Thus, at a physiological pH of 7.4, most molecules of AA exist as the monovalent anion ascorbate. This allows for considerable water solubility: 1 g AA dissolves in 3 ml of water at room temperature. Substances with similar high water solubility but that are un-ionized and smaller (e.g., ethanol or glycerol) diffuse readily throughout the body, including into and out of cells. This allows for rapid absorption of those compounds without any specific recognition or interaction between the solute and cell membranes.

Compounds that are charged and have a molecular weight higher than ~150 Da typically

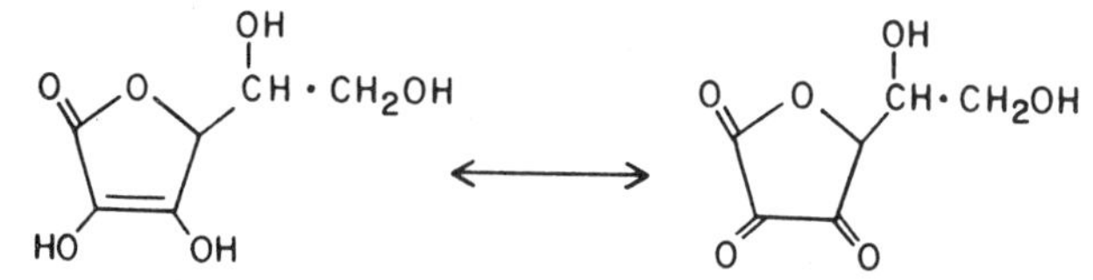

Figure 1 Structure of the reduced and oxidized forms of vitamin C.

permeate cell membranes very slowly by the process of simple diffusion. This is a consequence of membrane composition. Lipids account for 25–50% of the dry weight of membrane preparations. Erythrocyte ghosts contain >95% of the lipids present in the whole cells. Various fatty acid residues are found in lipids which range in carbon chain length from 16 to 22 carbon atoms. The range of unsaturation is from zero to four double bonds. As saturation increases, the fit between neighboring fatty acid side chains permits a closer molecular approach and an increase in intermolecular forces. Thus, fatty acid composition determines the physical properties of substrate permeation by dissolving in the biological membrane.

Simple diffusion through the lipid bilayer of the plasma membrane can account for a slow component of vitamin C entry into cells. Evidence concerning the diffusion mechanism was obtained by measuring the reduction of a spin label incorporated into dipalmitoylphosphatidylcholine vesicles by AA added to the incubation medium (2). It was observed that the protonated form of reduced vitamin C, namely AA, could not traverse the lipid membrane. However, data indicated that ascorbyl radicals bind cations such as Na^+ and the resulting electroneutral moieties are able to permeate lipid membranes (2).

Diffusion of the oxidized form of vitamin C, dehydro-L-ascorbic acid (DHAA), has also been investigated. It is chemically much different from AA by virtue of lacking the dissociable hydrogens at carbon positions 2 and 3 that allow AA to ionize and behave as a reductant. For many years DHAA was considered to be sufficiently lipid-soluble to diffuse readily through cell membranes. A more recent evaluation, however, showed oil/water distribution coefficients as follows: lauric acid $\gg$ mannitol $\approx$ DHAA > AA (3). In that mannitol is effectively used as an extracellular space marker (4), these findings do not support the concept that DHAA should be considered hydrophobic.

Carrier-Mediated Uptake of Ascorbate into Cells

Vitamin C can interact with specific membrane-bound proteins to enter or leave cells by facilitated diffusion or active transport. These transport mechanisms differ in that facilitated diffusion brings about net movement of the translocated solute only in the direction of an electrochemical gradient (e.g., down a concentration gradient in the case of DHAA), whereas active transport can move the solute against a concentration gradient (e.g., up an electrochemical gradient in the case of the ion ascorbate). Furthermore, active transport depends on cellular metabolic energy. For many cell types, concentrative uptake into cells is mediated by secondary active transport driven by the electrochemical gradient of Na^+ across the plasma membrane. When all extracellular vitamin C is in the reduced form (i.e., ascorbate), Na^+-dependent transport proceeds much faster than does simple diffusion and consequently mediates virtually all vitamin C uptake into cells. This secondary active transport mechanism can raise intracellular ascorbate concentration $\geq$10-fold higher than the extracellular concentration (see, for example, 5). Na^+-ascorbate cotransporters have not yet been cloned, but Na^+-dependent ascorbate transport has been induced in *Xenopus laevis* oocytes injected with poly(A) + ribonucleic acid (RNA) extracted from rabbit kidney (6) (see the section, Kidney).

Both facilitated diffusion and active transport display specificity and stereoselectivity. Initial rate of vitamin C uptake saturates with increasing external vitamin C concentration, reflecting a high affinity interaction that can be described by Michaelis–Menten kinetics. The concentration of vitamin C required for half-maximal vitamin C flux is the apparent K_m. The apparent K_m is not a direct measurement of the affinity of a solute for its binding site on the transporter because the transport cycle is not known to be a simple enzyme kinetic scheme. However, it is instructive to compare the apparent K_m to the extracellular vitamin C concentrations that occur under physiological or pathological circumstances. It is noteworthy that Na^+-dependent ascorbate uptake systems appear to possess an affinity for L-ascorbate (apparent K_m of 20–30 μM in many cell types expressing Na^+-ascorbate cotransporters) that is high enough for effective uptake in vivo, because plasma typically contains ascorbate concentrations of 10–160 μM.

Part of the metabolic energy requirement of Na^+-dependent ascorbate is associated with activity of sodium-potassium adenosine triphosphatase (Na^+,K^+-ATPase), which uses metabolic energy to keep the intracellular Na^+ concentration low. The resulting electro-chemical gradient of Na^+ favors the flow of Na^+ through the plasma membrane Na^+-ascorbate cotransporter and into the cell, providing the energy required to accumulate ascorbate against the ascorbate electrochemical gradient. Inhibition of Na^+,K^+-ATPase with ouabain eventually increases intracellular Na^+ concentration and inhibits ascorbate uptake (7,8).

Kinetic experiments suggest that two Na ions are required for the secondary active transport of each ascorbate molecule (7,9,10), indicating that the Na^+-ascorbate cotrans-porter is electrogenic. The ratio of cytoplasmic-to-extracellular ascorbate at steady state depends on the electrochemical gradients of Na^+ and ascorbate across the plasma mem-brane. It follows that membrane potential changes Na^+-ascorbate cotransport activity. From a thermodynamic viewpoint, this can be understood to result from changes in membrane potential altering the Na^+ electrochemical gradient and thus the free energy of the transport system.

Insight into the molecular mechanisms by which membrane potential affects Na^+-ascorbate transport may be gained by comparison with the high-affinity Na^+-glucose cotransporter SGLT1. Both cotransporters, Na^+-ascorbate (10) and SGLT1 (11), exhibit a stoichiometry of 2 Na ions per carbohydrate molecule transported. Studies of Na^+-glucose cotransport in LLC-PK epithelial cells indicate the rate of Na^+ binding to the extracellular site on the cotransporter is potential-dependent (12). Other steps, such as dissociation rates and rate of translocation of the free carrier across the plasma membrane, may also be potential-dependent.

A Na^+-ascorbate cotransporter stoichiometry of 2 Na^+:1 ascorbate can theoretically maintain an 80-fold intracellular accumulation of ascorbate in the cytoplasm (9). Given that extracellular ascorbate concentrations are typically about 0.1 mM, it follows that cells expressing the cotransporter can be expected to achieve cytoplasmic ascorbate concentra-tions of about 8 mM through this transport pathway alone. Total intracellular AA concentra-tion may be higher under steady-state conditions as a result of subcellular compartmenta-tion, for example, into secretory granules (13). Total intracellular content of vitamin C may also be augmented, at least transiently, by uptake of DHAA.

Cellular Transport and Reduction of Dehydro-L-Ascorbic Acid

Oxidation of AA produces DHAA, the reversibly oxidized form of vitamin C, and leads to potentially damaging effects on cells (1). Structurally DHAA is similar to the diabetogenic agent alloxan. Like alloxan, DHAA has three adjacent carbonyl groups in a ring structure, which is not seen elsewhere in biological systems. When given at low levels intravenously, both compounds destroy the pancreatic beta cells that produce insulin. Toxic effects of DHAA might be a consequence of damage to proteins that mediate cell transport and metabolism. Renal brush border membrane vesicles preincubated with DHAA have a loss of glucose transport activity (14). Erythrocytes incubated in buffer with DHAA at 1 mM lose membrane integrity as indicated by release of hemoglobin. The oxidized form of vitamin C also has short-term effects on inhibiting transport by surviving fragments of human placenta in vitro and by cultured corneal endothelial cells (15).

Reportedly DHAA is absent from normal human plasma (16) and presumably would occur only at very low concentrations in the extracellular fluid under physiological conditions. However, extracellular DHAA concentration may increase under pathological conditions involving oxidative stress. The DHAA can be taken into cells through carrier-mediated mechanisms and reduced to AA (17). For example, uptake of radioactivity by HL-60 cells incubated with [^{14}C]DHAA has been reported to be mediated by the Na$^+$-independent, facilitative hexose transporter glucose transporter-1 (GLUT1) (18,19), which appears to be selective for DHAA over ascorbate, because DHAA but not ascorbate inhibits GLUT1-mediated methylglucose uptake (19).

Because of certain steps in the hexose transport mechanism DHAA may transiently accumulate in cells. Kinetic experiments, studying transport of glucose and glucose analogues by erythrocytes, indicate that rapid translocation of sugars across the lipid bilayer of the plasma membrane is followed by slow sugar release into bulk cytoplasm, with the slowness of release due to reversible, intracellular binding of sugar (20). Drug treatments may target one or both steps of the two-step sugar uptake process. This makes it difficult to determine whether cells possess only one, or more than one, type of transporter mediating DHAA uptake.

Toxicity of DHAA is apparently kept minimal in most individuals under most circumstances because of the large number of tissues that have effective mechanisms for reducing DHAA to AA (1,17). Both plasma and pancreatic tissue are nearly devoid of DHAA in healthy individuals, but diabetic patients have persistently elevated levels. Interactions between glucose and DHAA may contribute in part to diabetic complications (21,22).

Recycling of DHAA to AA may depend on reducing equivalents derived from cell metabolism. Thus, metabolic energy may be required not only for secondary active transport of ascorbate but also for accumulation of intracellular AA from extracellular DHAA. It follows that any agents causing inhibition of cell metabolism are likely to interfere with both pathways (Na$^+$-ascorbate cotransport and the combination of DHAA uptake and reduction) by which most cells acquire intracellular AA.

Efflux of Vitamin C from Cells

Membrane proteins functioning as channels or carriers selectively increase membrane permeability to ascorbate. In cerebral astrocytes, for example, osmotic cell swelling causes release of cytoplasmic ascorbate into the extracellular medium (23). From the pharmacological properties of the efflux pathway, it can be inferred that ascorbate crosses the plasma membrane through volume-regulated anion channels (23). Adrenal chromaffin cells appear to release vitamin C from several intracellular compartments when stimulated by depolarizing concentrations of extracellular K^+ (24), but the efflux pathways involved have not been identified.

Extracellular vitamin C has been observed to stimulate efflux of radioactivity from various types of cells preloaded with L-[^{14}C]AA. For example, this effect has been reported for in vitro preparations of cat retinal pigment epithelial cells (25), rabbit iris-ciliary body (26), and bovine adrenal cortical cells (27). The underlying mechanism has not been conclusively identified but transstimulation of efflux through a homeoexchange system, in which uptake of new ascorbate is coupled to efflux of cellular ascorbate, appears likely.

Oxidation of intracellular AA accelerates efflux of vitamin C (28). Cytochalasin B, a drug which also inhibits facilitative hexose transporters, blocked 80% of radiolabel efflux from human erythrocytes that had been loaded with [^{14}C]AA and then exposed to oxidative stress by ferricyanide (28). Sensitivity to cytochalasin B suggests that facilitative hexose transporters constitute an efflux pathway for DHAA. However, it cannot be taken for granted that vitamin C is released from cells through the same carriers used for uptake because the carriers' affinities may be much lower for intracellular than for extracellular substrate. For example, the affinity of the Na^+-glucose cotransporter SGLT1 for at least some glucose analogs is an order of magnitude lower at its internal site than at its extracellular site (11).

VITAMIN C TRANSPORT IN ORGANS AND TISSUES OF SERVICE

Several organs of the body have specific processes for transporting or metabolizing vitamin C far beyond the needs of that tissue. These organs serve the rest of the body by delivering or preserving the vitamin.

Intestine

Intestinal absorption of ascorbate and other water-soluble vitamins was reviewed recently (29). Although the wall of the small intestine (functionally, the mucosal lining) is quite leaky to small monovalent electrolytes, it does not pass ascorbate to a significant extent. The advantage of this to the organism is that in times of an absence of AA in the diet, the body content of AA derived from a previous, more healthy diet does not leak down its concentration gradient from the blood into the intestinal content. That process would slowly drain the body of existing AA stores.

There is a potential problem with having an intestinal wall that is "tight" to AA: that is, if AA cannot diffuse from the blood into intestinal chyme, it also cannot diffuse from dietary sources into the blood. The same holds true for sugars, amino acids, and many other water-soluble nutrients. Thus, a rather elaborate protein has been genetically dispatched into the brush border membrane of the enterocyte (absorptive cell). This specific protein is the entire key to how vitamin C is absorbed in animal species that have lost the enzyme (another protein) for manufacturing AA. It is of interest that species which synthesize AA have very little capacity for absorption of it (29). It thus appears that only those animal species which have a dietary need for AA express high levels of Na^+-ascorbate cotransport activity in the intestinal mucosa.

The mechanism of AA transport has been studied in numerous preparations. It became apparent that one transport event occurs as AA enters the absorptive cell from the intestinal lumen. This event was studied in minute vesicles made from the brush border membrane. These spheres can be produced and then suspended in a buffer such that the electrolyte composition on the outside resembles extracellular fluid and the composition on the inside resembles intracellular fluid. In this way, each vesicle represents a cell having a Na^+ gradient from outside to inside and a K^+ gradient in the opposite direction; these gradients are dissipated by diffusion of Na^+ and K^+ (about 1–2 min). Because all of the cytoplasm is lost during vesicle preparation, there is no involvement of cellular metabolic energy or enzymatic metabolism of AA. When such vesicles are incubated in the presence of a low concentration (65 μM) of ^{14}C-labeled AA, there is rapid uptake of the substrate with a peak intravesicular content at 1–2 min. The $[^{14}C]AA$ content then declines to a lower steady-state level. When the study is performed in the absence of an initial transmembrane Na^+ gradient, the initial rate of uptake is slower and no "overshoot" of $[^{14}C]AA$ is seen.

These results and those of several other types of investigations have been used to support a model of AA transport by polarized epithelia originally presented by Crane (30). As applied to intestine, dietary vitamin C is consumed in foods that have a protective coating that shields the substance from light and atmospheric oxygen. The low pH of the gastric lumen also provides protection. The ease with which this vitamin is oxidized is discussed in preceding chapters of this text.

Upon reaching the proximal small intestine, AA is available for transport on the brush border carrier. In that the cellular content is normally maintained low in Na^+ by the Na^+,K^+-ATPase, a driving force exists for coupled cotransport of ascorbate and Na^+ into the cell. This continues until virtually all ascorbate is removed from the chyme, at which point a driving force exists in the form of a concentration gradient for ascorbate to diffuse across the basolateral cell membrane into the circulation. This latter process is brought about by a Na^+-independent carrier-mediated process. By this combination of events, dietary ascorbate is protected and absorbed; in this way it is made available not only to the intestinal mucosa for protection, for example, against dietary carcinogens, but also to all other components of the body.

Although most vitamin C in the primate diet is in the reduced form of the molecule, it is probably significant that transport mechanisms are present in both the brush border and basolateral membranes for uptake of the oxidized molecule DHAA (31). It appears likely that the brush border transporter functions to bring about the small amount of DHAA present in freshly harvested fruits and vegetables. More DHAA is present in foods that have been processed prior to consumption, especially by cooking.

The enterocyte is characteristic of several cell types that take up DHAA, often by unknown cellular mechanisms, and quickly reduce it. No consensus exists on the cellular mechanism of reduction, which possibly indicates that redundant processes contribute and these processes might differ among various cell types. Direct chemical reduction, as by interaction with glutathione, is considered to occur, especially in the ocular lens (discussed later). However, the intestine is characteristic of several tissues that show evidence of enzyme-mediated DHAA reduction. This entire question remains controversial (17,32).

A synopsis of one study is included here. Briefly, the small or large intestine of guinea pigs or rats (33) was obtained fresh and stripped of musculature. The mucosa was homogenized in buffer at a physiological pH. The homogenate was centrifuged and the supernatant was typically dialyzed overnight to remove low-molecular-weight compounds. The resulting supernatant was fractionated by ammonium sulfate precipitation; the 55–70% saturated fraction had most activity and was used in studies. This was dialyzed to remove ammonium sulfate. The resulting activity was processed through a Sephadex G-100 column. The tissue factor active in regenerating AA from DHAA is intermediate in size between cytochrome c and blue dextran. The assay for DHAA-reductase activity consisted of a 10 min incubation of the active preparation in the presence of ^{14}C-labeled or nonlabeled AA at 23°C with various combinations of reducing cofactors that might promote DHAA-reductase activity. Results indicated that intestinal mucosa reduces DHAA by a cytoplasmic enzyme that uses NADPH as a hydrogen donor.

The significance of these findings is not altogether clear. The intracellular concentration of DHAA in mucosa is maintained very low. Furthermore, in vitro uptake of DHAA was more rapid across the serosal surface of intestine than across the luminal surface (4). Thus, we speculated that DHAA is taken up from plasma into intestinal mucosa, reduced, and returned to the circulation as AA.

To the extent that AA acts as an antioxidant in the primate or guinea pig body, the need for a dietary source of it will vary with the animal's current need for protection against free radical species. Thus, the possibility was evaluated that the intestinal transport mechanism described might be regulated to adjust for the recent history of AA intake or consumption (34). The unidirectional influx of AA across the brush border into epithelial cells of guinea pig ileum was determined in vitro. Influx was reduced ~50% by supplementing the diet with 5 or 25 times the normal dose of AA. The rate of AA transport was also reduced by intramuscular administration of AA; that reduction suggests that the transport mechanism might respond to circulating levels of the vitamin. Aspects of this study were repeated, with similar conclusions (35).

Kidney

The kidney, like the intestine, has its own need for AA protection against reactive oxygen metabolites, such as renal disease or reperfusion injury. However, the kidney is a second example of an organ that processes many times more AA than it needs for its own use. In that AA is of low molecular weight and not bound to plasma proteins, it is filtered in the mammalian glomerulus. In the absence of a mechanism for reabsorption of filtered AA, the body would be effectively drained of the substance within a few hours.

The kidney and the intestine have very similar functions in terms of handling several organic substrates. The common feature is that they both are polarized transporting epithelia that serve to remove AA from the lumen of a physiological tube (intestine or renal tubule) and return it to the general circulation. Thus, the model of transport for reduced vitamin C in Figure 2 is also considered to be applicable to the kidney. This conclusion is based on studies in vesicles made from the brush border membrane of kidney cortex from rat, rabbit, and guinea pig tissue (36). Na^+-dependent uptake was shown with a K_m of ~0.2 mM ascorbate.

Metabolism of the oxidized form of vitamin C in kidney and intestine is also similar. Thus, a factor necessary for reduction of DHAA in renal cortex was found in the 55–70% ammonium sulfate fraction. It is retained by 12,000 molecular weight dialysis tubing; is heat-labile, pH-sensitive, and inhibited by thiol reagents; and has maximal reducing activity in the presence of NADPH and glutathione. It has a molecular weight similar to that of the intestinal preparation (37).

Intestinal AA transport in primates and guinea pigs has numerous similarities with AA transport in the kidney of several species. This appears to represent conservation of genetic material by using the same protein carrier in kidney as in intestine. Progress has recently

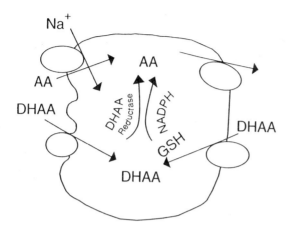

Figure 2 A summary of the transport and metabolic characteristics of animal cells: Some cells are polarized and bring about net vitamin C transport; the wavy border on the left represents the apical cell membrane of examples such as renal tubular reabsorptive cells and intestinal absorptive cells. Transport is brought about by the familiar secondary active transport process that moves ascorbic acid into the cytoplasm as Na^+ diffuses down its electrochemical gradient. A Na^+-independent carrier moves oxidized vitamin C (dehydro-L-ascorbic acid (DHAA)) into the cell by facilitated diffusion. DHAA is reduced either by direct chemical action of GSH or by an enzymatic process that makes use of GSH and/or NADPH as reducing factors. Astroglial cells of the brain, osteoblasts, and microvascular endothelial cells in culture are characterized also by having concentrative Na^+-dependent transport; in glial astrocytes this is blocked by classic anion transport inhibitors. Some nonpolarized cells such as the erythrocyte and lymphocyte preferentially take up DHAA and reduce it. This is also true for the polarized corneal endothelium, the human placental syncytiotrophoblast, and transport cells of the lacrimal gland. Exit of ascorbic acid from cells has been more difficult to study than the uptake process, but evidence exists in several systems for participation of a cell membrane carrier or channel. DHAA, dehydro-L-ascorbic acid; GSH, glutathione; NADPH, reduced nicotinamide-adenine dinucleotide phosphate.

been made in understanding the molecular nature of the ascorbate transport system through the strategy of expression cloning using *Xenopus* spp. oocytes (6). Cells were microinjected with poly(A)$^+$ RNA extracted from rabbit kidney cortex. Size fractionation of the cortex messenger RNA (mRNA) by sucrose gradient revealed that the active mRNA had a size of about 2.0 kilobases. Injection of this into the oocyte resulted in a >40-fold increase in ascorbate uptake. The expressed ascorbate transport properties included Na^+ dependence, substrate specificity, and saturation kinetics (K_m of 258 μM). This suggests that the transporter is derived from the brush border membrane of renal reabsorptive cells. The major importance of this study is that it provides evidence for the existence of Na^+-ascorbate cotransporter proteins.

Placenta

The placenta is considered a service organ along with intestine and kidney because it delivers AA and other nutrients from the maternal circulation to the fetus. It might also have a role in clearing DHAA from maternal blood. We currently consider only the human placenta because experimental animals have placentas with notably different histological and functional properties. Ascorbate present in incubation medium at a physiological concentration is taken up into surviving fragments of placenta by an energy-dependent and saturable process (38). Energy for the transport process came from either glycolysis or oxidative phosphorylation. Sodium and Na^+,K^+-ATPase activity was required for ascorbate uptake.

A possible role of Na^+-independent facilitative hexose (monosaccharide) transporters was investigated in vitamin C uptake by membrane vesicles made from the maternal surface of the placental syncytiotrophoblast (39). Oxidized vitamin C was taken up much more rapidly than the reduced form. It was convincingly shown that extravesicular DHAA and 3-O-methyl glucose at concentrations >2 mM blocked the uptake of each other with indistinguishable inhibitory constants (39). Thus, it seems unlikely that DHAA enters the placenta by facilitative hexose transporters under physiological conditions. The constant presence of 5–10 mM glucose in plasma and extracellular fluid would be expected to saturate hexose carriers, so that DHAA present at much lower concentrations would find little opportunity for transport.

The uptake and metabolism of AA and DHAA were reexamined in surviving fragments of placenta in vitro (40). This was done at a low extracellular concentration of radiolabeled vitamin C (10 μM) to evaluate whether a carrier that transports the vitamin at physiological concentration by a glucose-independent mechanism is present. It was confirmed that [^{14}C]DHAA is preferentially transported, compared to [^{14}C]AA. Most of the label in the tissue was present in the reduced form. From an evaluation of the radiolabeled molecules in the bath, it was concluded that ~25% of [^{14}C]AA formed by the tissue is released within 15 min. Uptake was dependent on intact cellular metabolic energy, but was not affected by the presence of Na^+ or glucose. It is concluded that the placenta helps to clear the toxic (oxidized) form of vitamin C from the blood and delivers the useful (reduced) form to the fetus.

Astroglial Syncytia in Brain

That mental depression is an early symptom of scurvy (41) indicates the importance of maintaining physiological levels of vitamin C in the central nervous system (CNS). Ascorbic acid is highly concentrated in the intracellular compartment of brain. In rat brain, for example, basal concentrations of the molecule are approximately 200 μM in extracellular fluid and average 10-fold higher in the intracellular compartment (42). Subcellular fractionation indicates that most cerebral AA is localized to the soluble cytosol fraction, with smaller amounts found in mitochondrial and nuclear fractions (43). It is not known whether various types of brain cells differ in their steady-state intracellular concentrations of AA.

Glial astrocytes are the most numerous cell type in mature brain. They participate in the regulation of extracellular ion concentrations, the formation of extracellular matrix, and the synthesis and clearance of transmitters and growth factors. These cells are extensively coupled to each other by gap junctions, forming astroglial syncytia both in vivo and in cell culture (44). It is not known whether ascorbate permeates gap junctions, but it is similar in molecular weight and charge to substrates, such as glucose-6-phosphate, which do pass from cell to cell through the junctions.

The characteristics of astroglial AA transport activity and the relationship between transport and intracellular AA concentration have been elucidated in cerebral astrocytes cultured from chicken, mouse, and rat brains. These cells cannot synthesize AA de novo (i.e., from glucose) but possess a concentrative ascorbate uptake system (7,10,45–49). This system is specific because glucose and organic acids (acetate, formate, lactate, malonate, oxalate, p-aminohippurate, pyruvate, and succinate) do not compete with ascorbate for uptake. Moreover, astroglial transport is stereoselective for L-ascorbate over D-isoascorbate. Uptake requires external Na^+. Kinetic experiments revealed an apparent K_m of 30 μM ascorbate in the presence of physiological Na^+ concentrations. Affinity for ascorbate is significantly decreased when the extracellular Na^+ concentration was lowered, indicating that Na^+ and ascorbate interact with the same transporter. Na^+-dependent [^{14}C]ascorbate uptake can be reversibly blocked by the anion transport inhibitors furosemide, 4-acetamido-4-4′-isothiocyanostilbene-2,2′-disulfonic acid (SITS) and 4,4′-diisothiocyanostilbene-2,2′-disulfonic acid (DIDS). The latter is an impermeant drug, so its inhibitory effect indicates the ascorbate transporter is located in the plasma membrane.

Astrocytes accumulate high concentrations of AA (~10 mM) when incubated with medium containing the vitamin at a level (200 μM) typical of brain extracellular fluid (23,45). Like initial rate of [^{14}C]ascorbate uptake, maintenance of cell ascorbate concentration at steady state depends on extracellular Na^+ and is sensitive to anion transport inhibitors. Taken together, these results provide extensive evidence that Na^+-ascorbate cotransporters located in the plasma membrane function to concentrate ascorbate in astrocytes.

Na^+-ascorbate cotransport activity in astrocytes is altered by several factors, including intracellular ascorbate, cyclic adenosine monophosphate (AMP), membrane depolarization, and cell swelling. For example, the rate of ascorbate influx into astrocytes slows as intracellular ascorbate concentration increases (49). This is an example of autoregulation of transport activity by the substrate ascorbate. The existence of this autoregulatory phenomenon suggests that, in the absence of neural or paracrine signals, Na^+-ascorbate cotransport activity tends to maintain intracellular ascorbate concentration at a constant value.

Astrocytes respond to transmitters and paracrine factors through receptors coupled to second messenger systems. For example, norepinephrine acts through β-adrenergic receptors to increase cyclic AMP concentration within astrocytes. Activation of cyclic AMP-dependent mechanisms changes astrocyte structure from polygonal to stellate (process-bearing) (45). This cyclic AMP-stimulated astroglial differentiation is associated with increased Na^+-ascorbate cotransport activity (7) and elevated intracellular ascorbate concentration at steady state (45).

Transient elevation of glutamate in brain extracellular fluid is associated with large increases in extracellular ascorbate (42). It has been suggested that glutamate uptake into brain cells is linked to ascorbate efflux through a heteroexchange transporter and that this is a mechanism which limits glutamate's receptor-mediated, excitotoxic effects on neurons (42,50). Astrocytes may be the sites of linked ascorbate and glutamate transmembrane fluxes, since both anions are stored at millimolar concentrations in astroglial cytoplasm. However, instead of the putative glutamate/ascorbate heteroexchanger, the apparent countertransport may result from the astroglial swelling and depolarization caused by glutamate uptake through the electrogenic Na^+-glutamate cotransporter. In this regard, osmotic cell swelling (23) and depolarizing agents (10) markedly inhibit ascorbate uptake by astrocytes. Moreover, osmotic swelling of cerebral astrocytes reversibly activates an ascorbate efflux pathway.

Swelling-induced ascorbate efflux is inhibited by the anion transport inhibitors, DIDS and 4,4′-dinitrostilbene-2,2′-disulfonic acid (DNDS). The pathway for ascorbate efflux is selective because a larger anion, 2′,7′-bis(carboxyethyl)-5(or-6)-carboxyfluorescein, is retained in the swollen astrocytes. Efflux appears to occur through volume-regulated anion channels which allow most intracellular ascorbate to be released within a few minutes of the onset of cell swelling (23). Many pathological conditions cause brain cell swelling and formation of reactive oxygen species. Ascorbate release during astroglial swelling may contribute to cellular osmoregulation and scavenging of reactive oxygen species.

Blood Vessels

Blood vessels require vitamin C in order to remain healthy. Ascorbic acid increases expression of endothelial markers and production of basement membrane proteins, while decreasing the permeability to macromolecules of monolayer endothelial cell cultures (51). Defective metabolism of vitamin C is associated with diabetic microangiopathy and capillary fragility.

The pathways by which vitamin C enters endothelial cells have been investigated using cell culture techniques. Experiments with a cell line derived from fetal bovine heart endothelium indicated that uptake of [^{14}C]vitamin C was inhibited by glucose (52). However, the incubation conditions employed may have allowed extensive oxidation of AA to DHAA in the medium, followed by cellular uptake of DHAA through glucose-sensitive facilitative hexose transporters. Corneal endothelial cells have been shown to take up DHAA and rapidly reduce it to AA (53) (see the section, The Eye). When AA oxidation is minimized, vitamin C uptake by endothelial cells is Na$^+$-dependent and glucose-insensitive. In microvascular endothelial cell cultures, intracellular ascorbate concentration can reach ~15 mM after incubation with a physiological concentration of extracellular ascorbate, as a result of Na$^+$-ascorbate cotransport activity (54).

VITAMIN C TRANSPORT IN ORGANS AND TISSUES OF CONSUMPTION

The Eye

Many organs or tissues provide little antioxidative protection to the rest of the body but derive important protection for themselves. A complex example is the eye. No organ of the body is more vulnerable to damage by reactive oxygen species. All components of the eye are subject to damage by solar radiation that is never experienced by other tissues of the body; thus, stratospheric ozone depletion is expected to be more damaging to the eye than to any other organ. Abrasion from sandstorms is an immediate threat to the eye. The cornea is unique in lacking a dermal covering for protection against atmospheric oxygen. Toxic actions of environmental chemicals thus affect the cornea much more rapidly than the stomach or heart. The retina is threatened by the high rate of oxygen consumption that promotes vision.

Antioxidant protection in the eye begins with production of aqueous humor by the ciliary body. This is the nutritive fluid of tissues in the anterior chamber, similar to blood in the rest of the body. Ascorbate is the primary water-soluble antioxidant described in texts on the eye (55). It is present in many animal species at a concentration up to 20 times that of plasma. Other species have little or no ascorbate in their aqueous humor. The difference between these groups is in their behavioral characteristics: diurnal animals have ocular ascorbate whereas nocturnal animals do not (56). The inference is that AA protects against radiation. The role of AA in protecting against ocular free radical damage has been reviewed from a comparative physiological perspective (57).

In the aqueous humor AA may have a function in protecting surrounding tissues from radiation damage. The ratios of lens/aqueous ascorbate concentrations ranged from 0.44 in the rabbit to 2.6 in the horse. Values of 1.0–2.0 are common for humans. A ~60 mV electrical potential difference is measured between fiber and aqueous humor, with lens interior negative. Because ascorbate is a monovalent anion at physiological pH, an active transport process is necessary to maintain the lens ascorbate concentration even 50% as high as the aqueous level. This could be brought about by transport through polarized cuboidal cells of the lens epithelium. The rate of entry of ascorbate into the epithelium is over 20 times greater than for L-glucose (the nontransported stereoisomer of D-glucose). Thus, a specific transport mechanism is anticipated, although its preferred form of vitamin C has not been determined.

In the aqueous humor AA might also have a function in protecting cornea. The properties of vitamin C uptake and metabolism in bovine corneal endothelial cells grown in culture have been evaluated (53). Dehydro-L-ascorbic acid was taken up approximately sevenfold more rapidly than was ascorbate. After a 30 s incubation with [^{14}C]DHAA, most labeled molecules in the cells were [^{14}C]AA. Corneal endothelium has transport and metabolic capacities to extract DHAA from aqueous humor and reduce it. This would help to maintain corneal vitamin C in the reduced state.

A review of corneal histological characteristics leaves one with the impression that although aqueous humor might be a good source for getting AA to the corneal endothelium, it probably is an unlikely source of AA for the corneal epithelium located at the anterior surface of the tissue. This is because the corneal stroma is quite thick and consists of nonpolarized cells that cannot promote net directional transport of AA. Thus, in the event of damage to the anterior surface of the eye through radiation, environmental chemicals, abrasion, or oxygen toxicity, the supply of AA by this path would have to depend on simple diffusion, which is a slow process. Threats to the epithelium might be met more quickly if there were a fluid with AA content that could be secreted directly onto this cell layer. Tear fluid is a candidate.

An unconfirmed report from the 1940s indicates tear fluid has high ascorbate content; no information on transport or metabolism of the lacrimal gland itself has been provided (58). Pig lacrimal glands were recently obtained from a local abattoir, washed in buffer, and sliced into thin sections (59). These were incubated in buffer in the presence of <12 μM ^{14}C-labeled ascorbate or DHAA. The oxidized molecule was taken up most rapidly. Carbon-14 label recovered from the tissue was at least 75% in the reduced form after incubation with either substrate. Uptake of ascorbate, but not DHAA, was blocked by the presence of nonlabeled ascorbate in the bath. It appears that the lacrimal gland provides a service to both the blood and the eye by taking DHAA from the circulation, reducing it, and delivering the product to the anterior surface of the eye.

Not all light rays that enter the eye reach the retina. Some photons interact with membranes of the cornea or lens. Other radiation interacts with water or various components of aqueous and vitreous humor. The reactive oxygen species thus generated may be scavenged by vitamin E in membranes or by water-soluble antioxidants in aqueous components of the eye. Albert Szent-Györgyi (60) made a bold prediction in the 1920s that his newly discovered hexuronic acid "might play a role in the oxidation mechanism of all animal tissues." This statement most certainly appears to apply to tissues of the eye.

Water-soluble antioxidants of the eye have recently been evaluated by high-performance liquid chromatography with electrochemical detection. Significant amounts of AA (0.73 μM), cysteine (0.12 μM), glutathione (14 μM), uric acid (41 μM), and tyrosine (100 μM) were found in human and rabbit aqueous humor (Richer and Rose, submitted). A possible significance of the presence of AA along with other antioxidants is the concept of a "pecking order" of scavengers, reviewed by Buettner (61). As this applies to the eye, the various antioxidants present might each scavenge a particular type of free radical. On the basis of one electron reduction potentials, AA is expected to maintain vitamin E and several of the other water-soluble antioxidants in the reduced state. A notable exception would appear to occur in the lens. Here the high concentration of glutathione is thought to bring about reduction of the low concentration of DHAA, simply by mass action.

The possibility that regeneration of DHAA is brought about by an enzyme that makes use of reducing cofactors such as NADPH and/or glutathione has been brought up in the literature for 30 years (62). This subject was reviewed recently (17). There are indications that several tissues of the body, including those of the eye (except lens), have a proteinlike substance that promotes regeneration of AA from DHAA. Such a substance was extracted from a homogenate of bovine iris-ciliary body by ammonium sulfate precipitation, with the primary activity appearing in the 50–75% ammonium sulfate fraction (63). Saturation kinetics of reduction are seen, with the activity being dependent on protein concentration, DHAA concentration, and glutathione concentration. The activity is sensitive to pH, high temperature, and digestion by trypsin. Activity is greatest in the presence of both gluta-thione and NADPH.

An enzyme with these or similar properties has been suggested to exist in erythrocytes (62), liver (62), intestine (33), brain (64,65), placenta (40), and several ocular tissues (66). Other investigators have not found evidence of enzyme participation. In these latter instances, however, it must be recalled that inappropriate assay conditions or loss of enzyme activity during tissue processing can lead investigators to overlook the participation of an enzyme.

Even among those who believe that AA recycling occurs enzymatically, there is no consensus about the properties or the identity of the enzyme. Activity of the known enzyme thioltransferase in reducing DHAA is documented (32). The issue remains as to how much of the DHAA-reductase activity in any particular tissue can be attributed to thioltransferase. The most recent and complete attempt at isolation and characterization of DHAA-reductase was made by an Italian group (67). A factor in rat liver cytosol was purified with an overall recovery of 27%; it required NADPH for activity. SDS-PAGE and gel filtration indicated a protein with an M_r of ~38,000; this is clearly larger than thioltransferase. The K_m for DHAA was 4.6 mM and for NADPH, 4.3 μM. Internal primary structure data identified the NADPH-dependent DHAA reductase as 3α-hydroxysteroid dehydrogenase. An additional glutathione-dependent DHAA reductase was purified by the same research group (68). The presence of at least three enzymatic pathways for catalyzing the recycling of cytoplasmic AA suggests it is of great physiological importance.

Blood Components

A great deal of the earliest work on vitamin C transport was performed on blood compo-nents. This was exceedingly important in laying the basis for more recent work on additional tissue and cell preparations. However, the methodology was not highly developed and consequently some of the major conclusions are suspect. Because of space limitations, this chapter focuses on more recent material.

Energy-dependent transport of vitamin C occurs in PML in vitro over a physiological range of vitamin C concentration (69). An AA concentration gradient is maintained with the intracellular level >10-fold the extracellular level. The uptake of vitamin C is competitively inhibited by glucose but not by fructose or galactose. The Ki for inhibition by glucose is 3.7 mM. It is concluded that granulocytes take up vitamin C by the same transport system as for glucose. The question of whether the millimolar concentration of glucose normally present in plasma provokes a local AA deficiency in leukocytes has not been addressed. It would also be of interest to know whether the energy dependence of vitamin C transport in these cells is associated with ascorbate uptake or DHAA reduction.

Elevated levels of both AA and DHAA are seen in lymphocytes of chronic lymphocytic leukemia (CLL) patients. The characteristics of DHAA uptake into lymphocytes of control subjects and CLL patients were compared. Kinetic evaluations indicated similar K_m values for DHAA uptake. However, the maximum velocity of DHAA uptake in normal cells was much greater than in CLL cells (70). That lymphocytes of CLL patients have a slower DHAA uptake but higher intracellular DHAA concentration than found in control subjects may indicate impaired reduction in CLL cells. Taken together, these findings suggest that differences in transport or metabolism of vitamin C contribute to the characteristics of these cells in disease.

Ascorbic acid is involved in the respiratory burst generated by human neutrophils for bacterial killing. At that time, vitamin C accumulates in neutrophils to as high as 10-fold the normal level. Levine and coworkers (71) hypothesized that extracellular AA is oxidized to DHAA, which is then transported into the neutrophil and reduced to the protective form of the molecule. If this is true, any mechanism of oxidizing AA should increase cellular AA. To test this, unstimulated neutrophils were incubated with 200 μM AA and the radical generating system xanthine/xanthine oxidase. Intracellular AA increased approximately fourfold more than cells incubated in AA without the oxidase enzyme. In additional studies (72), vitamin C uptake was seen to be dependent on the presence of calcium and magnesium in the bathing medium.

Accumulation of intracellular AA from extracellular DHAA occurs in human erythrocytes (73). These cells seem to lack a Na^+-ascorbate cotransporter and their processes of DHAA uptake and reduction are not affected by the anion transport inhibitor DIDS (73). Interestingly, the presence of DHAA uptake and reduction activities in human erythrocytes and erythrocyte ghosts leads to accumulation of ascorbate, but the steady-state internal ascorbate concentration is the same as the extracellular ascorbate concentration (25–100 μM) (28,73). Intracellular ascorbate concentration may be limited by the absence of a plasma membrane Na^+-ascorbate cotransporter and by inability of these cells to generate large amounts of reducing equivalents metabolically for DHAA reduction. Vitamin C must be kept reduced if it is to be trapped at high concentrations in the cytoplasm. As evidence of this requirement, it has been observed that oxidation of intracellular AA in human erythrocytes increases vitamin C efflux (28).

Mesenchymal Tissues

Ascorbic acid stimulates osteoblasts and myoblasts to produce a collagenous extracellular matrix and terminally differentiate. Rate of hydroxyproline synthesis (an indicator of collagen synthesis) and induction of alkaline phosphatase (a marker of cellular differentiation) both correlate with intracellular concentration of AA, indicating that the vitamin acts intracellularly to accelerate cell phenotype expression (5).

A specific ascorbate uptake system has been characterized in bone-derived, osteoblastic cells. Ascorbate enters osteoblasts by a Na^+-ascorbate cotransporter which can concentrate intracellular ascorbate 100-fold relative to the extracellular level (5,8,74–77). The cotransporter is stereoselective for L-ascorbate (apparent $K_m = 30$ µM) over the epimer, D-isoascorbate (apparent $K_m = 600$ µM), with the result that the steady-state intracellular concentration of ascorbate (9–11 mM) exceeds that of D-isoascorbic acid (5–7 mM) when cells are incubated with 0.1 mM extracellular ascorbate or D-isoascorbate (5). Ascorbate uptake does not involve facilitative hexose transporters since it is not acutely affected by agents which interact with hexose transporters, such as glucose, 2-deoxyglucose, or cytochalasin B. However, Na^+-ascorbate cotransport activity is regulated by ascorbate itself in that increasing intracellular ascorbate concentration slows uptake (77).

Paracrine factors of the transforming growth factor-β (TGF-β)/bone morphogenetic protein superfamily are modulators of osteoblast differentiation and potent stimulators of bone formation. Osteoblastic Na^+-ascorbate cotransport is stimulated by TGF-β (75), and the resulting increase in intracellular ascorbate concentration (76) may contribute to the paracrine factor's differentiating effects.

Stimulation of TGF-β of ascorbate transport in osteoblasts involves an increase in the maximum velocity of uptake without change in the apparent K_m of the cotransporter for the vitamin (75). A lack of effect on apparent K_m suggests that TGF-β has not changed the affinity of the transport process and is consistent with no change in the molecular identity of the transporter. Additional information aids in interpreting these kinetic results. For example, stimulation requires at least 6 h of exposure to the growth factor and is abolished by the protein synthesis inhibitor cycloheximide. Similarly, cycloheximide prevents the stimulatory effect of TGF-β on cellular steady-state ascorbate concentration (76). Taken together, these results suggest that TGF-β increases the rate of synthesis of either new Na^+-ascorbate cotransporters or regulatory proteins that interact with existing transporters to increase their turnover number.

CONCLUSIONS

Both the oxidized and reduced forms of vitamin C are transported by cells. Dehydro-L-ascorbic acid can be taken into cells by facilitated diffusion. The combination of DHAA uptake and reduction can rapidly elevate intracellular AA concentration. This process may require metabolic energy to provide the reducing equivalents which convert DHAA to AA. Both glucose-insensitive carriers and facilitative hexose transporters have been shown to mediate DHAA transport under experimental conditions. It is not clear to what extent facilitative hexose transporters contribute to DHAA uptake under physiological conditions when millimolar concentrations of glucose compete for micromolar DHAA concentrations at the uptake sites.

Many cells take up ascorbate through Na^+-ascorbate cotransport systems. These systems typically have apparent K_m for L-ascorbate of 20–30 µM and function by energy-requiring, secondary active transport to raise intracellular ascorbate concentration to millimolar levels. Ascorbate may subsequently exit cells passively through anion channels or other diffusion pathways. Ascorbate uptake and efflux pathways are regulated by ascorbate itself, paracrine factors, intracellular second messengers, membrane potential, and cell volume.

REFERENCES

1. Rose RC, Bode AM. Biology of free radical scavengers: an evaluation of ascorbate. FASEB J 1993; 7:1135–1142.
2. Lohmann W, Winzenburg J. Structure of ascorbic acid and its biological function. V. Transport of ascorbate and isoascorbate across artificial membranes as studied by the spin label technique. Z Naturforsch 1983; 38c:923–925.
3. Rose RC. Solubility properties of reduced and oxidized ascorbate as determinants of membrane permeation. Biochim Biophys Acta 1987; 924:254–256.
4. Rose RC, Choi J-L. Intestinal absorption and metabolism of ascorbic acid in rainbow trout. Am J Physiol 1990; 258:R1238–R1241.
5. Franceschi RT, Wilson JX, Dixon SJ. Requirement for Na$^+$-dependent ascorbic acid transport in osteoblast function. Am J Physiol 1995; 268:C1430–C1439.
6. Dyer DL, Kanai Y, Hediger MA, et al. Expression of a rabbit renal ascorbic acid transporter in *Xenopus laevis* oocytes. Am J Physiol 1994; 267:C301–C306.
7. Wilson JX. Ascorbic acid uptake by a high-affinity sodium-dependent mechanism in cultured rat astrocytes. J Neurochem 1989; 53:1064–1071.
8. Wilson JX, Dixon SJ. High-affinity sodium-dependent uptake of ascorbic acid by rat osteoblasts. J Membrane Biol 1989; 111:83–91.
9. Helbig H, Korbmacher C, Wohlfarth J, et al. Electrogenic Na+-ascorbate cotransport in cultured bovine pigmented ciliary epithelial cells. Am J Physiol 1989; 256:C44–C49.
10. Wilson JX, Jaworski EM, Dixon, SJ. Evidence for electrogenic sodium-dependent ascorbate transport in rat astroglia. Neurochem Res 1991; 16:73–78.
11. Chen X, Coady MJ, Jackson F, et al. Thermodynamic determination of the Na$^+$:glucose coupling ratio for the human SGLT1 cotransporter. Biophys J 1995; 69:2405–2414.
12. Bennett E, Kimmich GA. Na+-binding to the Na+-glucose cotransporter is potential dependent. Am J Physiol 1995; 262:C510–C516.
13. Zhou A, Matsumoto T, Farver O, Thorn NA. Uptake of ascorbic acid by freshly isolated cells and secretory granules from the intermediate lobe of ox hypophyses. Acta Physiol Scand 1990; 138:229–234.
14. Bianchi J, Rose RC. Dehydroascorbic acid and cell membranes: possible disruptive effects. Toxicology 1986; 40:75–82.
15. Rose RC, Choi J-L, Bode AM. Short term effects of oxidized ascorbic acid on bovine corneal endothelium and human placenta. Life Sci 1992; 50:1543–1549.
16. Wang Y-H, Dhariwal KR, Levine M. Ascorbic acid bioavailability in humans: ascorbic acid in plasma, serum, and urine. Ann NY Acad Sci 1992; 669:383–385.
17. Rose RC, Bode AM. Tissue mediated regeneration of ascorbic acid: is the process enzymatic? Enzyme 1992; 46:196–203.
18. Vera JC, Rivas CI, Fischbarg J, Golde DW. Mammalian facilitative hexose transporters mediate the transport of dehydroascorbic acid. Nature 1993; 364:79–82.
19. Vera JC, Rivas CI, Velasquez FV, et al. Resolution of the facilitated transport of dehydroascorbic acid from its intracellular accumulation as ascorbic acid. J Biol Chem 1995; 270:23706–23712.
20. Cloherty EK, Sultzman LA, Zottola RJ, Carruthers A. Net sugar transport is a multistep process: evidence for cytosolic sugar binding sites in erythrocytes. Biochemistry 1995; 34:15395–15406.
21. Cunningham JJ. Altered vitamin C transport in diabetes mellitus. Med Hypotheses 1988; 26:263–265.
22. Fay MJ, Bush MJ, Verlangieri AJ. Effects of cytochalasin B on the uptake of ascorbic acid and glucose by 3T3 fibroblasts: mechanism of impaired ascorbate transport in diabetes. Life Sci 1990; 46:619–624.
23. Siushansian R, Wilson JX, Dixon SJ. Osmotic swelling stimulates ascorbate efflux from cerebral astrocytes. J Neurochem 1996; 66:1227–1233.

24. Diliberto EJ, Menniti FS, Knoth J, et al. Adrenomedullary chromaffin cells as a model to study the neurobiology of ascorbic acid: from monooxygenation to neuromodulation. Ann NY Acad Sci 1987; 498:28–53.

25. Khatami M, Stramm LE, Rockey JH. Ascorbate transport in cultured rat retinal pigment epithelial cells. Exp Eye Res 1986; 43:607–615.

26. Socci RR, Delamere NA. Characteristics of ascorbate transport in the rabbit iris-ciliary body. Exp Eye Res 1988; 46:853–861.

27. Finn FM, Johns PA. Ascorbic acid transport by isolated bovine adrenal cortical cells. Endocrinology 1980; 106:811–817.

28. May JM, Qu Z, Whitesell RR. Ascorbate is the major electron donor for a transmembrane oxidoreductase of human erythrocytes. Biochim Biophys Acta 1995; 1238:127–136.

29. Rose RC. Water-soluble vitamin absorption and transport. In: EMM Quigley, MN Marsh, eds. The Small Intestine.

30. Crane RK. Hypothesis for mechanism of intestinal active transport of sugars. Fed Proc 1962; 21:891.

31. Bianchi J, Wilson FA, Rose RC. Dehydroascorbic acid and ascorbic acid transport in the guinea pig ileum. Am J Physiol 1986; 250:G461–G468.

32. Wells WW, Xu DP, Yang Y, Rocque PA. Mammalian thioltransferase glutaredoxin and protein disulfide isomerase have dehydroascorbate reductase activity. J Biol Chem 1990; 265:15361–15364.

33. Choi J-L, Rose RC. Regeneration of ascorbic acid by rat colon. Proc Soc Exp Biol Med 1989; 190:369–378.

34. Rose RC, Nahrwold DL. Intestinal ascorbic acid transport following diets of high or low ascorbic acid content. J Vitamin Nutr Res 1978; 48:382–386.

35. Karasov WH, Darken BW, Bottum MC. Dietary regulation of intestinal ascorbate uptake in guinea pigs. Am J Physiol 1991; 260:G108–G118.

36. Toggenburger G, Hausermann M, Mutsch B, et al. Na^+-dependent, potential-sensitive L-ascorbate transport across brush border membrane vesicles from kidney cortex. Biochim Biophys Acta 1981; 646:422–443.

37. Rose RC. Renal metabolism of the oxidized form of ascorbic acid (dehydro-L-ascorbic acid). Am J Physiol 1989; 256:F52–F56.

38. Streeter ML, Rosso P. Transport mechanisms for ascorbic acid in the human placenta. Am J Clin Nutr 1981; 34:1706–1711.

39. Ingermann RL, Stankove L, Bigley RH. Role of monosaccharide transporter in vitamin C uptake by placental membrane vesicles. Am J Physiol 1986; 250:C637–C641.

40. Choi J-L, Rose RC. Transport and metabolism of ascorbic acid in human placenta. Am J Physiol 1989; 257:C110–C113.

41. Hodges RE, Hood J, Canham JE, et al. Clinical manifestations of ascorbic acid deficiency in man. Am J Clin Nutr 1971; 24:432–443.

42. Grünewald RA. Ascorbic acid in the brain. Brain Res Rev 1993; 18:123–133.

43. Vatassery GT, Smith WE, Ouach HT. Distribution of vitamins C and E in subcellular fractions from rat brains. FASEB J 1994; 8:A8621.

44. Naus CCG, Bechberger JF, Caveney S, Wilson JX. Expression of gap junction genes in astrocytes and C6 glioma cells. Neurosci Lett 1991; 126:33–36.

45. Siushansian R, Wilson JX. Ascorbate transport and intracellular concentration in cerebral astrocytes. J Neurochem 1995; 65:41–49.

46. Wilson JX, Jaworski EM. Effect of oxygen on ascorbic acid uptake and concentration in embryonic chick brain. Neurochem Res 1992; 17:571–576.

47. Wilson JX. Regulation of ascorbic acid concentration in embryonic chick brain. Dev Biol 1990; 139:292–298.

48. Wilson JX, Dixon SJ. Ascorbic acid transport in mouse and rat astrocytes is reversibly inhibited by furosemide, SITS and DIDS. Neurochem Res 1989: 14:1169–1175.

49. Wilson JX, Jaworski EM, Kulaga A, Dixon SJ. Substrate regulation of ascorbate transport activity in astrocytes. Neurochem Res 1990; 15:1037–1043.

50. Rebec GV, Pierce RC. A vitamin as a neuromodulator: ascorbate release into the extracellular fluid of the brain regulates dopaminergic and glutaminergic transmission. Prog Neurobiol 1994; 43:537–565.

51. Utoguchi N, Ikeda K, Saeki K, et al. Ascorbic acid stimulates barrier function of cultured endothelial cell monolayer. J Cell Physiol 1995; 163:393–399.

52. Kapeghian JC, Verlangieri AJ. The effects of glucose on ascorbic acid uptake in heart endothelial cells: possible pathogenesis of diabetic angiopathies. Life Sci 1984; 34:577–584.

53. Bode AM, Vanderpool SS, Carlson EC, et al. Ascorbic acid uptake and metabolism by corneal endothelium. Invest Ophthalmol Vis Sci 1991; 32:2266–2271.

54. Wilson JX, Dixon SJ, Yu J, et al. Ascorbate uptake by microvascular endothelial cells of rat skeletal muscle. Microcirculation 1996; 54:211–221.

55. Lentner C. 1981 Geigy Scientific Tables.

56. Reiss GR, Werness PG, Zollman PE, Brubaker RF. Ascorbic acid levels in the aqueous humor of nocturnal and diurnal mammals. Arch Ophthalmol 1986; 104:753–755.

57. Rose RC, Bode AM. Ocular ascorbate transport and metabolism. Comp Biochem Physiol 1991; 100A:273–285.

58. Herrmann H, Hickman F. Exploratory studies on corneal metabolism. Bull Johns Hopkins Hosp 1948; 82:225.

59. Dreyer R, Rose RC. Lacrimal gland uptake and metabolism of ascorbic acid. Proc Soc Exp Biol Med 1993; 202:212–216.

60. Szent-Gyorgyi A. Observations on the function of peroxidase systems and the chemistry of the adrenal cortex. Biochem J 1928; 22:1387–1409.

61. Buettner GR. The pecking order of free radicals and antioxidants: lipid peroxidation, a-tocopherol, and ascorbate. Arch Biochem Biophys 1993; 300:535–543.

62. Hughes RE. Reduction of dehydroascorbic acid by animal tissues. Nature 1964; 203:1068–1069.

63. Bode AM. Metabolism and content of ascorbic acid and glutathione in the eye. Invest Ophthalmol Vis Sci 1994; 35:2133.

64. Grimble RF, Hughes RE. A "dehydroascorbic acid reductase" factor in guinea-pig tissues. Experientia 1967; 23:362.

65. Rose RC. Cerebral metabolism of oxidized ascorbate. Brain Res 1993; 628:49–55.

66. Bode AM, Green E, Yavarow CR, et al. Ascorbic acid regeneration by bovine iris-ciliary body. Curr Eye Res 1993; 12:593–601.

67. Del Bello B, Maellaro E, Sugherini L, et al. Purification of NADPH-dependent dehydroascorbate reductase from rat liver and its identification with 3a-hydroxysteroid dehydrogenase. Biochem J 1994; 304:385–390.

68. Maellaro E, Del Bello B, Sugherini L, et al. Purification and characterization of glutathione-dependent dehydroascorbate reductase from rat liver. Biochem J 1994; 301:421–426.

69. Moser U, Weber F. Uptake of ascorbic acid by human granulocytes. Int J Vitam Nutr Res 1984; 54:47–53.

70. Stahl RL, Farber CM, Liebes LF, Silber R. Relationship of dehydroascorbic acid transport to cell lineage in lymphocytes from normal subjects and patients with chronic lymphocytic leukemia. Cancer Res 1985; 45:6507–6512.

71. Washko PW, Wang Y, Levine M. Ascorbic acid recycling in human neutrophils. J Biol Chem 1993; 268:15531–15535.

72. Washko P, Rotrosen D, Levine M. Ascorbic acid accumulation in plated human neutrophils. FEBS Lett 1990; 260:101–104.

73. Wagner ES, White W, Jennings M, Bennett K. The entrapment of [^{14}C]ascorbic acid in human erythrocytes. Biochim Biophys Acta 1987; 902:133–136.

74. Dixon SJ, Kulaga A, Jaworski EM, Wilson JX. Ascorbate uptake by ROS 17/2.8 osteoblast-like

cells: substrate specificity and sensitivity to transport inhibitors. J Bone Miner Res 1991; 6: 623–629.

75. Dixon SJ, Wilson JX. Transforming growth factor-β stimulates ascorbate transport activity in osteoblastic cells. Endocrinology 1992; 130:484–489.

76. Wilson JX, Dixon SJ. Ascorbate concentration in osteoblastic cells is elevated by transforming growth factor-β. Am J Physiol 1995; 268:E565–E571.

77. Dixon SJ, Wilson JX. Adaptive regulation of ascorbate transport in osteoblastic cells. J Bone Miner Res 1992; 7:675–681.

9

Vitamin C as an Antiatherogen: Mechanisms of Action

BALZ FREI

*Whitaker Cardiovascular Institute, Boston University School of Medicine,
Boston, Massachusetts*

INTRODUCTION

The Role of Low-Density Lipoprotein Oxidation in the Pathogenesis of Atherosclerosis

Atherosclerosis, with its clinical manifestations of angina pectoris, myocardial infarction, and ischemic stroke, is the single most important cause of morbidity and mortality in the Western world (1). The earliest stages of atherosclerotic lesion development are characterized by local accumulation of plasma proteins, particularly low-density lipoprotein (LDL), in the arterial wall at lesion-prone sites (2). This local accumulation of LDL may be due to increased permeability of the vascular endothelial lining overlying the lesion-prone arterial sites (2,3), and/or to increased retention of LDL in the arterial wall by binding to proteoglycans and possibly lipoprotein lipase (4). In addition to lipoproteins, monocytes are preferentially recruited to the lesion-prone arterial areas by attachment to the endothelium and guided migration into the subendothelium (3,5,6). The monocyte–endothelial interactions are triggered by localized activation of the endothelium to express specific cellular adhesion molecules that interact with counterreceptors present on the surface of circulating monocytes (2,7,8). Once in the arterial wall, the monocytes undergo activation and differentiation to become resident macrophages and then gradually may be converted to lipid-laden foam cells. Foam cells are the hallmark of the earliest atherosclerotic lesion, called the fatty streak.

Localized LDL in the subendothelial space is subject to oxidative modification by endothelial cells (9), smooth muscle cells (10), and resident monocyte-macrophages (11). Mildly oxidized LDL (usually referred to as minimally modified LDL [mm-LDL]) and fully oxidized LDL (ox-LDL) can contribute to atherosclerosis through many different mechanisms (Tables 1 and 2). For example, both mm-LDL and ox-LDL can cause monocyte recruitment to the arterial wall by stimulating monocyte–endothelial interactions (12–

Table 1   Biological Properties by Which Minimally Modified Low-Density
Lipoprotein Differs from Native Low-Density Lipoprotein

Effect of minimally modified low-density lipoprotein (Refs.)	Significance for atherosclerosis
• Stimulation of monocyte adhesion to the endothelium (12)	Monocyte recruitment into the arterial wall
• Induction of monocyte chemotactic peptide-1 (MCP-1) in endothelial cells and smooth muscle cells (2,18)	Monocyte recruitment into the arterial wall by stimulation of transendothelial migration
• Induction of granulocyte and macrophage colony-stimulating factors (G-CSF and M-CSF) in endothelial cells (17).	Monocyte recruitment, monocyte/macrophage differentiation, and macrophage stability and replication in the arterial wall

14), likely as a result of up-regulation of cellular adhesion molecules on endothelial cells (15,16). Furthermore, mm-LDL stimulates expression of monocyte chemotactic peptide-1 and macrophage colony-stimulating factor by endothelial cells (17,18). Monocyte chemotactic peptide-1 plays an important role in the attraction and guided migration of monocytes into the arterial wall, while macrophage colony-stimulating factor stimulates the differentiation of monocytes into macrophages (Table 1). In addition, ox-LDL is directly chemotactic for monocytes (19), most likely because of intraparticle accumulation of lysophosphatidylcholine that is itself an effective chemotactic factor for monocytes (20). Finally, ox-LDL inhibits migration of resident tissue macrophages (19), thereby preventing their egress

Table 2   Some Biological Properties by Which Oxidatively Modified Low-Density
Lipoprotein Differs from Native Low-Density Lipoprotein

Effect of oxidatively modified LDL (Refs.)	Significance for atherosclerosis
• Stimulation of leukocyte adhesion to the endothelium (13,14)	Leukocyte recruitment into the arterial wall
• Chemotaxis of monocytes, T-lymphocytes, and smooth muscle cells (2,19,20)	Monocyte, T-lymphocyte, and smooth muscle cell recruitment into the arterial wall
• Inhibition of macrophage migration (19)	Trapping of macrophages in the arterial wall
• Recognition by macrophage scavenger receptors (9,21–26)	Foam cell genesis
• Immunogenicity, aggregation (27–29)	Immune responses, foam cell genesis
• Inhibition of endothelium-derived nitric oxide production and/or biological activity (30,31)	Inhibition of vasorelaxation; increased platelet aggregation, smooth muscle cell proliferation, etc.
• Stimulation of smooth muscle cell growth (37)	Neointimal smooth muscle cell proliferation
• Cytotoxicity (11,38,39)	Foam cell necrosis contributing to lesion progression; endothelial denudation triggering occlusive thrombosis and acute clinical events

from the arterial wall (Table 2). Thus, there exists a causal relationship between minimal as well as full oxidative modification of LDL and recruitment of monocytes to the arterial wall, the activation–differentiation of these monocytes into macrophages, and macrophage retention. The resulting colocalization of macrophages with subendothelial LDL provides a fertile environment for further LDL oxidation, thus perpetuating the atherosclerotic process.

In addition to the roles in arterial wall monocyte recruitment, maturation, and retention, ox-LDL present in the subendothelium can facilitate atherogenic progression by a number of other mechanisms (Table 2). Most prominent among these atherogenic properties of ox-LDL is its recognition by scavenger receptors on macrophages, leading to ox-LDL uptake and foam cell formation. Originally, two types of receptors that recognize ox-LDL (types I and II) were identified (21), but more recently several other scavenger receptors have been identified (22–24). The ox-LDL uptake by these scavenger receptors is 3- to 10-fold more efficient than native LDL uptake via the normal apolipoprotein B/E receptor (25) and, unlike native LDL uptake, is not subject to down-regulation by intracellular cholesterol (26). Consequently, macrophages in the subendothelial space become loaded with ox-LDL-derived lipids and are thus converted to foam cells (2). Foam cells may also arise from scavenger receptor-independent uptake of ox-LDL. For example, ox-LDL is immunogenic, stimulating formation of autoantibodies (27), and immune complexes of ox-LDL aggregates are efficiently internalized by macrophages via F_c receptors (28). In addition, ox-LDL aggregates can be internalized by macrophages via apolipoprotein B/E receptor-dependent phagocytosis (29).

Arterial formation and accumulation of ox-LDL may also be associated with local impaired production of endothelium-derived relaxing factor (EDRF; nitric oxide [NO]) (30) and/or inactivation of NO after its release from endothelium (31). Impairment of EDRF production and/or biological action can contribute to the progression of atherosclerosis through a number of mechanisms (32), as EDRF not only acts as a vasodilator, but also inhibits platelet aggregation, smooth muscle cell proliferation, and endothelial–leukocyte interactions (33). The ox-LDL also stimulates production of the vasoconstrictor molecule endothelin by endothelial cells (34) and contains increased amounts of free radical–derived prostaglandin F_2–like compounds (F_2-isoprostanes) (35,36), which can act as vasoconstrictors. More recently, it has also become evident that ox-LDL can stimulate smooth muscle cell migration and proliferation (37), events that critically contribute to lesion progression (2,5,6).

Furthermore, ox-LDL is cytotoxic as a result of its content of lipid hydroperoxide breakdown products and cholesterol oxidation products that can initiate lipid peroxidation in target cells (11,38,39). Cytotoxicity to foam cells may be particularly relevant to lesion progression, while cytotoxic damage and denudation of vascular endothelium may contribute to the acute thrombotic complications of atherosclerosis (2). Thrombosis may also be directly affected by mm-LDL and ox-LDL through enhanced synthesis of procoagulant tissue factor by endothelial cells (40,41). In addition, ox-LDL can abolish endothelial cell production of prostacyclin (42), an effective inhibitor of platelet thrombus formation. Finally, ox-LDL may inhibit fibrinolysis by enhanced endothelial synthesis of plasminogen activator inhibitor-1 (43).

By all these various mechanisms (Tables 1 and 2), mm-LDL and ox-LDL may play a pivotal role in atherosclerosis, from its initial stages characterized by monocyte recruitment and foam cell formation to its clinical manifestations many decades later. The notion that LDL is oxidized in vivo is supported by numerous findings. For example, antibodies to ox-LDL recognize material in aortic atherosclerotic lesions, but not normal aortic areas, and LDL extracted from human lesions cross-reacts with antibodies to ox-LDL (27,44,45). Lesion-derived LDL also contains oxidized lipids and apolipoprotein B fragments, is taken up at increased rates by macrophages, and is chemotactic for monocytes (44), all properties of ox-LDL. More recently, it has been reported that malondialdehyde-modified LDL, a form of ox-LDL, is detectable in human plasma, and that the levels of this modified lipoprotein are significantly elevated in patients with acute myocardial infarction or carotid atherosclerosis (46). In agreement with these observations, autoantibodies against ox-LDL can be found in human plasma, and the titers of these anti-ox-LDL antibodies are elevated in patients with carotid atherosclerosis (47).

Further indirect support for a role of ox-LDL in atherosclerosis comes from animal studies in which antioxidants such as probucol, butylated hydroxytoluene, and α-tocopherol (the chemically and biologically most active form of vitamin E) can slow the progression of atherosclerosis (48). However, the evidence from these animal studies for an anti-atherogenic effect of antioxidants is often mixed and inconsistent, and the data are difficult to interpret. For example, it is not clear whether beneficial antiatherosclerotic effects of α-tocopherol supplementation in cholesterol-fed rabbits are due to inhibition of LDL oxidation, lowering of plasma cholesterol levels, normalization of vascular reactivity, inhibition of vascular protein kinase C activity, or a combination of these factors. Other rabbit studies have found no effect of α-tocopherol supplementation on atherosclerotic lesion development, or even a proatherogenic effect (48).

Epidemiological and limited trial data suggest a protective role of dietary antioxidants against cardiovascular disease (CVD) in humans, including vitamins E and C (49). Currently there is quite consistent support for a protective effect against CVD of vitamin E supplementation with more than about 150 IU/day for at least 2 years, while the evidence for a beneficial effect of vitamin C is less convincing (49). The evidence in support of β-carotene to act as an antiatherogenic agent has been weakened substantially by recent trial data (50,51). A lack of an effect of β-carotene on CVD is also consistent with the finding that in vitro and in vivo supplementation with β-carotene does not inhibit LDL oxidation (52).

Mechanisms of Low-Density Lipoprotein Oxidation

Oxidative modification of LDL proceeds through a series of events involving formation of lipid hydroperoxides and modification of apolipoprotein B by lipid hydroperoxide breakdown products (Fig. 1). Usually, the initial event in LDL oxidation is lipid peroxidation, which is initiated by abstraction of a bis-allylic hydrogen atom from a polyunsaturated fatty acyl chain. Once lipid hydroperoxides have been formed in LDL, they may decompose to aldehydic breakdown products, including 4-hydroxynonenal and malondialdehyde (53), a process catalyzed by redox-active transition metal ions such as copper or iron. The aldehydic products are highly reactive and can react with ε-amino groups of lysine residues of apolipoprotein B, leading to formation of Schiff's bases (54). The formation of Schiff's bases results in an increased net-negative charge of apolipoprotein B, and as a consequence this modified LDL is no longer recognized by the apolipoprotein B/E LDL receptor (26), but instead is internalized by macrophages via the scavenger receptor pathway (21–24).

The nature of the initiating species in LDL oxidation is a matter of considerable debate. Recently, strong evidence has been presented that in vitro LDL oxidation is initiated by α-tocopheroxyl radicals formed in LDL upon attack by free radicals or other oxidant

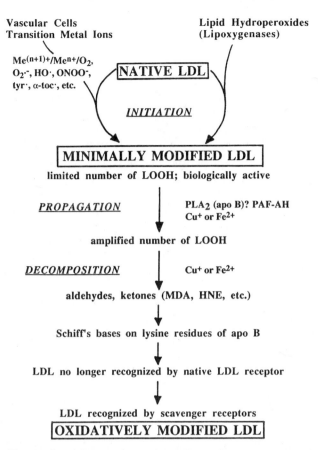

Figure 1 Mechanism of oxidative modification of human low-density lipoprotein (LDL). LDL can be oxidized by a number of mechanisms in vitro. Cultured vascular cells (endothelial cells, smooth muscle cells, macrophages) can oxidize LDL in the presence of medium-contained transition metal ions such as iron and/or copper. The molecular nature of the chemical species initiating LDL oxidation remains to be identified. Transition metal ion complexes with oxygen ($Me^{(n+1)+}/Me^{n+}/O_2$), cell-derived superoxide radicals ($O_2^{\cdot-}$), hydroxyl radicals (HO·), peroxynitrite ($ONOO^-$) formed by reaction of nitric oxide (NO) with $O_2^{\cdot-}$, myeloperoxidase-derived tyrosyl radicals (tyr·), and LDL-associated α-tocopheroxyl radicals (α-toc·) have all been implicated. Alternatively, lipid hydroperoxides formed by 15-lipoxygenase in plasma membranes of endothelial cells or macrophages may be transferred to native LDL. In the initial phase of LDL oxidation, a limited number of lipid hydroperoxides (LOOH) is formed, resulting in the transformation of native LDL into minimally modified LDL. Subsequently lipid peroxidation enters the propagation phase, which is catalyzed by cuprous (Cu^+) and/or ferrous (Fe^{2+}) ions. A phospholipase A_2 (PLA_2) activity intrinsic in apolipoprotein B (apo B) has also been suggested to be involved in this step. However, more recent evidence suggests that it is a platelet activating factor–acetyl hydrolase (PAF–AH) activity, which is associated with LDL and inhibits, rather than promotes, LDL oxidation. The propagation phase of lipid peroxidation is followed by the breakdown of lipid hydroperoxides in a metal-catalyzed (Cu^+, Fe^{2+}) reaction to malondialdehyde (MDA), 4-hydroxynonenal (HNE), and other aldehydes and ketones. These reactive lipid hydroperoxide degradation products can form Schiff's bases with lysine residues of apo B, resulting in loss of recognition of the modified LDL by the apolipoprotein B/E receptor. Instead, the oxidatively modified LDL is recognized by macrophage scavenger receptors, leading to internalization and foam cell formation.

species such as peroxyl radicals, hydroxyl radicals, or transition metal ions (55,56). Thus, α-tocopherol, which is naturally present in LDL, acts as a prooxidant, rather than an antioxidant, in LDL incubated in vitro under oxidizing conditions (55,57). This prooxidant activity of LDL-associated α-tocopherol may, however, be of limited relevance in vivo. One reason for this limited relevance is that vitamin C, which is present at high concentrations in human interstitial fluid and the arterial wall (58,59), can prevent the prooxidant activity of α-tocopherol by reducing the α-tocopheroxyl radical to α-tocopherol (60), thereby acting as a "coantioxidant" and inhibiting, rather than promoting, LDL oxidation (61).

In addition to LDL-associated α-tocopherol, redox-active metal ions seem to play a pivotal role in LDL oxidation in vitro. Low-density lipoprotein oxidation by cultured arterial wall cells, e.g., endothelial cells, smooth muscle cells, or monocyte/macrophages, is strictly dependent upon transition metal ions (10,62,63). Low-density lipoprotein can also be oxidatively modified by transition metal ions in the absence of cells to a form that is identical to cell-modified LDL (10,62). In addition, LDL can be oxidized by intact (non-proteolytically degraded) ceruloplasmin (64), a copper-binding protein which contains one redox-active copper ion per protein molecule. The potential biological relevance of metal ion-mediated LDL oxidation is emphasized by the observations that atherosclerotic lesions contain transition metal ions capable of stimulating lipid peroxidation (65), and that increased serum copper levels are associated with the progression of carotid atherosclerosis in humans (66). Similarly, serum ferritin levels, a measure of total body iron stores, are directly correlated with the degree of carotid atherosclerosis (67) and risk of myocardial infarction (68). However, other epidemiological studies did not find support for a role of body iron in atherosclerotic vascular disease (69,70), although intake of heme iron, mainly from red meat, was directly associated with an increased risk of CVD in one study (69). In vitro studies have demonstrated that human plasma and interstitial fluid have very high metal-binding capacities, which virtually abolish metal ion–dependent LDL oxidation by macrophages and in cell-free systems (58). As the availability of redox-active metal ions in vivo is uncertain, numerous investigators have proposed and investigated metal ion-independent mechanisms of LDL oxidation, particularly by myeloperoxidase-derived hypochlorous acid (71,72) and tyrosyl radicals (73).

ANTIOXIDANT PROTECTION OF LOW-DENSITY LIPOPROTEIN BY VITAMIN C

Molecular Mechanisms

If LDL oxidation plays a causal role in atherogenesis through the various mechanisms discussed (Tables 1 and 2), then antioxidants which can prevent LDL oxidation should prevent or slow the atherosclerotic process. As mentioned, this notion is supported in part by animal studies (48) as well as observational epidemiological studies and randomized trial data (49). Further clinical trials are needed and have been initiated to investigate whether dietary antioxidant supplementation can lower the risk of cardiovascular and cerebrovascular diseases (49,74). In addition, many basic research studies have investigated how effectively and by what mechanisms the endogenous antioxidants in human plasma and LDL can inhibit lipid peroxidation and oxidative modification of LDL (75,76).

Vitamin C (ascorbic acid) has been shown to be the most effective water-soluble antioxidant in human plasma. Physiological ascorbic acid concentrations in human plasma and interstitial fluid range from about 30 to 100 μM (58,77). Plasma exposed to a constant flux of aqueous or lipid-soluble peroxyl radicals (35,78–81), activated polymorphonuclear leukocytes (78), gas-phase cigarette smoke (82), or enzymatically generated superoxide radicals and hydrogen peroxide (83) is effectively protected against detectable lipid peroxidation by endogenous ascorbic acid. Indeed, ascorbic acid is the only plasma antioxidant capable of completely preventing initiation of lipid peroxidation (35,78,79). However, once ascorbic acid has been used up, detectable amounts of lipid hydroperoxides are formed, despite the continued presence of other antioxidants in plasma such as α-tocopherol and β-carotene (35,78,81).

Consistent with these in vitro data, in vivo studies have found increased plasma levels of thiobarbituric acid–relative substances (TBARS), an indirect marker of lipid peroxidation, in genetically scorbutic rats (84). These plasma TBARS were associated mainly with LDL. Conversely, when the rats were supplemented with vitamin C, the elevated TBARS levels decreased in a dose-dependent manner (84). These data suggest that vitamin C deficiency results in oxidative modification of LDL in vivo. Interestingly, plasma vitamin C levels in the marginally vitamin C–deficient rats remained above zero, yet TBARS levels were elevated (84). As no lipid peroxidation can be observed in plasma in the presence of vitamin C (78–80), it is conceivable that in these rat studies LDL became oxidized in microenvironments of the arterial wall devoid of ascorbic acid and was subsequently released into the circulation.

Studies using isolated human LDL, rather than plasma, have firmly established that vitamin C can protect the lipoprotein against oxidative modification (73,85–94). Vitamin C is much more effective than vitamin E and β-carotene at preventing LDL oxidation (Fig. 2), both at atmospheric and physiological oxygen partial pressures (94). We and other investigators have used many different types of oxidizing conditions to oxidize LDL. With only one exception (95), physiological concentrations of ascorbic acid effectively inhibited LDL oxidation by all the various mechanisms investigated. As illustrated in Fig. 3, 50–130 μM ascorbic acid strongly suppressed or abolished oxidative modification of LDL by endothelial cells (85; Martin and Frei, unpublished), macrophages (86,87), activated polymorphonuclear leukocytes (88), tyrosyl radicals (73), heme and hydrogen peroxide (89,90), aqueous peroxyl radicals (91,92), Fe^{3+} in Ham's F-10 medium (Martin and Frei, unpublished), and Cu^{2+} (86,91,93,94).

Several mechanisms of protection are responsible for these strong antioxidant effects of ascorbic acid against LDL oxidation.

Scavenging of Free Radicals and Other Oxidants in the Aqueous Milieu

Ascorbic acid has been shown to scavenge hypochlorous acid (96), tyrosyl radicals (97), aqueous peroxyl radicals (78,79), and superoxide radicals effectively (98). Direct trapping of these water-soluble oxidant species prevents them from attacking and oxidizing LDL. Such a mechanism likely explains the protective effects of ascorbic acid against activated polymorphonuclear leukocytes (88), which release copious amounts of hypochlorous acid capable of modifying LDL (71,72), and against aqueous peroxyl radicals and tyrosyl radicals, which can initiate lipid peroxidation in LDL (73,91), most likely via α-tocopheroxyl radical formation from α-tocopherol (55–57). Furthermore, superoxide radicals may play a role in endothelial cell–mediated LDL oxidation, and scavenging of these cell-generated superoxide radicals by ascorbic acid may explain, at least in part, the protective effect of ascorbic acid (85; Martin and Frei, unpublished).

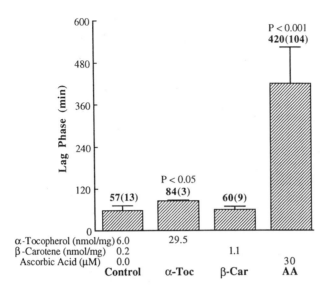

Figure 2 Relative protective effects of α-tocopherol, β-carotene, and ascorbic acid against lipid peroxidation in human low-density lipoprotein (LDL). Freshly isolated LDL (0.2 mg protein/ml) was incubated in 10 mM phosphate-buffered saline solution at 37°C with 2.5 μM Cu^{2+}, and the time course of lipid peroxidation (diene conjugation) was monitored at 234 nm. The lag phase plotted on the ordinate represents the length of the period during which lipid peroxidation was initially inhibited in LDL. The lag phase is a measure of the oxidative resistance of LDL. Control LDL containing 6.0 and 0.2 nmol/mg protein of α-tocopherol and β-carotene, respectively, exhibited a lag phase of 57 ± 13 min (n = 10); α-tocopherol supplementation in vitro led to an increase in LDL-associated α-tocopherol (α-Toc) to 29.5 nmol/mg protein and an increase in the lag phase to 84 ± 3 min (n = 4; p < 0.05 vs. control); β-carotene supplementation in vitro led to an increase in LDL-associated β-carotene (β-Car) to 1.1 nmol/mg protein, but the lag phase remained unchanged at 60 ± 9 min (n = 3; p = not significant vs. control); addition of a low physiological concentration of ascorbic acid (AA, 30 μM) led to an increase in the lag phase to 420 ± 104 min (n = 4; p < 0.001 vs. control). (Data from Refs. 90, 94.)

Regeneration of Low-Density Lipoprotein–Associated α-Tocopherol

Ascorbic acid may also inhibit LDL oxidation by regenerating LDL-associated α-tocopherol from the α-tocopheroxyl radical at the water–lipid interface (60,99). As mentioned, this is also the mechanism by which ascorbic acid prevents the prooxidant activity of LDL-associated α-tocopherol (61). When radicals are generated within the LDL particle by a lipid-soluble azo initiator (99), ascorbic acid cannot directly scavenge these radicals because it is not lipophilic and therefore cannot penetrate the lipoprotein particle. Instead, the lipid-soluble peroxyl radicals first react with LDL-associated α-tocopherol to form the α-tocopheroxyl radical. The latter is located at the surface of the LDL particle, where it can interact with ascorbic acid, leading to regeneration of α-tocopherol at the expense of vitamin C. Therefore, by this mechanism ascorbic acid can inhibit LDL oxidation initiated by lipid-soluble radicals (60,99). Although the synergistic interaction between vitamins C and E is well documented in vitro using liposomes or isolated LDL, there exists no convincing evidence for such a synergistic interaction in vivo.

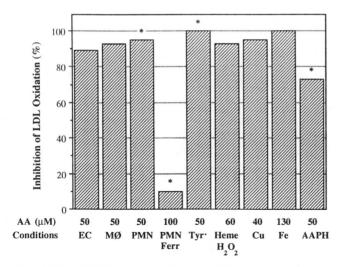

Figure 3 Inhibition of oxidative modification of human low-density lipoprotein (LDL) by ascorbic acid under different oxidizing conditions. Human LDL was oxidized by incubation with rabbit or human aortic endothelial cells (EC), mouse peritoneal or human monocyte-derived macrophages (MØ), activated human polymorpho-nuclear leukocytes (PMN), activated human PMN and ferritin (Ferr), tyrosyl radicals (tyr·) generated by a myeloperoxidase/hydrogen peroxide/tyrosine system, heme and hydrogen peroxide (H_2O_2), Cu^{2+} (Cu), Fe^{3+} in Ham's F-10 medium (Fe), or the aqueous radical initiator 2,2'-azobis(2-amidinopropane) hydrochloride (AAPH). LDL oxidation was assessed as increased electrophoretic mobility, which measures mod-ification of apolipoprotein B with lipid hydroperoxide degradation products (see Fig. 1), or lipid peroxidation (columns marked by asterisks). Ascorbic acid (AA) was added at the concentrations indicated, and the inhibition of LDL oxidation relative to the control incubation in the absence of AA is plotted on the ordinate. (Data from Refs. 73, 85–95; Martin and Frei, unpublished.)

Even in vitro, under most incubation conditions, regeneration of α-tocopherol is not the primary mechanism by which ascorbic acid prevents lipid peroxidation and LDL oxidation (79,80,90). As discussed, the protective effects of ascorbic acid are more readily explained by direct scavenging of reactive oxygen species and free radicals in the aqueous phase before they can attack the LDL particle. The contention that regeneration of α-tocopherol is not the primary mechanism of vitamin C's action is supported by the observation that the rate of ascorbic acid oxidation in human plasma exposed to oxidizing conditions is independent of the concentration of α-tocopherol; indeed, that rate of ascorbic acid oxida-tion in plasma exposed to a constant flux of aqueous peroxyl radicals is the same whether α-tocopherol is present or absent (Frei, unpublished observation; Stocker, personal com-munication). Furthermore, dehydroascorbic acid, the two electron oxidation product of ascorbic acid, can preserve α-tocopherol in LDL incubated with Cu^{2+} (90). Dehydro-ascorbic acid, however, has no direct reducing capability (91) and cannot reduce α-toco-pheroxyl radicals in LDL to α-tocopherol (Stocker and Witting, personal communication). Therefore, dehydroascorbic acid, like ascorbic acid, prevents α-tocopherol oxidation in the first place: i.e., vitamin C spares, rather than regenerates, α-tocopherol in plasma and LDL (90).

Inhibition of Metal Ion Binding to Low-Density Lipoprotein

Interestingly, ascorbic acid prevents metal ion–dependent LDL oxidation, either by vascular cells in culture or in cell-free systems containing Cu^{2+}, Fe^{3+}, or hemin (Fig. 3). This protective effect of ascorbic acid against metal ion–dependent LDL oxidation is paradoxical, because in vitro ascorbic acid is well known to act as a prooxidant, rather than an antioxidant, in the presence of transition metal ions (100). For example, Cu^{2+}-induced oxidative damage to deoxyribonucleic acid (DNA) bases is increased substantially by addition of ascorbic acid, not decreased (101). This prooxidant effect of ascorbic acid is due to its capacity to reduce transition metal ions (Me) and generate hydrogen peroxide (H_2O_2) by autooxidation [Eqs. (1) and (2), respectively]. Subsequently, reduced metal ions, such as cuprous or ferrous ions (Cu^+ or Fe^{2+}), can catalyze the production of hydroxyl radicals (HO·) from H_2O_2 [Eq. (3)].

$$AH^- + Me^{(n+1)+} \rightarrow A^{\cdot-} + Me^{n+} + H^+ \tag{1}$$

$$AH^- + O_2 + H^+ \rightarrow A + H_2O_2 \tag{2}$$

$$H_2O_2 + Me^{n+} \rightarrow HO^\bullet + HO^- + Me^{(n+1)+} \tag{3}$$

where AH^-, $A^{\cdot-}$, and A represent ascorbate, the ascorbyl radical, and dehydroascorbic acid, respectively. Equation (3) is called the Fenton reaction (100). Hydroxyl radicals are extremely reactive species that can initiate lipid peroxidation in LDL (102). Furthermore, the reduced metal ions can reinitiate lipid peroxidation by breakdown of existing lipid hydroperoxides to lipid alkoxy radicals (75). On the basis of these considerations, ascorbic acid should promote, rather than prevent, metal ion–dependent LDL oxidation.

In a partial explanation of the paradoxical protective effects of vitamin C against LDL oxidation, we observed that dehydroascorbic acid prevents metal ion–dependent LDL oxidation (90,91). In our experiments, both ascorbic acid and dehydroascorbic acid prevented the various stages of LDL oxidative modification (Fig. 1), i.e., consumption of endogenous antioxidants (except for ubiquinol-10), initiation of lipid peroxidation, apolipoprotein B modification leading to increased electrophoretic mobility, and degradation of LDL by macrophages via the scavenger receptor pathway (90,91). In addition, in LDL incubated with Cu^{2+} and ascorbic acid or dehydroascorbic acid, histidine residues of apolipoprotein B were oxidized to 2-oxo-histidine, and 2-oxo-histidine formation was associated with loss of bound Cu^{2+} from LDL (Retsky, Chen, and Frei, unpublished). These data are in agreement with findings showing that 2-oxo-histidine, in contrast to histidine, cannot bind Cu^{2+} (103). As Cu^{2+} binding to apolipoprotein B is a prerequisite for LDL oxidation (104), such limited, site-specific oxidative "damage" to the histidine residues of apolipoprotein B resulting in loss of bound Cu^{2+} could explain why vitamin C protects against Cu^{2+}-induced LDL oxidation.

Destruction of Preformed Lipid Hydroperoxides

In addition to the mechanisms discussed, ascorbic acid also prevents propagation of lipid peroxidation in LDL by rapid and complete destruction of preformed lipid hydroperoxides (90). This effect of ascorbic acid is dependent upon the presence of redox-active copper and is observed in LDL during the lag phase as well as the early stages of the propagation phase of lipid peroxidation (90). In contrast, in extensively oxidized LDL, ascorbic acid addition may have a prooxidant effect (87) due to metal ion reduction and stimulation of lipid peroxidation via lipid alkoxy radical formation (75). Prevention of Cu^{2+} binding to LDL may no longer be a critical factor in these advanced stages of LDL oxidation, where lipid peroxidation can occur by a self-propagating mechanism independently of initiating events.

In Vivo Studies

In an attempt to investigate whether the potent antioxidant protection of isolated LDL by ascorbic acid observed in vitro is relevant in vivo, some researchers have used vitamin C supplementation in humans (105–108). The LDL isolated from the plasma of these supplemented subjects was then examined for resistance to oxidation in vitro. However, this approach works only for lipid-soluble antioxidants that are naturally incorporated into LDL, e.g., α-tocopherol, but is not useful to test the possible in vivo effects of ascorbic acid against LDL oxidation. The trivial reason for this is that ascorbic acid is a water-soluble compound, which is not associated with LDL and thus is removed from LDL during isolation of the lipoprotein from plasma. Not surprisingly, therefore, vitamin C supplementation in humans has no effect on (106,107) or only moderately increases (105,108) the resistance of plasma-derived LDL to Cu^{2+}-induced or cell-mediated oxidation in vitro. The moderately increased oxidative resistance of LDL following vitamin C supplementation in some studies (105,108) was suggested to be due to preservation of LDL-associated vitamin E by vitamin C, but this notion could not be substantiated by measurement of the plasma levels of these vitamins: vitamin C supplementation increased plasma ascorbic acid levels, but left α-tocopherol levels unaffected (105).

It cannot be stressed enough that the preceding negative results from in vivo supplementation studies (105–108) cannot be interpreted to indicate that vitamin C has no protective effect against LDL oxidation in vivo, because the design of these studies is flawed. Low-density lipoprotein does not exist in isolated form in vivo, but is always bathed in a milieu containing various antioxidants, which can protect the lipoprotein from radical attack (35,58,78). Low-density lipoprotein and ascorbic acid coexist in plasma, interstitial fluid, as well as the arterial wall (58,59), and therefore vitamin C may very well protect LDL against oxidation in vivo.

As mentioned, epidemiological studies investigating the role of dietary vitamin C in reducing the risk of CVD are inconclusive (49,74,109), whereas several studies have found a significantly and substantially reduced risk of ischemic stroke with increased vitamin C consumption (49,109,110). Furthermore, it was reported recently that in men and women >55 years old the degree of carotid atherosclerosis is inversely correlated with vitamin C intake (111). Data from animal studies have shown that vitamin C deficiency is associated with accelerated atherosclerosis in guinea pigs (48,109). Consistent with this observation, the majority of studies investigating vitamin C supplementation in cholesterol-fed rabbits have found significant inhibition of the development of atherosclerosis (109). Although promising overall, the totality of the currently available scientific evidence is insufficient to conclude that vitamin C can act as an antiatherogen or to make specific recommendations with regard to optimal vitamin C intake in humans. Clearly, more studies are needed to answer the question of whether vitamin C can inhibit LDL oxidation and decrease the risk of cardiovascular and cerebrovascular disease in humans.

OTHER POTENTIAL MECHANISMS OF ANTIATHEROGENIC ACTION OF VITAMIN C

In addition to inhibiting LDL oxidation, ascorbic acid may affect a number of other processes that contribute to atherosclerosis and its clinical sequelae. These processes may themselves be related to oxidative stress or have no apparent causal relation to oxidative stress.

Lipoprotein Profile

Studies on coronary risk factors indicate that vitamin C may moderately improve lipoprotein profile and decrease total serum cholesterol levels in hypercholesterolemic subjects (112). In addition, vitamin C may increase high-density lipoprotein levels (113). The possible mechanisms by which ascorbic acid may affect lipoprotein profile have been investigated in numerous animal studies (109). Vitamin C was shown to affect cholesterol metabolism and to have a hypocholesterolemic effect by activation of the cytochrome P450-dependent enzyme cholesterol-7α-hydroxylase (114), which converts cholesterol to bile acids for disposal by the liver. Vitamin C also seems to affect triglyceride levels by modulation of lipoprotein lipase activity (115).

Extracellular Matrix

Effects on arterial wall integrity related to biosynthesis of collagen and glycosaminoglycans may be another mechanism by which vitamin C affects atherosclerosis. Vitamin C has long been known to serve as a cofactor for both prolyl and lysyl hydroxylases, enzymes that catalyze the posttranslational hydroxylation of procollagen (116). This hydroxylation reaction is essential for the stabilization of the mature collagen fiber. Glycosaminoglycan metabolism also is affected by vitamin C (116). Collagen and glycosaminoglycans are important components of the vascular wall extracellular matrix (2). The latter mediates a number of functions with significance to atherosclerosis, such as lipoprotein binding and retention, cell proliferation, and hemostasis (117). Therefore, loss of extracellular matrix integrity in conditions of vitamin C deficiency may promote the atherosclerotic process (109).

Leukocyte Adhesion and Platelet Aggregation

Ascorbic acid administration to hamsters has been shown to abolish cigarette smoke–induced or ox-LDL-induced leukocyte aggregation and adhesion to endothelium in vivo (118,119). These effects of ascorbic acid are likely due to scavenging of superoxide radicals, but the precise mechanism remains to be elucidated (14,118,119). As explained in the Introduction, adhesion of leukocytes to the endothelium is an important, initiating step in atherogenesis, and formation of leukocyte–platelet aggregates may critically contribute to clinical events such as myocardial infarction and ischemic stroke.

A role of ascorbic acid in inhibiting platelet function is also supported by some clinical studies. For example, supplementation of heart disease patients with 1 g of vitamin C twice a day for 6 months significantly reduced platelet adhesiveness; in addition, it enhanced fibrinolytic activity (120). Similarly, supplementation of patients with 3 g vitamin C/day for 10 days reduced platelet adhesiveness and aggregation (121). However, another study using lower levels of supplemental vitamin C (1 g/day for 3 months) did not find an effect on platelet adhesiveness and fibrinolysis (122).

There is also evidence from in vitro studies that physiological concentrations of ascorbic acid enhance formation of prostaglandin E_1 and prostaglandin I_2 (prostacyclin) in human platelets and vascular tissue, respectively, resulting in inhibition of platelet aggregation (123,124). Similarly, vitamin C may induce prostacyclin production by endothelial cells

(125). However, since prostacyclin production is not impaired in atherosclerosis, the relevance of these in vitro data is unclear.

Vascular Reactivity

With respect to clinical coronary events such as myocardial infarction and angina pectoris, it is becoming increasingly evident that not only arterial stenosis and plaque rupture but impaired vascular function and relaxation play important roles (126–128). Most interestingly, it has been demonstrated recently that ascorbic acid reverses endothelial vasomotor dysfunction in patients with coronary artery disease (128). In this placebo-controlled study, administration of 2 g of vitamin C to patients with severely impaired brachial artery dilatation led to a dramatic improvement of their vasodilatory response. Similar results were reported by a second group of researchers investigating the effects of vitamin C infusion on acetylcholine-induced dilation of coronary arteries in diabetic patients (129).

Several molecular mechanisms have been proposed for these beneficial effects of ascorbic acid on vasomotor activity. As mentioned, the agonist-induced release from endothelium and/or the activity of EDRF is inhibited by ox-LDL and superoxide radicals (30,31,130). In particular, superoxide radicals react rapidly with NO, which limits the biological activity of EDRF (131). Hence, it may be that ascorbic acid normalizes EDRF metabolism by preventing formation of ox-LDL and/or by scavenging superoxide radicals. It has also been speculated that ascorbic acid maintains intracellular levels of glutathione, which may improve EDRF action through increased synthesis of NO and/or stabilization of NO as an S-nitrosothiol species (128). High concentrations of native LDL also have been claimed to impair acetylcholine-induced EDRF responses in aortic tissue, and this effect was reversed by physiological concentrations of ascorbic acid (132). Consistent with these data, vitamin C has been shown to increase the hypotensive effect of acetylcholine and other agonists in a rat model (133). This finding may be related in part to the inverse correlation between blood pressure and vitamin C intake observed in some epidemiological studies (134,135).

SUMMARY AND CONCLUSIONS

According to the oxidative modification hypothesis of atherosclerosis, LDL entrapped in the subendothelial space of lesion-prone arterial sites becomes oxidized through the action of resident vascular cells. The accumulation of mm-LDL and ox-LDL is associated with the local recruitment of monocytes and macrophages that internalize ox-LDL, leading to foam cell formation (Tables 1 and 2). The continued presence of ox-LDL in the vascular wall contributes to foam cell necrosis and smooth muscle cell migration and proliferation, as well as abnormalities in the local control of platelet adhesion and vascular tone. All of these features combine to produce atherosclerotic progression and a fertile environment for the development of acute vascular syndromes such as angina pectoris, myocardial infarction, and ischemic stroke.

Human LDL and extracellular fluids contain a number of antioxidants that may inhibit these processes and thus may limit the development of atherosclerosis. Vitamin C is present in human plasma and interstitial fluid at comparable concentrations (58) and has also been detected in large amounts in the arterial wall (59). There is a large body of evidence showing that LDL oxidation in vitro is strongly inhibited by vitamin C. Physiological concentrations of ascorbic acid can prevent LDL oxidation by at least four different mechanisms: direct scavenging of water-soluble free radicals and other oxidants; regeneration of LDL-associated α-tocopherol; inhibition of metal ion binding to apolipoprotein B; and destruction of preformed lipid hydroperoxides. As a result of the limited understanding of the atherosclerotic process and the role and molecular mechanism of LDL oxidation in vivo, the data showing significant antioxidant protection of LDL by vitamin C in vitro can at present not be extrapolated to the in vivo situation in humans.

Epidemiological data and animal studies suggest that vitamin C supplementation may limit the development of atherosclerosis. However, in the studies showing a beneficial effect of vitamin C it is unclear whether the vitamin acts by inhibition of LDL oxidation or some other mechanism. In fact, emerging data from numerous animal studies suggest that antioxidants can act as antiatherogens without inhibiting LDL oxidation (136,137). In addition to preventing LDL oxidation, many other mechanisms of antioxidant or nonantioxidant action of vitamin C have to be considered, such as changes in lipoprotein profile, effects on thrombosis and fibrinolysis, and regulation of NO activity and vascular tone. Further investigations into these various mechanisms will be pivotal for a better understanding of the pathogenesis of atherosclerosis and a critical assessment of the ability of vitamin C to reduce morbidity and mortality from CVD in humans.

ACKNOWLEDGMENTS

The work in BF's laboratory is supported by the National Institutes of Health grants HL-49954, HL-56170, and ES-06593.

REFERENCES

1. Gotto AJ, Farmer JA. Risk factors for coronary artery disease. In: Braunwald E, ed. Heart Disease: A Textbook of Cardiovascular Medicine. 3rd ed. Philadelphia: Saunders, 1988:1153–1190.
2. Schwartz CJ, Valente AJ. The pathogenesis of atherosclerosis. In: Frei B, ed. Natural Antioxidants in Human Health and Disease. San Diego: Academic Press, 1994:287–302.
3. Gerrity RG, Naito HK, Richardson M, Schwartz CJ. Dietary induced atherogenesis in swine: morphology of the intima in prelesion stages. Am J Pathol 1979; 95:775–792.
4. Williams KJ, Tabas I. The response-to-retention hypothesis of early atherogenesis. Arterioscler Thromb Vasc Biol 1995; 15:551–561.
5. Ross R. The pathogenesis of atherosclerosis: an update. N Engl J Med 1986; 314:488–500.
6. Ross R. Rous-Whipple Award Lecture: atherosclerosis: a defense mechanism gone awry. Am J Pathol 1993; 143:987–1002.
7. Cybulsky MI, Gimbrone MA Jr. Endothelial expression of a mononuclear leukocyte adhesion molecule during atherogenesis. Science 1991; 251:788–791.
8. Li H, Cybulsky MI, Gimbrone MA Jr, Libby P. An atherogenic diet rapidly induces VCAM-1, a cytokine-regulatable mononuclear leukocyte adhesion molecule, in rabbit aortic endothelium. Arterioscler Thromb 1993; 13:197–204.
9. Henriksen T, Mahoney EM, Steinberg D. enhanced macrophage degradation of low density lipoprotein previously incubated with cultured endothelial cells: recognition by receptor for acetylated low density lipoproteins. Proc Natl Acad Sci USA 1981; 78:6499–6503.
10. Heinecke JW, Baker L, Rosen H, Chait A. Superoxide mediated modification of low density lipoprotein by human arterial smooth muscle cells in culture. J Clin Invest 1986; 77:757–761.
11. Cathcart MK, Morel DW, Chisolm GM. Monocytes and neutrophils oxidize low density lipoprotein making it cytotoxic. J Leukoc Biol 1985; 38:341–346.

12. Berliner JA, Territo MC, Sevanian A, et al. Minimally modified low density lipoprotein stimulates monocyte endothelial interactions. J Clin Invest 1990; 85:1260–1266.
13. Frostegard J, Haegerstrand A, Giglund M, Nilsson J. Biologically modified LDL increases the adhesive properties of endothelial cells. Atherosclerosis 1991; 90:119–126.
14. Lehr HA, Hübner C, Finckh B, et al. Role of leukotrienes in leukocyte adhesion following systemic administration of oxidatively modified human low density lipoprotein in hamsters. J Clin Invest 1991; 88:9–14.
15. Kim JA, Territo MC, Wayner E. Partial characterization of leukocyte binding molecules on endothelial cells induced by minimally oxidized LDL. Arterioscler Thromb 1994; 14: 427–433.
16. Sugiyama S, Kugiyama K, Ohgushi M, et al. Lysophosphatidylcholine in oxidized low-density lipoprotein increases endothelial susceptibility to polymorphonuclear leukocyte-induced endothelial dysfunction in porcine coronary arteries. Role of protein kinase C. Circ Res 1994; 74:565–575.
17. Rajavashisth TB, Andalibi A, Territo MC, et al. Induction of endothelial cell expression of granulocyte and macrophage colony-stimulating factors by modified low-density lipoproteins. Nature 1990; 344:254–257.
18. Parhami F, Fang ZT, Fogelman AM. Minimally modified low density lipoprotein-induced inflammatory responses in endothelial cells are mediated by cyclic adenosine monophosphate. J Clin Invest 1993; 92:471–478.
19. Quinn MT, Parthasarathy S, Fong LG, Steinberg D. Oxidatively modified low density lipoproteins: a potential role in recruitment and retention of monocyte/macrophages during atherogenesis. Proc Natl Acad Sci USA 1987; 84:2995–2998.
20. Quinn MT, Parthasarathy S, Steinberg D. Lysophosphatidylcholine: a chemotactic factor for human monocytes and its potential role in atherogenesis. Proc Natl Acad Sci USA 1988; 84: 1372–1376.
21. Krieger M, Herz J. Structures and functions of multiligand lipoprotein receptors: macrophage scavenger receptors and LDL receptor-related protein (LRP). Annu Rev Biochem 1994; 63: 601–637.
22. Stanton LW, White RT, Bryant CM, et al. A macrophage F_c receptor for IgG is also a receptor for oxidized low density lipoprotein. J Biol Chem 1992; 267:22446–22451.
23. Endemann G, Stanton LW, Madden KS, et al. CD36 is a receptor for oxidized low density lipoprotein. J Biol Chem 1993; 268:11811–11816.
24. Ottnad E, Parthasarathy S, Sambrano GR, et al. A macrophage receptor for oxidized low density lipoprotein distinct from the receptor for acetyl low density lipoprotein: partial purification and role in recognition of oxidatively damaged cells. Proc Natl Acad Sci USA 1995; 92:1391–1395.
25. Henriksen T, Mahoney EM, Steinberg D. Enhanced macrophage degradation of biologically modified low density lipoprotein. Arteriosclerosis 1983; 3:149–159.
26. Brown MS, Goldstein JL. A receptor-mediated pathway for cholesterol homeostasis. Science 1986; 232:34–47.
27. Palinski W, Rosenfeld ME, Ylä-Herttuala S, et al. Low density lipoprotein undergoes oxidative modification in vivo. Proc Nat Acad Sci USA 1989; 86:1372–1376.
28. Khoo JC, Miller E, Pio F, et al. Monoclonal antibodies against LDL further enhance macrophage uptake of LDL aggregates. Arterioscler Thromb 1992; 12:1258–1266.
29. Suits AG, Chait A, Aviram M, Heinecke JW. Phagocytosis of aggregated lipoprotein by macrophages: low density lipoprotein receptor-dependent foam-cell formation. Proc Natl Acad Sci USA 1989; 86:2713–2717.
30. Simon BC, Cunningham LD, Cohen RA. Oxidized low density lipoproteins cause contraction and inhibit endothelium-dependent relaxation in the pig coronary artery. J Clin Invest 1990; 86:75–79.

31. Chin JH, Azhar S, Hoffman BB. Inactivation of endothelial derived relaxing factor by oxidized lipoproteins. J Clin Invest 1992; 89:10–18.

32. Levine GN, Keaney JF Jr, Vita JA. Cholesterol reduction in cardiovascular disease: Clinical benefits and possible mechanisms. N Engl J Med 1995; 332:512–521.

33. Welch G, Loscalzo J. Nitric oxide and the cardiovascular system. J Cardiovasc Surg 1994; 9: 361–371.

34. Boulanger CM, Tanner FC, Bea ML, et al. Oxidized low density lipoproteins induce mRNA expression and release of endothelin from human and porcine endothelium. Circ Res 1992; 70:1191–1197.

35. Lynch SM, Morrow JD, Roberts LJ II, Frei B. Formation of non-cyclooxygenase-derived prostanoids (F_2-isoprostanes) in plasma and low density lipoprotein exposed to oxidative stress in vitro. J Clin Invest 1994; 93:998–1004.

36. Moore KP, Darley-Usmar V, Morrow J, Roberts LJ II. Formation of F_2-isoprostanes during oxidation of human low-density lipoprotein and plasma by peroxynitrite. Circ Res 1995; 77: 335–341.

37. Heery JM, Kozak M, Stafforini DM, et al. Oxidatively modified LDL contains phospholipids with platelet-activating factor-like activity and stimulates the growth of smooth muscle cells. J Clin Invest 1995; 96:2322–2330.

38. Hughes H, Mathews B, Lenz ML, Guyton JR. Cytotoxicity of oxidized LDL to porcine aortic smooth muscle cells is associated with the oxysterols 7-ketocholesterol and 7-hydroxy-cholesterol. Arterioscler Thromb 1994; 14:1177–1185.

39. Coffey MD, Cole RA, Colles SM, Chisolm GM. In vitro cell injury by oxidized low density lipoprotein involves lipid hydroperoxide-induced formation of alkoxyl, lipid and peroxyl radicals. J Clin Invest 1995; 96:1866–1873.

40. Drake TA, Hannani K, Fei HH, et al. Minimally oxidized low-density lipoprotein induces tissue factor expression in cultured human endothelial cells. Am J Pathol 1991; 138:601–607.

41. Weis JR, Pitas RE, Wilson BD, Rodgers GM. Oxidized low-density lipoprotein increases cultured human endothelial cell tissue factor activity and reduces protein C activation. FASEB J 1991; 5:2459–2465.

42. Thorin E, Hamilton CA, Dominiczak MH, Reid JL. Chronic exposure of cultured bovine endothelial cells to oxidized LDL abolishes prostacyclin release. Arterioscler Thromb 1994; 14:453–459.

43. Latron Y, Chautan M, Anfosso F, et al. Stimulating effect of oxidized low density lipoproteins on plasminogen activator inhibitor-1 synthesis by endothelial cells. Arterioscler Thromb 1991; 11:1821–1829.

44. Ylä-Herttuala S, Palinski W, Rosenfeld ME, et al. Evidence for the presence of oxidatively modified low density lipoprotein in atherosclerotic lesions of rabbit and man. J Clin Invest 1989; 84:1086–1095.

45. Jürgens G, Chen Q, Esterbauer H, et al. Immunostaining of human autopsy aortas with antibodies to modified apolipoprotein B and apoprotein(a). Arterioscler Thromb 1993; 13: 1689–1699.

46. Holvoet P, Perez G, Zhao Z, et al. Malondialdehyde-modified low density lipoproteins in patients with atherosclerotic disease. J Clin Invest 1995; 95:2611–2619.

47. Salonen JT, Ylä-Herttuala S, Yamamoto R, et al. Autoantibody against oxidised LDL and progression of carotid atherosclerosis. Lancet 1992; 339:883–887.

48. Lynch SM, Frei B. Antioxidants as antiatherogens: animal studies. In: Frei B, ed. Natural Antioxidants in Human Health and Disease. San Diego: Academic Press, 1994:353–385.

49. Gaziano MJ, Manson JE, Hennekens CH. Natural antioxidants and cardiovascular disease: observational epidemiologic studies and randomized trials. In: Frei B, ed. Natural Antioxidants in Human Health and Disease. San Diego: Academic Press, 1994:387–410.

50. The Alpha-Tocopherol, Beta Carotene Cancer Prevention Study Group: The effect of vitamin

E and beta carotene on the incidence of lung cancer and other cancers in male smokers. N Engl J Med 1994; 330:1029–1035.

51. Marwick C. Trials reveal no benefit, possible harm of beta carotene and vitamin A for lung cancer prevention. JAMA 1996; 275:422–423.

52. Gaziano JM, Hatta A, Flynn M, et al. Supplementation with β-carotene in vivo and in vitro does not inhibit low density lipoprotein oxidation. Atherosclerosis 1995; 112:187–195.

53. Esterbauer H, Jürgens G, Quehenberger O, Koller E. Autoxidation of human low density lipoprotein: loss of polyunsaturated fatty acids and vitamin E and generation of aldehydes. J Lipid Res 1987; 28:495–509.

54. Haberland ME, Olch CL, Fogelman AM. Role of lysines in mediating interaction of modified low density lipoproteins with the scavenger receptor of human monocyte macrophages. J Biol Chem 1984; 259:11305–11311.

55. Bowry V, Ingold KU, Stocker R. Vitamin E in human low-density lipoprotein: when and how this antioxidant becomes a pro-oxidant. Biochem J 1992; 288:341–344.

56. Ingold KU, Bowry VW, Stocker R, Walling C. Autoxidation of lipids and antioxidation by α-tocopherol and ubiquinol in homogeneous solution and in aqueous dispersions of lipids: unrecognized consequences of lipid particle size as exemplified by oxidation of human low density lipoprotein. Proc Natl Acad Sci USA 1993; 90:45–49.

57. Bowry VW. Stocker R. Tocopherol-mediated peroxidation: the prooxidant effect of vitamin E on the radical-initiated oxidation of human low-density lipoprotein. J Am Chem Soc 1993; 115:6029–6044.

58. Dabbagh AJ, Frei B. Human suction blister interstitial fluid prevents metal ion-dependent oxidation of low density lipoprotein by macrophages and in cell-free systems. J Clin Invest 1995; 96:1958–1966.

59. Suarna C, Dean RT, May J, Stocker R. Human atherosclerotic plaque contains both oxidized lipids and relatively large amounts of alpha-tocopherol and ascorbate. Arterioscler Thromb Vasc Biol 1995; 15:1616–1624.

60. Kagan VE, Serbinova EA, Forte T, et al. Recycling of vitamin E in human low density lipoproteins. J Lipid Res 1992; 33:385–397.

61. Bowry VW, Mohr D, Cleary J, Stocker R. Prevention of tocopherol-mediated peroxidation in ubiquinol-10-free human low density lipoprotein. J Biol Chem 1995; 270:5756–5763.

62. Steinbrecher UP, Parthasarathy S, Leake DS, et al. Modification of low density lipoprotein by endothelial cells involves lipid peroxidation and degradation of low density lipoprotein phospholipids. Proc Natl Acad Sci USA 1984; 81:3883–3887.

63. Parthasarathy S, Printz DJ, Boyd D, et al. Macrophage oxidation of low density lipoprotein generates a modified form recognized by the scavenger receptor Arteriosclerosis 1986; 6: 505–510.

64. Ehrenwald E, Chisolm GM, Fox PL. Intact human ceruloplasmin oxidatively modifies low density lipoprotein. J Clin Invest 1994; 93:1493–1501.

65. Smith C, Mitchinson MJ, Aruoma OI, Halliwell B. Stimulation of lipid peroxidation and hydroxyl-radical generation by the contents of human atherosclerotic lesions. Biochem J 1992; 286:901–905.

66. Salonen JT, Salonen R, Seppänen K, et al. Interactions of serum copper, selenium, and low density lipoprotein cholesterol in atherogenesis. Br Med J 1991; 302:756–760.

67. Kiechl S, Aichner F, Gerstenbrand F, et al. Body iron stores and presence of carotid atherosclerosis: results from the Bruneck Study. Arterioslcer Thromb 1994; 14:1625–1630.

68. Salonen JT, Nyyssönen K, Korpela H, et al. High stored iron levels are associated with excess risk of myocardial infarction in eastern Finnish men. Circulation 1992; 86:803–811.

69. Ascherio A, Willett WC, Rimm EB, et al. Dietary iron intake and risk of coronary disease among men. Circulation 1994; 89:969–974.

70. Moore M, Folsom AR, Barnes RW, Eckfeldt JH. No association between serum ferritin and

asymptomatic carotid atherosclerosis: The Atherosclerosis Risk in Communities (ARIC) Study. Am J Epidemiol 1995; 141:719–723.

71. Hazell LJ, Stocker R. Oxidation of low-density lipoprotein with hypochlorite causes transformation of the lipoprotein into a high-uptake form for macrophages. Biochem J 1993; 290: 165–172.

72. Hazell LJ, van den Berg JJ, Stocker R. Oxidation of low-density lipoprotein by hypochlorite causes aggregation that is mediated by modification of lysine residues rather than lipid oxidation. Biochem J 1994; 302:297–304.

73. Savenkova MI, Mueller DM, Heinecke JW. Tyrosyl radical generated by myeloperoxidae is a physiological catalyst for the initiation of lipid peroxidation in low density lipoprotein. J Biol Chem 1994; 269:20394–20400.

74. Jha P, Flather M, Lonn E, et al. The antioxidant vitamins and cardiovascular disease. A critical review of epidemiologic and clinical trial data. Ann Intern Med 1995; 123:860–872.

75. Keaney JF Jr, Frei B. Antioxidant protection of low-density lipoprotein and its role in the prevention of atherosclerotic vascular disease. In: Frei B, ed. Natural Antioxidants in Human Health and Disease. San Diego: Academic Press, 1994:303–351.

76. Frei B. Cardiovascular disease and nutrient antioxidants: Role of low-density lipoprotein oxidation. Crit Rev Food Sci Nutr 1995; 35:83–98.

77. Stocker R, Frei B. Endogenous antioxidant defences in human blood plasma. In: Sies H, ed. Oxidative Stress: Oxidants and Antioxidants, Orlando, FL: Academic Press, 1991:213–243.

78. Frei B, Stocker R, Ames BN. Antioxidant defenses and lipid peroxidation in human blood plasma. Proc Natl Acad Sci USA 1988; 85:9748–9752.

79. Frei B, England L, Ames BN. Ascorbate is an outstanding antioxidant in human blood plasma. Proc Natl Acad Sci USA 1989; 86:6377–6381.

80. Frei B, Stocker R, England L, Ames BN. Ascorbate: the most effective antioxidant in human blood plasma. Adv Exp Med Biol 1990; 264:155–163.

81. Neuzil J, Stocker R. Free and albumin-bound bilirubin are efficient co-antioxidants for α-tocopherol inhibiting plasma and low density lipoprotein lipid peroxidation. J Biol Chem 1994; 269:16712–16719.

82. Frei B, Forte T, Ames BN, Cross CE. Gas-phase oxidants of cigarette smoke induce lipid peroxidation and changes in lipoprotein properties in human blood plasma: protective effects of ascorbic acid. Biochem J 1991; 277:133–138.

83. Frei B, Stocker R, Ames BN. Small molecule antioxidant defenses in human extracellular fluids. In: Scandalios J, ed. The Molecular Biology of Free Radical Scavenging Systems. Cold Spring Harbor, NY: Cold Spring Harbor Laboratory Press, 1992:23–45.

84. Kimura H, Yamada Y, Morita Y, et al. Dietary ascorbic acid depresses plasma and low density lipoprotein lipid peroxidation in genetically scorbutic rats. J Nutr 1992; 122:1904–1909.

85. Steinbrecher UP. Role of superoxide in endothelial-cell modification of low-density lipoproteins. Biochim Biophys Acta 1988; 959:20–30.

86. Jialal I, Grundy SM. Preservation of the endogenous antioxidants in low density lipoprotein by ascorbate but not probucol during oxidative modification. J Clin Invest 1991; 87:597–601.

87. Stait SE, Leake DS. Ascorbic acid can either increase or decrease low density lipoprotein modification. FEBS Lett 1994; 341:263–267.

88. Stocker R, Bowry VW, Frei B. Ubiquinol-10 protects human low density lipoprotein more efficiently against lipid peroxidation than does α-tocopherol. Proc Natl Acad Sci USA 1991; 88:1646–1650.

89. Balla G, Jacob HS, Eaton JW, et al. Hemin: a possible physiological mediator of low density lipoprotein oxidation and endothelial injury. Arterioscler Thromb 1991; 11:1700–1711.

90. Retsky KL, Frei B. Vitamin C prevents metal ion-dependent initiation and propagation of lipid peroxidation in human low density lipoprotein. Biochim Biophys Acta 1995; 1257: 279–287.

91. Retsky KL, Freeman MW, Frei B. Ascorbic acid oxidation product(s) protect human low

density lipoprotein against atherogenic modification: anti- rather than prooxidant activity of vitamin C in the presence of transition metal ions. J Biol Chem 1993; 268:1304–1309.

92. Ma YS, Stone WL, LeClair IO. The effects of vitamin C and urate on the oxidation kinetics of human low-density lipoprotein. Proc Soc Exp Biol Med 1994; 206:53–59.

93. Jialal I, Vega GL, Grundy SM. Physiologic levels of ascorbate inhibit oxidative modification of low density lipoprotein. Atherosclerosis 1990; 82:185–191.

94. Hatta A, Frei B. Oxidative modification and antioxidant protection of human low density lipoprotein at high and low oxygen partial pressures. J Lipid Res 1995; 36:2383–2393.

95. Abdalla DSP, Campa A, Monteiro HP. Low density lipoprotein oxidation by stimulated neutrophils and ferritin. Atherosclerosis 1992; 97:149–159.

96. Halliwell B, Wasil M, Grootveld M. Biologically significant scavenging of the myeloperoxidase-derived oxidant hypochlorous acid by ascorbic acid. Implications for antioxidant protection in the inflamed rheumatoid joint. FEBS Lett 1987; 213:15–17.

97. Hunter EPL, Desrosiers MF, Simic MG. The effect of oxygen, antioxidants and superoxide radical on tyrosine phenoxyl radical dimerization. Free Radical Biol Med 1989; 6:581–585.

98. Nishikimi M. Oxidation of ascorbic acid with superoxide anion generated by the xanthine-xanthine oxidase system. Biochim Biophys Res Commun 1975; 63:463–468.

99. Sato K, Niki E, Shimasaki H. Free radical-mediated chain oxidation of low density lipoprotein and its synergistic inhibition by vitamin E and C. Arch Biochem Biophys 1990; 279:402–405.

100. Samuni A, Aronovitch J, Godinger D, et al. On the cytotoxicity of vitamin C and metal ions: a site-specific Fenton mechanism. Eur J Biochem 1983; 137:119–124.

101. Aruoma OI, Halliwell B, Gajewski E, Dizdaroglu M. Copper-ion-dependent damage to the bases in DNA in the presence of hydrogen peroxide. Biochem J 1991; 273:601–604.

102. Bedwell S, Dean RT, Jessup W. The action of defined oxygen-centered free radicals on human low-density lipoprotein. Biochem J 1989; 262:707–712.

103. Uchida K, Kawakishi S. Site-specific oxidation of angiotensin I by copper(II) and L-ascorbate: conversion of histidine residues to 2-imidazolones. Arch Biochem Biophys 1990; 283:20–26.

104. Kuzuya M, Yamada K, Hayashi T, et al. Role of lipoprotein–copper complex in copper catalyzed-peroxidation of low-density lipoprotein. Biochim Biophys Acta 1992; 1123: 334–341.

105. Harats D, Ben-Naim M, Dabach Y, et al. Effect of vitamin C and E supplementation on susceptibility of plasma lipoproteins to peroxidation induced by acute smoking. Atherosclerosis 1990; 85:47–54.

106. Belcher JD, Balla J, Balla G, et al. Vitamin E, LDL, and endothelium: brief oral vitamin supplementation prevents oxidized LDL-mediated vascular injury in vitro. Arterioscler Thromb 1993; 13:1779–1789.

107. Reaven PD, Khouw A, Beltz WF, et al. Effect of dietary antioxidant combinations in humans: protection of LDL by vitamin E but not beta-carotene. Arterioscler Thromb 1993; 13:590–600.

108. Rifici VA, Khachadurian AK. Dietary supplementation with vitamins C and E inhibits in vitro oxidation of lipoproteins. J Am Coll Nutr 1993; 12:631–637.

109. Lynch SM, Gaziano JM, Frei B. Ascorbic acid and atherosclerotic cardiovascular disease. In: Harris JR, ed. Ascorbic Acid: Biochemistry and Biomedical Cell Biology. New York: Plenum Press, 1996:331–367.

110. Gale CR, Martyn CN, Winter PD, Cooper C. Vitamin C and risk of death from stroke and coronary heart disease in a cohort of elderly people. Br Med J 1995; 310:1563–1566.

111. Kritchevsky SB, Shimakawa T, Tell GS, et al. Dietary antioxidants and carotid artery wall thickness: The ARIC Study. Circulation 1995; 92:2142–2150.

112. Simon JA. Vitamin C and cardiovascular disease: a review. J Am Coll Nutr 1992; 11:107–125.

113. Hallfrisch J, Singh VN, Muller DC, et al. High plasma vitamin C associated with high plasma HDL- and HDL_2 cholesterol. Am J Clin Nutr 1994; 60:100–105.

114. Bjorkhem I, Kallner A. Hepatic 7alpha-hydroxylation of cholesterol in ascorbate-deficient and ascorbate-supplemented guinea pigs. J Lipid Res 1976; 17:360–365.

115. Bobek P, Ginter E. Serum triglycerides and post-heparin lipolytic activity in guinea-pigs with latent vitamin C deficiency. Experientia 1978; 34:1554–1555.

116. Levine M. New concepts in the biology and biochemistry of ascorbic acid. N Engl J Med 1986; 314:892–902.

117. Robert L, Jacob MP, Labat-Robert J. Cell-matrix interactions in the genesis of arteriosclerosis and atheroma: effect of aging. Ann NY Acad Sci 1992; 673:331–341.

118. Lehr HA, Frei B, Arfors KE. Vitamin C prevents cigarette smoke-induced leukocyte aggregation and adhesion to endothelium in vivo. Proc Natl Acad Sci USA 1994; 91:7688–7692.

119. Lehr HA, Frei B, Olofsson M, et al. Protection from oxidized LDL-induced leukocyte adhesion to micro- and macrovascular endothelium in vivo by vitamin C but not by vitamin E. Circulation 1995; 91:1525–1532.

120. Bordia AK. The effect of vitamin C on blood lipids, fibrinolytic activity and platelet adhesiveness in patients with coronary heart disease. Atherosclerosis 1980; 35:181–187.

121. Bordia A, Verma SK. Effect of vitamin C on platelet adhesiveness and platelet aggregation in coronary artery disease patients. Clin Cardiol 1985; 8:552–554.

122. Crawford GP, Warlow CP, Bennett B, et al. The effect of vitamin C supplements on serum cholesterol coagulation, fibrinolysis and platelet adhesiveness. Atherosclerosis 1975; 21:451–454.

123. Beetens JR, Herman AG. Vitamin C increases the formation of prostacyclin by aortic rings from various species and neutralizes the inhibitory effect of 15-hydroperoxy-arachidonic acid. Br J Pharmacol 1983; 80:249–254.

124. Srivastava KC. Ascorbic acid enhances the formation of prostaglandin E1 in washed human platelets and prostacyclin in rat aortic rings. Prostaglandins Leukotrienes Med 1985; 18:227–233.

125. Toivanen JL. Effects of selenium, vitamin E and vitamin C on human prostacyclin and thromboxane synthesis in vitro. Prostaglandins Leukotrienes Med 1987; 26:265–280.

126. Vita JA, Treasure CB, Nabel EG, et al. Coronary vasomotor response to acetylcholine relates to risk factors for coronary artery disease. Circulation 1990; 81:491–497.

127. Anderson TJ, Meredith IT, Yeung AC, et al. The effect of cholesterol-lowering and antioxidant therapy on endothelium-dependent coronary vasomotion. N Engl J Med 1995; 332:488–493.

128. Levine GN, Frei B, Koulouris SN, et al. Ascorbic acid reverses endothelial vasomotor dysfunction in patients with coronary artery disease. Circulation 1996; 93:1107–1113.

129. Ting HH, Timimi FK, Boles KS, et al. Vitamin C improves endothelium-dependent vasodilation in patients with non-insulin-dependent diabetes mellitus. J Clin Invest 1996; 97:22–28.

130. Kugiyama K, Kerns SA, Morrisett JD, et al. Impairment of endothelium-dependent arterial relaxation by lysolecithin in modified low-density lipoproteins. Nature 1990; 344:160–162.

131. Gryglewski RJ, Palmer RM, Moncada S. Superoxide anion is involved in the breakdown of endothelium-derived vascular relaxing factor. Nature 1986; 320:454–456.

132. Plane F, Jacobs M, McManus D, Bruckdorfer KR. Probucol and other antioxidants prevent the inhibition of endothelium-dependent relaxation by low density lipoproteins. Atherosclerosis 1993; 103:73–79.

133. Laursen JB, Boesgaard S, Poulsen HE, Aldershvile J. Vitamin C and thiol supplementation potentiate receptor stimulated nitric oxide release in vivo. Circulation 1994; 90:A1301.

134. Moran JP, Cohen L, Greene JM, et al. Plasma ascorbic acid concentrations relate inversely to blood pressure in human subjects. Am J Clin Nutr 1993; 57:213–217.

135. Jacques PF. A cross-sectional study of vitamin C intake and blood pressure in the elderly. Int J Vitam Nutr Res 1992; 62:252–255.

136. Keaney JF Jr, Gaziano JM, Xu A, et al. Dietary antioxidants preserve endothelium-dependent vessel relaxation in cholesterol-fed rabbits. Proc Natl Acad Sci USA 1993; 90:11880–11884.

137. Shaish A, Daugherty A, O'Sullivan F, et al. Beta-carotene inhibits atherosclerosis in hyper-cholesterolemic rabbits. J Clin Invest 1995; 96:2075–2082.

10

Protection of Human Low-Density Lipoprotein from Oxidative Modification by Vitamin C

ETSUO NIKI and NORIKO NOGUCHI
Research Center for Advanced Science and Technology,
University of Tokyo, Tokyo, Japan

OUTLINE OF ANTIOXIDANT ACTION OF VITAMIN C

Vitamin C, ascorbic acid or ascorbate, acts as an electron donor and/or hydrogen atom donor; that characteristic makes it a potent antioxidant (1–5). It rapidly reduces superoxide and nitroxide radicals and scavenges hydroxyl, alkoxyl, and peroxyl radicals. It also reacts with nonradical species such as singlet oxygen and hypochlorous acid. It is water-soluble and plays an important role, especially in the plasma. It has been observed in in vitro experiments that vitamin C acts as the first defense in the plasma (6–8). When the peroxyl radicals are generated in the blood (6) or plasma (7) from a water-soluble azo compound, 2,2'-azo-bis(2-amidinopropane) dihydrochloride (AAPH), vitamin C is consumed faster than other antioxidants, such as uric acid, bilirubin, and vitamin E, and lipid hydroperoxides are formed appreciably only after vitamin C is completely depleted (Fig. 1). A similar function of ascorbic acid has been also observed in the oxidation of plasma challenged by activated neutrophils (7) and cigarette smoke (9). It also suppresses the aqueous peroxyl radical–induced hemolysis of erythrocytes (10).

In the preceding examples, vitamin C scavenges peroxyl radicals before the radicals attack the target molecules such as lipids and proteins. Vitamin C scavenges peroxyl radicals with a rate constant of 7.5×10^4 M^{-1}s^{-1} (11). The peroxyl radicals are less reactive and more selective than hydroxyl and alkoxyl radicals. Because vitamin C is more reactive than polyunsaturated lipids by a factor of about 10^3 (11), it competes well with polyunsaturated lipids against peroxyl radicals. However, it should be borne in mind that vitamin C, like vitamin E (12), can scavenge neither hydroxyl nor alkoxyl radicals effectively in competition with lipids and/or proteins. The stoichiometric number of radicals scavenged by each molecule of vitamin C varies between 2 and 0, depending on conditions, especially concentration (13).

Another important issue that should be appreciated is the hydrophilicity of vitamin C: it

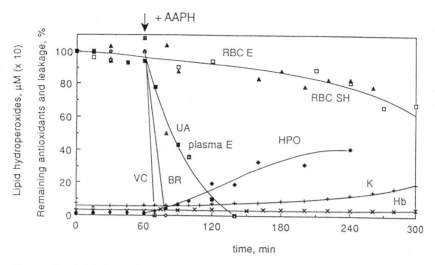

Figure 1 Oxidation of human blood induced by AAPH at 37°C in air. The blood from a healthy donor (diluted four times with physiological saline solution) was incubated with 309 mM AAPH (added at 60 min after incubation) and the consumption of vitamin C (VC), bilirubin (BR), uric acid (UA), vitamin E in plasma and erythrocytes (Plasma E and RBC E, respectively), and total thiol in erythrocytes (RBC SH) was measured. The formation of lipid hydroperoxides (HPO) and leakage of potassium (K) and hemoglobin (Hb) were also followed. AAPH, 2,2'-azo-bis(2-amidinoprorane) dihydrochloride.

scavenges aqueous radicals rapidly but is much less efficient in scavenging lipophilic radicals present within the lipophilic compartment of the membranes and lipoproteins. Accordingly, vitamin C suppresses the oxidation of phospholipid liposomal membranes induced by aqueous AAPH efficiently, but it can only retard the oxidation of membranes when it is initiated by radicals generated within the membranes. Such an effect of location of radicals on the scavenging efficacy of vitamin C can be clearly shown by experiments using a spin label. N-Oxyl-4,4'-dimethyloxazolidine derivatives of stearic acid (NS), **1**,

$$CH_3-(CH_2)_m-C-(CH_2)_{n-2}-COOH$$
$$O \qquad N-{}^{\bullet}O$$
$$CH_2-C-CH_3$$
$$CH_3$$

1 n-NS (m + n) = 17

have been used as a spin label. A nitroxide group is attached at various positions along the fatty acid chain in order to situate it at different depths in the hydrophobic interior of the membranes. In solution, the nitroxide radicals are reduced very rapidly by vitamin C independently of the position of the nitroxide group. However, when the spin label is incorporated into phosphatidylcholine liposomal membranes, it is still reduced by vitamin C present in the aqueous phase but the rate of reduction is markedly reduced and decreased in the order 5-NS > 12-NS > 16-NS, suggesting that it becomes less efficient for vitamin C to scavenge the radical as it goes deeper into the interior of the membranes (14).

Another interesting feature of the antioxidant action of vitamin C is its synergistic interaction with vitamin E. It was suggested by Tappel in 1968 that vitamins C and E may act synergistically in the inhibition of oxidation (15). It was experimentally established by flash photolysis experiment (16) that vitamin C reduces the vitamin E radical formed from vitamin E when it scavenges the radical. This was confirmed later by electron spin resonance (ESR) study (17). As mentioned above, vitamin C cannot scavenge radicals within the lipophilic compartment of the membranes efficiently and vitamin E scavenges such radicals to break the chain propagation. The resulting vitamin E radical is reduced by vitamin C to regenerate vitamin E and thus vitamin C spares vitamin E (11). It was not known whether vitamin C present in the aqueous phase could reduce the vitamin E radical in the membranes as efficiently as it did in homogeneous solution. It was confirmed by in vitro experiment by controlling the site of radical generation that such interaction can in fact take place efficiently even in the membrane system, where the two vitamins are present at the different sites (18,19). This synergistic inhibtion of oxidation by a combination of vitamin C and vitamin E has since been observed in many in vitro studies (20–25). However, it is still a matter of controversy whether such interaction is important in vivo (26).

Cysteine (27) and glutathione (17) also reduce the vitamin E radical to give vitamin E, but they are both much less efficient than vitamin C (28). The interaction between vitamin C and β-carotene appears not to be important (12,29).

INHIBITION OF OXIDATION OF LOW-DENSITY LIPOPROTEIN BY VITAMIN C

A number of antioxidants with different functions protect membranes and tissues from oxidative damage induced by free radicals (12). As described previously, vitamin C acts as the primary defense in the plasma against the oxidation induced by aqueous peroxyl radicals. It has been reported that vitamin C protects LDL from oxidative modification induced by endothelial cells (30), macrophages (31), copper ion (31–36), and AAPH (37,38). Esterbauer (32) has shown that ascorbic acid suppresses the oxidation of LDL induced by copper and prolongs the lag phase in a concentration-dependent manner.

As indicated, vitamin C probably acts as the first defense in the plasma by scavenging aqueous radicals before they attack membranes and lipoproteins. However, as pointed out previously, vitamin C is not capable of scavenging lipophilic radicals located within the lipophilic compartment. The efficiency of lipophilic radical scavenging within LDL by vitamin C can also be measured by a spin label technique.

The spin prove, N-oxyl-4,4'-dimethyloxazolidine derivatives of stearic acid 1, has the paramagnetic nitroxide moiety at different positions of the stearic acid chain, thus making it possible to situate the stable radical at different distances from the LDL surface (Fig. 2). The ESR spectra of five doxyl stearic acids are shown in Figure 3 together with the ESR order parameters measured at 37°C (38). The number before NS indicates the carbon number from the LDL surface on which the nitroxide is attached. For example, 5-NS indicates that the nitroxide group is on the fifth carbon from the LDL particle surface. The 16-doxyl stearic acid ester of cholesterol (16-NSC) has been also synthesized and incorporated into LDL. Its ESR spectra observed in benzene solution and in LDL are shown in Figure 4 together with the ESR parameters. These figures show that the LDL surface is quite hard and it becomes more fluid as it goes from the surface to the interior of the outer monolayer and that the LDL core is more fluid than the outer monolayer. The rate of reduction of the nitroxide radical by ascorbate becomes slower as the radical goes deeper

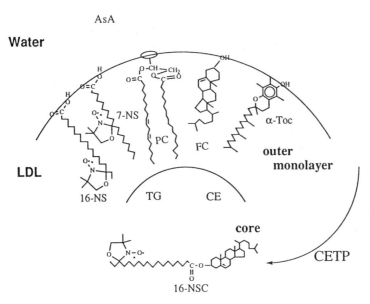

Figure 2 Spin labels incorporated into LDL particles. LDL, low-density lipoprotein; ASA, ascorbate; α-Toc, α-tocopherol; FC, free cholesterol; PC, phosphatidylcholine; CE, cholesterol ester; TG, triglyceride; CETP, cholesterol ester transfer protein; NS, spin label doxyl stearate; NSC, spin label, cholesterol ester of doxyl stearic acid.

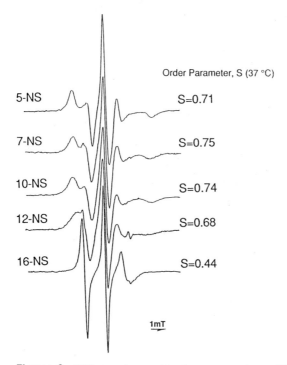

Figure 3 ESR spectra and order parameters of five different NS spin labels incorporated into human LDL at 37°C. ESR, electron spin resonance; NS, spin label doxyl stearate; LDL, low-density lipoprotein.

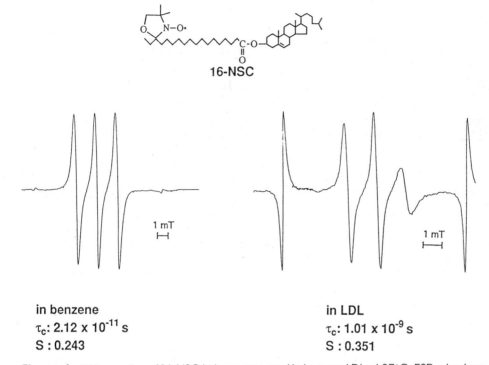

Figure 4 ESR spectra of 16-NSC in benzene and in human LDL at 37°C. ESR, electron spin resonance; 16-NSC, 16-doxyl stearic acid ester of cholesterol; LDL, low-density lipoprotein.

into the interior, and, interestingly, 16-NSC is not reduced at an appreciable rate, suggesting that the scavenging of radicals present in the LDL core by ascorbate is quite difficult. This also implies that the reduction of phenoxyl radicals derived from antioxidants such as vitamin E and probucol takes place efficiently only when the phenoxyl radicals are present at or near the LDL surface.

The synergistic inhibition of oxidation of LDL by a combination of vitamin C and vitamin E has been observed (36,38,39). As shown in Figure 5, both ascorbic acid and uric acid suppress the oxidation of LDL induced by aqueous radical initiator and spare vitamin E. On the other hand, when the LDL oxidation is induced by a lipophilic radical initiator, uric acid, which does not reduce the tocopheroxyl radical, does not spare vitamin E, whereas ascorbic acid efficiently spares vitamin E. The reduction of the vitamin E radical in LDL by ascorbic acid has been confirmed by ESR spectroscopy (35,39). Kalyanaraman et al. (35) have observed that the incubation of LDL and lipoxygenase produced an ESR spectrum due to endogenous α-tocopherol and that the addition of ascorbic acid reduced this radical to regenerate α-tocopherol with concomitant formation of the ascorbate radical. Kagan et al. (39) have observed similar results. Furthermore, they have demonstrated that although dihydrolipoic acid is not efficient in direct reduction of the chromanoxyl radical, it is capable of recycling vitamin E by synergistically interacting with ascorbate; that is, dihydrolipoic acid reduces dehydroascorbate, thus maintaining the steady-state concentration of ascorbate (39).

Ubiquinol acts as a potent antioxidant by itself (40) and can also reduce the α-tocopheroxyl radical to regenerate α-tocopherol (41,42). Ascorbic acid and ubiquinol compete to react

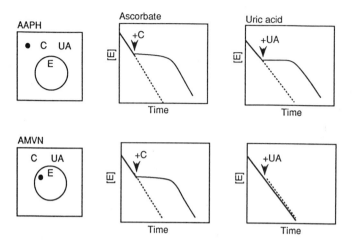

Figure 5 Sparing of α-tocopherol (E) by ascorbate (C) and uric acid (UA) in the oxidation of LDL induced by either hydrophilic AAPH or lipophilic AMVN. LDL, low-density lipoprotein; AAPH, 2,2′-azo-bis(2-amidinopropane) dihydrochloride; AMVN, 2,2′-azo-bis(2,4-dimethyl-valeronitrile).

with the α-tocopheroxyl radical. It has been found that when α-tocopherol, ascorbic acid, and ubiquinol are all present in the oxidation of phospholipid liposomal membranes induced by hydrophilic AAPH, ascorbic acid is consumed first, followed by ubiquinol, and α-tocopherol is spared, while ubiquinol is consumed faster than ascorbic acid in the oxidations induced by lipophilic 2,2′-azobis-(2,4-dimethylvaleronitrile) (AMVN) incorporated into liposomal membranes (Fig. 6) (43). Ascorbic acid does not reduce the radical derived from ubiquinol (44). Ascorbic acid is not capable of sparing ubiquinol as it does α-tocopherol in the oxidation of liposomal membranes. These data suggest that although ubiquinol present at high concentration effectively suppresses the oxidations of both lipids and proteins in mitochondria (40) and suppresses the oxidation of LDL efficiently when it is present (45,46), practically ubiquinol may not play an important role against the oxidative modification of LDL, since ubiquinol concentration is so low that not all LDL particles contain the ubiquinol molecule.

Recently, it has been argued that α-tocopherol acts as a prooxidant rather than an antioxidant in the oxidation of LDL (47–50). Stocker and his colleagues have observed that LDL oxidation induced by a hydrophilic or lipophilic azo initiator or by a transition metal ion is accelerated by increasing the concentration of α-tocopherol in LDL. They interpreted such a prooxidant effect of α-tocopherol as accelerated incorporation of aqueous radical into LDL particle and the chain initiation of lipid peroxidation by a hydrogen atom abstraction from LDL lipids by the α-tocopheroxyl radical and called the effect "tocopherol-mediated peroxidation" (47–50). The simulation of lipid peroxidation in LDL by a kinetic model shows that this α-tocopherol–mediated peroxidation can take place under certain conditions, but it also shows that nevertheless the oxidation proceeds faster than without α-tocopherol (49,51,52). Therefore, it is open to question whether it is appropriate to call it a "prooxidant" effect of α-tocopherol. It may be noteworthy, however, that the absolute rate constants for the relevant elementary reactions have been measured in solution but that

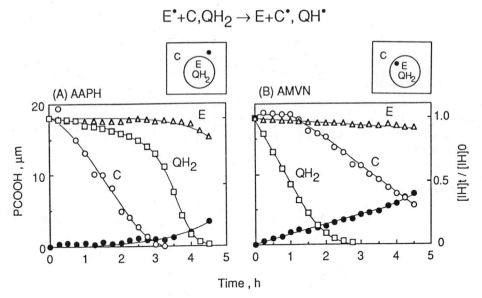

Figure 6 Consumption of α-tocopherol (E), ascorbate (C), and ubiquinol (QH$_2$) in the oxidation of soybean phosphatidylcholine (PC) induced by hydrophilic AAPH or lipophilic AMVN. Accumulation of PC hydroperoxide (PCOOH) has been also measured. AAPH, 2,2′-azobis(2-amidinopropane) di-hydrochloride; AMVN, 2,2′-azobis (2,4-dimethylvaleronitrile).

those in LDL are not accurately known. The prooxidant effect of α-tocopherol or vitamin E in vivo or against atherosclerosis has never been observed. In this context, the reduction of the α-tocopheroxyl radical by ascorbate or ubiquinol is important for maintaining α-tocopherol and for inhibiting tocopherol-mediated peroxidation, if any (38,43,49,50). It has been observed previously that the prooxidant effect of α-tocopherol seen in the spontaneous oxidation of lipids, especially at high concentration, is inhibited almost completely by ascorbate (53,54).

INTERACTION OF VITAMIN C WITH PROBUCOL

Probucol 4,4′-(isopropylidenedithio)bis(2,6-di-*tert*-butylphenol) is known to be a drug which prevents atherogenesis by acting as an antioxidant and suppressing the oxidative modification of LDL; in addition it lowers cholesterol levels. It was found that LDL isolated from plasma of hypercholesterolemic patients under treatment with conventional dosages of probucol was highly resistant to oxidative modification either by incubation with endothelial cells or by cupric ion (55). The treatment of diabetic rats with probucol inhibited both in vivo oxidation and in vitro cytotoxicity without altering hyperglycemia (56). As with α-tocopherol, a phenoxyl radical is formed from probucol when it scavenges the radical. This probucol radical is reduced rapidly by ascorbate and also by α-tocopherol (57,58).

CONCLUDING REMARKS

Ascorbate, or vitamin C, is a potent radical scavenger especially for aqueous radicals and acts as a reductant for the phenoxyl radical derived from lipophilic antioxidants. It was shown previously that ascorbate reduces the α-tocopheroxyl radical in LDL efficiently to spare α-tocopherol and to inhibit tocopherol-mediated peroxidation, although it has not been proved how important such an enhancing effect of α-tocopherol is in vivo. It may be safely concluded that ascorbate plays a very important role as an antioxidant against oxidative modification of LDL by scavenging active radicals per se and by reducing the α-tocopheroxyl radical.

REFERENCES

1. Bendich A, Machlin LJ, Scandurra O, et al. The antioxidant role of vitamin C. Adv Free Radical Biol Med 1986; 2:419–444.
2. Burns JJ, Rivers JM, Machlin LJ, eds. Third Conference on Vitamin C. Ann NY Acad Sci 1987; 498:1–538.
3. Niki E. Vitamin C as an antioxidant. World Rev Nutr Diet 1991; 64:1–30.
4. Block G, Henson DE, Levine M, eds. Ascorbic acid: biologic functions and relation to cancer. Am J Clin Nutr 1991; 54:1113S–1327S.
5. Frei B, ed. Natural Antioxidants. San Diego: Academic Press, 1994.
6. Niki E, Yamamoto Y, Takahashi M, et al. Free radical–mediated damage of blood and its inhibition by antioxidants. J Nutr Sci Vitaminol 1988; 34:507–512.
7. Frei B, Stocker R, Ames BN. Antioxidant defenses and lipid peroxidation in human blood plasma. Proc Natl Acad Sci USA 1988; 85:9748–9752.
8. Frei B, England L, Ames BN. Ascorbate is an outstanding antioxidant in human blood plasma. Proc Natl Acad Sci USA 1989; 86:6377–6381.
9. Frei B, Forte TM, Ames BN, Cross CE. Gas phase oxidants of cigarette smoke induce lipid peroxidation and changes in lipoprotein properties in human blood plasma. Biochem J 1991; 277:133–138.
10. Niki E. Antioxidants in relation to lipid peroxidation. Chem Phys Lipids 1987; 44:227–253.
11. Niki E, Saito T, Kawakami A, Kamiya T. Inhibition of oxidation of methyl linoleate in solution by vitamin E and vitamin C. J Biol Chem 1984; 259:4177–4182.
12. Niki E, Noguchi N, Tsuchihashi H, Gotoh N. Interaction among vitamin C, vitamin E, and β-carotene. J Am Clin Nutr 1995; 62(suppl):1322S–1326S.
13. Wayner DDM, Burton GW, Ingold KU. The antioxidant efficiency of vitamin C is concentration-dependent. Biochim Biophys Acta 1986; 884:119–123.
14. Takahashi M, Tsuchiya J, Niki E, Urano S. Action of vitamin E as antioxidant in phospholipid liposomal membranes as studied by spin label technique. J Nutr Sci Vitaminol 1988; 34:25–34.
15. Tappel AL. Will antioxidant nutrients slow aging processes? Geriatrics 1968; 23:97–105.
16. Packer JE, Slater TF, Willson RL. Direct observation of a free radical interaction between vitamin E and vitamin C. Nature 1979; 278:737–738.
17. Niki E, Tsuchiya J, Tanimura R, Kamiya Y. Regeneration of vitamin E from α-chromanoxy radical by glutathione and vitamin C. Chem Lett 1982; 789–792.
18. Niki E, Kawakami A, Yamamoto Y, Kamiya Y. Synergistic inhibition of oxidation of vitamin E and vitamin C. Bull Chem Soc Jpn 1985; 58:1971–1975.
19. Doba T, Burton GW, Ingold KU. Antioxidant and co-antioxidant activity of vitamin C: the effect of vitamin C, either alone or in the presence of vitamin E or a water-soluble vitamin E analogue, upon the peroxidation of aqueous multilamellar phospholipid liposomes. Biochim Biophys Acta 1985; 835:298–303.

20. McCay PB. Vitamin E: interactions with free radicals and ascorbate. Annu Rev Nutr 1985; 5: 323–340.

21. Chen LH. Interaction of vitamin E and ascorbic acid (review). In Vivo 1989; 3:199–210.

22. Wefers H, Sies H. The protection by ascorbate and glutathione against microsomal lipid peroxidation is dependent on vitamin E. Eur J Biochem 1988; 174:353–357.

23. Mukai K, Nishimura M, Kikuchi S. Stopped-flow investigation of the reaction of vitamin E with tocopheroxyl radical in aqueous triton X-100 micellar solutions. J Biol Chem 1991; 266: 274–278.

24. Chen H, Tappel AL. Protection by vitamin E, selenium, trolox C, ascorbic acid palmitate, acetylcysteine, coenzyme Q, beta-carotene, canthaxanthin, and (+)-catechin against oxidative damage to liver slices measured by oxidized heme proteins. Free Radical Bio Med 1994; 16: 437–444.

25. Packer L. Interactions among antioxidants in health and disease: vitamin E and its redox cycle. Proc Soc Exp Biol Med 1992; 200:271–276.

26. Burton GW, Hughes L, Foster DO, et al. Antioxidant mechanisms of vitamin E and β-carotene. In: Poli G, Albano E, Dianzani MU, eds. Free Radicals: From Basic Science to Medicine. Basel, Switzerland: Birkhauser Verlag, 1993:388–399.

27. Motoyama T, Miki M, Mino M, et al. Synergistic inhibition of oxidation in dispersed PC liposomes by a combination of vitamin E and cysteine. Arch Biochem Biophys 1989; 270: 655–661.

28. Tsuchiya J, Yamada T, Niki E, Kamiya Y. Interaction of galvinoxyl radical with ascorbic acid, cysteine, and glutathione in homogeneous solution and in aqueous dispersions. Bull Chem Soc Jpn 1985; 58:326–330.

29. Tsuchihashi H, Kigoshi M, Iwatsuki M, Niki E. Action of β-carotene as an antioxidant against lipid peroxidation. Arch Biochem Biophys 1995; 323:137–147.

30. Steinbrecher UP. Role of superoxide in endothelial-cell modification of low-density lipoproteins. Biophys Biochim Acta 1988; 959:20–30.

31. Jialal I, Grundy SM. Preservation of the endogenous antioxidants in low density lipoprotein by ascorbate but not probucol during oxidative modification. J Clin Invest 1991; 87:597–601.

32. Esterbauer H, Striegl G, Puhl H, Rotheneder M. Continuous monitoring of in vitro oxidation of human low density lipoprotein. Free Radical Res Commun 1989; 6:67–75.

33. Esterbauer H, Striegl G, Puhl H, et al. The role of vitamin E and carotenoids in preventing oxidation of low density lipoprotein. Ann NY Acad Sci 1989; 570:254–267.

34. Jialal I, Vega GL, Grundy SM. Physiologic levels of ascorbate inhibit oxidative modification of low density lipoprotein. Atherosclerosis 1990; 82:185–191.

35. Kalyanaraman B, Darley-Usmar VM, Wood J, et al. Synergistic interaction between the probucol phenoxyl radical and ascorbic acid in inhibiting the oxidation of low density lipoprotein. J Biol Chem 1992; 267:6789–6795.

36. Sato K, Niki E, Shimasaki H. Free radical–mediated chain oxidaion of low density lipoprotein and its synergistic inhibition by vitamin E and vitamin C. Arch Biochem Biophys 1990; 279: 402–405.

37. Retsky KL, Freeman MW, Frei B. Ascorbic acid oxidation product(s) protect human low density lipoprotein against atherogenic modification: anti- rather than prooxidant activity of vitamin C in the presence of transition metal ions. J Biol Chem 1993; 268:1304–1309.

38. Gotoh N, Noguchi N, Tsuchiya J, et al. Inhibition of oxidation of low density lipoprotein by vitamin E and related compounds. Free Radical Res 1996; 24:123–134.

39. Kagan VE, Serbinova EA, Forte T, et al. Recycling of vitamin E in human low density lipoproteins. J Lipid Res 1992; 33:385–397.

40. Forsmark-Andree P, Dallner G, Ernster L. Endogenous ubiquinol prevents protein modification accompanying lipid peroxidation in beef heart submitochondrial particles. Free Radical Biol Med 1995; 19:749–757.

41. Yamamoto Y, Komuro E, Niki E. Antioxidant activity of ubiquinol in solution and phosphatidylcholine liposome J. Nutr Sci Vitaminol 1990; 36:505–511.

42. Mukai K, Kikuchi S, Urano S. Stopped-flow kinetic study of the regeneration reaction of tocopheroxyl radical by reduced ubiquinone-10 in solution. Biochim Biophys Acta 1990; 1035: 77–82.

43. Niki E, Noguchi N, Gotoh N. Inhibition of oxidative modification of low density lipoprotein by antioxidants. J Nutr Sci Vitaminol 1993; 39:S1–S8.

44. Frei B, Kim MC, Ames BN. Ubiquinol-10 is an effective lipid-soluble antioxidant at physiological concentrations. Proc Natl Acad Sci USA 1990; 87:4879–4883.

45. Stocker R, Bowry VW, Frei B. Ubiquinol-10 protects human low density lipoprotein more efficiently against lipid peroxidation than does α-tocopherol. Proc Natl Acad Sci USA 1991; 88:1646–1650.

46. Yamamoto Y, Kawamura M, Tatsuno K, et al. Formation of lipid hydroperoxides in the cupric ion–induced oxidation of plasma and low density lipoprotein. In: Davies KJA, ed. Oxidative Damage and Repair: Chemical Biological and Medical Aspects. New York: Pergamon Press, 1991:287–291.

47. Bowry VW, Ingold KU, Stocker R. Vitamin E in human low-density lipoprotein. Biochem J 1992; 288:341–344.

48. Ingold KU, Bowry VW, Stocker R, Walling C. Autoxidation of lipids and antioxidation by α-tocopherol and ubiquinol in homogeneous solution and in aqueous dispersions of lipids: unrecognized consequences of lipid particle size as exemplified by oxidation of human low density lipoprotein. Proc Natl Acad Sci USA 1993; 90:45–49.

49. Bowry VW, Stocker R. Tocopherol-mediated peroxidation: the prooxidant effect of vitamin E on the radical-initiated oxidation of human low-density lipoprotein. J Am Chem Soc 1993; 115:6029–6044.

50. Thomas SR, Neuzil J, Mohr D, Stocker R. Coantioxidants make α-tocopherol an efficient antioxidant for low-density lipoprotein. Am J Clin Nut 1995; 62:1357S–1364S.

51. Esterbauer H, Jurgens G. Mechanistic and genetic aspects of susceptibility of LDL to oxidation. Curr Opin Lipidology 1993; 4:114–124.

52. Abuja PM, Esterbauer H. Simulation of lipid peroxidation in low-density lipoprotein by a basic "skeleton" of reactions. Chem Res Toxicol 1995; 8:753–763.

53. Terao J, Matsushita S. The peroxidizing effect of α-tocopherol on autoxidation of methyl linoleate in bulk phase. Lipids 1986; 21:255–260.

54. Takahashi M, Yoshikawa Y, Niki E. Oxidation of lipids. XVII. Crossover effect of tocopherols in the spontaneous oxidation of methyl linoleate. Bull Chem Soc Jpn 1989; 62:1885–1890.

55. Parthasarathy S, Young SG, Witztum JL, et al. Probucol inhibits oxidative modification of low density lipoprotein. J Clin Invest 1986; 77:641–644.

56. Breugnot C, Maziere C, Salmon S, et al. Phenothiazines inhibit copper and endothelial cell–induced peroxidation of low density lipoprotein—a comparative study with probucol, butylated hydroxytoluene and vitamin E. Biochem Pharmacol 1980; 40:1975–1980.

57. Kagan VE, Freisleben H-J, Tsuchiya M, et al. Generation of probucol radicals and their reduction by ascorbate and dihydrolipoic acid in human low density lipoproteins. Free Radical Res Commun 1991; 15:265–276.

58. Gotoh N, Shimizu K, Komuro E, et al. Antioxidant activities of probucol against lipid peroxidations. Biochim Biophys Acta 1992; 1128:147–154.

11

Diet and Oxidative Damage to DNA: The Importance of Ascorbate as an Antioxidant

ALAN ANTHONY WOODALL and BRUCE N. AMES
University of California, Berkeley, California

INTRODUCTION

Increasing evidence suggests that oxidative stress is a major factor that causes aging and degenerative diseases associated with it, including arthritis, cancer, cardiovascular disease, cataractogenesis, macular degeneration, neurodegenerative disorders, and autoimmune diseases (1). There appears to be a critical balance between the oxidative stress experienced by cells and tissues and their level of antioxidant defense that determines the extent and rate of tissue injury. Almost all cellular biomolecules are susceptible to free radical–mediated damage, but oxidative damage to DNA is of particular importance in somatic cells because of the risk of mutations that could lead to cancer (2). Damage to germline cell DNA (i.e., spermatozoan and ovum DNA) is also of particular importance as this may be a causal factor in the formation of subsequent birth defects and childhood cancer in offspring (3–5).

A variety of epidemiological, biochemical, and nutritional studies demonstrate that ascorbate (vitamin C) is an important component of cellular antioxidant defenses and that an adequate dietary intake of ascorbate is required to limit oxidative damage to DNA (6–10). In this chapter we summarize the evidence that supports the role for ascorbate as a protective antioxidant against oxidative DNA damage and draw attention to its possible importance in prevention of DNA mutations in the male germline.

THE IMPORTANCE OF OXIDATIVE DAMAGE TO DNA

Oxidative Damage to DNA Can Lead to Deleterious Mutations

The process of natural selection is driven by the subtle differences between individuals which arise via mutations in the gene pool (11). However, most mutations in established genes lead to the malfunction of the gene product with often catastrophic consequences for the cell. The molecular structure of DNA is such that it contains bases which are highly susceptible to free radical attack (12), and as mutations to the gene pool generally have harmful effects; in cells, mechanisms to minimize the effects of oxidative stress have evolved.

It has been estimated that the number of oxidative lesions to DNA formed per cell per day is about 10^4 in the human and 10^5 in the rat (13). Over 20 different oxidative adducts have been identified through radiolysis of DNA in vitro and a number of these can be isolated from cellular DNA; that suggests that oxidative damage to DNA in vivo occurs continuously (1,13–16). Most of the oxidative lesions are efficiently repaired by specific glycosylases (e.g., 8-oxoguanine-DNA glycosylase, uracil DNA glycosylase) (17,18) but the lesion level in DNA increases with age, reaching about 1 million per rat cell. When the cell divides, the lesions may be converted to mutations, some of which can lead to cancer.

Perhaps the best known oxidative adduct to DNA is the 8-hydroxy-guanine adduct, which forms the basis for a widely used assay for measurement of oxidative damage to DNA (18–21). Formation of ·OH radical in close proximity to DNA (e.g., by radiation or by presence of transition metals and peroxide) leads to the formation of oxo^8dG, one of about 20 major oxidative lesions, many of which are mutagenic. Guanine normally base pairs with cytosine (G–C), but oxo^8dG adopts a different stereochemical conformation about the glycosidic bond in DNA which allows the formation of a oxo-8-guanine–adenine base pair (oxo8G-A) (22). After a further round of replication a mutation of the genetic sequence from G–C to A–T can result. If this base is in a critical position, in a critical gene such as the tumor suppressor gene, *p53*, then there is no *p53*-driven cell cycle checkpoint block or apoptotic cell death and a tumor may result (23–25).

Formation of Free Radicals in Vivo: Can These Interact with DNA?

Free radicals are highly reactive molecules that possess at least one unpaired electron in an molecular orbital (e.g., ·OH, O_2^-, NO·) and are normally short-lived species (26). Free radicals can be formed both externally to the organism, which then enter tissues or body fluids (e.g., free radicals formed in cigarette smoke and exhaust pollutants) (27–28), and by absorption of ionizing radiation within cells (e.g., ·OH formed by hemolytic cleavage of H_2O_2) (29–32). Free radicals are also formed as a consequence of metabolism. Electron leakage during oxidative phosphorylation in mitochondria is estimated to lead to up to 2% of molecular oxygen's being converted to O_2^- (33). Detoxification of xenobiotics such as paracetamol by the cytochrome P450 enzymes can lead to free radical production in the liver (34,35). Chronic inflammation (due to persistent infections such as schistosomiasis or hepatitis B) stimulates leukocytic oxidant production that can damage host tissues (36–39). In most cases these oxidants cannot diffuse far before they react, so it seems unlikely, for example, that ·OH formed in the mitochondria would interact directly to promote oxidative damage to nuclear DNA (40). However, initiation of oxidative damage to lipids (lipid peroxidation) leads to a chain reaction, so there is the possibility that some diffusion of free radical oxidation will proceed from the primary reaction site. Two factors are worth noting: a lipid hydroperoxide in a plasma membrane can rapidly diffuse the length of the cell (41), facilitating the spread of intracellular oxidation, and cellular organelles are dynamic and constantly interact (42–46). Hence, although nuclear DNA is removed from primary cellular sites of oxidant production (such as mitochondria, peroxisomes, and endoplasmic reticulum), the formation of free radicals in close proximity to DNA can occur by absorption of ionizing radiation and by chain reactions of lipid peroxidation, particularly in the presence of Fe^{2+} or Cu^+.

Protection of DNA from Oxidative Attack

Under normal circumstances cellular DNA is protected from free radical attack by a number of defenses. First, when not undergoing active expression or replication, cellular DNA is tightly supercoiled with histone proteins which may serve to limit the accessibility of reactive sites on DNA to free radical attack (47–49). In addition, nuclear DNA is compartmentalized within the nucleus away from the major sites of intracellular oxidant production such as the mitochondria, endoplasmic reticulum, and peroxisomes (50–51). Second, redox-active transition metals which can promote the formation of free radicals are sequestered within proteins to limit free radical formation. Iron is stored within ferritin (52) and transferrin (53), and copper within ceruloplasmin (54). Thus, the availability of free transition metals to catalyze free radical formation is reduced (55). In addition, those proteins which associate with DNA to modulate expression, the zinc finger proteins, utilize a transition metal that in the ionic form cannot undergo redox reactions. One benefit of utilizing zinc in these proteins could be that this element cannot initiate free radical formation in close proximity to the cellular DNA (56). Third, a range of enzymes have evolved, such as catalase (57), superoxide dismutase (58), and glutathione peroxidase (59), which catalytically remove oxidants from the cell. Fourth, a range of other biomolecules are either obtained from the diet or formed as metabolites which act as scavengers of oxidants in both the water- and lipid-soluble environments of the cell. These include glutathione, ubiquinol, ascorbate, bilirubin, carotenoids, urate, and tocopherols (60–64).

ASCORBIC ACID: A POWERFUL INTRACELLULAR AND EXTRACELLULAR ANTIOXIDANT

Ascorbic acid is a water-soluble, low-molecular-weight compound that is synthesized from glucose in most mammals (65). However, three mammalian groups, the primates, guinea pigs, and fruit bats, have lost the ability to synthesize ascorbic acid de novo through a gene mutation that has rendered inactive a key ascorbate biosynthetic enzyme, L-gulono-lactone oxidase (66), and hence these mammals must obtain ascorbate from dietary sources, particularly fruits and vegetables.

Nonantioxidant Functions of Ascorbate

The most well-known function of ascorbate is the prevention of the deficiency disease scurvy, which was first documented in 1536 in sailors (67). It was soon recognized that scurvy could be prevented by daily inclusion in the diet of fresh fruits and vegetables. Indeed, scurvy had become such a problem for some maritime nations that in 1793 the Royal Navy of Britain made it a punishable offense for any sailor to refuse his daily ration of lemon or lime juice (68)! Once this policy was adopted, the incidence of scurvy among British ratings and officers dramatically declined. Ascorbate was finally identified as the active antiscorbutic agent and the pathological basis of the deficiency determined (69). Ascorbate, an excellent reducing agent, is required to maintain the Fe atom in the active site of prolyl hydroxylase in a reduced (Fe^{2+}) state (70). Prolyl hydroxylase is required to synthesize hydroxyproline, a key modified amino acid in collagen biosynthesis. Collagen synthesized in the absence of ascorbate is insufficiently hydroxylated, and this characteris-

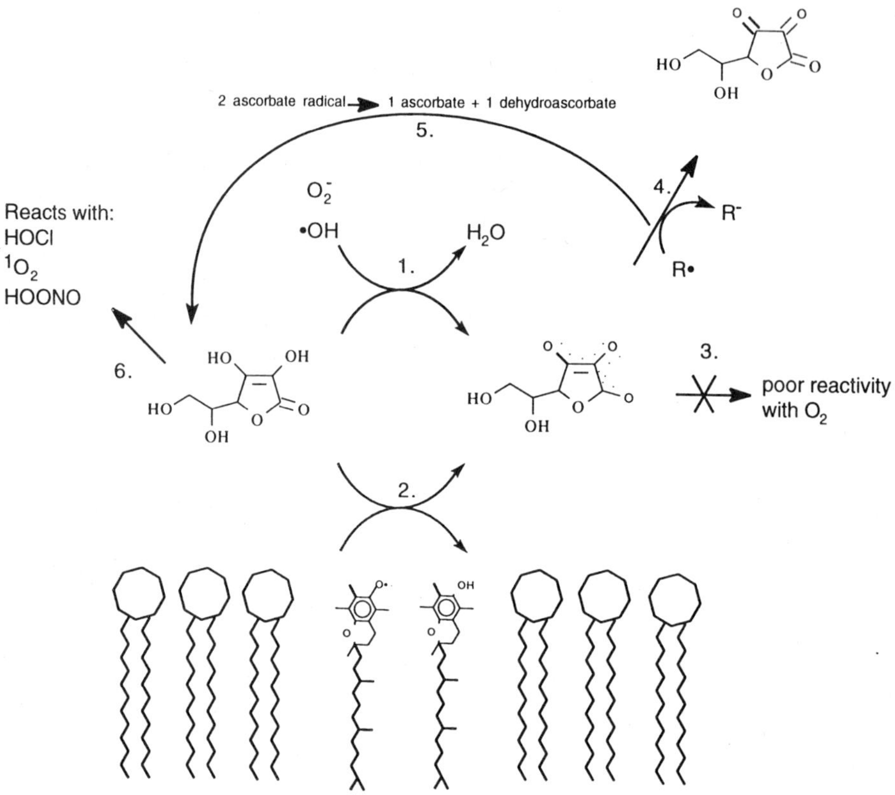

Figure 1 Antioxidant properties of ascorbate in cells and plasma. Ascorbate is present in both the intracellular and extracellular compartments and acts as an excellent hydrogen atom donor to oxygen free radicals such as hydroxyl radical at diffusion limiting rates in the water soluble compartment (1). Ascorbate can also regenerate tocopherol from the tocopheroxyl radical in the lipid phase of membranes and lipoproteins, thus aiding in the limitation of membrane lipid peroxidation (2). The semidehydroascorbate radical that is formed reacts poorly with oxygen and is insufficiently reactive to abstract hydrogen from other radicals (2), thus contributing to the efficacy of ascorbate as an antioxidant. This radical can further reduce radicals to form dehydroascorbate (4). Ascorbate can also be regenerated by dismutation of two semidehydroascorbate anion radicals (5). Ascorbate also acts as an excellent reducing agent, quenching oxidizing species that are produced from inflammatory reactions, such as hypochlorous acid and peroxynitrite (6).

tic leads to the inability of the fibrous protein to form fibers, leading to the clinical symptoms of blood vessel fragility and skin disease that manifest clinically as scurvy (71).

Diet and Bioavailability of Ascorbate

Ascorbate is obtained in the diet of humans primarily from fresh fruits and vegetables, particularly citrus fruits, potato, and tomato, and increasingly ascorbate is added to convenience foods and drinks (e.g., breakfast cereals and some carbonated drinks) (72). The minimum daily requirement for prevention of clinical symptoms of ascorbate deficiency is

10 mg, but the current recommended daily allowance (RDA) for both men and women is 60 mg per day, which solely reflects the level estimated to allow normal collagen synthesis (i.e., prevent scurvy) (73). Typical plasma ascorbate levels are between 30 and 150 μM, but the concentrations in some other tissues are much higher (74). However, recent experimental evidence obtained from both human kinetic studies and studies examining the antioxidant functions of ascorbate suggests that the level of ascorbate required to prevent deficiency may not be the optimal level to prevent oxidative damage to tissues (75). There has been some reluctance to raise the RDA for ascorbate resulting from evidence obtained in vitro that ascorbate can exhibit prooxidant activity in the presence of transition metal ions (76,77). However, it is unlikely that in vivo this is observed in healthy organisms, since almost all transition metals are sequestered in proteins and are unavailable to promote radical reactions (78).

Antioxidant Activity of Ascorbate

Ascorbic acid is an excellent free radical scavenger (79–82). In vitro studies where plasma is stressed with peroxyl radicals or exposed to polymorphonuclear leukocytes demonstrate that ascorbate is an outstanding antioxidant in human plasma, since oxidation of other plasma components (e.g, lipoproteins, protein thiols, tocopherols) is retarded until all ascorbate is depleted (83). Ascorbate is able to trap aqueous free radicals before they can diffuse into the lipid compartments of the plasma (84). Only ascorbate was able to inhibit completely lipid peroxidation in human plasma, unlike tocopherols, urate, and protein thiols, which were only able to lower the rate of lipid peroxidation but were unable to prevent initiation of detectable lipid peroxidation by aqueous peroxyl radicals (85).

Ascorbate appears to function as an excellent antioxidant in four main ways. First, it is an excellent scavenger of radicals including ˙OH, O_2^-, reacting at almost diffusion limiting rates (86,87). Second, the ascorbate radical formed is neither strongly oxidizing nor reducing and reacts poorly with molecular oxygen by one electron reduction or addition, producing little superoxide or peroxyl radical (88). Third, ascorbate is also an excellent quencher of other oxidants produced in vivo, including HOCl (89), $^1O_2$ (90), and peroxynitrite (91), all of which cause inflammatory damage to tissues (92). Fourth, ascorbate can also help to limit any oxidation in the membranous compartment of cells (in addition to the aqueous and extracellular compartments) by regenerating tocopherol from the tocopheryl radical (93–95). Thus, maintenance of an adequate cell and tissue fluid ascorbate level in the body allows the tissues to be optimally protected against oxidative stress, and hence limits oxidation to DNA by both scavenging oxidants directly and limiting lipid peroxidation, which can lead to DNA oxidation or mutation indirectly. The importance of ascorbate as an antioxidant in preventing DNA damage can be seen in the following example.

Prevention of Oxidative Damage to Sperm DNA: A Possible Cause of Birth Defects and Childhood Cancer

Most current public health policy suggests that women who are trying to conceive or have become pregnant should refrain from smoking, limit alcohol intake, and try to obtain a balanced diet containing high proportions of fruits and vegetables to limit risk of damage to the unborn child (96–99). However, the risk of genetic injury which can be passed on to the offspring is more likely to have been passed on from the male parent (3,100). Epidemiological evidence suggests that oxidative damage to the male germline can contribute to subsequent risk of childhood birth defects and cancer in offspring (101,102). Male sperm are produced at high rates from puberty throughout life (unlike ova, which are produced when the female is herself in utero and stored in a mitotically inactive state until ovulation). The spermatozoan plasma membrane contains an unusually high proportion of unsaturated fatty acids (103), and the sperm DNA is tightly packed without the presence of histone proteins or active DNA repair enzymes which could protect it against oxidative damage (104). Sperm cells are thus unusually prone to oxidative damage. However, seminal fluid contains a high concentration of ascorbate, typically around 400 μM, which is eight times the level in the plasma (105). Free-living males with lowered seminal plasma ascorbate had elevated oxo[8]dG in sperm DNA (106). Hospitalized volunteers maintained on a strict diet which was depleted of ascorbate had elevated oxo[8]dG compared to that before the start of the diet, and repletion with ascorbate again lowered the observed levels of damage to sperm DNA. In a separate study, male smokers had both lowered seminal plasma ascorbate and elevated 8-OHdG in sperm DNA compared with nonsmokers, suggesting that smoking, which depletes plasma ascorbate, can lead to depletion of other ascorbate body pools that may lead to elevated damage to germline DNA (107). Finally, a recent study has shown that lowered seminal plasma ascorbate concentrations are associated with decreased sperm cell number, an elevated percentage of sperm cells with tail defects, and elevated levels of seminal plasma hexanal, a toxic aldehyde marker for mutagenic aldehydes which is an end product of lipid peroxidation (Woodall et al., unpublished data). Hence, it is likely that depletion of ascorbate in the seminal plasma (and probably in the testicular cells and prostate) leads to decreased protection of sperm against oxidative stress. This will result in increased oxidation to lipids, producing toxic aldehydes, lower male fertility, and an increase in the risk of mutation to DNA that can manifest as birth defects.

Dietary Requirements for Ascorbate: A Reevaluation Is Necessary

Evidence gathered from epidemiological and biochemical sources clearly demonstrates a role for ascorbate in the prevention of oxidative damage. Current U.S. guidelines suggest an intake of 60 mg per person for adults as an adequate source to prevent scurvy, but this may be an insufficient amount to optimize antioxidant status in adults. Undoubtedly, the most important factor is the steady-state ascorbate concentration in both plasma and tissues, and maintaining a particular blood plasma concentration (e.g., 60 μM) may be a better goal to aim for, although more difficult for the public to conceptualize. Furthermore, smokers require two to three times the intake of ascorbate of nonsmokers to maintain comparable plasma ascorbate levels; that suggests maintenance of a specific plasma concentration rather than a set dietary intake should be promoted since two individuals with the same body mass will have different dietary ascorbate requirements depending on their daily exposure to oxidants (such as are present in cigarette smoke) (108). Clearly, some members of the population are at greater risk of ascorbate depletion and consequent risk of DNA mutations that manifests as cancer and birth defects in offspring. Public acceptance of plasma concentrations of other important biomolecules (e.g., plasma cholesterol, plasma glucose) has been readily achieved in recent years, and thus a move to promote this idea should be developed for ascorbate and other antioxidants. Undoubtedly, the development of a simple commerical test to quantitate plasma antioxidant capacity for ascorbate and other antioxidants that could be performed at a pharmacy would increase public awareness of the role of antioxidant status in preventing disease.

CONCLUSIONS

The evidence to support the role of oxidative stress as a cause of aging and degenerative disease and the importance of maintaining an adequate dietary intake of antioxidants have become accepted in recent years by both the scientific community and the public at large. As we probe further into the role of mutation to DNA it is becoming apparent that oxidation is of major importance. Knowledge that ascorbate can protect somatic and germline tissues against oxidative stress points to prevention strategies of routinely measuring and optimizing ascorbate in plasma.

ACKNOWLEDGMENTS

We are indebted to the National Cancer Institute (Outstanding Investigator Grant CA 39910) and to the National Institute of Environmental Health Sciences (Grant ESO1896).

REFERENCES

1. Ames BN, Shigenaga MK, Hagen TM. Oxidants, antioxidants and the degenerative diseases of aging. Proc Natl Acad Sci USA 1993; 90:7915–7922.
2. Ames BN, Gold LS, Willett WC. The causes and prevention of cancer. Proc Natl Acad Sci USA 1995; 92:5258–5265.
3. Crow J. How much do we know about spontaneous human mutation rates? Environ Mol Mutagen 1993; 21:122–129.
4. Dryja TP, Shizuo M, Petersen R, et al. Parental origin of mutations of the retinoblastoma gene. Nature 1989; 339:556–558.
5. Ames BN, Motchnik P, Fraga CG, et al. Antioxidant prevention of birth defects and cancer. In: Mattison DR, Olshan A, eds. Male-Mediated Developmental Toxicity. New York: Plenum Press, 1994.
6. Green MH, Lowe JE, Waugh AP, et al. Effect of diet and vitamin C on DNA strand breakage in freshly-isolated human white blood cells. Mutat Res 1994; 316:91–102.
7. Anderson D, Yu TW, Phillips BJ, Schmezer P. The effect of various antioxidants and other modifying agents on oxygen-radical-generated DNA damage in human lymphocytes in the COMET assay. Mutat Res 1994; 307:261–271.
8. Dreosti I, McGown M. Antioxidants and UV-induced genotoxicity. Res Commun Chem Pathol Pharmacol 1992; 75:251–254.
9. Smit MJ, Anderson R. Biochemical mechanisms of hydrogen peroxide– and hypochlorous acid–mediated inhibition of human mononuclear leukocyte functions in vitro: protection and reversal by anti-oxidants. Agents Actions 1992; 36:58–65.
10. Fischer-Nielsen A, Loft S, Jensen KG. Effect of ascorbate and 5-aminosalicylic acid on light-induced 8-hydroxydeoxyguanosine formation in V79 Chinese hamster cells. Carcinogenesis 1993; 14:2431–2433.
11. Sueoka N. Directional mutation pressure, mutator mutations, and dynamics of molecular evolution. J Mol Evol 1993; 37:137–153.
12. Lindahl T. Instability and decay of the primary structure of DNA. Nature 1993 342:709–715.
13. Ames BN, Shigenaga MK. Oxidants are a major contributor to aging. Ann NY Acad Sci 1992; 663:85–96.
14. Zastawny TH, Altman SA, Randers-Eichhorn L, et al. DNA base modifications and membrane damage in cultured mammalian cells treated with iron ions. Free Radical Biol Med 1995; 18:1013–1022.
15. Dizdaroglu M. Chemical determination of oxidative DNA damage by gas chromatography-mass spectrometry. Methods Enzymol 1994; 234:3–16.

16. Girault I, Molko D, Cadet J. Ozonolysis of thymidine: isolation and identification of the main oxidation products. Free Radical Res 1994; 20:315–325.

17. Slupphaug G, Markussen FH, Olsen LC, et al. Nuclear and mitochondrial forms of human uracil–DNA glycosylase are encoded by the same gene. Nucleic Acid Res 1993; 21:25792584.

18. Bessho T, Tano K, Kasai H, et al. Evidence for two DNA repair enzymes for 8-hydroxyguanine (7,8-dihydro-8-oxoguanine) in human cells. J Biol Chem 1993; 268:19416–19421.

19. Fraga CG, Shigenaga MK, Park JW, et al. Oxidative damage to DNA during aging: 8-hydroxy-2'-deoxyguanosine in rat organ DNA and urine. Proc Natl Acad Sci USA 1990; 87: 4533–4537.

20. Shigenaga MK, Aboujaoude EN, Chen Q, Ames BN. Assay of oxidative DNA damage biomarkers 8-oxo-2'-deoxyguanosine and 8-oxoguanine in nuclear DNA and biological fluids by high-performance liquid chromatography with electrochemical detection. Methods Enzymol 1994; 234:16–33.

21. Park EM, Shigenaga MK, Degan P, et al. Assay of excised oxidative DNA lesions: isolation of 8-oxoguanine and its nucleoside derivatives from biological fluids with a monoclonal antibody column. Proc Natl Acad Sci USA 1992; 89:3375–3379.

22. Guyton KZ, Kensler TV. Oxidative mechanisms of carcinogenesis. Br Med Bull 1993; 49: 523–544.

23. Nelson WG, Kastan MB. DNA strand breaks: the DNA template alterations that trigger p53-dependent DNA damage response pathways. Mol Cell Biol 1994; 14:1815–1823.

24. Meikrantz W, Schlegel R. Apoptosis and the cell cycle. J Cell Biochem 1995; 58:160–174.

25. Evan G. Why we live and why we die. Chem Biol 1994; 1:137–141.

26. Halliwell B, Gutteridge JMC. Free Radicals in Biology and Medicine. 2d ed. Oxford: Clarendon Press, 1989.

27. Church F, Pryor WA. The free-radical chemistry of cigarette smoke and its toxicological implications. Environ Health Perspect 1985; 64:111–126.

28. Blaurock B, Hippeli S, Metz N, Elstner EF. Oxidative destruction of biomolecules by gasoline engine exhaust products and detoxifying effects of the three-way catalytic converter. Arch Toxicol 1992; 66:681–687.

29. Mori T, Hori Y, Dizdaroglu M. DNA base damage generated in vivo in hepatic chromatin of mice upon whole body gamma-irradiation. Int J Radiat Biol 1993; 64:645–650.

30. Stevens RG, Kalkwarf DR. Iron, radiation, and cancer. Environ Health Perspect 1990; 87: 291–300.

31. Nygren J, Ljungman M, Ahnstrom G. Chromatin structure and radiation-induced DNA strand breaks in human cells: soluble scavengers and DNA-bound proteins offer a better protection against single- than double-strand breaks. Int J Radiat Biol 1995; 68:11–18.

32. Isabelle V, Prevost C, Spotheim-Maurizot M, et al. Radiation-induced damages in single- and double-stranded DNA. Int J Radiat Biol 1995; 67:169–176.

33. Chance B, Sies H, Boveris A. Hyperoxide metabolism in mammalian organs. Physiol Rev 1979 59:527–605.

34. Wendel A, Feuerstein S, Konz KH. Acute paracetamol intoxication of starved mice leads to lipid peroxidation "in vivo." Biochem Pharmacol 1979 28:2051–2055.

35. Poli G. Liver damage due to free radicals. Br Med Bull 1995; 49:604–620.

36. Winrow VR, Winyard PG, Morris CJ, Blake DR. Free radicals in inflammation: second messengers and mediators of tissue destruction. Br Med Bull 1995; 49:506–522.

37. Rodenas J, Mitjavila MT, Carbonell T. Simultaneous generation of nitric oxide and superoxide by inflammatory cells in rats. Free Radical Biol Med 1995; 18:869–875.

38. Halliwell B, Hoult JR, Blake DR. Oxidants, inflammation, and anti-inflammatory drugs. FASEB J 1988; 2:2867–2873.

39. Blake DR, Allen RE, Lunec J. Free radicals in biological systems: a review orientated to inflammatory processes. Br Med Bull 1987; 43:371–385.

40. Pryor WA, Dooley MM, Church DF. The mechanism of the inactivation of human α-1-pro-

teinase inhibitor by gas-phase cigarette smoke. Adv Free Radical Biol Med 1986; 48:161–188.

41. el Hage Chahine JM, Cribier S, Devaux PF. Phospholipid transmembrane domains and lateral diffusion in fibroblasts. Proc Natl Acad Sci USA 1993; 90:447–451.

42. Koning AJ, Lum PY, Williams JM, Wright R. DiOC6 staining reveals organelle structure and dynamics in living yeast cells. Motil Cytoskeleton 1993; 25:111–128.

43. Couchman JR, Rees DA. Organelle–cytoskeleton relationships in fibroblasts: mitochondria, Golgi apparatus, and endoplasmic reticulum in phases of movement and growth. Eur J Cell Biol 1982; 27:47–54.

44. Chemes HE, Fawcett DW, Dym M. Unusual features of the nuclear envelope in human spermatogenic cells. Anat Rec 1978; 192:493–512.

45. Djaldetti M, Lewinski UH. Origin of intranuclear inclusions in myeloma cells. Scand J Haematol 1973; 20:200–205.

46. Flickinger CJ. Metabolic requirements for interactions between nuclear and cytoplasmic membranes in the repair of damaged Amoeba nuclei. J Cell Sci 1976; 21:291–302.

47. Enright HU, Miller WJ, Hebbel RP. Nucleosomal histone protein protects DNA from iron-mediated damage. Nucleic Acid Res 1992; 20:3341–3346.

48. Ljungman M, Hanawalt PC. Efficient protection against oxidative DNA damage in chromatin. Mol Carcinogenesis 1992; 5:264–269.

49. Elia MC, Bradley MO. Influence of chromatin structure on the induction of DNA double strand breaks by ionizing radiation. Cancer Res 1992; 52:1580–1586.

50. Shigenaga MK, Hagen TM, Ames BN. Oxidative damage and mitochondrial decay in aging. Proc Natl Acad Sci USA 1994; 91:10771–10778.

51. Sohal RS, Ku HH, Agarwal S, et al. Mitochondrial damage, mitochondrial oxidant generation and antioxidant defenses during aging and in response to food restriction in the mouse. Mech Age Dev 1994; 74:121–133.

52. Joshi JG, Clauberg M. Ferritin: an iron storage protein with diverse functions. Biofactors 1988; 1:207–212.

53. Maguire JJ, Kellogg EW III, Packer L. Protection against free radical formation by protein bound iron. Toxicol Lett 1982; 14:27–34.

54. Gutteridge JMC, Stocks J. Ceruloplasmin: physiological and pathological perspectives. CRC Crit Rev Clin Lab Sci 1981; 14:257–329.

55. Halliwell B, Gutteridge JMC. Iron and free radical reactions: two aspects of antioxidant protection. Trends Biochem Sci 1986; 11:372–375.

56. Chevion M. A site-specific mechanism for free radical induced biological damage: the essential role of redox-active transition metals. Free Radical Biol Med 1988; 5:27–37.

57. Deisseroth A, Dounce AL. Catalase: physical and chemical properties, mechanism of catalysis and physiological role in mammals. Physiol Rev 1970 50:319–375.

58. McCord JM, Fridovich I. Superoxide dismutase: an enzymic function for erythrocuperin (hemocuprein). J Biol Chem 1969; 244:6049–6056.

59. Wendel A. Glutathione peroxidase. In: Jakoby WB, Bend WR, Caldwell J, eds. Enzymatic Basis of Detoxification. New York: Academic Press, 1980.

60. Frei B, England L, Ames BN. Ascorbate is an outstanding antioxidant in human blood plasma. Proc Natl Acad Sci USA 1989; 86:6377–6381.

61. Stocker R, Yamamoto Y, McDonagh AF, et al. Bilirubin is an antioxidant of possible physiological importance. Science 1987; 235:1043–1045.

62. Hennekens CH. Antioxidant vitamins and cancer. Am J Med 1994; 97:2–4.

63. Sevanian A, Davies KJ, Hochstein P. Serum urate as an antioxidant for ascorbic acid. Am J Clin Nutr 1991; 54:1129S–1134S.

64. Meister A. Glutathione–ascorbic acid antioxidant system in animals. J Biol Chem 1994; 269: 9397–9400.

65. Grollman AP, Lehninger AL. Enzymic synthesis of vitamin C in different animal species. Arch Biochem Biophys 1957; 69:458–467.

66. Nishikimi M, Yagi K. Molecular basis for the deficiency in humans of gulonolactone oxidase, a key enzyme for ascorbic acid biosynthesis. Am J Clin Nutr 1991; 54S:1203S–1208S.

67. Carpenter KJ. The history of scurvy and vitamin C. New York: Cambridge University Press, 1986.

68. Lind J. Nutrition classics: a treatise of the scurvy by James Lind, MDCCLIII. Nutr Rev 1983; 41:155–157.

69. Dickman SR. The search for the specific factor in scurvy. Perspect Biol Med 1981; 24: 382–395.

70. Pihlajaniemi T, Myllyla R, Kivirikko KI. Prolyl 4-hydroxylase and its role in collagen synthesis. J Hepatol 1991; 13:S2–7.

71. Reuler JB, Broudy VC, Cooney TG. Adult scurvy. JAMA 1985; 253:805–807.

72. Block G. Vitamin C and cancer prevention: the epidemiologic evidence Am J Clin Nutr 1991; 53:270S–282S.

73. Chinoy NJ. Ascorbic acid levels in mammalian tissues and its metabolic significance. Comp Physiol Biochem A 1972; 42:945–952.

74. Bui MH, Sauty A, Collet F, et al. Dietary vitamin C intake and concentrations in the body fluids and cells of male smokers and nonsmokers. J Nutr 1992; 122:312–316.

75. Bendich A, Langseth L. 1995. Health effects of vitamin C supplementation: a review. J Am Coll Nutr 1995; 14:124–136.

76. Prabhu HR, Krishnamurthy S. Ascorbate-dependent formation of hydroxyl radicals in the presence of iron chelates. Int J Biochem Biophys 1993; 30:289–292.

77. Giulivi C, Cadenas E. The reaction of ascorbic acid with different heme iron redox states of myoglobin: antioxidant and prooxidant aspects. FEBS Lett 1993; 332:287–290.

78. Chevion M. Protection against free radical–induced and transition metal–mediated damage: the use of "pull" and "push" mechanisms. Free Radical Res Commun 1991; 12–13(Pt 2): 691–696.

79. Sharma MK, Buettner GR. Interaction of vitamin C and vitamin E during free radical stress in plasma: an ESR study. Free Radical Med 1993; 14:649–653.

80. Beyer RE. The role of ascorbate in antioxidant protection of biomembranes: interaction with vitamin E and coenzyme Q. J Bioenerg Biomembr 1994; 26:349–358.

81. Frei B, Stocker R, England L, Ames BN. Ascorbate: the most effective antioxidant in human blood plasma. Adv Exp Biol Med 1990; 264:155–163.

82. Packer JE, Slater TF, Willson RL. Direct observation of a free radical interaction between vitamin E and vitamin C. Nature 1979; 278:737–738.

83. Frei B. Ascorbic acid protects lipids in human plasma and low-density lipoprotein against oxidative damage. Am J Clin Nutr 1991; 54:1113S–1118S.

84. Frei B, Forte TM, Ames BN, Cross CE. Gas phase oxidants of cigarette smoke induce lipid peroxidation and in lipoprotein properties in human blood plasma: protective effects of ascorbic acid. Biochem J 1991; 277:133–138.

85. Frei B, England L, Ames BN. Ascorbate is an outstanding antioxidant in human blood plasma. Proc Natl Acad Sci USA 1985; 86:6377–6381.

86. Anbar M, Neta P. A compilation of specific biomolecular rate constants for the reactions of hydrated electrons, hydrogen atoms and hydroxyl radicals with inorganic and organic compounds in aqueous solution. Int J Appl Radiat Isotopes 1967; 78:493–523.

87. Lal M, Schoneich C, Monig J, Asmus KD. Rate constants for the reactions of halogenated organic radicals. Int J Radiat 1988; 54:773–785.

88. Buettner GR. The pecking order of free radicals and antioxidants: lipid peroxidation, alpha-tocopherol, and ascorbate. Arch Biochem Biophys 1993; 300:535–543.

89. Smit MJ, Anderson R. Biochemical mechanisms of hydrogen peroxide– and hypochlorous acid–mediated inhibition of human mononuclear leukocyte functions in vitro: protection and reversal by anti-oxidants. Agents Actions 1992 36:58–65.

90. Wagner JR, Motchnik PA, Stocker R, et al. The oxidation of blood plasma and low density

lipoprotein components by chemically generated singlet oxygen. J Biol Chem 1993; 268: 18502–18506.

91. Bartlett D, Church DF, Bounds PL, Koppenol WH. The kinetics of the oxidation of L-ascorbic acid by peroxynitrite. Free Radical Biol Med 1995; 18:85–92.

92. Rosen GM, Pou S, Ramos CL, et al. Free radicals and phagocytic cells. Faseb J 1995; 9: 200–209.

93. Bisby RH, Parker AW. Reaction of ascorbate with the alpha-tocopheroxyl radical in micellar and bilayer membrane systems. Arch Biochem Biophys 1995; 317:170–178.

94. Kagan VE, Serbinova EA, Forte T, et al. Recycling of vitamin E in human low density lipoproteins. J Lipid Res 33:385–397.

95. Scarpa M, Rigo A, Maiorino M, et al. Formation of alpha-tocopherol radical and recycling of alpha-tocopherol by ascorbate during peroxidation of phosphatidylcholine liposomes: an electron paramagnetic resonance study. Biochim Biophys Acta 1984; 801:215–219.

96. Randall CL, Ekblad U, Anton RF. Perspectives on the pathophysiology of fetal alcohol syndrome. Alcohol Clin Exp Res 1990; 14:807–812.

97. Van den Eeden SK, Karagas MR, Daling JR, Vaughan TL. A case-control study of maternal smoking and congenital malformations. Paediatr Perinatal Epidemiol 1990; 4:147–155.

98. Goldberg GR, Prentice AM. Maternal and fetal determinants of adult diseases. Nutr Rev 1994; 52:191–200.

99. Vergel RG, Sanchez LR, Heredero BL, et al. Primary prevention of neural tube defects with folic acid supplementation: Cuban experience. Prenatal Diagn 1990; 10:149–152.

100. Woodall AA, Ames BN. Nutritional prevention of DNA damage to sperm and consequent birth defects and cancer in offspring. In: Bendich A, Deckelbaum R, eds. New York: Preventative Nutrition. In press.

101. Olshan AF, Schnitzer PG, Baird PA. Paternal age and the risk of congenital heart defects. Teratology 1994; 50 80–84.

102. Zhang J, Savitz DA, Schwingl PJ, Cai WW. A case-control study of paternal smoking and birth defects. Int J Epidemiol 1992; 21:273–278.

103. Wolf DE. Lipid domains in sperm plasma membranes. Mol Membr Biol 1994; 12:101–104.

104. Matsuda Y, Seki N, Utsugi-Takeuchi T, Tobari I. X-ray- and mitomycin C (MMC)–induced chromosome aberrations in spermiogenic germ cells and the repair capacity of mouse eggs for the X-ray and MMC damage. Mutat Res 1989; 211:65–75.

105. Srivastava A, Chopra SK, Dasgupta PR. Biochemical analysis of human seminal plasma. I. Fructose, ascorbate, cholesterol, adenosine triphosphatase and lactic dehydrogenase. Andrologia 1983; 15:431–435.

106. Fraga CG, Motchnik PA, Shigenaga MK, et al. Ascorbic acid protects against endogenous oxidative DNA damage in human sperm. Proc Natl Acad Sci USA 1991; 88:11003–11006.

107. Fraga CG, Motchnik PA, Wyrobek AJ, et al. Smoking and low antioxidant levels increase oxidative damage to sperm DNA. Mutat Res. In press.

108. Duthie GG, Arthur JR, James WP. Effects of smoking and vitamin E on blood antioxidant status. Am J Clin Nutr 1991; 53(suppl 4):1061S–1063S.

12

Vitamin C, Collagen Biosynthesis, and Aging

CHARLOTTE L. PHILLIPS
University of Missouri, Columbia, Missouri

HEATHER N. YEOWELL
Duke University Medical Center, Durham, North Carolina

INTRODUCTION

Aging is a natural and progressive process. In the United States the most rapidly growing segment of the population are those individuals more than 65 years of age (1). In 1900, when the average life expectancy was 47 years, there were only three million people in the United States who were over 65 years old. By 1990 the average life expectancy had increased to 75 years, and consequently there has been a dramatic increase in the aging population to more than 32 million individuals over the age of 65 (1). Researchers and physicians have only recently become aware of and begun to address the impact of this shift in demographics on human health issues.

Connective tissues, in particular, undergo dramatic alterations during the aging process, demonstrating pronounced age-related changes not only in the more obvious outward appearance (such as seen with skin), but in physiological, biochemical, and mechanical properties as well (2–5). The extracellular matrix is the foundation of the connective tissue in the body and collagens are the major component of this matrix. The predominant collagen in the human body is type I collagen, which is a major component of many tissues, including bone, skin, tendon, ligament, sclera, cornea, blood vessels, and hollow organs. Type I collagen serves different structural and functional roles in different tissues. It provides tensile strength to bone, skin, and tendon; in bones and teeth it serves as the template for mineralization; in the eye it allows or facilitates the transparency of the cornea as well as the opaqueness of the sclera; and it forms the solid structures of tendons as well as the hollow tubes of blood vessels (6).

The importance of ascorbic acid to connective tissue and type I collagen in particular has been evident for centuries (as described in Chap. 1); descriptions of scurvy, a disorder resulting from ascorbic acid deficiency, are found in ancient Roman, Greek, and Egyptian writings. Scurvy, which is associated with bleeding gums, poor wound healing, petechiae, anemia, arthralgia, and joint effusions, fatigue, depression, and sudden death, appears to result primarily from decreased collagen synthesis (7–9). As collagen synthesis is dependent on ascorbic acid, adequate amounts of this vitamin are essential for maintenance of healthy connective tissue. The objective of this chapter is to present what is known of the role of ascorbic acid in collagen biosynthesis, in vivo (skin and bone) and in vitro (fibroblasts and osteoblasts), and the relationship of ascorbic acid and collagen (connective tissue) during the aging process and wound healing.

COLLAGEN
Protein Structure

Collagens belong to a superfamily of proteins initially characterized as heterotrimeric or homotrimeric extracellular matrix proteins whose polypeptide chains contain long regions of a repeating [Glycine-X-Y-] motif, where X and Y are usually any amino acid other than cysteine and tryptophan, which are folded into a tight triple helical structure (6,10). The use of genomic and complementary deoxyribonucleic acid (cDNA) libraries spawned the search for and identification of the diverse group of collagens, of which some do not have the traditional structure of long uninterrupted triple helices but have very short repeats and triple helical domains. There are now at least 19 defined types of collagens and over 30 genes for these have been identified (6,11,12) (Table 1). Collagens can be divided into several classes on the basis of structure: (1) fibrillar (types I, II, III, V, and XI), (2) basement membrane (type IV), (3) fibrillar associated collagens with interrupted triple helices (types IX and XII), (4) network collagens (types VIII and X), (5) microfibrils (type VI), and (6) long-chain anchoring fibrils with interrupted triple helix (type VII). This chapter will focus on the fibrillar collagens. Quantitatively, types I, II, and III account for greater than 70% of the collagen in the body (13), and of these type I collagen is by far the most abundant and best characterized. Fibrillar collagens are characterized by an uninterrupted triple helical domain of approximately 300 nm in length. They are synthesized as individual proα collagen chains of approximately 1000 amino acids in which nearly a third of the residues are glycine, with a high content of proline and hydroxyproline and fewer residues of hydroxylysine.

Type I collagen is a heterotrimer composed of two α1(I) chains and one similar but genetically distinct α2(I) chain. The precursor polypeptide chains of the type I procollagen can be divided into seven domains: a signal sequence, N-terminal propeptide globular domain, N-terminal propeptide triple helical domain, N-terminal telopeptide, triple helical domain, C-terminal telopeptide, and C-terminal propeptide globular domain (6) (Fig. 1).

Gene Structure

The basic structure of the fibrillar collagen genes is very similar; they contain 52 exons, with the uninterrupted triple helical region coded by 42 exons that contain either 45, 54, 99, 108, or 162 base pairs (11,14). In addition, the exons of the triple helical region always begin with a complete codon for glycine and end with a complete codon for a Y amino acid; the exons code for a discrete number of Glycine-X-Y repeats. The relative size and pattern of the exons appear to be conserved. The type I collagen genes, COL1A1 coding for proα1(I)collagen and COL1A2 coding for proα2(I) collagen, are respectively, 18 kb and 38 kb in length and located on different chromosomes, 17 and 7 (Table 1). The difference in size between these two genes is primarily due to differences in size of their intronic

Table 1   Collagen Types and the Location of Their Genes on Human Chromosomes

Type	Gene	Chromosome	Expression
I	COL1A1	17q21.3–q22	Most connective tissues
	COL1A2	7q21.3–q22	
II	COL2A1	12q13–q14	Cartilage, vitreous humor
III	COL3A1	2q24.3–q31	Extensible connective tissue, e.g., skin, lung, vascular system
IV	COL4A1	13q34	Basement membranes
	COL4A2	13q34	
	COL4A3	2q35–q37	
	COL4A4	2q35–q37	
	COL4A5	Xq22	
	COL4A6	Xq22	
V	COL5A1	9q34.2–q34.3	Tissues containing collagen I, quantitatively minor component
	COL5A2	2q24.3–q31	
	COL5A3		
VI	COL6A1	21q22.3	Most connective tissues
	COL6A2	21q22.3	
	COL6A3	2q37	
VII	COL7A1	3p21	Anchoring fibrils
VIII	COL8A1	3q12–q13.1	Many tissues, especially endothelium
	COL8A2	1p32.3–p34.3	
IX	COL9A1	6q12–q14	Tissues containing collagen II
	COL9A2	1p32	
	COL9A3		
X	COL10A1	6q21–q22	Hypertrophic cartilage
XI	COL11A1	1p21	Tissues containing collagen II
	COL11A2	6p21.2	
	COL2A1	12q13–q14	
XII	COL12A1	6	Tissues containing collagen I
XIII	COL13A1	10q22	Many tissues
XIV	COL14A1		Tissues containing collagen I
XV	COL15A1	9q21–22	Many tissues
XVI	COL16A1	1p34–35	Many tissues
XVII	COL17A1	10q24.3	Skin hemidesmosomes
XVIII	COL18A1	21q22.3	Many tissues, especially liver and kidney
XIX	COL19A1	6q12–q14	Rhabdomyosarcoma cells

Source: Ref. 11.

sequences. Throughout evolution there appears to be a high degree of conservation of this exon structure between different fibrillar collagens and between species, which supports the concept of a common ancestry in the evolution of collagen's gene structure (11,14).

COLLAGEN BIOSYNTHESIS

Ascorbic acid plays a crucial role as a cofactor for the hydroxylating enzymes that are essential for the synthesis of a stable collagen molecule (15). The following section

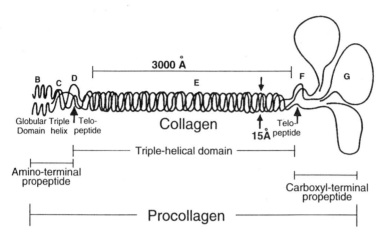

Figure 1 A schematic of a type I procollagen molecule with the major domains of the molecule indicated: A, The signal sequence (not shown); B, N-terminal propeptide globular domain; C, N-terminal propeptide triple helical domain; D, N-terminal telopeptide; E, triple helical domain; F, C-terminal telopeptide; G, C-terminal propeptide globular domain. (Adapted from Ref. 6 with permission.)

describes the biosynthesis of type I collagen, the prototype of the fibrillar collagens, exemplifying many of the common features of collagen biosynthesis. Each collagen chain is synthesized as a precursor proα type I collagen chain, and these chains assemble into mature collagen molecules via a complex series of cotranslational and posttranslational processing steps, including association of the correct proα collagen chains, hydroxylation of specific prolyl and lysyl residues, glycosylation, cleavage of propeptides, and intra-molecular and intermolecular cross-linking, to form the mature collagen fibrils in the extracellular matrix. This entire biosynthetic process involves at least 10 different enzymes.

Intracellular Events

Nucleus (Transcription)

The expression of collagen genes can be regulated by a variety of growth factors (15–19) and ascorbic acid (15,20,21). In type I collagen the expression of the COL1A1 and COL1A2 genes is almost always coordinately regulated. These genes are present in equal number, one copy per haploid genome. Researchers have determined that to achieve the normal heterotrimeric composition of type I collagen, two α1(I) chains to a single α2(I) chain, the COL1A1 and COL1A2 genes are transcribed at different efficiencies. Transcription of the COL1A1 gene produces twice the amount of steady-state messenger ribonucleic acid (mRNA) as the COL1A2 gene (22). This is independent of the stability of the mRNA, and the translation efficiencies appear similar. Type I collagen genes are transcribed by a similar process to that of other eukaryotic mRNAs which encode secreted proteins. They undergo coordinate normal transcription of precursor heteronuclear RNA by RNA polymerase II, followed by splicing out of intronic sequences, 5′ capping, and 3′ end polyadenylation (23). The mRNAs are transported into the cytoplasm and associate with ribosomes to begin the translational process.

Cytoplasm (Translation and Processing)

The individual collagen chains are synthesized on the ribosomes of the rough endoplasmic reticulum (RER), and the signal sequences of preproα1(I) and preproα2(I) collagen chains are cleaved as the elongated chains are transported into the lumen of the RER (Fig. 2).

Certain prolyl and lysyl residues that are immediately amino terminal to a glycine in the newly synthesized polypeptide chains are hydroxylated by the enzymes prolyl 4-hydroxylase (P 4-H) and lysyl hydroxylase (LH), respectively. In addition, some prolyl residues are hydroxylated by prolyl 3-hydroxylase (P 3-H). The reaction mechanisms of all three hydroxylating enzymes are similar, and as described in the section, Prolyl and Lysyl Hydroxylases, each enzyme requires ascorbate, α-ketoglutarate, molecular oxygen, and ferrous iron as cofactors. The substrate for all three enzymes must be an unfolded (i.e., nonhelical) procollagen chain. Both P 4-H and LH are influenced by adjacent amino acids and by peptide chain length (24–26).

The enzyme P 4-H exists as a tetramer of two α subunits and two β subunits (26,27). The β subunit is identical to protein disulfide isomerase (PDI), which facilitates disulfide exchange in folding proteins (28–30). The enzyme P 4-H catalyzes the formation of 4-hydroxyproline in collagen by the hydroxylation of proline residues in the -X-Pro-Gly- sequence. These residues are essential for the folding and stabilization of the newly synthesized procollagen chains into triple helical molecules under physiological conditions. If the majority of the prolyl residues are not correctly hydroxylated, then at 37°C, a stable collagen molecule will not form (24).

The enzyme P 3-H is highly sequence specific, catalyzing the hydroxylation of prolyl residues at the X position of Gly-X-Y- triplets, and only when Y is occupied by a 4-hydroxyprolyl residue (31). The function of 3-hydroxyproline, the major product of this reaction, is unknown.

The enzyme LH catalyzes the hydroxylation of lysyl residues in the triplet sequence -X-Lys-Gly-. The function of the hydroxylysyl residues formed by the action of LH is twofold: forming specific covalent intermolecular cross-links that are essential for the tensile strength of the collagen fibril and for the attachment of carbohydrate residues (24,25,32).

The glycosylation of certain hydroxylysine residues within the triple helix requires the activity of two enzymes, hydroxylysyl galactosyltransferase and galactosylhydroxylysyl glucosyltransferase (33). These enzymes transfer galactose to position 5 of some of the hydroxylysines and glucose to position 2 of some of the galactosylhydroxylysine residues, respectively. Requirements for activity include Mn^{2+} as the preferred divalent cation and a free ε-amino group of hydroxylysine. The extent of glycosylation is variable and the function of the carbohydrate moieties is unknown. They may influence fibril formation, as suggested by the inverse relationship that exists between carbohydrate content and collagen fibril diameter (33).

Following synthesis and modification, the proα collagen chains associate at the carboxyl terminal to form trimers that are stabilized by interchain disulfide bond formation, catalyzed by PDI (12). In the example of type I collagen, a heterotrimer is formed by the association of two proα1(I) chains with one proα2(I) chain. The folding of the helical domain proceeds from the carboxy terminal to the amino terminal end of the molecule with a rate that is limited by cis–trans isomerization of peptidyl prolyl bonds (34). As suggested by recent reports, chain association and folding of type I and IV collagens may involve colligin, a specific molecular chaperone protein (35). Cross-linking studies have shown that this protein binds specifically to type I procollagen and that this association is

ROUGH ENDOPLASMIC
RETICULUM

Synthesis and modification
of procollagen chains

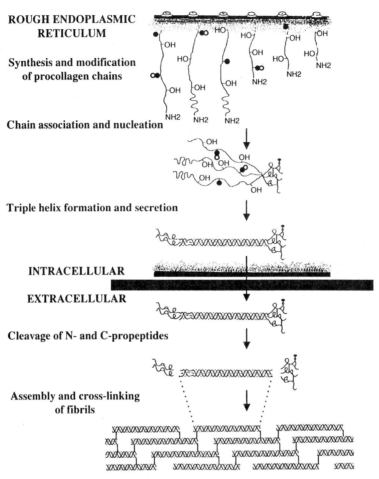

Chain association and nucleation

Triple helix formation and secretion

INTRACELLULAR

EXTRACELLULAR

Cleavage of N- and C-propeptides

Assembly and cross-linking
of fibrils

Figure 2 Schematic representation of the intracellular and extracellular steps involved in the synthesis, processing, and assembly of type I collagen molecules into fibrils. The individual collagen polypeptide chains are synthesized on the ribosomes of the rough endoplasmic reticulum and secreted into the lumen, where they undergo complex enzymic modifications, including prolyl and lysyl hydroxylation, prior to chain association and triple helix formation. The newly formed procollagen molecules are then secreted to the extracellular space, where they undergo further modification by specific proteinases which cleave off the N- and C-propeptides. The collagen molecules thus formed may participate in fibril formation by aligning in a characteristic staggered array which is subsequently stabilized by covalent cross-linking. -OH, prolyl and lysyl hydroxylation; —•, galactosylhydroxylysine; —•○, glucosylgalactosylhydroxylysine. (Adapted from Ref. 10 with permission.)

increased when cells are either heat shocked or treated with an inhibitor of hydroxylation of prolyl residues, α,α'-dipyridyl (36). The procollagen molecules are then secreted by the classical pathway (37) that involves translocation to the Golgi complex and packaging into secretory vesicles that fuse with the membrane prior to secretion.

Extracellular Events

Following secretion, the soluble procollagen is enzymatically processed to an insoluble collagen by proteolytic cleavage of both amino- and carboxy-terminal propeptide extensions. These propeptides must be cleaved by specific proteinases for the proteins to self-assemble into fibrils under physiological conditions. The N-propeptides of both types I and II procollagens are cleaved by the same specific procollagen N-proteinase. In patients with Ehlers-Danlos syndrome type VII (EDS VII) (6,38) in which the N-propeptides of type I collagen are retained, as a result of either mutations at the enzyme cleavage site in the COLIA1 (EDS VIIA) (39) or COLIA2 genes (EDS VIIB) (40) or a lack of the enzyme itself (EDS VIIC) (41), abnormal fibrillar collagen is observed and also skin fragility (in EDS VIIC) (41). Presumably, the presence of partially processed procollagen I molecules prevents normal fibril growth, and therefore fibrillogenesis is affected (39).

The normally processed collagen monomers then spontaneously aggregate into fibrils in a regular staggered array (42) such that the telopeptide regions of one collagen monomer interact with the triple helical region of adjacent molecules. These associations are stabilized by intermolecular cross-links that provide the collagen fibrils with extraordinary tensile strength and structural integrity (43). Lysyl oxidase (LO) is a copper-requiring, extracellular posttranslational modifying enzyme that catalyzes the initial reaction in the formation of lysine- or hydroxylysine-derived cross-links via oxidative deamination of the ε-amino group of specific lysine or hydroxylysine residues in the collagen telopeptide region to form the aldehyde precursors of the cross-links (44). The resulting aldehydes, allysine and hydroxyallysine, can then, by an aldol condensation reaction, spontaneously form intermolecular cross-links by condensation with other lysine or hydroxylysine residues in the triple helical regions of adjacent molecules (45). This divalent cross-linking precedes the formation of a more complex cross-linking process in which nonreducible cross-links are formed. One of these stable cross-links, histidinohydroxylysinonorleucine, the major nonreducible trifunctional cross-link in skin, has been shown to increase steadily with chronological aging (46).

Although there is a relatively slow turnover of extracellular collagen in the adult body and the average half-life of mature collagen is estimated to be in the range of several months (47), synthesis and degradation of collagen fibers are continually in progress (48). Collagenase is the rate-limiting enzyme in the degradative pathway of collagen (49,50). This enzyme is one of a family of matrix metalloproteinases that plays a major role in the proteolysis of components of the extracellular matrix (51). Collagenase cleaves collagen specifically at Gly-Leu or Gly-Ileu sequences in an initial step that allows the molecule to unwind so that it can be cut by less specific proteases. Stromelysins 1 and 2 have a broader substrate capacity, targeting matrix proteins such as fibronectin, proteoglycan core protein, nonhelical regions of elastin, and laminin, as well as some collagen types (52).

Elastin is another major component of the extracellular matrix and plays an important role in the changes associated with aging skin (53). The basic polypeptide chains of the precursor of elastin, tropoelastin, form a fiber network linked by specific intermolecular cross-links, desmosines and isodesmosines, that are only found in the elastin structure. In a similar process to collagen, the mRNA is translated on the RER and transferred to the extracellular space, where the elastin polypeptides align to form a fibrillar structure stabilized by desmosine cross-links. These cross-links are initiated via the conversion of some lysine residues to aldehydes in a reaction catalyzed by lysyl oxidase; three of these aldehydes spontaneously condense with an unmodified lysyl residue to give a desmosine that stabilizes the elastin network. A group of proteases, collectively called elastases, catalyze the degradative pathway of elastin (48).

ROLE OF ASCORBIC ACID IN CONNECTIVE TISSUE REGULATION

Type I Collagen

Ascorbic acid affects the biosynthesis of collagen at several levels from collagen gene transcription to expression, including the regulation of the processing enzymes. Ascorbic acid has been shown by several laboratories to increase collagen synthesis in vitro in several different kinds of cell lines including fibroblasts (15,19,54,55), osteoblasts (56–58), and chondrocytes (59). The stimulation of collagen synthesis appears to occur at the transcriptional level (21,54,60). In addition to demonstrating that ascorbic acid and its long-acting derivative, ascorbic acid 2-PO_4, increased type I collagen RNA by stimulating transcription in cultured human dermal fibroblasts, Kurata et al. showed that in fibroblasts incubated in the presence of the protein synthesis inhibitor, cycloheximide, ascorbic acid, and ascorbic acid 2-PO_4 were still able to increase type I collagen RNA levels. This suggests that there may be cis-regulatory elements present in or near the collagen genes which are responsible for activation of the genes by ascorbic acid (54). There is also some evidence that ascorbic acid may act to stabilize collagen mRNA (21). Additional studies on the mechanism of collagen responsiveness to ascorbic acid are still required in order to define their relationship further.

When considering the mechanism of action of ascorbic acid, we know that ascorbic acid increases collagen gene transcription and that it is necessary for the hydroxylation of prolyl and lysyl residues. In various biological systems it also functions as a reducing agent. However, its ability to stimulate proliferation of fibroblasts and to increase collagen synthesis cannot be due simply to its reducing activity since the same concentration of another reducing agent, dithiothreitol, is incapable of either stimulating fibroblast proliferation or increasing type I collagen production (61). There is some evidence that in the presence of transitional metal ions, ascorbic acid induces lipid peroxidation, resulting in the formation of reactive aldehydes; this makes peroxide a candidate as an intracellular mediator for the actions of ascorbate. Both ascorbic acid–induced peroxidation in cultured fibroblasts and addition of malondialdehyde, a product of lipid peroxidation, to culture medium of human fibroblasts are capable of stimulating transcription of the COL1A1 gene (60). Retinoids or other inhibitors of lipid peroxidation (propyl gallate, cobalt chloride, α-naphthol) inhibit ascorbate-induced peroxidation and collagen synthesis (62). However, studies by Darr et al. suggest that increased lipid peroxidation is coincidental with increased collagen synthesis in ascorbate-treated dermal fibroblasts and that lipid peroxidation and collagen synthesis are not related (63). Further studies are needed to define clearly the mechanisms and the cis- and trans-transcription factors involved in the regulation of collagen by ascorbic acid.

Prolyl and Lysyl Hydroxylases

In the body, one function of ascorbate is to act as cofactor for several metal-dependent oxidation reactions catalyzed by both monooxygenases and dioxygenases (64). Other cofactors required by the dioxygenases are Fe^{2+}, α-ketoglutarate, and O_2, whereas the two monooxygenases described to date require Cu^+ and O_2 for activity (8). In addition to the three dioxygenases, P 4-H, P 3-H, and LH required in collagen biosynthesis, other ascorbate-dependent dioxygenases include butyrobetaine hydroxylase and 6-N-trimethyl-L-lysine hydroxylase, both required in the biosynthesis of carnitine (64). The reaction mechanism of P 4-H and LH involves a stoichiometric decarboxylation of α-ketoglutarate in which one atom of the O_2 molecule is incorporated into the succinate and the other is incorporated into the hydroxyl group formed on the prolyl or lysyl residue (Fig. 3A) (65). Extensive kinetic studies show that there is a systematic binding of cofactors Fe^{2+}, α-ketoglutarate, O_2, and the peptide substrate to the enzyme, followed by an ordered release of products (24,66). Although ascorbate is not consumed stoichiometrically in this process and the hydroxylation reaction may occur without it for a few cycles, ascorbate is specifically required by the hydroxylating enzymes (67,68). One of its functions may be to act as an alternative oxygen acceptor in the uncoupled decarboxylation of α-ketoglutarate in which it is consumed stoichiometrically (Fig. 3B) (66). In the complete reaction with the

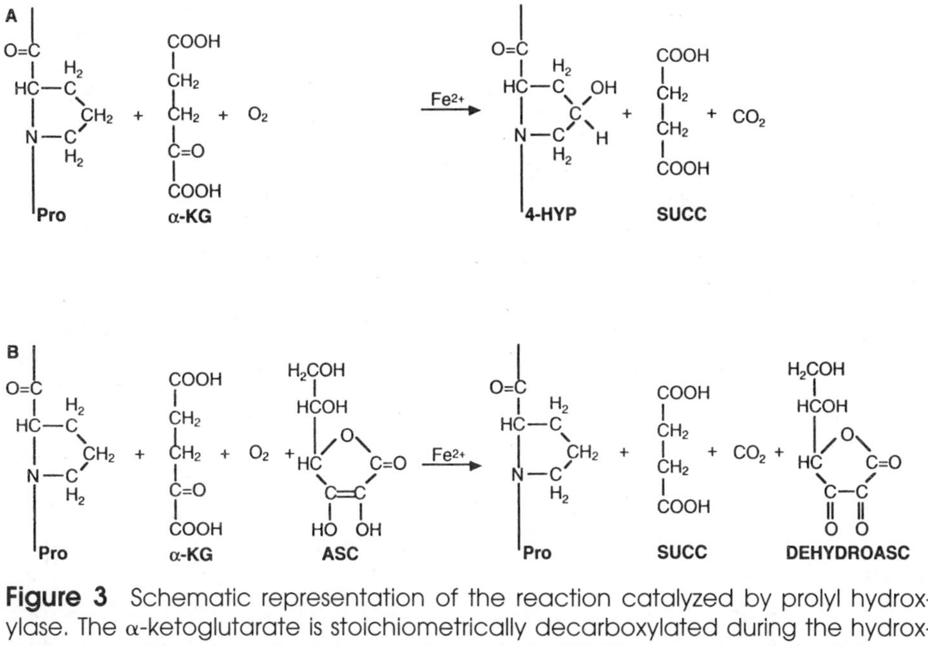

Figure 3 Schematic representation of the reaction catalyzed by prolyl hydroxylase. The α-ketoglutarate is stoichiometrically decarboxylated during the hydroxylation reaction, which does not need ascorbate (A). The enzymes also catalyze an uncoupled decarboxylation of α-ketoglutarate without subsequent hydroxylation of the peptide substrate. Ascorbate serves as a stoichiometrically consumed alternative oxygen acceptor in the uncoupled reaction cycles, which may take place either in the presence (B) or absence of the peptide substrate. Pro, proline; 4-Hyp, 4-hydroxyproline; α-KG, α-ketoglutarate; SUCC, succinate; ASC, ascorbate; DEHYDROASC, dehydroascorbate. (Adapted from Ref. 24 with permission.)

peptide substrate, the decarboxylation of α-ketoglutarate probably results in the formation of an iron-oxo complex (ferryl ion) that acts as the active intermediate in oxygen transfer and hydroxylates the peptide-bound prolyl or lysyl residue (69). In the uncoupled reaction that can take place in the presence or absence of substrate, the reactive iron-oxo complex is probably converted to $[Fe^{3+\cdot}O^-]$ with the Fe^{3+} ion remaining bound to the active site and therefore inactivating the enzyme (66). Ascorbate is then required to reactivate the enzyme by reducing the oxy iron complex to a ferrous ion (70). Derivatives of ascorbate that differ only in their side chain, such as D-isoascorbate and 5,6-O-isopropylidene L-ascorbate, can effectively replace ascorbate (71–73). However, modifications of the ring atoms that abolish the capacity to bind iron deactivate the molecule (71).

The active P 4-H in vertebrates is a tetramer (α2 β2) of M_r 240,000 consisting of the α-subunit (M_r 64,000) and the β-subunit (M_r 60,000) (26). These subunits are the products of different genes (28,74). Binding experiments with suicide inactivators and other compounds indicate that the α-subunit may be the principal contributor to the active site of P 4-H. But some parts of the catalytic sites, including the ascorbate binding site that resembles the binding site of α-ketoglutarate, may be built up of both α- and β-subunits (24). The β-subunit of P 4-H has been shown to be an unusual multifunctional polypeptide. The cDNA sequence demonstrates its identity with PDI and also with a cellular thyroid hormone binding protein (75). The presence of the tetrapeptide sequence -Lys-Asp-Glu-Leu (-KDEL-), which is essential for the retention of a polypeptide within the lumen of the RER, in the carboxy terminus of the β-subunit suggests that one of its functions is to retain the enzyme within the RER (28). The β-subunit is synthesized in excess of the α-subunit so that it can both associate with the α-subunit for hydroxylase activity and be available as free β-subunit for disulfide isomerase (PDI) activity (24). In contrast to the available pool of free β-subunit, all of the α-subunit appears to become incorporated into the tetramer directly after its synthesis. Hybridization analysis indicates that in untreated cells, the concentration of the α-subunit mRNA is about 25% that of the β-subunit mRNA (76). Administration of hydralazine, an antihypertensive drug, to cultured skin fibroblasts increased the mRNA levels for the α-subunit immediately, whereas the mRNA for the β-subunit was maximally stimulated at 72 h (76). The earlier induction of the α-subunit mRNA may indicate that the regulation of P 4-H activity may be mediated by the regulation of the α-subunit of P 4-H. Unlike the β-subunit, the α-subunit does not contain the -KDEL- retention signal; it is presumably retained in the RER by binding to the β-subunit (77,78). The α-subunit contains five cysteine residues, of which some are likely to be involved in the binding of Fe^{2+} at the catalytic site of the enzyme.

The enzyme LH is a homodimer of identical subunits, each of M_r 85,000 (24). Recent cloning and sequencing of the cDNA from placenta (79) and human skin fibroblasts (80,81) have shown that although there is marked similarity between the kinetic properties of the two enzymes, there is no significant sequence homology between LH and the two subunits of P 4-H. Unlike the β-subunit of P 4-H, LH lacks the retention signal typical of the luminal or transmembrane proteins of the endoplasmic reticulum (ER). It has recently been shown to reside loosely bound to the ER via weak electrostatic bonds (82). The protein contains nine cysteine residues, of which at least one is likely to be involved in the binding of the iron atom at a catalytic site. The catalytic site of LH is not known, but there is considerable sequence homology between the chick and human amino acid sequences at the carboxy terminal of the enzyme, suggesting that this region may be important for activity (83). The recent development of a baculovirus system to express LH in an active form should facilitate the analysis of the catalytic site of the enzyme (84).

Previous work has shown that treatment of human skin fibroblasts with ascorbate for 3 h prior to harvest increases the level of P 4-H activity threefold (85), in contrast to the decrease in P 4-H reported after a longer exposure of cells (72 h) to ascorbate (15). After a similar 72-h treatment, however, LH activity was stimulated approximately threefold by ascorbate (15). The stimulation of LH by administration of ascorbate was recently confirmed at a pretranslational level in a study demonstrating the upregulation of the mRNA and activity of LH by administration of ascorbate to fibroblasts from both a normal donor and a patient with EDS VI (86). Patients with EDS VI, who have features of extreme joint hypermobility and hyperextensible skin, are biochemically characterized by a deficiency of LH (38,87). Mutations characterized in the LH cDNA from the patient in this study (88) appeared to be responsible for the decreased LH activity (24% of normal) in the skin fibroblasts. Administration of ascorbate resulted in a twofold increase in LH activities in both EDS VI and normal cells which paralleled the increase in their steady-state LH mRNAs. Ascorbate also increased total collagen production twofold from a similar basal level of collagen synthesis in each cell type (86). This was confirmed by protein gel analysis, which showed increases in proα1(I), proα2(I), and proα1(III) collagen chains in both normal and EDS VI cells (Fig. 4). Earlier studies showed that administration of pharmacological amounts of ascorbate to this patient significantly improved his wound healing and muscle strength (89). These results suggest that the mechanism for the favorable response may involve an ascorbate-mediated stimulation of the mRNAs for LH and α1(I) collagen, which, in turn, produces a parallel increase in LH activity and collagen production. A similar response to ascorbate was reported in another EDS VI patient (90), and this treatment protocol is used on a regular basis for EDS VI patients (6).

Somewhat surprisingly, ascorbic acid does not exert the same effect on elastin, another major component of the extracellular matrix. Several reports show reduced elastin secretion and accumulation by cultured cells after ascorbic acid treatment (91,92). In addition, it

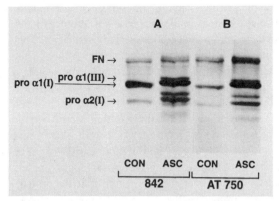

Figure 4   Levels of proα1(I), proα2(I), and proα1(III) collagens in fibroblasts from both (A) a normal donor (842) and (B) an EDSVI patient (AT750) are stimulated twofold by treatment with 100 μM ascorbate (ASC) for 72 h, compared with controls (CON). Tritiated samples from a collagen synthesis experiment, in which cells were labeled with L-(2,3-³H) proline (86), were electrophoresed on a 5% polyacrylamide -SDS gel prior to autoradiography. The collagen bands were quantitated by laser densitometry. Note: The proα1(III) collagen is only visible in the ascorbate-treated samples in both cell types. SDS, sodium dodecyl sulfate. (Adapted from Ref. 86 with permission.)

was shown that even though in vivo ascorbic acid did not appear to inhibit LO activity, high doses inhibited this enzyme in vitro (93).

ASCORBIC ACID AND AGING CONNECTIVE TISSUE

Aging may be defined as a progressive time-dependent deterioration in organ function and increased vulnerability to disease (3–5). The maturation and aging process is complex and induces pronounced changes in biochemical and mechanical parameters of connective tissue. From investigations in several species and different tissues, the general scenario indicates that during the maturation process there is an increase in strength and quality of connective tissue which is reversed as senescence (aging) approaches. The following sections will present current in vivo (skin and bone) and in vitro (fibroblasts and osteo-blasts) investigations characterizing the effects of aging and ascorbic acid on collagen and the extracellular matrix.

Skin (In Vivo)

In the skin, the results of aging arise from a complex situation in which several independent factors contribute to the pathogenesis of degenerative changes. These factors may be grouped into two major biologically different, but interractive processes, determined by intrinsic and extrinsic events. Intrinsic or chronological aging is an endogenous process that probably reflects the biological aging affecting other organs as well. This form of aging is clinically characterized by fine wrinkling, atrophy of the dermis, and loss of subcutaneous fat (2). There is also evidence of poor wound healing and fragility of the dermal connective tissue. In contrast, the extrinsic process of aging is a result of exposure to environmental elements (5). The differences between these pathways have been well described (3), and the extracellular matrix is variously affected in aging, depending on the extent of exposure to extrinsic factors.

The extracellular matrix is a complex integrated system composed of several macro-molecules that can be divided into four major classes: collagens, elastins, proteoglycans, and structural glycoproteins. Changes in the external appearance of aging skin are accompanied by dramatic changes in the architecture of the extracellular matrix. Although the dermis is more strikingly affected by aging, changes in the epidermal layers include a decrease in the numbers of melanocytes and Langerhans cells (2,94). This is accompanied by a marked reduction of the protective function of dermis. The dermal–epidermal junction is markedly changed as the skin ages: it becomes flattened and the resulting decrease in the surface area between the layers lessens the adhesion between them. As a result, elderly skin becomes more susceptible to the effects of shearing forces and is more easily torn. The major tissue component of human dermis is collagen, which comprises approximately 70% to 80% of the dry weight of dermis. Collagen fibers, therefore, constitute the primary fibrillar structures in dermis providing tensile properties that allow skin to protect against external trauma. Elastic fibers in normal adult skin occupy a much smaller volume of the dermal volume, in the range of 2% to 4%. With aging, the connective tissue becomes disorganized, with a loss of collagen content, destruction of elastin fiber architecture, and a decrease in glycosoaminoglycans and fibronectin (95). The loss of collagen decreases the tensile strength of the skin, making it more vulnerable to tearing and external forces and the changes in elastin responsible for loss of elasticity result in sagging and wrinkling.

In studies conducted on the effect of aging on collagen and elastin fiber content in the dermis, collagen levels have been shown to vary only slightly with age, whereas elastin fibers display the most prominent changes associated with both the intrinsic and extrinsic pathways of aging. Skin collagen content, expressed per unit area of skin surface (96) or tissue section (97), have been shown in both sexes to decrease linearly with aging at a rate of about 1% annually from adulthood to old age. This results from both a thinning of dermis and a decline of collagen density. The rate of collagen synthesis in skin decreases markedly with age. Using markers of hydroxyproline production, prolyl hydroxylase activity, and solubility of newly synthesized collagen to measure collagen synthesis, a significant decrease was observed in the age range from birth to about 30 to 40 years, after which the rate stayed approximately the same (Fig. 5) (98). Morphological studies have shown that collagen fibers become thinner and more widely spaced in aging skin (99). A recent study showed a similar trend in both sexes, in which collagen fiber density began to decrease at the age of 30 to 40 years in a reversal of the increasing density reported during the younger years (100).

Although a study of 14 enzymes involved in major metabolic pathways in the epidermis of normal human donors showed no difference in activity with age (101), there have been reports that some of the posttranslational modifying enzymes of collagen biosynthesis, including P 4-H and LH, decrease in aging human skin (95). Fornieri et al. reported decreased LO activity in the skin from old rats (102), although this pattern of activity was later shown to be tissue-dependent (103). However, these changes were not reflected in a study of the steady-state levels of the mRNAs of LH and LO in fibroblasts from human donors of differing ages (104). Another study reported no correlation between the extent of collagen hydroxylation and age (105). However, one study in rats suggested a marked increase in collagen degradation in all tissues with age (106) and one explanation for this could be the presence of underhydroxylated collagen that is susceptible to degradation.

The ratio of genetically distinct collagen types also changes with increasing age. During early fetal development type III collagen is the major form and consequently the ratio of type III to type I collagen is the reverse of that in adult skin, which has a sixfold excess of type I to type III collagen (95,107).

The sagging and loss of elasticity observed in both sun-protected and sun-damaged skin with aging can probably be explained on the basis of loss of functional elastic fibers (108). In biological aging the elastin fibers disintegrate, and spontaneous and progressive degeneration of the elastin fibers has occurred in most people by the age of 70. Elastin biosynthesis declines dramatically with biological aging (95). Elastin fibers are stabilized by the formation of the intermolecular cross-links desmosine and isodesmosine, which are initiated by the enzyme LO. However, there is no clear correlation between the levels of LO and desmosine cross-links in skin; in fact LO appears to decrease in aging rat skin.

An examination of the relationship of vitamin C to aging shows that ascorbate levels in blood and tissue decrease in proportion to age, but they can be increased by ascorbate supplementation. As ascorbate is required by both P 4-H and LH for activity, its deficiency results in the synthesis of an underhydroxylated collagen that is structurally unstable. Skin appears to be particularly vulnerable to ascorbate deficiency, and many of the undesirable effects of aging skin can be attributed to the loss of connective tissue. The stimulation of collagen synthesis in elderly persons by pharmacological means would appear to have beneficial effects on skin physiological mechanisms. Although ascorbic acid does not appear significantly to affect elastin biosynthesis, it enhances collagen biosynthesis at the transcriptional and posttranslational levels and may restore some of the properties which

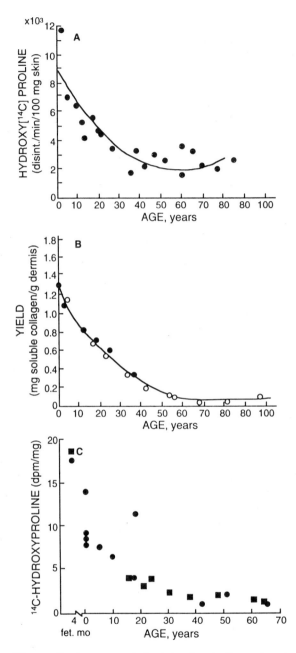

Figure 5 Age-associated decline in the rate of collagen synthesis in human skin. The results indicate that collagen production, measured by the synthesis of radio-labeled hydroxyproline (A), collagen solubility in acid extraction (B), and activity of prolyl hydroxylase (C), progressively decreases from high levels in the neonatal and early postnatal periods to relatively low levels beyond the fourth decade. (Reprinted from Ref. 98 with permission.)

deteriorate in aging skin, such as vulnerability to external trauma and poor wound healing. This is described in more detail in Chapter 29.

Dermal Fibroblasts (In Vitro)

Studies have clearly shown that the chronological age of donor tissue is strongly reflected in the behavior of cultured skin-derived cells (22,109), thus making in vitro studies using cultured dermal fibroblasts a very useful system for evaluating the cellular manifestations of aging and the effect of ascorbic acid. One of the well characterized manifestations of aging is a loss of a cell's ability to proliferate (104,110,111). For example, Takeda et al. showed that growth rates of cultured fibroblasts decreased with the increasing age of the donor (in vivo–aged) and after passage 20 of fetal fibroblasts (in vitro–aged) (112). It is hypothesized that the loss of proliferative capacity is due to decreased responsiveness to growth factors. It has been suggested by certain investigators that ascorbic acid itself may function as a growth factor (19,20,104,113). In one study examining ascorbic acid's growth-factor-like activity, a comparison of cultured dermal fibroblasts derived from three newborn donors and three elderly donors (78–93 years) demonstrated that the addition of ascorbic acid stimulated both the newborn and the elderly cells to grow faster and reach higher densities than its absence (104). Without ascorbate the newborn cells grew faster and reached higher densities than cells from elderly donors. These elderly cell lines reached a plateau in cell growth within a few divisions and were no longer dividing. Administration of ascorbic acid overcame the reduced proliferative capacity of the elderly cell lines. Ascorbic acid's growth-factor-like activity therefore appears to act via mechanisms which are unrelated to age.

It has been well documented that there is an inverse relationship between collagen synthesis and the age of the cells, that is independent of whether the cells have been aged in vivo (based on donor age) or in vitro (based on doublings in culture) (20,104,114). In a study of in vivo aged cultured dermal fibroblasts, the levels of type I and type III collagen from women aged between 19 and 68 years showed a linear decrease in secretion of both collagen types with increasing donor age (114). A comparative study of the changes in extracellular matrix components, including collagen, proteoglycans, and glycoproteins, in in vitro and in vivo aged skin showed that the rates of collagen and proteoglycan synthesis also decreased in both types of aging (112). The decreased collagen synthesis correlated with decreased levels of both proα1(I) collagen and proα2(I) collagen mRNAs, although this regulation was not coordinate. Levels of type III collagen mRNA also declined in both forms of aging. However, in another study in which in vivo aged cultured fibroblasts (from newborn and elderly donors) were examined the basal levels of collagen synthesis of the elderly cell lines decreased to about half the levels of synthesis in newborn cells (Table 2) (104). In this study the difference in levels of collagen expression appeared to result from a posttranslational event, since the steady-state proα1(I)collagen and proα1(III) collagen mRNA levels appeared similar; the differences in steady-state mRNA levels between the newborn and elderly cell lines were no greater than the variability within the specific age classes. Although the basal level of collagen synthesis was less in the elderly cell lines than in the newborn, administration of ascorbic acid increased the levels of collagen synthesis in both cell types to the same extent (Table 2). A similar age-independent effect was observed with the steady-state mRNA levels of LH: ascorbate administration resulted in small equivalent increases in LH mRNA in both young and elderly cell lines. In contrast the level of steady-state LO mRNA was unchanged by administration of ascorbic acid to

Table 2 Effect of Ascorbic Acid on Relative Collagen Synthesis
in Dermal Fibroblasts from Newborn and Elderly Donors

Cell strain	% Collagen[a]				Fold increase over control	
	−ASC[b]		+ASC (100 μM)[c]			
Newborn		Mean ± SD		Mean ± SD		Mean ± SD
3 Day (671)	10.2		19.0		1.9	
3 Day (672)	11.5	10.5 ± 0.9	19.7	19.9 ± 1.0	1.7	1.9 ± 0.2
8 Day (722)	9.8		20.9		2.1	
Elderly						
78 Year (882)	6.3		10.4		1.7	
88 Year (663)	5.2	6.2 ± 1.2	12.2	12.4 ± 2.0	2.4	2.0 ± 0.3
93 Year (655)	7.5		14.4		1.9	

[a]Expressed as proportion of total protein synthesis devoted to collagen. Data have been corrected
to take into account the increased proline content.
[b]Cells cultured under nonproliferating conditions, in DMEM, supplemented with 0.5% dialyzed
fetal calf serum for 72 h. ASC, ascorbic acid; DMEM, Dulbecco's modified eagle medium.
[c]Cells cultured under nonproliferating conditions, in DMEM, supplemented with 0.5% dialyzed
fetal calf serum in the presence of 100 μM ascorbic acid for 72 h.
Source: Ref. 104.

fibroblasts from either newborn or elderly donors (104). A comparison of age-related
collagen secretion from fibroblasts from exposed (facial) and unexposed (mammary) skin
showed that secretion of both type I and type III collagen was decreased to a greater extent
in exposed than protected dermis, and that this effect was even more pronounced with the
secretion of type III collagen (114). The mechanisms by which collagen expression is
decreased with age appear complex and under different circumstances may involve pretranslational and/or posttranslational events.

Bone (In Vivo)

The predominant organic component of bone is type I collagen, which is identical to soft
tissue type I collagen (115) in primary structure (amino acid sequence) and the result of the
same gene products. Even though there are only minor compositional differences between
bone and soft tissue type I collagen, which result from slight differences in posttranslational
modifications of some lysine residues (115–118), there are significant differences in physical and biochemical properties. Bone collagen does not swell in dilute acid and is relatively
insoluble in its native state as compared to soft tissue type I collagen.

The predominant parameter for evaluating age-related changes in bone has been biomechanical. Bone exhibits a generalized decrease in material strength and stiffness with
age. In humans of both sexes, between ages 35 and 70 years, decreases in cortical bone
strength in bending (15%–20%) and decreases in cancellous bone compression (50%) are
accompanied by an increase in bone brittleness (119). The age-related changes in mechanical properties of bone are hypothesized to be the result of age-related changes in local
microstructural factors, which include porosity (fraction of the volume occupied by soft
tissue spaces), geometric and histological effects, mineralization, collagen fiber orientation,
and fatigue microdamage (119).

Collagen fiber orientation has been shown to affect cortical bone strength; more longitudinally oriented fibers enhance tensile strength (120). Martin and Ishida demonstrated, using linear regression analysis, that collagen fiber orientation was consistently the best predictor of strength (120). This orientation becomes less longitudinal in bones of elderly individuals. It is uncertain whether this actually decreases or simply exacerbates reduction in material strength caused by other factors.

Bone is not a static organ; it is continuously being remodeled by the removal of old and damaged bone by osteoclasts and the formation of new bone by osteoblasts. The constituent collagen of bone is continuously renewed by remodeling and adaptive changes to mechanical loading (119,121). During aging there are changes in the structural and functional properties of connective tissues (2–5,119,121,122). There is an increase in collagen insolubility, which is believed to result from increased cross-link formation including non-enzymatic cross-linking, as a result of the formation of advanced glycosylation end products (123). The homeostatic balance in remodeling of bone appears altered with age; the bone formation rate and resorption rate become uncoupled (124). Bone formation does not keep pace with bone resorption and there is a net loss of bone tissue. In addition the unremodeled bone accumulates fatigue damage (122). Old bone that has not been re-modeled for many years accumulates an excess number of loading cycles so that fatigue damage increases with the occurrence of microfractures. The stability of the cancellous bone collagen deteriorates with age, with a decline in trabecular number and increase in trabecular separation, so that the cancellous bone becomes progressively disconnected and subsequently weakens (125). Vertebral trabecular connectivity correlates well with vertebral compression strength, and the progressive age-related disruption of trabecular network is a major factor in vertebral fragility (126).

In vivo studies are difficult to undertake because of the complexity of bone formation and the difficulty in obtaining bone samples, in addition to controlling and distinguishing between environmental, mechanical, physiological, and biochemical influences. As a result, the majority of studies addressing the role of ascorbic acid in collagen synthesis and bone formation have been performed in vitro using cultured primary and established osteoblast cell lines.

Osteoblasts (In Vitro)

In vitro studies investigating collagen synthesis in cultured primary bone cells derived from donors of various ages (fetal to 60 years) demonstrated that collagen biosynthesis rates and extractability of collagen followed a temporal sequence (127). The rate of collagen synthesis increased prenatally through birth and reached a maximum between 10 and 15 years (a doubling of the collagen synthetic rate occurs between fetal development and puberty), then by age 20 declined to one-third of the maximum rate at the pubertal peak, and further declined to one-quarter of the maximum rate after the fourth decade (Fig. 6). The percentage of extractable collagen from the cell layer doubled between fetal age and 15 years, and after 22 years it remained constant. There are two periods of known rapid bone growth in humans, which are the third trimester in utero and at 10–16 years during puberty. Collagen synthesis rates and the percentage of extractable collagen from the cell layer measured in primary osteoblast cultures from specific aged donors correlated very well with the documented periods of rapid bone growth.

Several laboratories investigating collagen and matrix formation by osteoblasts, the cells responsible for bone matrix deposition, have clearly demonstrated a dependence of cultured osteoblasts on ascorbic acid and collagen synthesis for normal osteoblast function

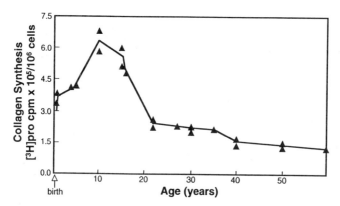

Figure 6   Rate of collagen synthesis by human osteoblasts as a function of donor age. Osteoblast cultures were incubated in the presence of (^{3}H) proline (20% to 30% of the residues in collagen are prolines) and the collagen biosynthetic rates were determined by quantitating the amount of collagenase digestible material in the medium and the cell layer. (Adapted from Ref. 127 with permission.)

and differentiation (56–58). Franceschi et al. demonstrated, using MC3T3-El cell lines, that ascorbic acid plays an important role in osteoblast differentiation (58). The clonal murine MC3T3-El calvarial-derived cell line provides a model for the study of differentiation of osteoblasts. These MC3T3-El cell lines are a nontransformed population of osteoprogenitor cells which can undergo a developmental sequence similar to that of osteoblasts in bone tissue (128). They exhibit early proliferation of undifferentiated MC3T3-El cells followed by postmitotic expression of alkaline phosphatase, formation of extracellular matrix, osteocalcin production, and generation of mineralized nodules. Incubation with ascorbic acid altered the matrix production by posttranslationally increasing collagen production through the stimulation of hydroxylation, secretion, and processing of type I procollagen, in addition to increasing collagen synthesis at the transcriptional level. In the absence of ascorbic acid there is very little expression of osteoblast markers (alkaline phosphatase or osteocalcin). When collagen synthesis was inhibited, osteoblasts were unable to differentiate or express alkaline phosphatase and osteocalcin even in the presence of ascorbic acid (129). Ascorbic acid is essential in vitro for collagen matrix, alkaline phosphatase, and osteocalcin accumulation as well as mineralization.

ASCORBIC ACID AND WOUND HEALING

Both clinical and animal studies have clearly demonstrated that wounds in the elderly heal more slowly (130). Researchers see not only decreases in cell proliferation, but also an overall decrease in wound repair, as indicated by decreased inflammatory response, delayed angiogenesis, delayed remodeling, and slower reepithelialization, with increasing age (131). Using Syrian hamsters, Bruce and Deamond demonstrated an inverse relationship between age, as represented by in vitro fibroblast life span, and wound repair (131). Dermal fibroblasts cultured from young animals exhibited a higher number of cumulative doublings before reaching in vitro senescence than the fibroblasts cultured from older animals. The number of cumulative doublings was inversely related to the rate of wound closure; wounds healed more rapidly in the younger animals. Collagen synthesis and degradation (remodeling) are also greater in younger animals; this condition is thought to be due to increased levels of collagenase (132). With increasing age, not only is slightly less collagen produced and less collagen remodeling occurring in healing wounds, but the quality of the collagen is different (130,133). These differences may reflect a different pattern of collagen cross-links as well as variations in other components of the extracellular matrix. In addition, the growth of capillaries into wounds decreases with increasing age (134). In one study in which the biomechanical properties of wounds were examined, the mean breaking strengths of healing incisional wounds were shown to be significantly stronger in younger rats than older rats (135). In a small study using human volunteers from age 22 to 87, the individuals received 5-cm incisions on their forearms, which were assayed for tensile strength at 5 days post incision (136). Although no statistical analysis was presented, the wounds in individuals above 70 years of age had less tensile strength than the wounds from younger individuals. Contraction rates measured in older animals and elderly individuals showed a delay in both contracture and closure of superficial wounds (137).

It has been well documented both historically, by examination of the pathogenicity of scurvy, and clinically, in scorbutic animal studies, that wound healing can be severely compromised under conditions of ascorbic acid deficiency. Studies using ascorbic acid–deficient guinea pigs with laparotomy wounds and skin incisions showed significantly impaired wound healing in the scorbutic animals, which exhibited increased hemorrhaging, reduced collagen formation, and decreased wound strength (138,139). In an early human study in 1940, a healthy young male volunteer was placed on an ascorbic acid–free diet, which was otherwise nutritionally complete, for 6 months (140). His serum levels of ascorbic acid dropped to zero after 42 days, whereas the ascorbic acid levels in his white blood cells took 122 days to reach zero. At 3 months and 6 months from the start of this experiment, 2-in. incisional wounds were made and evaluated for healing performance by gross appearance and histological characteristics of a wound biopsy specimen. The incision performed at 3 months healed normally. The incision performed at 6 months exhibited compromised wound healing with failure of the wound edges to unite below the skin, and histologically there was reduction in the vasculature and decreased intracellular substance (later shown to be collagen).

Wound tissue appears more metabolically active than normal connective tissue and this state may last for a long period (years) (139). Greater concentrations of ascorbic acid appear to be required for maintenance of wound integrity than for collagen development (139). In one study, in which guinea pigs that were on adequate dietary amounts of ascorbic acid underwent laparotomies, normal wound healing was observed for 6 weeks (138). After the initial 6 weeks these animals were placed on an ascorbic acid–free diet which resulted in a gradual progressive loss of new collagen, hemorrhaging, greater fragility of capillaries, and wounds which appeared more immature and increasingly weakened with the development of hernias.

Under conditions of ascorbic acid deficiency there is not only impaired wound healing, but increased wound susceptibility to infections, which are often more severe (139). It has been hypothesized that this could result from impaired collagen synthesis interfering with the walling off process to isolate the infection, thereby disrupting neutrophil antibacterial function (ascorbic acid's role in reducing oxygen to superoxide) and/or impairing complement-dependent immune reactions (ascorbic acid is necessary for synthesis of some of the components of complement) (139).

It is now known that higher levels of ascorbic acid accumulate at wound sites than in surrounding tissue. After severe acute trauma, such as extensive third-degree burns, the ascorbic acid levels in the plasma from a patient previously in good nutritional status drop to zero (141). These patients become "biochemical scorbutic," like uninjured individuals who become scorbutic as a result of prolonged ascorbic acid deficiency. Only after large quantities of daily ingestion of ascorbic acid (2 g/day) do the biochemical parameters begin to approach normal levels. This phenomenon was also demonstrated in a well documented study using guinea pigs (142). Similar responses have been reported in burns of less severity (139). Although the mechanisms involved in this response are unknown, these studies suggest that physicians should be aware of the nutritional status of their patients, particularly with the elderly and during times of trauma and surgery.

SUMMARY

Aging is an important, natural, and inevitable part of the organismal existence. Its manifestations can be observed in all tissues, functions, and processes in the body. Connective tissues, in particular, undergo many alterations physiologically, biochemically, and mechanically. This chapter demonstrates the important role that ascorbic acid plays in the production and maintenance of healthy connective tissue and its relationship to aging. Type I collagen, the predominant protein of the extracellular matrix, is the foundation of this connective tissue, and ascorbic acid is a key to its regulation and biosynthesis. We have reviewed the most recent biochemical studies concerning the role of ascorbic acid in the regulation of collagen gene expression and its processing enzymes, as well as the influence ascorbic acid may have at the level of the whole animal (skin and bone tissue) during the aging process and wound healing. Studies by several investigators and laboratories, looking at many different cell lines, tissues, and whole animals as well as humans, have clearly demonstrated that ascorbic acid is essential to maintaining healthy functioning connective tissue throughout the aging process.

REFERENCES

1. Aging American: Trends and Projections. 1991 ed. U.S. Department of Health and Human Services, Washington, DC, 1991.
2. West MD. The cellular and molecular biology of skin aging. Arch Dermatol 1994; 130:87–95.
3. Yaar M, Gilchrest BA. Cellular and molecular mechanisms of cutaneous aging. Dermatol Surg Oncol 1990; 16:915–922.
4. Balin AK, Allen RE. Mechanisms of biologic aging. Dermatol Clin 1986; 4:37–58.
5. Uitto J, Fazio MJ, Olsen DR. Molecular mechanisms of cutaneous aging: age-associated connective tissue alterations in the dermis. J Am Acad Dermatol 1989; 21:614–622.
6. Byers PH. Disorders of collagen biosynthesis and structure. In: Scriver CR, Baudet AL, Sly WS, Valle D, eds. The Metabolic and Molecular Bases of Inherited Disease. Vol. III. 7th ed. New York: McGraw-Hill, 1995:4029–4077.
7. Berg R, Kerr J. Nutritional aspects of collagen metabolism. Annu Rev Nutr 1992; 12:369–390.
8. Padh H. Vitamin C: Newer insights into its biochemical functions. Nutr Rev 1991; 49:65–70.
9. Sauberlich H. Pharmacology of vitamin C. Annu Rev Nutr 1994; 14:371–391.
10. Kielty C, Hopkinson I, Grant M. Collagen: the collagen family: structure, assembly, and organization in the extracellular matrix. In: Royce PM, Steinmann B, eds. Connective Tissue and Its Heritable Disorders. New York:Wiley-Liss, 1993:103–147.
11. Prockop D, Kivirikko K. Collagens: molecular biology, diseases, and potentials for therapy. Annu Rev Biochem 1995; 64:403–434.

12. Olsen BR. New insights into the function of collagens from genetic analysis. Curr Opin Cell Biol 1995; 7:720–727.

13. Kuhn K. The classical collagens: types I, II and III. In: Mayne R, Burgeson RE, eds. Structure and Function of Collagen Types. Orlando, FL: Academic Press, 1987; 1–42.

14. Chu M, Prockop D. Collagen: gene structure. In: Royce PM, Steinmann B. eds. Connective Tissue and Its Heritable Disorders. New York: Wiley-Liss, 1993:149–165.

15. Murad S, Grove D, Lindberg KA, et al. Regulation of collagen synthesis by ascorbic acid. Proc Natl Acad Sci USA 1981; 78:2879–2882.

16. Roberts AB, Sporn MB, Assoian RK, et al. Transforming growth factor type-β: rapid induction of fibrosis and angiogenesis in vivo and stimulation of collagen formation in vitro. Proc Natl Acad Sci USA 1986; 83:4167–4171.

17. Raghow R, Postlethwaite AE, Keski-Oja J, et al. Transforming growth factor-β increases steady state levels of type 1 procollagen and fibronectin messenger RNAs posttranscriptionally in cultured human dermal fibroblasts. J Clin Invest 1987; 79:1285–1288.

18. Phillips CL, Tajima S, Pinnell SR. Ascorbic acid and transforming growth factor-β1 (TGF-β1) increase collagen biosynthesis via different mechanisms: coordinate regulation of proα1(I) and proα1(III) collagens. Arch Biochem Biophys 1992; 295:397–403.

19. Hata R, Sunada H, Arai K, et al. Regulation of collagen metabolism and cell growth by epidermal growth factor and ascorbate in cultured human skin fibroblasts. J Biochem 1988; 173:261–267.

20. Chan D, Lamande S, Cole W, Bateman J. Regulation of procollagen synthesis and processing during ascorbate-induced extracellular matrix accumulation in vitro. Biochem J 1990; 269:175–181.

21. Lyons B, Schwarz R. Ascorbate stimulation of PAT cells causes an increase in transcription rates and a decrease in degradation rates of procollagen mRNA. Nucleic Acids Res 1984; 5:2569–2579.

22. Hata R. Transfection of normal human skin fibroblasts with human α1(I) and α2(I) collagen gene constructs and evidence for their coordinate expression. Cell Biol Int 1995; 19:735–741.

23. Rothwell NV. Understanding Genetics: A Molecular Approach. New York: Wiley-Liss, 1993:273–308.

24. Kivirikko KI, Myllylä R, Pihlajaniemi T. Hydroxylation of proline and lysine residues in collagens and other animal and plant proteins. In: Harding JJ, Crabbe MJC, eds. Post-translational modifications of proteins. Boca Raton, FL: CRC Press, 1992:1–51.

25. Kivirikko KI, Myllylä R. Post translational processing of procollagens. Ann NY Acad Sci 1985; 460:187–201.

26. Kivirikko KI, Myllylä R, Pihlajaniemi T. Protein hydroxylation: prolyl 4-hydroxylase, an enzyme with four cosubstrates and a multifunctional subunit. FASEB 1989; 3:1609–1617.

27. Pihlajaniemi T, Myllylä R, Kivirikko KI. Prolyl 4-hydroxylase and its role in collagen synthesis. J Hepatol 1991; 13 (suppl 3):52–57.

28. Pihlajaniemi T, Helaakoski T, Tasanen K, et al. Molecular cloning of the β-subunit of human prolyl 4-hydroxylase: this subunit and protein disulfide isomerase are products of the same gene. EMBO J 1987; 6:643–649.

29. Koivu J, Myllylä R, Helaakoski T, et al. A single polypeptide acts as the subunit of prolyl 4-hydroxylase and as a protein disulfide-isomerase. J Biol Chem 1987; 262:6447–6449.

30. John DCA, Grant ME, Bulleid NJ. Cell-free synthesis and assembly of prolyl 4-hydroxylase: the role of the β-subunit (PDI) in preventing misfolding and aggregation of the α1-subunit. EMBO J 1993; 12:1587–1595.

31. Tryggvason K, Majamaa K, Risteli J, Kivirikko KI. Prolyl 3-hydroxylase and 4-hydroxylase activities in certain rat and chick-embryo tissues and age-related changes in their activities in the rat. Biochem J 1979; 178:127–131.

32. Pinnell SR, Murad S. In: Stanbury JB, Wyngaarden JB, Frederickson DS, et al., eds. The Metabolic Basis of Inherited Disease. 5th ed. New York: McGraw Hill, 1983:1425–1449.

33. Kivirikko KI, Myllylä R. Collagen glycosyltransferases. Int Rev Connect Tissue Res 1979; 8:23–72.

34. Bächinger HP. The influence of peptidyl-prolyl cis-trans isomerase on the in vitro folding of type III collagen. J Biol Chem 1987; 262:17144–17148.

35. Hu G, Gura T, Sabsay B, et al. Endoplasmic reticulum protein Hsp47 binds specifically to the N-terminal globular domain of the amino-propeptide of the procollagen Iα1(I)-chain. J Cell Biochem 1995; 59:350–367.

36. Kivirikko KI, Myllylä R. Posttranslational enzymes in the biosynthesis of collagen: intracellular enzymes. Methods Enzymol 1982; 82:245–304.

37. Prockop DJ, Berg RA, Kivirikko KI, Uitto J. Intracellular steps in the biosynthesis of collagen. In: Ramachandran GN, Reddi AH, eds. Biochemistry of Collagen. New York: Plenum, 1976: 163–273.

38. Yeowell HN, Pinnell SR. The Ehlers–Danlos syndromes. Semin Dermatol 1993; 12:229–240.

39. Cole WG, Evans R, Sillence DO. The clinical features of Ehlers–Danlos syndrome type VII due to a deletion of 24 amino acids from the proα1(I) chain of type I procollagen. J Med Genet 1987; 24:698–701.

40. Weil D, D'Alessio M, Ramirez F, et al. Temperature-dependent expression of a collagen splicing defect in the fibroblasts of a patient with Ehlers–Danlos syndrome type VII. J Biol Chem 1989; 264:16804–16809.

41. Smith LT, Wertelecki W, Milstone LM, et al. Human dermatosparaxis: a form of Ehlers–Danlos syndrome that results from failure to remove the amino-terminal propeptide of type I procollagen. Am J Hum Genet 1992; 51:235–244.

42. Trelstad RL. Multistep assembly of type I collagen fibrils. Cell 1982; 28:197–198.

43. Light ND, Bailey AJ. The chemistry of the collagen cross-links: purification and characterization of cross-linked polymeric peptide material from mature collagen containing unknown amino acids. Biochem J 1980; 185:373–381.

44. Kagan HM. Characterization and regulation of lysyl oxidase. In: Mecham RP, ed. Regulation of Matrix Accumulation: Biology of the Extracellular Matrix. Vol. 1. Orlando, FL: Academic Press, 1986:321–398.

45. Eyre D: Collagen cross-linking amino acids. Methods Enzymol 1987; 114:115–139.

46. Yamauchi M, Woodley DT, Mechanic GL: Aging and cross-linking of skin collagen. Biochem Biophys Res Commun 1988; 152:898–903

47. Kivirikko KI. Urinary excretion of hydroxy proline in health and disease. Int Rev Connect Tissue Res 1970; 5:93–163.

48. Murphy G, Reynolds JJ. Extracellular matrix degradation. In: Royce PM, Steinmann B, eds. Connective Tissue and Its Heritable Disorders. New York: Wiley-Liss, 1993:287–316.

49. Birkedahl-Hansen H. Catabolism and turnover of collagens–collagenases. Methods Enzymol 1987; 144D:140–171.

50. Welgus HG, Jeffery JJ, Eisen AZ. The collagen substrate specificity of human skin fibroblast collagenase. J Biol Chem 1981; 256:9511–9515.

51. Matrisian LM. Metalloproteinases and their inhibitors in matrix remodeling. Trends Genet 1990; 6:121–125.

52. Quinones S, Saus J, Otani Y, et al. Transcriptional regulation of human stromelysin. J Biol Chem 1989; 264:8339–8344.

53. Rosenbloom J. Elastin. In: Royce PM, Steinmann B, eds. Connective Tissue and Its Heritable Disorders. New York: Wiley-Liss, 1993:167–188.

54. Kurata S, Senoo H, Hata R. Transcriptional activation of type I collagen genes by ascorbic acid 2-phosphate in human skin fibroblasts and its failure in cells from a patient with α_2 (I)-chain-defective Ehlers–Danlos syndrome. Exp Cell Res 1993; 206:63–71.

55. Geesin J, Hendricks LJ, Falkenstein PA, et al. Regulation of collagen synthesis by ascorbic acid: characterization of the role of ascorbate-stimulated lipid peroxidation. Arch Biochem Biophys 1991; 290(1):127–132.

56. Whitsom S, Whitsom M, Bowers D, Falk M. Factors influencing synthesis and mineralization of bone matrix from fetal bovine bone cells grown in vitro. J Bone Miner Res 1992; 7:727–741.

57. Denis I, Pointillart A, Lieberherr M. Cell stage–dependent effects of ascorbic acid on cultured porcine bone cells. Bone Miner 1994; 25:149–161.

58. Franceschi R, Iyer B, Cui Y. Effects of ascorbic acid on collagen matrix formation and osteoblast differentiation in murine MC3T3-E1 cells. J Bone Miner Res 1994; 9:843–854.

59. Sandell L, Daniel J. Effects on ascorbic acid on collagen mRNA levels in short term chondrocyte cultures. Connect Tissue Res 1988; 17:11–22.

60. Chojkier M, Houglum K, Solis-Herruzo J, Brenner D. Stimulation of collagen gene expression by ascorbic acid in cultured human fibroblasts. J Biol Chem 1989; 264:16957–16962.

61. Hata R, Senoo H. L-Ascorbic acid 2-phosphate stimulates collagen accumulation, cell proliferation, and formation of a three-dimensional tissuelike substance by skin fibroblasts. J Cell Physiol 1989; 138:8–16.

62. Geesin J, Gordon J, Berg R. Retinoids affect collagen synthesis through inhibition of ascorbate-induced lipid peroxidation in cultured human dermal fibroblasts. Arch Biochem Biophys 1990; 278:350–355.

63. Darr D, Combs S, Pinnell S. Ascorbic acid and collagen synthesis: rethinking a role for lipid peroxidation. Arch Biochem Biophys 1993; 307:331–335.

64. England S, Seifter S. The biochemical functions of ascorbic acid. Annu Rev Nutr 1986; 6: 365–406.

65. Rhoads RE, Udenfriend S. Decarboxylation of α-ketoglutarate coupled to collagen proline hydroxylase. Proc Natl Acad Sci USA 1968; 60:1473–1478.

66. Myllylä R, Majamaa K, Günzler V, Hanauske-Abel HM, Kivirikko KI. Ascorbate is consumed stoichiometrically in the uncoupled reactions catalyzed by prolyl 4-hydroxylase and lysyl hydroxylase. J Biol Chem 1984; 259:5403–5405.

67. Puistola U, Turpeenniemi-Hujanen TM, Myllylä R, Kivirikko KI. Studies on the lysyl hydroxylase reaction II: inhibition kinetics and the reaction mechanism. Biochim Biophys Acta 1980; 611:51–60.

68. Myllylä R, Kuutti-Savolainen ER, Kivirikko KI. The role of ascorbate in the prolyl hydroxylase reaction. Biochem Biophys Res Commun 1978; 83:441–448.

69. Hanauske-Abel HM, Günzler V. A stereochemical concept for the catalytic mechanism of prolyl hydroxylase: applicability to classification and design of inhibitors. J Theor Biol 1982; 94:421–455.

70. Günzler V, Brocks D, Henke S, et al. Syncatalytic inactivation of prolyl 4-hydroxylase by synthetic peptides containing the unphysiologic amino acid 5-oxaproline. J Biol Chem 1988; 263:19498–19504.

71. Hutton JJ, Tappel AL, Udenfriend S. Cofactor and substrate requirements of collagen proline hydroxylase. Arch Biochem Biophys 1967; 118:231–240.

72. Tschank G, Sanders J, Baringhaus KH, et al. Structural requirements for the utilization of ascorbate analogues in the prolyl 4-hydroxylase reaction. Biochem J 1994; 300:75–79.

73. Majamaa K, Günzler V, Hanauske-Abel H, et al. Partial identity of the 2-oxoglutarate and ascorbate binding sites of prolyl 4-hydroxylase. J Biol Chem 1986; 261:7819–7823.

74. Pajunen L, Jones TA, Helaakoski T, et al. Assignment of the gene coding for the α-subunit of prolyl 4-hydroxylase to human chromosome region 10q21.3-23.1. Am J Hum Genet 1989; 45: 829–834.

75. Parkkonen T, Kivirikko KI, Pihlajaniemi T. Molecular cloning of a multifunctional chicken protein acting as the prolyl 4-hydroxylase β-subunit, protein disulfide isomerase and a cellular thyroid hormone binding protein: comparison of cDNA-deduced amino acid sequences with those in other species. Biochem J 1988; 256:1005–1011.

76. Yeowell HN, Murad S, Pinnell SR. Hydralazine differentially increases mRNAs for the α and β subunits of prolyl 4-hydroxylase whereas it decreases proα(I) collagen mRNAs in human skin fibroblasts. Arch Biochem Biophys 1991; 289:399–404.

77. Helaakoski T, Vuori K, Myllylä R, et al. Molecular cloning of the α-subunit of human prolyl 4-hydroxylase: the complete cDNA derived amino acid sequence and evidence for alternative splicing of RNA transcripts. Proc Natl Acad Sci USA 1989; 86:4392–4396.

78. Bassuk JA, Kao WW-Y, Herzer P, et al. Prolyl 4-hydroxylase: molecular cloning and the primary structure of the α subunit from chicken embryo. Proc Natl Acad Sci USA 1989; 86:7382–7386.

79. Hautala T, Byers MG, Eddy RL, et al. Cloning of human lysyl hydroxylase: complete cDNA-derived amino acid sequence and assignment of the gene (PLOD) to chromosome 1p36.3-p36.2. Genomics 1992; 13:62–69.

80. Yeowell HN, Ha V, Walker LC, et al. Characterization of a partial cDNA for lysyl hydroxylase from human skin fibroblasts: lysyl hydroxylase mRNAs are regulated differently by minoxidil derivatives and hydralazine. J Invest Dermatol 1992; 99:864–869.

81. Yeowell HN, Ha VT, Clark LW, et al. Sequence analysis of a cDNA for lysyl hydroxylase isolated from human skin fibroblasts from a normal donor: differences from human placental lysyl hydroxylase cDNA. J Invest Dermatol 1994; 102:382–384.

82. Kellokumpu S, Sormunen R, Heikkinen J, Myllylä R. Lysyl hydroxylase, a collagen processing enzyme, exemplifies a novel class of luminally-oriented peripheral membrane proteins in the endoplasmic reticulum. J Biol Chem 1994; 269:30524–30529.

83. Myllylä R, Pihlajaniemi T, Pajunen L, et al. Molecular cloning of chick lysyl hydroxylase. J Biol Chem 1991; 266:2805–2810.

84. Krol BJ, Murad S, Walker LC, et al. The expression of a functional secreted human lysyl hydroxylase in a baculovirus system. J Invest Dermatol 1996; 106:11–16.

85. Murad S, Sivarajah A, Pinnell SR. Prolyl and lysyl hydroxylase activities of human skin fibroblasts: effect of donor age and ascorbate. J Invest Dermatol 1980; 75:404–407.

86. Yeowell HN, Walker LC, Marshall MK, et al. The mRNA and activity of lysyl hydroxylase are upregulated by the administration of ascorbate and hydralazine to human skin fibroblasts from a patient with Ehlers Danlos syndrome type VI. Arch Biochem Biophys 1995; 321:510–516.

87. Pinnell SR, Krane SM, Kenzora JE, Glimcher MJ. A heritable disorder of connective tissue: hydroxylysine-deficient collagen disease. N Engl J Med 1972; 886:1013–1020.

88. Ha VT, Marshall MK, Elsas LJ, et al. A patient with Ehlers–Danlos syndrome type VI is a compound heterozygote for mutations in the lysyl hydroxylase gene. J Clin Invest 1994; 93:1716–1721.

89. Dembure PP, Janko AR, Priest JH, Elsas LJ. Ascorbate regulation of collagen biosynthesis in Ehlers Danlos Syndrome, type VI. Metab Clin Exp 1987; 36:687–691.

90. Miller RL, Elsas LJ, Priest RE. Ascorbate action on normal and mutant human lysyl hydroxylases from cultured dermal fibroblasts. J Invest Dermatol 1979; 72:241–247.

91. Faris B, Ferrera R, Toselli P, et al. Effect of varying amounts of ascorbate on collagen, elastin and lysyl oxidase synthesis in aortic smooth muscle cell cultures. Biochim Biophys Acta 1984; 797:71–75.

92. Dunn DM, Franzblau C. Effects of ascorbate on insoluble elastin accumulation and cross-link formation in rabbit pulmonary artery smooth muscle cultures. Biochemistry 1982; 21:4195–4202.

93. Quaglino D, Fornieri C, Botti B, et al. Opposing effects of ascorbate on collagen and elastin deposition in the neonatal rat aorta. Eur J Cell Biol 1991; 54:18–26.

94. Fenske NA, Lober CW. Structural and functional changes of normal and aging skin. J Am Acad Dermatol 1986; 15:571–586.

95. Uitto J. Connective tissue biochemistry of the aging dermis: age-related alterations in collagen and elastin. Dermatol Clin 1986; 4:433–446.

96. Shuster S, Black MM, McVitie E. The influence of age and sex on skin thickness, skin collagen and density. Br J Dermatol 1975; 93:639–643.

97. Branchet MC, Boisnic S, Frances C, et al. Morphometric analysis of dermal collagen fibers in normal human skin as a function of age. Arch Gerontol Geriat 1991; 13:1–14.

98. Uitto J. Cellular and molecular basis of skin aging-lessons for understanding the aging of oral mucosa. In: Squier CA, Hill MW, eds. The Effect of Aging in Oral Mucosa and Skin. Boca Raton, FL: CRC Press, 1995:58–64.

99. Smith L. Histopathologic characteristics and ultrastructure of aging skin. Cutis 1989; 43:414–424.

100. Vitellaro-Zuccarello L, Cappelletti S, Dal Pozzo Rossi V, Sari-Gorla M. Stereological analysis of collagen and elastic fibers in the normal human dermis: variability with age, sex, and body region. Anat Rec 1994; 238:153–162.

101. Yamasawa S, Cerimele D, Serri F. The activity of human epidermis in relationship to age. Br J Dermatol 1972; 86:134–140.

102. Fornieri C, Quaglino D, Mori G. Correlations between age and rat dermis modifications: Ultrastructural-morphometric evaluations and lysyl oxidase activity. Aging 1989; 1:127–138.

103. Quaglino D, Fornieri C, Nanney LB, Davidson JM. Extracellular matrix modification in rat tissues of different ages. Matrix 1993; 13:481–490.

104. Phillips CL, Combs SB, Pinnell SR. Effects of ascorbic acid on proliferation and collagen synthesis in relation to the donor age of human dermal fibroblasts. J Invest Dermatol 1994; 103:228–232.

105. Barnes MD, Constable BJ, Morton LF, Royce PM. Age-related variations in hydroxylation of lysine and proline in collagen. Biochem J 1974; 139:461–468.

106. Mays PK, McAnulty RJ, Campa JS, Laurent GJ. Age-related changes in collagen synthesis and degradation in rat tissues: importance of degradation of newly synthesized collagen in regulating collagen production. Biochem J 1991; 276:307–313.

107. Epstein EH. [αI(III)$_3$ Human skin collagen: release by pepsin digestion and preponderance in fetal life. J Biol Chem 1974; 249:3225–3231.

108. Bouissou H, Pieraggi MT, Julian M, Savit T. The elastic tissue of the skin: a comparison of spontaneous and actinic (solar) aging. Int J Dermatol 1988; 27:327–335.

109. Praeger B. In vitro studies of aging. Dermatol Clin 1986; 4:359–369.

110. Plisko A, Gilchrest BA. Growth factor responsiveness of cultured human fibroblasts declines with age. J Gerontol 1983; 38:513–518.

111. Phillips PD, Kaji K, Cristofalo VJ. Progressive loss of the proliferative response of senescing WI-38 cells to platelet-derived growth factor, epidermal growth factor, insulin, transferrin and dexamethasone. J Gerontol 1984; 39:11–17.

112. Takeda K, Gosiewska A, Peterkofsky B. Similar, but not identical, modulation of expression of extracellular matrix components during in vitro and in vivo aging of human skin fibroblasts. J Cell Physiol 1992; 153:450–459.

113. Rowe D, Starman B, Fujimoto W, Williams R. Differences in growth response to hydrocortisone and ascorbic acid by human diploid fibroblasts. In Vitro 1977; 13:824–830.

114. Dumas M, Chaudagne C, Bonte F, Meybeck A. In vitro biosynthesis of type I and III collagens by human dermal fibroblasts from donors of increasing age. Mech Ageing Dev 1994; 73: 179–187.

115. Stoltz M, Furthmayr H, Timpl R. Increased lysine hydroxylation in rat bone and tendon collagen and localization of the additional residues. Biochim Biophys Acta 1973; 310:461–468.

116. Fowler LJ, Bailey AJ. Current concepts of the crosslinking in bone collagen. Clin Orthop 1972; 85:193–206.

117. Eyre D, Glimcher M. The dissolution of bovine and chicken bone collagens in concentrated formic acid. Calcif Tissue Res 1974; 15:125–132.

118. Eyre D, Oguchi H. The hydroxypyridinium crosslinks of skeletal collagens: their measurement, properties and a proposed pathway of formation. Biochem Biophys Res Commun 1980; 92:403–410.

119. Martin B. Aging and strength of bone as a structural material. Calcif Tissue Int 1993; 53(suppl 1):S34–S40.

120. Martin RB, Ishida J. The relative effects of collagen fiber orientation, porosity, density, and mineralization on bone strength. J Biomechanics 1989; 22:419–426.

121. Danielsen C, Mosekilde L, Svenstrup B. Cortical bone mass, composition, and mechanical properties in female rats in relation to age, long-term ovariectomy, and estrogen substitution. Calcif Tissue Int 1993; 52:26–33.

122. Schnitzler C. Bone quality: a determinant for certain risk factors for bone fragility. Calcif Tissue Int 1993; 53(suppl 1):S27–S31.

123. Tomasek J, Meyers S, Basing J, et al. Diabetic and age-related enhancement of collagen-linked fluorescence in cortical bones of rats. Life Sci 1994; 55:855–861.

124. Kiebzak G. Age-related bone changes. Exp Gerontol 1991; 26:171–187.

125. Schnitzler CM, Pettifor JM, Mesquita JM, et al. Histomorphometry of iliac crest bone in 346 normal black and white South African adults. Bone Miner 1990; 10:183–199.

126. Mellish R, Ferguson-Pell M, Cochran G, et al. A new manual method for assessing two-dimensional cancellous bone structure: comparison between iliac crest and lumbar vertebra. J Bone Miner Res 1991; 6:689–696.

127. Fedarko NS, Vetter UK, Weinstein S, Robey P. Age-related changes in hyaluronan, proteoglycan, collagen, and osteonectin synthesis by human bone cells. J Cell Physiol 1992; 151:215–227.

128. Quarles L, Yohay D, Lever L, et al. Distinct proliferative and differentiated stages of murine MC3T3-E1 cells in culture: an in vitro model of osteoblast development. J Bone Miner Res 1992; 7:683–693.

129. Franceschi R, Iyer B. Relationship between collagen synthesis and expression of the osteoblast phenotype in MC3T3-E1 cells. J Bone Miner Res 1992; 7:235–246.

130. Gerstein D, Phillips T, Rogers G, Gilchrest B. Wound healing and aging. Dermatol Clin 1993; 11:749–757.

131. Bruce S, Deamond S. Longitudinal study of in vivo wound repair and in vitro cellular senescence of dermal fibroblasts. Exp Gerontol 1991; 26:17–27.

132. Platt D, Ruhl W. An age-dependent determination of lysosomal enzyme activities, as well as the measurements of the incorporation of 14-C-proline and 14-C-glucosamine in a subcutaneously implanted polyether sponge. Gerontologia 1972; 18:96–112.

133. Boucek R, Noble N, Kao K, Elden H. The effects of age, sex and race upon the acetic acid fractions of collagen (human biopsy-connective tissue). J Gerontol 1958; 13A:2–9.

134. Yamaura H, Matsuzawa T. Decrease in capillary growth during aging. Exp Gerontol 1980 15:145–150.

135. Sussman M. Aging of connective tissue: physical properties of healing wounds in young and old rats. Am J Physiol 1973; 224:1167–1171.

136. Sandblom PH, Petersen P, Muren A. Determination of the tensile strength of the healing wound as a clinical test. Acta Chir Scand 1953; CV:252–257.

137. Orentreich N, Selmanowitz V. Levels of biological functions with aging. Trans NY Acad Sci 1969; 2:992–1012.

138. Pirani C, Levenson S. Effect of vitamin C deficiency on healed wounds: Scurvy and healed wounds. Proc Soc Exp Biol Med 1953; 82:95–99.

139. Levenson S, Demetriou A. Metabolic factors. In: Cohen, Diegelmann, Lindblad, eds. Wound Healing: Biochemical and Clinical Aspects, Philadelphia: Saunders, 1992:248–273.

140. Crandon J, Lund C, Dill D. Experimental human scurvy. N Engl J Med 1940; 223:353–369.

141. Levenson SM, Green RW, Taylor FHL, et al. Ascorbic acid, riboflavin, thiamin, and nicotinic acid in relation to severe injury, hemorrhage, and infection in the human. Ann Surg 1946; 124:840–856.

142. Levenson S, Upjohn H, Preston J, Steer A. Effect of thermal burns on wound healing. Ann Surg 1957; 146:357–368.

13

Oxidative Stress and Ascorbate in Relation to Risk for Cataract and Age-Related Maculopathy

ALLEN TAYLOR, C. K. DOREY, and THOMAS NOWELL
Jean Mayer USDA Human Nutrition Research Center on Aging, Tufts University, Boston, Massachusetts

INTRODUCTION

The number of associations among nutriture, eye lens cataract, and age-related macular degeneration (AMD) has burgeoned in the last decade, inspired in part by early studies regarding antioxidant properties of nutrients (1). Such studies include laboratory, clinical, and epidemiological investigations, as well as human intervention trials. Since this volume has as its focus relationships of ascorbate, health, and disease, data regarding associations between ascorbate and eye health are given most thorough treatment in this chapter. For a review of data regarding relationships between other nutrients and visual function or with respect to animal studies, readers can refer to other recent summaries and the rich body of pioneering work, which is, of necessity, given limited coverage here (2–11). Cataract is discussed first; discussion of retinopathy follows.

Cataract as a Public Health Issue

Cataract is one of the major causes of blindness throughout the world (12–14). In the United States, the prevalence of visually significant cataract increases from approximately 5% at age 65 to about 50% for persons older than 75 years (14a–16). In less developed countries, such as India (17), China (18), and Kenya (19), cataracts are more common and develop earlier in life than in more developed countries. For example, by age 60 cataract with low vision or aphakia (i.e., absence of the lens, which is usually the result of cataract extraction) is approximately five times more common in India than in the United States (16,17). The impact of cataract on impaired vision is much greater in less developed countries, where more than 90% of the cases of blindness and visual impairment are found (14,20–24) and where there is a dearth of ophthalmologists to perform lens extractions. Such surgery is routinely successful in restoring sight.

Given both the extent of disability caused by age-related cataract and its costs, $5

253

270

billion/year* in the United States, it is urgent that we elucidate causes of cataract and identify strategies to slow the development of this disorder. It is estimated that a delay in cataract formation of about 10 years would reduce the prevalence of visually disabling cataract by about 45% (12). Such a delay would enhance the quality of life for much of the world's older population and substantially reduce the economic burden due to cataract-related disability and cataract surgery. Such data provide the impetus for this research.

Age-Related Macular Degeneration as a Public Health Issue

Age-related macular degeneration (AMD) affects almost 30% of Americans over age 65 (25–27), and the proportion of affected persons increases with age (28). It is the primary cause of new blindness for Americans over age 65. Clinicians estimate that by the year 2011 over 8 millon Americans will experience some visual loss due to AMD (29). There are two forms of the disorder. The vast majority of the cases have the "dry" form characterized by a slow, insidious atrophy of the photoreceptors, retinal pigment epithelium (RPE), and choriocapillaris (the rich capillary bed that serves the avascular outer retina, i.e., the photoreceptors, outer plexiform layer, and the RPE). This atrophy severely compromises normal visual tasks such as reading, facial recognition, and depth perception. The atrophied area expands with time (over 100 μm in any one direction per year) but rarely leads to total blindness (i.e., no perception of light). At present there is no prevention or treatment for the dry type of AMD.

Almost 90% of severe visual loss in AMD occurs in the 10% of cases with "wet or exudative AMD," characterized by subretinal neovascularization, an aggressive growth of blood vessels from the choriocapillaris up through the retina that causes hemorrhage and scarring in the retina. Careful monitoring and laser ablation slow the course of the exudative disease (30–32), but this treatment may cause some immediate loss of vision, and it usually does not prevent the ultimate loss of central vision.

CATARACT

Age-Related Changes in Lens Function

The primary function of the eye lens is to collect and focus light on the retina (Fig. 1). To do so it must remain clear throughout life. The lens is located posterior to the cornea and iris and receives nutriture from the aqueous humor. Although the lens appears to be free of structure it is exquisitely designed. A single layer of epithelial cells is found directly under the anterior surface of the collagenous membrane in which it is encapsulated (Fig. 2). The epithelial cells at the germinative region divide, migrate posteriorly, and differentiate into lens fibers. The fibers elaborate, as their primary gene products, the predominant proteins of the lens, called crystallins. They also lose their organelles. New cells are formed throughout life, but older cells are usually not lost. Instead, they are compressed into the center or nucleus of the lens. There is a coincident dehydration of the proteins and of the lens itself. Consequently, protein concentrations rise to hundreds of milligrams per milliliter (mg/ml) (33). Together with other age-related modifications of the protein (noted later) and other constituents, these changes result in a less flexible lens with limited accommodative capability.

---

*Congressional Testimony of S. J. Ryan, May 5, 1993.

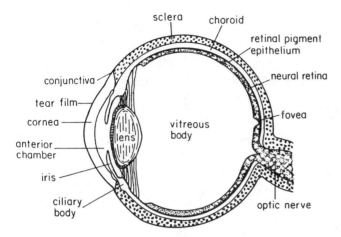

Figure 1 Cross section of the eye.

In addition, as the lens ages the proteins are photooxidatively damaged, aggregate, and accumulate in lens opacities. Dysfunction of the lens due to opacification is called cataract. The term *age-related cataract* is used to distinguish lens opacification associated with old age from opacification associated with other causes, such as congenital and metabolic disorders (34).

Clinical Features of Cataract

There are several systems for evaluating and grading cataracts. Most of these employ an assessment of extent, or density, and location of the opacity (35). Usually evaluated are opacities in the posterior subcapsular, nuclear, cortical, and multiple (mixed) locations

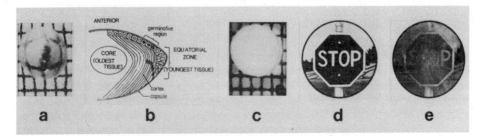

Figure 2 Clear and cataractous lens: (a) Clear lens allows an unobstructed view of the wire grid placed behind it. (b) Cartoon of the structure of the lens: The anterior surface of the lens has a unicellular layer of epithelial cells (youngest tissue). Cells at the anterior equatorial region divide and migrate to the cortex as they are overlaid by less mature cells. These cells produce a majority of the crystallins. As development and maturation proceed, the cells denucleate and elongate. Tissue originally found in the embryonic lens is found in the core or nucleus (oldest tissue). (c) The cataractous lens prohibits viewing the wire grid behind it. (d) Artist's view through a clear uncolored young lens. The image is clear and crisp. (e) Artist's view through a lens with developing cataract. The image is partially obscured, and the field is darkened as a result of browning of the lens which accompanies aging.

(Fig. 2). However, it is not established that cataract has completely different causes at each location. Coloration or brunescence is also quantified, since these diminish visual function (36,37).

Cataractogenic Insult Due to Exposure to Ultraviolet High-Energy Radiation, Oxidation, Smoking, and Failure of Primary and Secondary Defense Systems

The solid mass of the lens is about 98% protein. These proteins undergo minimal turnover as the lens ages. Accordingly, upon aging they are subject to the chronic stresses of exposure to light or other high-energy radiation and oxygen.

Various epidemiological studies show associations between elevated risk of various forms of cataract and exposure to higher intensities of incident and/or reflected ultraviolet light (14a,38–54). Greater light exposure was (weakly) associated with increased risk for cortical opacity in Chesapeake Bay watermen (45) and in men (but not women) in Wisconsin (55). Light-related risk for cataract was also increased among Italians but not among residents of Massachusetts (56). Risk for posterior subcapsular cataract was weakly related to light exposure in Chesapeake Bay watermen and (nonsignificantly) in residents of Wisconsin. Other studies (Massachusetts and Italy) did not find associations between posterior subcapsular cataract risk and light exposure. Nuclear cataract appears unrelated to risk for cataract in most studies.

Geographical data provide some support for purported relationships between light exposure and cataract risk (38). Persons living closer to the equator (40) and living at higher

Table 1 Selected Correlations Between Risk for Cataract and Extent of Light Exposure

Study and location	Exposure	Prevelance ratio[a]	95% CI
USA-35 areas NHANES survey data[b] (232)	Daily of sunlight in area ages 65–74		
	<6.6 h	1.0	
	7.1–7.7 h	1.7	1.2–2.7
	>8.2	2.7	1.6–4.6
Australia (166)	Daily hours of sunshine in area		
	8 or less	1.0	
	8.5–9	2.9	0.6–13.2
	9.5 or more	4.2	0.9–18.9
	Average mean erythemal dose of area		
	2000	1.0	
	2500	1.3	0.8–2.3
	3000	1.8	1.0–3.4
Nepal (42)	Average hours of sunlight		
	Low (7–9 h)	1.0	
	Medium (10–11 h)	1.2	0.9–1.4
	High (12+ h)	2.5	2.1–3.0

[a]The prevalence ratios and 95% confidence intervals in this table were calculated from the published data.
[b]These data were originally reported as annual light exposure. To obtain daily exposure, the annual light exposure (<2400 h, 2600–2800 h, >3000 h, for each of the three prevalence groups) was divided by 365.

elevations appear to have an elevated risk of various forms of cataract (42,50,57,58). Indeed, one of the strongest predictors of cataract surgery likelihood in a Medicare beneficiary is a person's latitude of residence (59). Although not uniformly observed (2,60,61), these epidemiological data have been corroborated or anticipated by exposure of squirrels to ultraviolet light in vivo (62) and in many experiments in vitro (6–8,40,63–68). As an aggregate, the latter references indicate that exposure of lens constituents to various wavelengths of light results in alterations which are quite similar to those found in cataract. They also indicate that structural proteins, proteases, and many other enzymes are inactivated upon exposure to ultraviolet light.

Cataractogenesis is also clearly related to exposure to higher-energy radiation. Taylor et al. showed a dose–response relationship between Cs135 radiation and risk for cataract in rats (69). In a study with 99 patients, in the 89 who received whole body irradiation (10 g) cataract developed in <4 years (70). The 10 patients who were treated for aplastic anemia and did not receive radiation treatment did not show evidence of cataractogenesis.

There is also ample evidence to support a role for oxidation in cataractogenesis. Nuclear cataract was observed in patients treated with hyperbaric oxygen therapy (71). Markedly elevated levels of mature cataract were observed in mice that survived exposure to 100% oxygen twice weekly for 3 h (72). A decline in glutathione (GSH) and increase in glutathione disulfide (oxidative changes normally related to aging or cataract) were also noted. A higher incidence of cataract was noted in lenses exposed to hyperbaric oxygen in vitro (73). Giblin also noted very early stages of cataract in guinea pigs exposed to hyperbaric oxygen (74), but there was difficulty in repeating these results (Taylor et al., unpublished). Damage to membrane lipids in fiber cells is also associated with lens opacities (75).

Smoking appears to induce oxidative stress and has been associated with both diminished levels of antioxidants, ascorbate, and carotenoids (76–81) and enhanced rate of cataract at a younger age (82–84). Of interest are recent observations that (1) for male smokers there appears to be an inverse relationship between serum levels of α-carotene, β-cryptoxanthin, lutein, and severity of nuclear sclerosis (85) (but the reverse may be true for women), and (2) there is diminished risk for cataract in smokers who use multivitamins (24).

Protection against photooxidative insult can be conceived as due to two interrelated processes. Primary defenses offer protection of proteins and other constituents by lens antioxidants and antioxidant enzymes. Secondary defenses include proteolytic and repair processes which degrade and eliminate damaged proteins and other biomolecules in a timely fashion (86). A schematic summary of insults and protective species, along with a proposal of their interactions, are indicated in Figure 3.

The major aqueous antioxidants in the lens are ascorbate (87) and GSH (3,88,89). Both are present in the lens at millimolar (mM) concentrations (90–92).

Ascorbate is probably the most effective, least toxic antioxidant identified in mammalian systems (93,94). Interest in the function of ascorbate in the lens was prompted by teleological arguments, which suggested age-related compromises in ascorbate and compromises in lens function might be related. Thus, it was observed that (1) the lens concentrates ascorbate >10-fold the level found in human plasma (87,95,96) (Fig. 4); (2) in the lens core (Fig. 2b), the oldest part of the lens and the region involved in much senile cataract, the concentration of ascorbate is only 25% that of the surrounding cortex (97); (3) lens ascorbate concentrations are lower in cataract than in the normal lens (98); and (4) ascorbate levels in the lens are significantly lower in old guinea pigs than in young

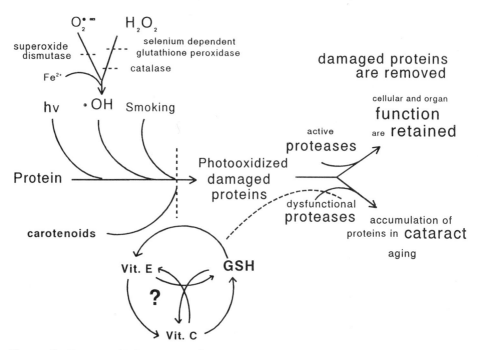

Figure 3 Proposed interaction among lens proteins, oxidants, light, smoking, anti-oxidants, antioxidant enzymes, and proteases. Lens proteins are extremely long lived. Lens (and retina) proteins are subject to alteration by light and various forms of oxygen. They are protected indirectly by antioxidant enzymes: superoxide dismutase, catalase, and glutathione reductase/peroxidase. These enzymes convert active oxygen to less damaging species. Direct protection is offered by antioxidants: glutathione (GSH), ascorbate (vitamin C), tocopherol (vitamin E), and carotenoids. Levels of reduced and oxidized forms of some, but perhaps not all, of these molecules are determined by interaction among the three and with the environment (227–230). Proteins which are damaged may accumulate and precipitate in cataract if there is insufficient proteolytic capability. When the proteolytic capability is sufficient, obsolete and damaged proteins may be reduced to their constituent amino acids. Upon aging some of the eye antioxidant supplies are diminished, antioxidant enzymes inactivated, and proteases less active. This appears to be related to the accumulation, aggregation, and eventual precipitation in cataractous opacities of damaged proteins.

animals with the same dietary intake of ascorbate (87,95,99). The same pertains in Emory mice (92). These data suggest either that there is age-related depletion of ascorbate in the lens or that the bioavailability of this compound changes with age. Enthusiasm for nutrient antioxidants has been fueled by observations that ocular levels of ascorbate are related to dietary intake in humans and animals that require exogenous ascorbate (Fig. 4) (87,95,96). Thus, the concentration of vitamin C in the lens was increased with dietary supplements beyond levels achieved in persons who already consumed more than two times the required daily allowance (RDA) (60 mg/day) for vitamin C (87,99). Even more dramatic increases are observed in guinea pigs fed high-, as compared with low-, ascorbate-containing diets (96).

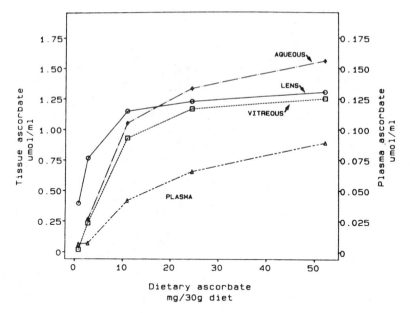

Figure 4 Total ascorbate in guinea pig eye tissues versus total ascorbate in 30 g diet. (From Ref. 96.)

Feeding an elevated level of ascorbate delayed progress of—or prevented—galactose cataract in guinea pigs (100) and rats (101), selenite-induced cataracts in rats (102), and lens opacification in GSH-depleted chick embryos (103) and delayed ultraviolet- (UV)-induced protein and protease damage in guinea pig lenses (8,9,104). Increasing lens ascorbate concentrations only twofold is associated with protection against cataractlike damage (8).

Although biochemically plausible and the subject of considerable contemporary work, there are no data to demonstrate that vitamin C induces damage in the lens in vivo (7,105, 106). In mice fed 8% of the weight of their diet as ascorbate cataract did not develop (107).

Levels of GSH are severalfold the levels found in whole blood and orders of magnitude greater than the concentration observed in the plasma. They also diminish in the older and cataractous lens (89). There have been several attempts to exploit the reducing capabilities of GSH. Injection of GSH-OMe was associated with delayed buthionine sulfoxamine–induced (108) and naphthalene cataract (89,109,110). Preliminary evidence from studies with galactose-induced cataract also indicates some advantage of maintaining elevated GSH status in rats (90). However, it is not clear that feeding GSH is associated with higher ocular levels of this antioxidant (90). Other compounds, such as pantetheine, which also include sulfhydryls, are under investigation as anticataractogenic agents. However, the results have not been encouraging (111).

Pharmacological opportunities are suggested by observations that incorporating the industrial antioxidant 0.4% butylated hydroxytoluene in diets of galactose-fed (50% of diet) rats diminished prevalence of cataract (112).

Although beyond the purview of this chapter, it is appropriate to appreciate that tocopherols and carotenoids are lipid-soluble antioxidants (113,114) with probable roles in maintaining membrane integrity (115) and GSH recycling (116). Concentrations of tocopherol in the whole lens are in the micromolar range (117). Since most of the compound is found in the membranes, the concentrations can be orders of magnitude higher. Age-related changes in levels of tocopherol and carotenoids have not been documented. Tocopherol is reported to be effective in delaying a variety of induced cataracts in animals, including galactose- (34,118,119) and aminotriazole-induced cataracts in rabbits (120).

Elevated carotenoid intake is frequently associated with health benefits. However, little experimental work has been done regarding lens changes in response to variations in levels of this nutrient. Given current discussion regarding health benefits of β-carotene and other carotenoids, it is intriguing that β-carotene levels in the lens are limited (117). Instead, major lens carotenoids are lutein/zeaxanthin. Also present are retinol and retinol ester, and tocopherols.

The lens also contains antioxidant enzymes—glutathione peroxidase/reductase, catalase, and superoxidase dismutase—and enzymes of the glutathione redox cycle (63,64, 109,121,122). These interact via the forms of oxygen, as well as with the nonenzymic antioxidants; i.e., GSH is a substrate for glutathione peroxidase. The activities of many antioxidant enzymes are compromised upon development, aging, and cataract formation (75).

Most of these secondary defense capabilities, such as proteolytic systems, exist in young lens tissue (2,86,100,123–129), and damaged proteins are usually maintained at harmless levels by primary and secondary defense systems.

Two studies indicate interactions between primary and secondary defense systems. A direct sparing effect of ascorbate on photooxidatively induced compromise of proteolytic function has been demonstrated (7). In addition, GSH spares activity of enzymes involved in conjugation of ubiquitin to substrates. Ubiquitin conjugation is required for selective targeting of substrates for degradation (Jahngen-Hodge, manuscript submitted). However, upon aging most of these enzymatic capabilities are found in a state of reduced activity (86) (Table 2). The observed accumulation of (photo)oxidized (and/or otherwise modified) proteins in older lenses is consistent with the failure of these protective systems to keep pace with the insults that damage lens proteins. This occurs in part because like bulk proteins, enzymes that compose some of the protective systems are damaged by photooxidation (2,7).

From these data it is clear that the young lens has significant primary and secondary protection. However, age-related compromises in the activity of antioxidant enzymes, concentrations of the antioxidants, and activities of secondary defenses may lead to diminished protection against oxidative insults. This diminished protection leaves the long-lived proteins and other constituents vulnerable. Lens opacities develop as the damaged proteins aggregate and precipitate (2). Current data predict that elevated antioxidant intake can be exploited to extent function of some of these proteolytic capabilities.

Restriction of caloric intake extends youth and delays age-related cataract (as well as many other late-life diseases) in these animals. Since cataract is associated with oxidative stress, it might be anticipated that the delay in cataract would be accompanied by elevated ascorbate levels in the protected animals. Nevertheless, in young and old animals, plasma-ascorbate concentrations were lower than in the nonrestricted mice (87,91,92).

Associations Among Ascorbate, Other Antioxidants, and Cataract

As noted, dietary ascorbate intake is related to eye tissue ascorbate levels. Given potential anticataractogenic and putative procataractogenic roles for ascorbate, it is useful to review

Table 2   Effect of Aging and Development on
Proteolytic Activities in Lens Tissues and Cultured Lens
Cells[a]

Activity	Source	Effect
Neutral proteinase/proteasome/high molecular weight protease (233–235)	Tissue	↓
Endopeptidase (123)	BLEC[b]	↓
LAP (123, 236)	Tissue	↓
	BLEC	
Cathepsins (123)	BLEC	↓
Calpain (237, 238)	Tissue	↑
	BLEC	N.D.[c]

[a]In cultured cells—aging was simulated by progressive passage of cells in culture.
[b]BLEC beef lens epithelial cells.
[c]Not determined.

available epidemiological data regarding ascorbate intake and risk for cataract. More than 10 epidemiological studies have examined the associations between cataract and antioxidant nutrients (24,51,53,54,56,130–135). Seven of the studies were retrospective case-control studies comparing the nutrient levels of cataract patients with those of similarly aged individuals with clear lenses (51,53,54,56,130,131,133). Our ability to interpret data from retrospective studies such as these is limited by the concurrent assessment of lens status and nutrient levels. Prior diagnosis of cataract might influence behavior of cases including diet and it might also bias reporting of usual diet. Three other studies assessed nutrient levels and/or supplement use, and then followed individuals with intact lenses for 8 years (132,135), and 5 years (24), respectively. Prospective studies such as these are less prone to bias because assessment of exposure is performed before the outcome is present. These latter studies did not directly assess lens status, but used cataract extraction or reported diagnosis of cataract as a measure of cataract risk. Extraction may not be a good measure of cataract incidence (development of new cataract), because it incorporates components of both incidence and progression in severity of existing cataract. However, extraction is the result of visually disabling cataract and is the endpoint that we wish to prevent. Although Hankinson et al. (132) measured nutrient intake over a 4-year period, Knekt et al. (135) used only one measure of serum antioxidant status, and Seddon et al. (24) used only one measure of supplement use. One measure may not provide an accurate assessment of usual, long-term nutrient levels. Multiple measures may be the best nutritional correlate of cataract since cataract develops over many years (96,99,136). Another study ($n = 367$), which monitored cataract in vivo and cataract extraction but did not find associations between nutriture and cataract, is not further described because the cataract classifications do not match those used on other work (49). In addition to the different study designs noted, the various studies used different lens classification schemes, different definitions of high and low levels of nutrients, and different age groups of subjects.

Vitamin C was considered in eight published studies (52–54,56,130–133) and one preliminary report (134) and observed to be inversely associated with at least one type of cataract in seven of these studies (Fig. 5). Jacques and Chylack (130) observed that persons with high plasma vitamin C levels ($>90\ \mu M$) had less than one-third the prevalence of early

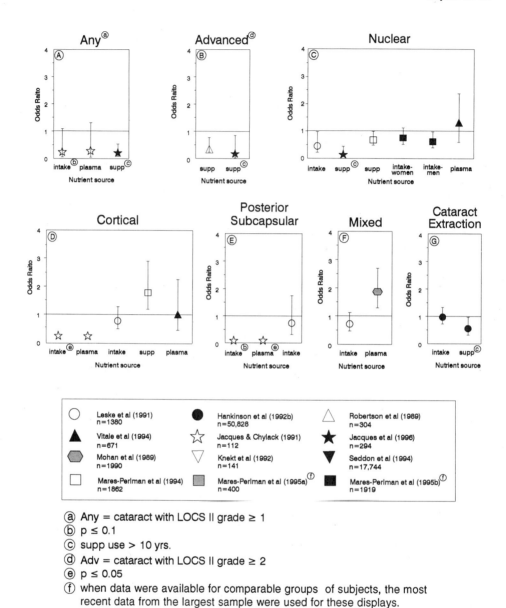

Figure 5 Cataract risk ratio, high vs. low intake (with or without supplements), and plasma levels for vitamin C.

cataract of persons with low plasma vitamin C (<40 μM) although this difference was not statistically significant (risk ratio [RR]: 0.29; 95% confidence interval [CI]: 0.06–1.32) after adjustment for age, sex, race, and history of diabetes (Fig. 5A). They observed similar relationships between intake of vitamin C and cataract prevalence. Among persons with higher vitamin C intakes (>490 mg/day), the prevalence of cataract was 25% of the prevalence among persons with lower intakes (<125 mg/day) (RR: 0.25; CI: 0.06–1.09).

This relationship is corroborated by data from other studies. Robertson and coworkers

(53) compared cases (with cataracts that impaired vision) to age- and sex-matched controls who either were free of cataract or had minimal opacities that did not impair vision. Results indicated that the prevalence of cataract in persons who consumed vitamin C supplements of >300 mg/day was approximately one-third that in persons who did not consume vitamin C supplements (RR: 0.30; CI: 0.24–0.77, Fig. 5B). Leske and coworkers (54) observed that persons with vitamin C intake in the highest 20% of their population group had a 52% lower prevalence for nuclear cataract (RR: 0.48; CI: 0.24–0.99) compared with persons who had intakes among the lowest 20% after controlling for age and sex (Fig. 5C). Weaker inverse associations were noted for other types of cataract (Figs. 5D–F).

After controlling for nine potential confounders including age, diabetes, smoking, and energy intake, Hankinson and coworkers (132) did not observe an association between total vitamin C intake and rate of cataract surgery (RR: 0.98; CI: 0.72–1.32) in a large prospective study when they compared women with high intakes (median = 705 mg/day) to women with low intakes (median = 70 mg/day) (Fig. 5G). However, they did note that women who consumed vitamin C supplements for >10 years had a 45% reduction in rate of cataract surgery (RR: 0.55; CI: 0.32–0.96). Age-adjusted analyses (99) based on 165 women with high vitamin C intake (mean = 294 mg/day) and 136 women with low vitamin C intake (mean = 77 mg/day) demonstrated that the women who took vitamin C supplements ⩾10 years had >70% lower prevalence of early opacities (RR: 0.27; CI: 0.11–0.67) (Fig. 5D) and >80% lower risk of advanced opacities (RR: 0.19; CI: 0.05–0.80) at any site compared with women who did not use vitamin C supplements.

In comparison to the data noted, Mares-Perlman and coworkers (51) report that past use of supplements containing vitamin C was associated with a reduced prevalence of nuclear cataract (RR: 0.7; CI: 0.5–1.0) (Fig. 5C), but an increased prevalence of cortical cataract (adjusted RR: 1.8; CI: 1.2–2.9) after controlling for age, sex, smoking, and history of heavy alcohol consumption (Fig. 5D). Mohan et al. (131) also noted an 87% (RR: 1.87; CI: 1.29–2.69) increased prevalence of mixed cataract with posterior subcapsular and nuclear involvement for each standard deviation increase in plasma vitamin C levels. Vitale and coworkers (133) observed that persons with plasma levels greater than 80 μM and below 60 μM had similar prevalences of both nuclear (RR: 1.31; CI: 0.61–2.39) and cortical (RR: 1.01; CI: 0.45–2.26) cataract after controlling for age, sex, and diabetes. Similarly, no differences in cataract prevalence were observed between persons with high (>261 mg/day) and low (<115 mg/day) vitamin C intakes. One other study (56) observed no association between prevalence of cataract and vitamin C intake.

Vitamin E and carotenoids provide another rich source and resource of natural lipid-soluble antioxidants which can inhibit lipid peroxidation (115) and, possibly, stabilize cell membranes (137). Ascorbate may affect vitamin E (see legend to Fig. 3), as well as enhance glutathione recycling, perhaps helping to maintain reduced glutathione levels in the lens and aqueous humor (116). Three studies assessing plasma vitamin E levels also reported significant inverse associations with cataract (Fig. 6).

β-Carotene is the best known carotenoid because of its importance as a vitamin A precursor. It exhibits particularly strong antioxidant activity at low partial pressures of oxygen (15 torr) (138). Partial pressure of oxygen in the core of the lens is approximately 20 torr (139). However, it is only one of ≈400 naturally occurring carotenoids (140), and other carotenoids may have similar or greater antioxidant potential (114,115,141,142). In addition to β-carotene, α-carotene, lutein, and lycopene are important carotenoid components of the human diet (143). Carotenoids have been identified in the lens in ≈10 ng/g wet weight concentrations (117,144), but there are no laboratory data relating carotenoids to cataract

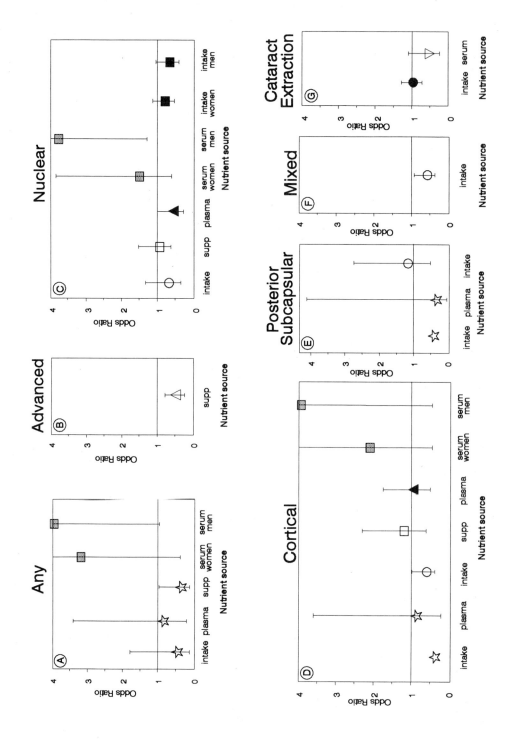

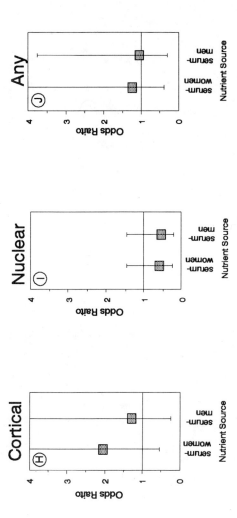

Figure 6 Same as Figure 5, but in levels for vitamin E:A–G, including α-tocopherol, and H–J γ-tocopherol.

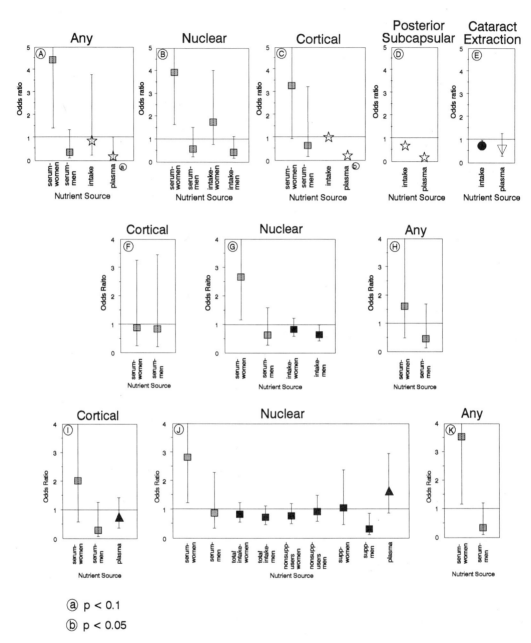

Figure 7 Same as Figure 5, but in levels for carotenoids, including α-carotene, β-carotene, lycopene, β-cryptoxanthin, and lutein: A–E, total carotenoids; F–H, γ-carotene; I–K, β-carotene; L–N, lycopene; O–Q, β-cryptoxanthin; R–T, lutein.

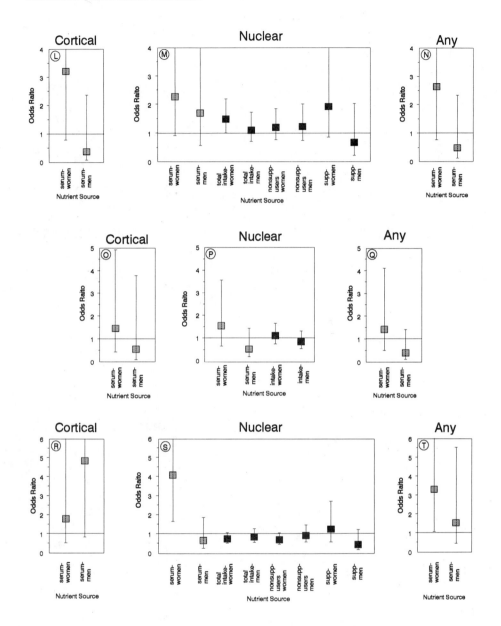

formation. Carotenoids have been associated with some levels of protection against cataract (Fig. 7). The impression created by the literature is that carotenoids other than β-carotene may confer the health advantages observed (99).

Antioxidant Nutrient Combinations

Combinations of multiple antioxidant nutrients were also considered because of possible synergistic effects of the antioxidant nutrients on cataract risk (Fig. 8). The first, and perhaps most important, study in terms of revealing the utility of diet indicates a significant

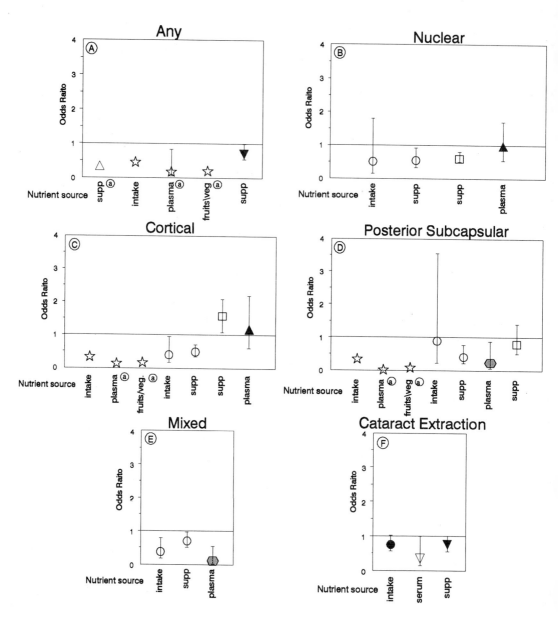

@ p ≤ 0.05

Figure 8 Same as Figure 5, but for antioxidant nutrient index, including multivitamin supplements.

fivefold decrease in risk ratio for cataract between persons consuming ⩾1.5 servings of fruits and/or vegetables (130). Jacques and Chylack (130) also found that the adjusted prevalence of all types of cataract was 40% (RR: 0.62; CI: 0.12–1.77) and 80% (RR: 0.16; CI: 0.04–0.82) lower for persons with moderate- and high-antioxidant index scores (based on combined plasma vitamin C, vitamin E, and carotenoid levels), as compared with persons with low scores. Using a similar index based on combined antioxidant nutrient intakes (vitamin C, vitamin E, and carotene, as well as riboflavin), Leske and coworkers (54) found that persons with high scores had 60% lower adjusted prevalence of cortical (RR: 0.42; CI: 0.18–0.97) and mixed (RR: 0.39; CI: 0.19–0.80) cataract compared to those who had low scores. However, Robertson and coworkers (53) found no enhanced benefit to persons taking both vitamin E and vitamin C supplements compared with persons who only took either vitamin C or vitamin E. Mohan and coworkers (131) constructed a somewhat more complex antioxidant scale which included red blood cell levels of glutathione peroxidase, glucose-6-phosphate dehydrogenase, and plasma levels of vitamin C and vitamin E. Even though they did not see any protective associations with any of these individual factors and even reported a positive association between plasma vitamin C and prevalence of cataract, they found that persons with high-antioxidant index scores had a substantially lower prevalence of cataracts involving the posterior subcapsular region (RR: 0.23, CI: 0.06–0.88) or mixed cataract with posterior subcapsular and nuclear components (RR: 0.12; CI: 0.03–0.56) after multivariate adjustment. Hankinson and coworkers (132) calculated an antioxidant score based on intakes of carotene, vitamin C, vitamin E, and riboflavin and observed a 24% reduction in the adjusted rate of cataract surgery among women with high-antioxidant scores relative to women with low scores (RR: 0.76; CI: 0.57–1.03). Knekt and coworkers (135) observed that the rate of cataract surgery for persons with high levels of both serum vitamin E and β-carotene concentrations appeared lower than the rate for persons with either high vitamin E or high β-carotene levels. Persons with high serum levels of either nutrient had a rate of cataract surgery that was 40% less than persons with low levels of both nutrients (RR: 0.38; CI: 0.15–1.0). Vitale and coworkers (133) also examined the relationship between antioxidant scores (based on plasma concentrations of vitamin C, vitamin E, and β-carotene) and prevalence of cataract, but did not see evidence of any association. The age-, sex-, and diabetes-adjusted risk ratios were close to 1 for both nuclear (RR: 0.96; CI: 0.54–1.70) and cortical (RR: 1.17; CI: 0.62–2.20) cataract. Relationships between multiple antioxidant nutrients and cataract risk are further supported by multivitamin use data. Leske and coworkers (54) found that use of multivitamin supplements was associated with decreased prevalence for each type of cataract: 60%, 48%, 45%, and 30%, respectively, for posterior subcapsular (RR: 0.40; CI: 0.21–0.77) (Fig. 8D), cortical (RR: 0.52; CI: 0.36–0.72), nuclear (RR: 0.55; CI: 0.33–0.92), and mixed (RR: 0.70; CI: 0.51–0.97) cataracts. Seddon and coworkers (24) also observed a reduced risk for incident cataract for users of multivitamins (RR: 0.73; CI: 0.54–0.99).

To date only one intervention trial designed to assess the effect of vitamin supplements on cataract risk has been completed. Sperduto and coworkers (145) took advantage of two ongoing randomized, double-blinded vitamin and cancer trials to assess the impact of vitamin supplements on cataract prevalence. The trials were conducted among almost 4000 participants aged 45 to 74 years from rural communes in Linxian, China. Participants in one trial received either a multinutrient supplement or a placebo. In the second trial, a more complex factorial design was used to evaluate the effects of four different vitamin/mineral combinations: retinol (5000 IU) and zinc (22 mg); riboflavin (3 mg) and niacin (40 mg); vitamin C (120 mg) and molybdenum (30 μg); and vitamin E (30 mg), β-carotene (15 mg), and selenium (50 μg). At the end of the 5- to 6-year follow-up period, the investigators conducted eye examinations to determine the prevalence of cataract.

In the first trial there was a significant 43% reduction in the prevalence of nuclear cataract for persons aged 65 to 74 years for those receiving the multinutrient supplement (RR: 0.57; CI: 0.36–0.90) (Fig. 9C). The second trial demonstrated a significantly reduced prevalence of nuclear cataract in persons receiving the riboflavin/niacin supplement relative to those persons not receiving this supplement (RR: 0.59; CI: 0.45–0.79). The effect

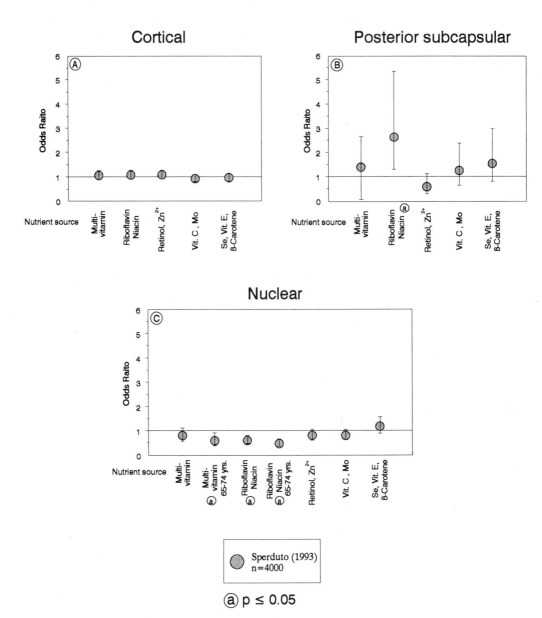

Figure 9 Cataract risk ratio: intervention trials.

was strongest in those aged 65 to 74 years (RR: 0.45; CI: 0.31–0.64). However, the riboflavin/niacin supplement appeared to increase the risk of posterior subcapsular cataract (RR: 2.64; CI: 1.31–5.35). The results further suggested a protective effect of the retinol/zinc supplement (RR: 0.77; CI: 0.58–1.02) and the vitamin C/molybdenum supplement (RR: 0.78; CI: 0.59–1.04) on prevalence of nuclear cataract.

AGE-RELATED MACULAR DEGENERATION

The degenerative process of AMD begins in the macula, a ≈1.5-mm-diameter area in the posterior fundus. In the center of the macula—and initially spared from degeneration—is the fovea, the ≈0.35-mm-diameter locus of both best-visual acuity and color vision. For most clinicians, the first clinical evidence of AMD includes pigmentary changes in the RPE and soft drusen, which are lipoidal deposits in the extracellular matrix (Bruch's membrane) lying under the RPE cells (146–150).

Specializations of the fovea include the densely packed cone photoreceptors and the absence of rod photoreceptors, blood vessels, and layers of the inner retina (ganglion cells, inner plexiform, and inner nuclear layers). In life the fovea and surrounding macula are yellowish as a result of the accumulation of the polar carotenoids, lutein, and zeaxanthin (151,152). Elevated levels of the latter give the fovea a deeper color (152). The concentration of the two carotenoids reaches 35–120 ng/retina (151,152).

Because carotenoids absorb blue light, their high concentration in the fovea may serve to (1) increase visual acuity by reducing chromatic aberration due to the more highly scattered blue light (153) and (2) protect against blue light damage to the retina (154) and/or RPE (155–157). Carotenoids can also quench activated photosensitizers (142,158–160). However, they are found in highest concentrations in the proximal end of the cones, well removed from the cone photopigments (161). This location may attenuate some quenching activity.

Putative Associations Among Light Exposure, Oxidation, Smoking, and Age-Related Macular Degeneration

Although the pathogenesis of age-related macular degeneration has not been elucidated, it is widely believed that the primary lesion lies within the RPE cells (162,163) and that excessive exposure to light and active forms of oxygen are involved (164). This is because the photoreceptors and RPE cells reside in a highly oxygenated environment subject to bright illumination (165).

Support for a deleterious role for light comes from epidemiological studies. Taylor et al. found that the risk for more advanced cases in the older subjects was significantly correlated with a history of greater exposure to blue light (166). The same study noted no relationship with UV exposure (46). The prevalence of AMD was found to be significantly higher among those with light-colored irides than among those with dark irides (167–171). This suggested that the retina of a person whose iris absorbed less light (e.g., blue or gray eyes) might be chronically exposed to more damaging light. Missing from these circumstantial arguments relating light exposure and AMD are significant data proving that the amount of light entering eyes with dark irides is different from that of those with light irides. Moreover, recent retrospective analyses of data from two large eye studies have found no difference in the risk for AMD among whites and blacks (172) and no correlation between AMD and iris color among diabetics (173). A role for light as a cause of AMD is also indicated by human studies, which show that the retina is photooxidatively damaged by short periods of exposure to intense light (174–177).

A substantial body of laboratory evidence also documents the damaging consequences to the retina of excessive light. The amount of damage is influenced by many features, including antioxidant capacity of the exposed retina (178), duration and intensity of light (155,179), time in diurnal cycle (180), ocular pigmentation (181–183), and antioxidants in the retina or diet—particularly ascorbate (179,184,185), vitamin E, (164,186), and β-carotene (187). Previous light history, which also influences the antioxidant capacity of the retina, also affects damage (188,189).

There are also laboratory and epidemiological data that suggest relationships between oxidative insult and elevated risk for AMD. In the metabolically active photoreceptor cells, free radicals and reactive species of oxygen are also produced as metabolic by-products of mitochondrial respiration, production of prostaglandins, glucose oxidation, nucleic acid breakdown, phagocytosis, etc. Superoxide is released when RPE phagocytose artificial particles (190), although perhaps not outer segment tips. Chronic oxidative damage to the photoreceptors can be inferred from the massive accumulation of lipofuscin found in 60-, 70-, and 80-year-old RPE (191–193).

Lipofuscin is considered to be a by-product of oxidative damage to the photoreceptors. It progressively accumulates in—and appears to erode—the RPE cells (164,192). That lipofuscin accumulation is related to oxidation is implied by observations that the amount of lipofuscin in the RPE increases in antioxidant-deficient rats (194,195) and decreases with loss of photoreceptors (196,197).

The hypothesis that lipofuscin contributes to the pathogenesis of AMD (Fig. 10) is supported by the strong parallels between the patterns of lipofuscin accumulation and the natural history of the disease: (1) the earliest signs of AMD (especially soft drusen) and of atrophy occur in retinal regions that have the highest level of lipofuscin (191,192,198); (2) the amount of lipofuscin in the RPE is highly correlated both with the amount of drusenoid material in Bruch's (199) and with the loss of photoreceptors in the human fovea (200); (3) atrophy advances in directions (201) that parallel the patterns of greatest lipofuscin accumulation. The damaging consequences of lysosomal accumulation of lipofuscinlike material can be confirmed in several types of inherited retinal degeneration (202–204). Finally, monkeys fed vitamin E-deficient diets for 2 years developed macular degeneration characterized by massive disruption of the macular photoreceptors and RPE distended with lipofuscin developed (205). Similar accumulations of lipofuscin were found in the RPE of vitamin E–deficient dogs (206).

Compromises to the RPE have many ramifications. Without the RPE, both the photoreceptors and the choriocapillaris atrophy. The RPE participates in the turnover and renewal of the photoreceptor itself. Each day the RPE phagocytoses and digests the worn-out distal tips of the photoreceptors, which, being enriched in polyunsaturated fatty acids (especially 22:6 docosahexenoic acid), are especially vulnerable to oxidative damage (207,208). Residues from damaged lipids and proteins appear to accumulate as lipofuscin (209). It is also possible that lipofuscin is produced in response to decreased lysosomal protease activity (210). Recent discovery of an intrinsic rod ubiquitin dependent proteolytic pathway (129,211,212) and demonstration of a connection between glutathione status and function of this pathway (Jahngen-Hodge, manuscript submitted) suggest further correlations between oxidation and accumulation (rather than the timely degradation) of damaged or obsolete proteins, and an association of these phenomena with AMD.

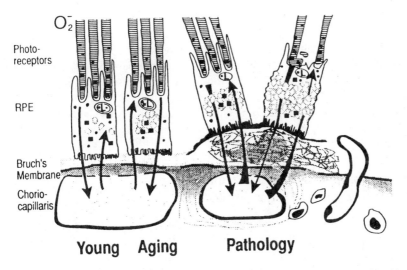

O_2^-

Photo-
receptors

RPE

Bruch's
Membrane

Chorio-
capillaris

Young   Aging   Pathology

Figure 10   Schematic representation of the changes hypothesized to contribute to aging-related macular degeneration (AMD). Only the tips of the photoreceptors (PR) and single cells of the retinal pigment epithelium (RPE) monolayer are illustrated. Exposed to light, high levels of oxygen and free radicals (e.g., O_2^-), the PR are vulnerable to oxidative damage (■). These fragile structures are maintained by high levels of antioxidants and by daily renewal. Each day, the worn out and oxidatively damaged tips of the PR are phagocytosed by the RPE and digested in lysosomes (L). Oxidative damage in the PR produces indigestible residues which accumulate in the lysosomes as lipofuscin (shaded circles in the RPE). Lipofuscin is the dominant feature of older RPE cells and is dramatically increased in experimental antioxidant deficiency. Some antioxidants in the RPE and PR decrease with aging. The RPE side of Bruch's membrane also exhibits age-related changes, including patches of thick collagen fiber and accumulation of lipids (231). Bruch's membrane is an acellular matrix through which nutrients and oxygen diffuse to supply both the RPE and the PR (upward arrows); wastes and water move in the opposite direction (downward arrows), the latter being actively pumped. Pathological changes in eyes with AMD, first seen in Bruch's membrane, include continuous basal linear deposits of thick collagen fibers and more extensive lipoidal debris (pathological). In foci called drusen, these accumulations elevate the RPE. The amount of debris in Bruch's membrane is correlated with lipofuscin content of the overlying RPE, and with elevated risk for neovascularization. Moreover, the accumulated lipofuscin and the hydrophobic lipoidal material in Bruch's membrane may impede the flow of nutrients, wastes, and/or water across Bruch's membrane—putting the RPE and PR at risk for atrophy and/or detachment from Bruch's membrane by accumulated fluid. Impeded flow of RPE factors may explain both the age-related shrinkage of the choriocapillaris and its atrophy where the RPE is lost. In nonatrophic areas the rod PR become longer and bent, and debris is found between PR and the RPE (possibly involving impaired phagocytosis). In more advanced stages of AMD, macrophages are frequently found eroding the altered Bruch's membrane and may be accompanied by neovascular fronds that extend through Bruch's membrane into the retina and form scars, the most common cause of blindness in AMD.

As in the lens, antioxidant enzymes appear to play critical roles in maintaining function. A potential role for catalase in lowering risk for AMD is indicated by a recent report that catalase activity in human RPE cells declines with age, that the rate of decline is more rapid in the macula than in the periphery, and that catalase (but not superoxide dismutase) activity was significantly lower in RPE cells from eyes with drusen and pigmentary changes consistent with AMD (213).

Smoking, an oxidative insult, is also identified as a risk factor for AMD in case-control studies (167,214) and is also negatively correlated with plasma carotenoid and ascorbate concentrations (76,77).

Associations Between Antioxidant Status and Age-Related Macular Degeneration

If the pathogenesis of AMD involves oxidative damage, then it is plausible that antioxidants that decrease this damage might provide protection. Recent reports indicate correlations between administered ascorbate and retinal levels of ascorbate (215), dietary levels and retinal levels of other antioxidants (216,217) and interrelationships between ascorbate and tocopherol intake and retinal glutathione levels (218). In addition there have been some preliminary reports regarding influences of carotenoids, vitamin A, vitamin E, and/or zinc on the risk for or progression of AMD. In order to appreciate the results reviewed later, it is useful to understand that among the problems with existing epidemiological research on AMD is that different studies utilized different diagnostic criteria to distinguish normal subjects from those with "early" AMD. As the cause of AMD is elucidated and better grading schemes are devised, this should recede as a problem.

An inverse correlation between the neovascular form of AMD and carotenoids was reported recently (219). A 5-year multicenter case-control study compared plasma levels of vitamin C, vitamin E, carotenoids, and selenium in 356 cases and 520 controls (without obvious AMD). Logistic regression accounting for influence of age, sex, clinic, and patient source demonstrated a 43% lower risk for AMD (OR: 0.57; CI: 0.35, 0.92) for higher carotenoid levels but not vitamin E, vitamin C, or selenium alone (Table 3). These data also suggest that carotenoids lower the individual risk for advanced AMD and that they impede progression of AMD into the fovea. The positive influence of carotenoids would be consistent with the proposed carotenoid basis of foveal sparing in AMD (220), and with the observed relationship between exposure to blue light and risk for advanced stages of AMD (166). Interestingly, like the protective relationships between carotenoids in spinach and cataract risk (130,132), lutein and zeaxanthin, as opposed to β-carotene, are also associated with diminished risk for retinopathy (219). Spinach contains lutein and zeaxanthin, whereas carrots are primary sources of β-carotene.

A negative correlation between AMD and consumption of vitamin A rich fruits and vegetables was found in data from the first National Health and Nutrition Examination Survey (221). Carotenoids are present in foods rich in vitamin A.

The vitamin E content of human RPE and neural retina increases significantly with aging, perhaps partitioning into the nonpolar lipofuscin (186,223). Such partitioning could mean that the vitamin E requirement of the aging retina would increase. However, no differences in plasma levels of vitamin E or C were found in a case-control study of 85 Italians who had soft drusen (early evidence of AMD) or hard drusen (a nonspecific change with aging) (223).

Table 3   Odds Ratios for Exudative Age-Related Macular
Degeneration by Highest vs. Lowest Quintile of Energy-Adjusted
Nutrient Intake

Nutrient	Quintiles			
	1	5		P (Trend)
Alpha carotene				
Median intake, IU	152.5	1830		
Multivariate OR (95% CI)[a]	1.0	0.79	(0.5–1.3)	0.14
Beta carotene				
Median intake, IU	1143	8053		
Multivariate OR (95% CI)[a]	1.0	0.59	(0.4–0.96)	0.03
Beta cryptoxanthin				
Median intake, IU	17.44	224		
Multivariate OR (95% CI)[a]	1.0	0.89	(0.5–1.4)	0.84
Lycopene				
Median intake, IU	217.7	3450		
Multivariate OR (95% CI)[a]	1.0	1.16	(0.7–1.8)	0.96
Lutein/zeaxanthin				
Median intake, IU	560.8	5757		
Multivariate OR (95% CI)[a]	1.0	0.43	(0.2–0.7)	0.001
Carotenoids				
Median intake, IU	3154	19250		
Multivariate OR (95% CI)[a]	1.0	0.57	(0.35–0.92)	0.02

[a]Included forms for age (continuous), sex, clinic (Massachusetts, New York, Illinois, Wisconsin, Maryland), education ($>$, $<$, or $=$ 12th grade), systolic blood pressure (mm Hg), self-reported physical activity level (average, below average, above average), alcohol intake (grams per day), body mass index, and smoking status (never smoker, former smoker, current smoker). Adapted from Ref. 219.

CONCLUSION

Light and oxygen appear to be both a boon and a bane. While necessary for physiological function, when present in excess or in uncontrolled circumstances, they appear to be related, probably causally, to cataractogenesis and AMD. Upon aging, compromised function of the lens and retina are exacerbated by depleted or diminished primary antioxidant reserves and antioxidant enzyme capabilities and diminished secondary defenses such as proteases. Smoking appears to provide an oxidative challenge and is also associated with an elevated risk of cataract and AMD.

Is there a clear correlation between nutriture and risk for cataract and/or AMD? The impression created by the literature is that there is some benefit to enhanced antioxidant, particularly ascorbate, intake with respect to diminished risk for cataract. However, more information is essential prior to describing optimal nutriture vis-à-vis cataract. It is difficult to compare the various studies. That the correlations were not always with the same form of cataract may indicate, in addition to the conclusions reached, that the cataracts were graded differently and/or that there are common etiological features of each of the forms of cataract described. It may also be that insufficient data have been gathered. Most of the studies noted utilized case-control designs, and most assessed nutrient status only once. Since nutrient intake or nutrient status measures are highly variable and the effects of diet are likely to be cumulative, studies should be performed on populations for which long-term dietary records are available. Thus, hindsight suggests a need for more uniform methods of lens and retina evaluation, diet recording, blood testing, etc., and a need for longitudinal and natural history studies.

Optimization of nutriture can be achieved through better diets and supplement use once appropriate levels of specifically beneficial nutrients are defined. In addition to quantifying optimal intake, it is essential to know for how long or when intake of the nutrient would be useful with respect to delaying cataract. It is possible to adjust normal dietary practice to obtain close-to-saturating levels of plasma ascorbate (less than 250 mg/day) (87,99,132, 224). Because the bioavailability of ascorbate may decrease with age, slightly higher intakes may be required in the elderly. Two studies indicated that persons who consumed supplements of ascorbate for over 10 years have decreased risk for cataract or cataract extraction. Monitoring correlations between nutrient status and intermediate markers of cataract (when they are defined) may allow anticipation of relationships between nutrient status and cataract. Thus, the overall impression created by these data suggests that further research in this field will yield significant health benefits.

Poor education and lower socioeconomic status also markedly increase risk for these debilities (54,131,225,226). These are related to poor nutrition. Since cost–benefit analysis regarding remediation clearly indicates that prevention is preferable for cataract and essential for AMD, it is not premature to contemplate the value of intervention for populations at risk. The work available, albeit preliminary, indicates that nutrition may provide the least costly and most practicable means to attempt the objectives of delaying cataract and AMD.

ACKNOWLEDGMENTS

We acknowledge the assistance of Dr. Xin Gong in the preparation of figures and Ms. E. Epstein in the preparation of the manuscript.

REFERENCES

1. Muller HK, Buschke W. Vitamin C in linse, kammerwasser und blut normalem und pathologischem linsentstoffwech. Arch F Augenh 1934; 108:368–390.
2. Taylor A, Jacques PF, Dorey CK. Oxidation and aging: impact on vision. J Toxicol Ind Health 1993; 9349–9371.
3. Bunce GE, Kinoshita J, Horwitz J. Nutritional factors in cataract. Annu Rev Nutr 1990; 10:233–254.
4. Jacques PF, Chylack LT Jr, Taylor A. Relationships between natural antioxidants and cataract formation. In: Frei B, ed. Natural Antioxidants in Human Health and Disease. Orlando, FL: Academic Press, 1994:513–533.
5. Taylor A. Vitamin C. In: Hartz SC, Russell RM, Rosenberg IH, eds. Nutrition in the Elderly: The Boston Nutritional Status Survey. London: Smith Gordon, 1992:147–150.
6. Taylor A. Cataract: relationships between nutrition and oxidation. J Am Coll Nutr 1993; 12: 138–146.
7. Blondin J, Taylor A. Measures of leucine aminopeptidase can be used to anticipate UV-induced age-related damage to lens proteins: ascorbate can delay this damage. Mech Ageing Dev 1987; 41:39–46.

8. Blondin J, Baragi VJ, Schwartz E, et al. Delay of UV-induced eye lens protein damage in guinea pigs by dietary ascorbate. Free Radical Biol Med 1986; 2:275–281.

9. Taylor A, Jacques PF. Relationships between aging, antioxidant status, and cataract. Am J Clin Nutr 1995; 62:1439S–1447S.

10. Taylor A. Oxidative stress and antioxidant function in relation to risk for cataract. In: Sies H, ed. Antioxidants in Disease Mechanisms and Therapeutic Strategies. San Diego: Academic Press. In press.

11. Taylor A, Jacques P. Antioxidant status and risk for cataract. In: Bendich A, Deckelbaum RJ, eds. Preventive Nutrition. Totawa NJ: Humana Press. In press.

12. Kupfer C. The conquest of cataract: a global challenge. Trans Ophthal Soc UK 1984; 104: 1–10.

13. Schwab L. Cataract blindness in developing nations. Int Ophthalmol Clin 1990; 30:16–18.

14. World Health Organization. Use of intraocular lenses in cataract surgery in developing countries. Bull WHO 1991; 69:657–666.

14a. Klein BEK, Klein R, Linton KLP. Prevalence of age-related lens opacities in a population: The Beaver Dam Eye Study. Ophthalmology 1992; 99:546–552.

15. Klein R, Klein BE, Linton KL, DeMets DL. The Beaver Dam Eye Study: the relation of age-related maculopathy to smoking. Am J Epidemiol 1993; 137:190–200.

16. Leibowitz H, Krueger D, Maunder C, et al. The Framingham Eye Study Monograph. Surv Ophthalmol (Suppl) 1980; 24:335–610.

17. Chatterjee A, Milton RC, Thyle S. Prevalence and etiology of cataract in Punjab. Br J Ophthalmol 1982; 66:35–42.

18. Wang G-M, Spector A, Luo C-Q, et al. Prevalence of age-related cataract in Ganzi and Shanghai: The Epidemiological Study Group. Chin Med J 1990; 103:945–951.

19. Whitfield R, Schwab L, Ross-Degnan D, et al. Blindness and eye disease in Kenya: ocular status survey results from the Kenya Rural Blindness Prevention Project. Br J Ophthalmol 1990; 74:333–340.

20. Chan CW, Billson FA. Visual disability and major causes of blindness in NSW: a study of people aged 50 and over attending the Royal Blind Society 1984 to 1989. Aust NZ J Ophthalmol 1991; 19:321–325.

21. Dana MR, Tielsch JM, Enger C, et al. Visual impairment in a rural Appalachian community: prevalence and causes. JAMA 1990; 264:2400–2405.

22. Salive ME, Guralnik J, Christian W, et al. Functional blindness and visual impairment in older adults from three communities. Ophthalmology 1992; 99:1840–1847.

23. Wormald RPL, Wright LA, Courtney P, et al. Visual problems in the elderly population and implications for services. Br Med J 1992; 304:1226–1229.

24. Seddon JM, Christen WG, Manson JE, et al. The use of vitamin supplements and the risk of cataract among US male physicians. Am J Public Health 1994; 84:788–792.

25. Ganley JP, Roberts J. Eye conditions and related need for medical care. Vital and Health Statistics, Data from the National Health Survey, 1983 Series 11, No 228.

26. Kahn HA, Leibowitz HM, Ganley JP, et al. The Framingham Eye Study: outline and major prevalence findings. Am J Epidemiol 1977; 106:17–32.

27. Murphy RP. Age-related macular degeneration. Ophthalmology 1986; 93:969–971.

28. Hyman L. Epidemiology of eye disease in the elderly. Eye 1987; 1:213–227.

29. Pizzarello LD. The dimensions of the problem of eye disease among the elderly. Ophthalmology 1987; 94:1191–1195.

30. Macular Photocoagulation Study Group. Argon laser photocoagulation for senile macular degeneration: results of a randomized clinical trial. Arch Ophthalmol 1982; 100:912–918.

31. Macular Photocoagulation Study Group. Argon laser photocoagulation for neovascular maculopathy after five years: results from randomized clinical trials. Arch Ophthalmol 1991; 109: 1109–1114.

32. Macular Photocoagulation Study Group. Laser photocoagulation of subfoveal neovascular

lesions in age-related macular degeneration: results of a randomized clinical trial. Arch Oph-thalmol 1991; 109:1220–1231.

33. Taylor A, Tisdell FE, Carpenter FH. Leucine aminopeptidase (bovine lens): synthesis and kinetic properties of ortho, meta, and para substituted leucyl-anilides. Arch Biochem Biophys 1981; 210:90–97.

34. Jacques PF, Taylor A. Micronutrients and age-related cataracts. In: Bendich A, Butterworth CE, eds. Micronutrients in Health and in Disease Prevention. New York: Marcel Dekker, 1991; 359–379.

35. Chylack LT Jr, Wolfe JK, Singer DM, et al. The lens opacities classification system III. Arch Ophthalmol 1993; 111:831–836.

36. Chylack LT Jr, Wolfe JK, Friend J, et al. Nuclear cataract: relative contributions to vision loss of opalescence and brunescence (abstr). Invest Ophthalmol Vis Sci 1994; 35:42632.

37. Wolfe JK, Chylack LT Jr, Leske MC, et al. Lens nuclear color and visual function (abstr). Invest Ophthalmol Vis Sci 1993; 34:4,2550.

38. Dolin P. Assessment of the epidemiological evidence that exposure to solar ultraviolet radia-tion causes cataract. Doc Ophthalmol 1995; 88:327–337.

39. West SK, Valmadrid CT. Epidemiology of risk factors for age-related cataract. Surv Ophthal-mol 1995; 39:323–334.

40. Zigman S. Effects of near ultraviolet radiation on the lens and retina. Doc Ophthalmol 1983; 55:375–391.

41. Bochow TW, West, SK, Azar A, et al. Ultraviolet light exposure and risk of posterior subcapsular cataracts. Arch Ophthalmol 1989; 107:369–372.

42. Brilliant LB, Grasset NC, Pokhrel RP, et al. Associations among cataract prevalence, sunlight hours, and altitude in the Himalayas. Am J Epidemiol 1983; 118:250–264.

43. Christen WG, Manson JE, Seddon JM, et al. A prospective study of cigarette smoking and risk of cataract in men. JAMA 1992; 268:989–993.

44. Hankinson SE, Willett WC, Colditz GA, et al. A prospective study of cigarette smoking and risk of cataract surgery in women. JAMA 1992; 268:994–998.

45. Taylor HR, West SK, Rosenthal FS, et al. Effect of ultraviolet radiation on cataract formation. N Engl J Med 1988; 319:1429–1433.

46. West SK, Rosenthal FS, Bressler NM, et al. Exposure to sunlight and other risk factors for age-related macular degeneration. Arch Ophthalmol 1989; 107:875–879.

47. West SK, Munoz B, Emmett EA, Taylor HR. Cigarette smoking and risk of nuclear cataracts. Arch Ophthalmol 1992; 107:1166–1169.

48. Zigman S, Datiles M, Torczynski E. Sunlight and human cataract. Invest Ophthalmol Vis Sci 1979; 18462–18467.

49. Wong L, Ho SC, Coggon D, et al. Sunlight exposure, antioxidant status, and cataract in Hong Kong fishermen. J Epidemiol Community Health 1993; 47:46–49.

50. Hirvela H, Luukinen H, Laatikainen L. Prevalence and risk factors of lens opacities in the elderly in Finland: a population-based study. Ophthalmology 1995; 102:108–117.

51. Mares-Perlman JA, Klein BEK, Klein R, Ritter LL. Relationship between lens opacities and vitamin and mineral supplement use. Ophthalmology 1994; 1.01:315–355.

52. Mares-Perlman JA, Brady WE, Klein BEK, et al. Diet and nuclear lens opacities. Am J Epi-demiol 1995; 141:322–334.

53. Robertson JM, Donner AP, Trevithick JR. Vitamin E intake and risk for cataracts in humans. Ann NY Acad Sci 1989; 570:372–382.

54. Leske MC, Chylack LT Jr, Wu S. The lens opacities case-control study risk factors for cataract. Arch Ophthalmol 1991; 109:244–251.

55. Cruickshanks KJ, Klein BE, Klein R. Ultraviolet light exposure and lens opacities: The Beaver Dam Eye Study. Am J Public Health 1992; 82:1658–1662.

56. The Italian-American Cataract Study Group. Risk factors for age-related cortical, nuclear, and posterior subcapsular cataracts. Am J Epidemiol 1991; 133:541–553.

57. Guo-min W, Spector A, Lus C-q, et al. Prevalence of age-related cataract in Ganzi and Shanghai. Chin Med J 1990; 103:945–951.

58. Klein BE, Cruickshanks KJ, Klein R. Leisure time, sunlight exposure and cataracts (review). Doc Ophthalmol 1994–95; 88:295–305.

59. Javitt JC, Taylor HR. Cataract and latitude (1995). Doc Ophthalmol 1995; 88:307–325.

60. Minassian DC, Baasanhu J, Johnson GJ, Burendei G. Acta Ophthalmol 1994; 72:490–495.

61. Wolff SP. Cataract and UV radiation. Doc Ophthalmol 1995; 88:201–204.

62. Zigman S, Paxhia T, McDaniel T, et al. Effect of chronic near-ultraviolet radiation on the gray squirrel lens in vivo. Invest Ophthalmol Vis Sci 1991; 32:1723–1732.

63. Zigler JS, Goosey JD. Singlet oxygen as a possible factor in human senile nuclear cataract development. Curr Eye Res 1984; 3:59–65.

64. Varma SD, Chand O, Sharma YR, et al. Oxidative stress on lens and cataract formation: role of light and oxygen. Curr Eye Res 1984; 3:35–57.

65. Taylor A, Jahngen-Hodge J, Huang LL, Jaques P. Aging in the eye lens: roles for proteolysis and nutrition in formation of cataract. AGE 1991; 14:65–71.

66. Rao CM, Qin C, Robison WG Jr, Zigler JS Jr. Effect of smoke condensate on the physiological integrity and morphology of organ cultured rat lenses. Curr Eye Res 1995; 14:295–301.

67. Shalini VK, Luthra M, Srinivas L, et al. Oxidative damage to the eye lens caused by cigarette smoke and fuel smoke condensates. Ind J Biochem Biophys 1994; 31:261–266.

68. Zigman S, McDaniel T, Schultz JB, et al. Damage to cultured lens epithelial cells of squirrels and rabbits by UV-A (99.9%) plus UV-B (0.1%) radiation and alpha tocopherol protection. Mol Cell Biochem 1995; 143:35–46.

69. Smith D, Palmer V, Kehyias J, Taylor A. Induction of cataracts by X-ray exposure of guinea pig eyes. Lab Anim 1993; 22:34–39.

70. Calissendorff BM, Lonnqvist B, el Azazi M. Cataract development in adult bone marrow transplant recipients. Acta Ophthalmol Scand 1995; 73:52–154.

71. Palmquist BM, Phillipson B, Barr PO. Nuclear cataract and myopia during hyperbaric oxygen therapy. Br J Ophthalmol 1984; 60:113–117.

72. Schocket SS, Esterson J, Bradford B, et al. Induction of cataracts in mice by exposure to oxygen. Isr J Med 1972; 8:1596–1601.

73. Giblin FJ, Schrimscher L, Chakrapani B, Reddy VN. Exposure of rabbit lens to hyperbaric oxygen in vitro: regional effects on GSH level. Invest Ophthalmol Vis Sci 1988; 29:1312–1319.

74. Giblin FJ, Padgaonkar VA, Leverenz VR, et al. Nuclear light scattering, disulfide formation and membrane damage in lenses of older guinea pigs treated with hyperbaric oxygen. Exp Eye Res 1995; 60:219–235.

75. Berman ER. In: Biochemistry of the Eye. New York: Plenum Press, 1991:210–308.

76. Schectman G, Byrd JC, Gruchow HW. The influence of smoking on vitamin C status in adults. Am J Health 1989; 79:158–162.

77. Russell-Briefel R, Bates MW, Kuller LH. The relationship of plasma carotenoids to health and biochemical factors in middle-aged men. Am J Epidemiol 1985; 122:741–749.

78. Giraud DW, Martin HD, Driskell JA. Plasma and dietary vitamin C and E levels of tobacco chewers, smokers, and nonusers. J Am Diet Assoc 1995; 95:798–800.

79. Chow CK, Thacker RR, Changchit C, et al. Lower levels of vitamin C and carotenes in plasma of cigarette smokers. J Am Coll Nutr 1986; 5:305–312.

80. Mezzetti A, Lapenna D, Pierdomenico SD, et al. Vitamins E, C, and lipid peroxidation in plasma and arterial tissue of smokers and non-smokers. Atherosclerosis 1995; 112:91–99.

81. Bolton-Smith C, Casey CE, Gey KF, et al. Antioxidant intakes assessed using a food-frequency questionnaire: correlation with biochemical status in smokers and non-smokers. Br J Nutr 1991; 65:337–346.

82. Flaye DE, Sullivan KN, Cullinan TR, Silver JH, Whitelocke RAF. Cataracts and cigarette smoking: the City Eye Study. Eye 1989; 3:379–384.

83. West SK, Munoz B, Emmett EA, Taylor HR. Cigarette smoking and risk of nuclear cataracts. Arch Ophthalmol 1989; 107:1166–1169.

84. West S. Does smoke get in your eyes? JAMA 1992; 268:1025–1026.

85. Mares-Perlman JA, Brady WE, Klein BEK, et al. Serum carotenoids and tocopherols and severity of nuclear and cortical opacities. Invest Ophthalmol Vis Sci 1995; 36:276–288.

86. Taylor A, Davies KJA. Protein oxidation and loss of protease activity may lead to cataract formation in the aged lens. Free Radical Biol Med 1987; 3:371–377.

87. Taylor A, Jacques PF, Nadler D, et al. Relationship in humans between ascorbic acid consumption and levels of total and reduced ascorbic acid in lens, aqueous humor, and plasma. Curr Eye Res 1991; 10:751–759.

88. Kuck JFR Jr. Composition of the lens. In: Bellows JG, ed. Cataract and Abnormalities of the Lens. New York: Grune & Stratton, 1974:69–96.

89. Reddy VN. Glutathione and its function in the lens: an overview. Exp Eye Res 1990; 150:771–778.

90. Sastre J, Meydani M, Martin A, et al. Effect of glutathione monoethyl ester administration on galactose-induced cataract in the rat. Life Chem Rep 1994; 12:89–95.

91. Taylor A, Jahngen-Hodge J, Smith D, et al. Dietary restriction delays cataract and reduces ascorbate levels in Emory mice. Exp Eye Res 1995; 61:55–62.

92. Taylor A, Lipman RD, Jahngen-Hodge J, et al. Dietary calorie restriction in the Emory Mouse: effects on lifespan, eye lens cataract prevalence and progression, levels of ascorbate, glutathione, glucose, and glycohemoglobin, tail collagen breaktime, DNA and RNA oxidation, skin integrity, fecundity and cancer. Mech Ageing Dev 1995; 79:33–57.

93. Levine M. New concepts in the biology and biochemistry of ascorbic acid. N Engl J Med 1986; 314:892–902.

94. Frei B, Stocker R, Ames BN. Antioxidant defenses and lipid peroxidation in human blood plasma. Proc Natl Acad Sci USA 1988; 85:9748–9752.

95. Berger J, Shepard D, Morrow F, Taylor A. Relationship between dietary intake and tissue levels of reduced and total vitamin C in the guinea pig. J Nutr 1989; 119:1–7.

96. Berger J, Shepard D, Morrow F, et al. Reduced and total ascorbate in guinea pig eye tissues in response to dietary intake. Curr Eye Res 1988; 7:681–686.

97. Nakamura B, Nakamura O. Ufer das vitamin C in der linse und dem Kammerwasser der menschlichen katarakte. Graefes Arch Clin Exp Ophthalmol 1935; 134:197–200.

98. Wilczek M, Zygulska-Machowa H. Zawartosc witaminy C W. roznych typack zaem. J Klin Oczna 1968; 38:477–480.

99. Jacques P, Taylor A, Lahav M, et al. Associations between risk for cataract and long-term ascorbate supplementation (abstr). Invest Ophthal Vis Sci 1996; 37:S236.

100. Kosegarten DC, Mayer TJ. Use of guinea pigs as model to study galactose-induced cataract formation. J Pharm Sci 1978; 67:1478–1479.

101. Vinson JA, Possanza CJ, Drack AV. The effect of ascorbic acid on galactose-induced cataracts. Nutr Rep Int 1986; 33:665–668.

102. Devamanoharan PS, Henein M, Morris S, et al. Prevention of selenite cataract by vitamin C. Exp Eye Res 1991; 52:563–568.

103. Nishigori H, Lee JW, Yamauchi Y, Iwatsuru M. The alteration of lipid peroxide in glucocorticoid-induced cataract of developing chick embryos and the effect of ascorbic acid. Curr Eye Res 1986; 5:37–40.

104. Blondin J, Baragi VJ, Schwartz E, et al. Dietary vitamin C delays UV-induced age-related eye lens protein damage. Vitamin C. Ann NY Acad Sci 1987; 498:460–463.

105. Garland DD. Ascorbic acid and the eye. Am J Clin Nutr 1991; 54:1198S–1202S.

106. Naraj RM, Monnier VM. Isolation and characterization of a blue fluorophore from human eye lens crystallins: in vitro formation from Maillard action with ascorbate and ribose. Biochim Biophys Acta 1992; 1116:34–42.

107. Bensch KG, Fleming EE, Lohmann W. The role of ascorbic acid in senile cataract. Proc Natl Acad Sci USA 1985; 82:7193–7196.

108. Martenssen J, Steinhertz R, Jain A, Meister A. Glutathione ester prevents buthionine sulfox-imine-induced cataracts and lens epithelial cell damage. Biochemistry 1989; 86:8727–8731.

109. Rathbun WB, Holleschau AM, Murray DL, et al. Glutathione synthesis and glutathione redox pathways in naphthalene cataract in the rat. Curr Eye Res 1990; 9:45–53.

110. Vina J, Perez C, Furukawa T, et al. Effect of oral glutathione on hepatic glutathione levels on rats and mice. Br J Nutr 1989; 62:683–691.

111. Clark JI, Steele JE. Phase-separation inhibitors and prevention of selenite cataract. Proc Natl Acad Sci USA 1992; 89:1720–1724.

112. Srivastava SK, Ansari NH. Prevention of sugar induced cataractogenesis in rats by butylated hydroxytoluene. Diabetes 1988; 37:1505–1508.

113. Tinkler JH, Bohm F, Schalch W, Truscott TG. Dietary carotenoids protect human cells from damage. J Photochem Photobiol B Biology 1994; 26:283–285.

114. Schalch W, Weber P. Vitamins and carotenoids: a promising approach to reducing the risk of coronary heart disease, cancer and eye diseases. Adv Exp Med Biol 1994; 366:335–350.

115. Machlin LJ, Bendich A. Free radical tissue damage: protective role of antioxidant nutrients. FASEB J 1987; 1:441–445.

116. Costagliola C, Iuliano G, Menzione M, et al. Effect of vitamin E on glutathione content in red blood cells, aqueous humor and lens of humans and other species. Exp Eye Res 1986; 43:905–914.

117. Yeum K-J, Taylor A, Tang G, Russell RM. Measurement of carotenoids, retinoids, and tocopherols in human lenses. Invest Ophthalmol Vis Sci 1995; 36:2756–2761.

118. Creighton MO, Ross WM, Stewart-DeHaan PJ, et al. Modeling cortical cataractogenesis. VII. Effects of vitamin E treatment on galactose induced cataracts. Exp Eye Res 1985; 40:213–222.

119. Bhuyan DK, Podos SM, Machlin LT, et al. Antioxidant in therapy of cataract. II. Effect of all-roc-alpha-tocopherol (vitamin E) in sugar-induced cataract in rabbits. Invest Ophthalmol Vis Sci 1983; 24:74.

120. Bhuyan KC, Bhuyan DK. Molecular mechanism of cataractogenesis. III. Toxic metabolites of oxygen as initiators of lipid peroxidation and cataract. Curr Eye Res 1984; 3:67–81.

121. Fridovich I. Oxygen: aspects of its toxicity and elements of defense. Curr Eye Res 1984; 3:1–2.

122. Giblin FJ, McReady JP, Reddy VN. The role of glutathione metabolism in detoxification of H_2O_2 in rabbit lens. Invest Ophthalmol Vis Sci 1992; 22:330–335.

123. Eisenhauer DA, Berger JJ, Peltier CZ, Taylor A. Protease activities in cultured beef lens epi-thelial cells peak and then decline upon progressive passage. Exp Eye Res 1988; 46:579–590.

124. Jahngen-Hodge J, Laxman E, Zuliani A, Taylor A. Evidence for ATP ubiquitin-dependent degradation of proteins in cultured bovine lens epithelial cells. Exp Eye Res 1991; 52:341–347.

125. Shang F, Taylor A. Oxidative stress and recovery from oxidative stress are associated with altered ubiquitin conjugating and proteolytic activities in bovine lens epithelial cells. Biochem J 1995; 307:297–303.

126. Huang LL, Jahngen-Hodge J, Taylor A. Bovine lens epithelial cells have a ubiquitin-dependent proteolysis system. Biochim Biophys Acta 1993; 1175:181–187.

127. Jahngen JH, Lipman RD, Eisenhauer DA, et al. Aging and cellular maturation cause changes in ubiquitin-eye lens protein conjugates. Arch Biochem Biophys 1990; 276:32–37.

128. Jahngen-Hodge J, Cyr D, Laxman E, Taylor A. Ubiquitin and ubiquitin conjugates in human lens. Exp Eye Res 1992; 55:897–902.

129. Obin MS, Nowell T, Taylor A. The photoreceptor G-protein transducin (G_t) is a substrate for ubiquitin-dependent proteolysis. Biochem Biophys Res Commun 1994; 200:1169–1176.

130. Jacques PF, Chylack LT Jr. Epidemiologic evidence of a role for the antioxidant vitamins and carotenoids in cataract prevention. Am J Clin Nutr 1991; 53:352S–355S.

131. Mohan M, Sperduto RD, Angra SK, et al. India-US case-control study of age-related cataracts. Arch Ophthalmol 1989; 107:670–676.

132. Hankinson SE, Stampfer MJ, Seddon JM, et al. Nutrient intake and cataract extraction in women: a prospective study. Br Med J 1992; 305:335–339.

133. Vitale S, West S, Hallfrisch J, et al. Plasma antioxidants and risk of cortical and nuclear cataract. Epidemiology 1994; 4:195–203.

134. Jacques PF, Lahav M, Willett WC, Taylor A. Relationship between long-term vitamin C intake and prevalence of cataract and macular degeneration (abstr). Exp Eye Res 1992; 55(suppl 1):S152.

135. Knekt P, Heliovaara M, Rissanen A, et al. Serum antioxidant vitamins and risk of cataract. Br Med J 1992; 305:1392–1394.

136. Taylor A, Jacques P, Lahav M, et al. Relationship between long-term dietary and supplement ascorbate intake and risk of cataract (abstr). Exp Eye Res 1994; 59(suppl 1):S133.

137. Libondi T, Menzione M, Auricchio G. In vitro effect of alpha-tocopherol on lysophosphatidyl-choline-induced lens damage. Exp Eye Res 1985; 40:661–666.

138. Burton W, Ingold KU. Beta-carotene: an unusual type of lipid antioxidant. Science 1984; 224:569–573.

139. Kwan M, Niinikoski J, Hunt TK. In vivo measurement of oxygen tension in the cornea, aqueous humor, and the anterior lens of the open eye. Invest Ophthalmol 1972; 11:108–114.

140. Erdman J. The physiologic chemistry of carotenes in man. Clin Nutr 1988; 7:101–106.

141. Di Mascio P, Murphy ME, Sies H. Antioxidant defense systems: the role of carotenoids, tocopherols and thiols. Am J Clin Nutr 1991; 53:194S–200S.

142. Krinsky NI, Deneke SS. Interaction of oxygen and oxy-radicals with carotenoids. J Natl Cancer Inst 1982; 69:205–210.

143. Micozzi MS, Beecher GR, Taylor HR, Khachik F. Carotenoid analyses of selected raw and cooked foods associated with a lower risk for cancer. J Natl Cancer Inst 1990; 82:282–285.

144. Daicker B, Schiedt K, Adnet JJ, Bermond P. Canthaxamin retinopathy: an investigation by light and electron microscopy and physiochemical analyses. Graefes Arch Clin Exp Ophthalmol 1987; 225:189–197.

145. Sperduto RD, Hu T-S, Milton RC, et al. The Linxian Cataract Studies: two nutrition intervention trials. Arch Ophthalmol 1993; 111:1246–1253.

146. Sarks SH. Ageing and degeneration in the macular region: a clinicopathologic study. Br J Ophthalmol 1976; 60:324–341.

147. Sarks SH. Drusen and their relationship to senile macular degeneration. Aust J Ophthalmol 1980; 8:117–130.

148. Green WR, Key SN. Senile macular degeneration: a histopathologic study. Trans Am Ophthalmol Soc 1977; 75·180–254.

149. Gass JDM. Pathogenesis of macular detachment and degeneration. Ophthalmic Forum 1984; 2:8–17.

150. Bressler NM, Bressler SB, Fine SB. Age-related macular degeneration. Surv Ophthalmol 1988; 32:375–413.

151. Bone R, Landrum JT, Fernandez L, Tarsis SL. Analysis of the macular pigment by HPLC: retinal distribution and age study. Invest Ophthalmol Vis Sci 1988; 29:843–849.

152. Handelman GJ, Dratz EA, Reay CC, van Kuijk JG. Carotenoids in the human macula and whole retina. Invest Ophthalmol Vis Sci 1988; 29:850–855.

153. Walls GL, Judd HD. The intraocular colour filters of vertebrates. Br J Ophthalmol 1983; 17:641.

154. Haegerstrom-Portnoy G. Short-wavelength sensitive cone sensitivity loss with aging: a protective role for macular pigment? J Opt Soc Am 1988; 5:2140–2144.

155. Noell WK. There are different kinds of retinal light damage. In: Williams TP, Baker N, eds. The Effects of Constant Light on Visual Processes. New York: Plenum Press, 1980:3–18.

156. Pautler EL, Morita M, Beezley D. Reversible and irreversible blue light damage to the isolated, mammalian pigment epithelium. Prog Clin Biol Res 1989; 314:555–567.

157. Dorey CK, Akeo K, Delori FC. Growth of cultured RPE cells and endothelial cells is inhibited by blue light, but not green or red light. Curr Eye res 1990; 9:549–559.

158. Krinsky NI. Photobiology of carotenoid protection. In: Regen JD, Parrish JA, eds. The Science of Photomedicine. New York: Plenum Press, 1982:397–403.

159. Matthews-Roth MM, Wilson T, Fujimori E, Krinsky NI. Carotenoid chromophore length and protection against photosensitization. Photochem Photobiol 1974; 18:217.

160. Terao J. Antioxidant activity of β-carotene related carotenoids in solution. Lipids 1989; 24:659.

161. Snodderly DM, Auran JD, Delori FC. The macular pigment. II. Spatial distribution in primate retinas. Invest Ophthalmol Vis Sci 1984; 25:674–685.

162. Hogan MJ. Role of the retinal pigment epithelium in macular disease. Trans Am Acad Ophthalmol Otolaryngol 1972; 76:61–80.

163. Young RW. Pathophysiology of age-related macular degeneration. Surv Ophthalmol 1987; 31:291–306.

164. Eldred GE. Vitamins E and A in RPE lipofuscin formation and implications for age-related macular degeneration. Prog Clin Biol Res 1989; 314:113–129.

165. Young RW. Solar radiation and age related macular degeneration. Surv Ophthalmol 1988; 32:252–269.

166. Taylor HR, West S, Munoz B, Rosenthal FS, Bressler SB, Bressler NM. The long-term effects of visible light on the eye. Arch Ophthalmol 1992; 110:99–104.

167. Hyman LG, Lilienfeld AM, Ferris FL III. Senile macular degeneration: a case-control study. Am J Epidemiol 1983; 18:213–227.

168. Weiter JJ, Delori FC, Wing GL, Fitch KA. Relationship of senile macular degeneration to ocular pigmentation. Am J Ophthalmol 1985; 99:185–187.

169. Das BN, Thompson JR, Patel R, Rosenthal AR. Prevalence of eye disease in the elderly Asians in an English city. Invest Ophthalmol Vis Sci 1989; 30(suppl):438.

170. Matsui M. Macular diseases in the elderly person. Nippon Ganka Gakkai Zasshi 1989; 93: 893–907.

171. Hoshino M, Mizuno K, Ichikawa H. Aging alterations of retina and choroid of Japanese: light microscopic study of macular region of 176 eyes. Jpn J Ophthalmol 1984; 28:89–102.

172. Klein BE, Klein R. Cataracts and macular degeneration in older Americans. Arch Ophthalmol 1982; 100:571–573.

173. Moss SE, Klein R, Meuer MB, Klein BEK. The association of iris color with eye disease in diabetes. Ophthalmology 1987; 94:1226–1231.

174. Jaffe GJ, Irvine AR, Wood IS, et al. Retinal phototoxicity from the operating microscope: the role of inspired oxygen. Ophthalmology 1988; 95:1130–1141.

175. Zheltov G, Glazkov V, Podoltzef A, et al. Retinal damage from intense visible light. Health Phys 1989; 56:625–630.

176. Penner R, McNair JN. Eclipse blindness: report of an epidemic in the military population of Hawaii. Am J Ophthalmol 1966; 61:1452–1457.

177. Green WR, Robertson DM. Pathologic findings of photic retinopathy in the human eye. Am J Ophthalmol 1991; 112:518–525.

178. Andley UP. Photodamage to the eye. Photochem Photobiol 1987; 46:1057–1066.

179. Organisciak DT, Jiang YL, Wang HM, Bicknell I. The protective effect of ascorbic acid in retinal light damage of rats exposed to intermittent light. Invest Ophthalmol Vis Sci 1990; 31:1195–1202.

180. Duncan TE, O'Steen WK. The diurnal susceptibility of rat retinal photoreceptors to light-induced damage. Exp Eye Res 1985; 41:497–507.

181. Rapp LM, Williams TP. The role of ocular pigmentation in protecting against retinal light damage. Vis Res 1980; 20:1127–1131.

182. LaVail MM. Eye pigmentation and constant light damage in the rat retina. In: Williams TP, Baker BN, eds. Effects of Constant Light on Visual Processes. New York: Plenum, 1980: 357–387.

183. LaVail MM, Gorrin GM. Protection from light damage by ocular pigmentation: analysis using experimental chimeras and translocation mice. Exp Eye Res 1987; 44:877–889.

184. Noell WK, Organisciak DT, Ando H, et al. Ascorbate and dietary protective mechanisms in

retinal light damage of rats: electrophysiological, histological and DNA measurements. Prog Clin Biol Res 1987; 247:469–483.

185. Organisciak DT, Wang HM, Li ZY, Tso MO. The protective effect of ascorbate in retinal light damage of rats. Invest Ophthalmol Vis Sci 1985; 26:1580–1588.

186. Organisciak DT, Berman ER, Wang H, Feeney-Burns L. Vitamin E in human neural retina and retinal pigment epithelium: effect of age. Curr Eye Res 1987; 6:1051–1055.

187. Tso MOM. Experiments on visual cells by nature and man: in search of treatment for photoreceptor degeneration. Friedenwald Lecture. Invest Ophthalmol Vis Sci 1989; 30:2430–2454.

188. Penn JS, Naash MI, Anderson RE. Effect of light history on retinal antioxidants and light damage susceptibility in the rat. Exp Eye Res 1987; 44:779–788.

189. Naash MI, LaVail MI, Anderson RE. Factors affecting the susceptibility of the retina to light damage. Prog Clin Biol Res 1989; 314:513–522.

190. Dorey CK, Ghouri GC, Syniuta LA, et al. Superoxide production by porcine retinal pigment epithelium in vitro. Invest Ophthalmol Vis Sci 1989; 30:1047–1054.

191. Wing GL. Blanchard GC, Weiter JJ. The topography and age-relationship of lipofuscin concentration in the retinal pigment epithelium. Invest Ophthalmol Vis Sci 1978; 17:601–607.

192. Feeney-Burns L, Hilderbrand ES, Eldridge S. Aging human RPE: analysis of macular, equatorial and peripheral cells. Invest Ophthalmol Vis Sci 1984; 25:195–200.

193. Weiter JJ, Delori FC, Wing GL, Fitch KA. Retinal pigment epithelial lipofuscin and melanin and choroidal melanin in human eyes. Invest Ophthalmol Vis Sci 1986; 27:145–152.

194. Katz ML, Stone WL, Dratz EA. Fluorescent pigment accumulation in retinal pigment epithelium of antioxidant deficient rats. Invest Ophthalmol Vis Sci 1978; 17:1049–1058.

195. Robison WG Jr, Kuwubara T, Bieri JG. Deficiencies of vitamins E and A in the rat: retinal damage and lipofuscin accumulation. Invest Ophthalmol Vis Sci 1980; 19:1030–1037.

196. Katz ML, Drea CM, Eldred GE, et al. Influence of early photoreceptor degeneration on lipofuscin in the retinal pigment epithelium. Exp Eye Res 1986; 43:561–573.

197. Katz ML, Eldred GE. Retinal light damage reduced autofluorescent pigment deposition in the retinal pigment epithelium. Invest Ophthalmol Vis Sci 1989; 30:37–43.

198. Feeney-Burns L, Burns RP, Gao CL. Age-related macular changes in humans over 90 years old. Am J Ophthalmol 1990; 109:265–278.

199. Feeney-Burns L, Ellersieck MR. Age-related changes in the ultrastructure of Bruch's membrane. Am J Ophthalmol 1985; 100:686–697.

200. Dorey DK, Wu G, Ebenstein D, et al. Cell loss in the aging retina: relationship to lipofuscin accumulation and macular degeneration. Invest Ophthalmol Vis Sci 1989; 30:1047–1054.

201. Schatz H, McDonald HR. Atrophic macular degeneration. Rate of spread of geographic atrophy and visual loss. Ophthalmology 1989; 96:1541–1551.

202. Eagle RC Jr, Lucier AC, Bernadino VB Jr, Yanoff M. Retinal pigment epithelial abnormalities in fundus flavimaculatus. Ophthalmology 1980; 87:1189–1200.

203. Armstrong D, Koppang N, Rider J. Ceroid Lipofuscinosis (Batten's Disease). Amsterdam: Elsevier, 1982.

204. O'Gorman S, Flaherty WA, Fishman GA, Berson EL. Histopathologic findings in Best's viteliform macular dystrophy. Arch Ophthalmol 1988; 106:1261–1268.

205. Hayes KC. Retinal degeneration in monkeys induced by deficiencies of vitamins E or A. Invest Ophthalmol Vis Sci 1974; 13:499–510.

206. Hayes KC, Rousseau JE Jr, Hegstead DM. Plasma tocopherol concentrations and vitamin E deficiency in dogs. J Am Vet Med Assoc 1970; 157:64–71.

207. Handelman GJ, Dratz EA. The role of antioxidants in the retina and retinal pigment epithelium and the nature of prooxidant-induced damage. Adv Free Radical Biol Med 1986; 2:1–89.

208. Feeney-Burns L, Eldred GE. The fate of the phagosome: conversion to age pigment and impact in human retinal pigment epithelium. Trans Ophthalmol Soc UK 1984; 103:416–421.

209. Eldred GE, Katz ML. The autofluorescent products of lipid peroxidation may not be lipofuscin-like. Free Radical Biol Med 1989; 7:157–163.

210. Katz ML, Shanker MJ. Development of lipofuscin-like fluorescence in the retinal pigment epithelium in response to protease inhibitor treatment. Mech Ageing Dev 1989; 49:23–40.

211. Obin M, Nowell T, Taylor A. A comparison of ubiquitin-dependent proteolysis of rod outer segment proteins in reticulocyte lysate and a retinal pigment epithelial cell line. Curr Eye Res 1995; 14:751–760.

212. Obin MS, Jahngen-Hodge J, Nowell T, Taylor A. Ubiquitinylation and ubiquitin-dependent proteolysis in vertebrate photoreceptors (rod outer segments): evidence for ubiquitinylation of G_t and rhodopsin. J Biol Chem 1996; 271:14473–14484.

213. Liles MR, Newsome DA, Oliver PD. Antioxidant enzymes in the aging human retinal pigment epithelium. Arch Ophthalmol 1991; 109:1285–1288.

214. Maltzman BA, Mulvhill MN, Greenvaum A. Senile macular degeneration and risk factors: A case-control study. Ann Ophthalmol 1979; 11:1197–1201.

215. Organisciak DT, Bicknell IR, Darrow RM. The effects of L- and D-ascorbic acid administration on retinal tissue levels and light damage in rats. Curr Eye Res 1992; 11:231–241.

216. Nishida A, Togari H. Effect of vitamin E administration on α-tocopherol concentrations in the retina, choroid, and vitreous body of human neonates. J Pediatr 1986; 108:150–153.

217. Mojon D, Boscaboinik D, Haas A, et al. Vitamin E inhibits retinal pigment epithelium cell proliferation in vitro. Ophthalmic Res 1994; 26:304–309.

218. Kowluru R, Kern TS, Engerman RL. Abnormalities of retinal metabolism in diabetes or galactosemia. II. Comparison of γ-glutamyl transpeptidase in retina and cerebral cortex, and effects of antioxidant therapy. Curr Eye Res 1994; 13:891–896.

219. Seddon JM, Ajani UA, Sperduto RD, et al. Dietary carotenoids, vitamins A, C, and E, and advanced age-related macular degeneration: Eye Disease Case-Control Study Group. JAMA 1994; 272:1413–1420.

220. Weiter JJ, Delori FC, Dorey CH. Annular macular degeneration: an explanation for the central sparing. Am J Ophthalmol 1988; 106:286–292.

221. Goldberg J, Flowerdew G, Smith E, et al. Factors associated with age-related macular degeneration: an analysis of data from the first National Health and Nutrition Examination Survey. Am J Epidemiol 1988; 128:700–710.

222. Organisciak DT, Feeney-Burns L, Bridges CD. On the measurement of vitamin E in human ocular tissues (letter). Curr Eye Res 1987; 6:1487–1488.

223. Staurenghi G. Serum levels of vitamins C and E and lipids in patients with hard and soft drusen. Invest Ophthalmol Vis Sci 1992; 33(suppl 4):2690.

224. Jacob RA, Otradovec CL, Russell RM, et al. Vitamin C status and nutrient interactions in a healthy elderly population. Am J Clin Nutr 1988; 48:1436–1442.

225. Harding JJ, van Heyningen R. Epidemiology and risk factors for cataract. Eye 1987; 1:537–541.

226. McLaren DS. Nutritional Ophthalmology. 2d ed. London: Academic Press, 1980.

227. Wefers H, Sies H. The protection by ascorbate and glutathione against microsomal lipid peroxidation is dependent on vitamin E. FEBS 1988; 174:353–357.

228. Burton GW, Wronska U, Stone L, et al. Biokinetics of dietary RRR-α-tocopherol in the male guinea pig at three dietary levels of vitamin C and two levels of vitamin E: evidence that vitamin C does not "spare" vitamin E in vivo. Lipids 1990; 25:199–210.

229. Sasaki H, Giblin FJ, Winkler BS, et al. A protective role for glutathione-dependent reduction of dehydroascorbic acid in lens epithelium. Invest Ophthalmol Vis Sci 1995; 36:1804.

230. Johnston CS, Meyer CG, Srilakshmi JC. Vitamin C elevates red blood cell glutathione in healthy adults. Am J Clin Nutr 1993; 58:103–105.

231. Pauleikhoff D, Narper CA, Marshall J, Bird AC. Aging changes in Bruch's membrane: a histochemical and morphologic study. Ophthalmol 1990; 97:171–178.

232. Hiller R, Giacometti L, Yuen K. Sunlight and cataract: an epidemiologic investigation. Am J Epidemiol 1977; 105:450–459.
233. Fleshman KR, Wagner BJ. Changes during aging in rats lens endopeptidase activity. Exp Eye Res 1984; 39:543–551.
234. Ray K, Harris H. Purification of neutral lens endopeptidase: close similarity to a neutral proteinase in pituitary. Proc Natl Acad Sci USA 1985; 82:7545–7549.
235. Murakami K, Jahngen JH, Lin S, et al. Lens proteasome shows enhanced rates of degradation of hydroxyl radical modified alpha-crystallin. Free Radical Biol Med 1990; 8:217–222.
236. Taylor A, Brown MJ, Daims MA, Cohen J. Localization of leucine aminopeptidase in hog lenses using immunofluorescence and activity assays. Invest Ophthalmol Vis Sci 1983; 24:1172–1181.
237. Varnum MD, David LL, Shearer TR. Age-related changes in calpain II and calpastatin in rat lens. Exp Eye Res 1989; 49:1053–1065.
238. Yoshida H, Yumoto N, Tsukahara I, Murachi T. The degradation of alpha-crystallin at its carboxyl-terminal portion by calpain in bovine lens. Invest Ophthalmol Vis Sci 1986; 27:1269–1273.

14

Antioxidant Action of Vitamin C in the Lung

LOU ANN S. BROWN and DEAN P. JONES

Emory University, Atlanta, Georgia

INTRODUCTION

Ascorbate (ASC) is a central redox-active molecule in the lung, functioning as an antioxidant in extracellular and intracellular compartments and also in protein processing that is required for normal differentiation and recovery from oxidant-induced injury. Although significant gaps remain in our understanding of the cell biological mechanisms of ASC, evidence continues to accumulate that adequate nutritional supply of ASC is important in protection against a variety of oxidative disease processes in the lung. In this review, we briefly discuss the redox properties of ASC as they relate to the cell biological and biochemical characteristics of the lung and survey some of the studies where ASC appears to be important in protection against oxidant-induced injury.

REDOX PROPERTIES OF ASCORBATE

Its redox potential makes ASC appropriate to play a central role in redox balance between cells and extracellular compartments and also between the cytoplasmic compartment and other intracellular compartments. The midpoint potential for the $2e^-$ oxidation of ASC to dehydroASC (DHA) is $+76$ mV (1), which means that DHA can be reduced by most of the important biological reductants in cells, e.g., reduced nicotinamide-adenine dinucleotide (NADH), reduced nicotinamide-adenine dinucleotide phosphate (NADPH), glutathione (GSH), provided that a suitable mediator or catalyst is present. Ascorbate can reduce many biologically important oxidants because it can also undergo a $1e^-$ oxidation. The midpoint potential at pH 7.0 for the 1-electron oxidation of ASC monoanion is 282 mV, a value that allows ASC to reduce oxidizing free radicals, such as $HO^\cdot$, $RO^\cdot$, $LOO^\cdot$, $GS^\cdot$, and tocopheroxyl radical (2). The semidehydroASC (SDA) formed in this $1e^-$ oxidation of ASC is relatively nonreactive (2), rapidly disproportionates to form ASC and DHA (2), and is reducible by an NADH-dependent semidehydroASC reductase system (3). Thus, under usual intracellular conditions, ASC is maintained in a highly reduced state and can function efficiently as a 1e$^-$ carrier.

ASCORBATE POOLS

Cellular Versus Extracellular Ascorbate

Within the cytoplasm of cells, the redox potential of the NADH/NAD$^+$ couple is in the range of -240 mV while that of the NADPH/NADP$^+$ couple is approximately -400 mV (4). Thus, the energetics of these pools are very high and are appropriate for maintenance of ASC/DHA. Winkler (5) has shown that GSH reacts nonenzymatically to reduce DHA to ASC and has presented strong arguments against the involvement of enzymes in this process in animal tissues (6). Because glutathione disulfide (GSSG) reductase utilizes NADPH to maintain GSH/GSSG, the NADPH pool is ultimately responsible for keeping ASC at a very highly reduced state. The rate of NADPH supply is in the range of 20% to 40% of the rate of O_2 consumption or 10% to 20% of the rate of NADH supply so that the capacity to maintain ASC is adequate under conditions where toxicity is mediated via radical species derived from O_2. Because the redox potential for GSH/GSSG (-230 mV) is so much more negative than that for ASC/DHA ($+76$), even if GSH were 90% oxidized, most of the ASC would be maintained in the reduced state.

In contrast, the extracellular redox state is considerably more oxidized than the cytoplasm. Hwang and Sinskey (7) showed that a variety of cell lines controlled their extracellular redox state in the range of -60 mV as measured by a potentiometric electrode. If the in vivo extracellular redox state is similar, one can expect that ASC/DHA is lower in extracellular fluids than in the cytoplasm. Of great interest, the thiol concentrations are much lower in the extracellular pools; GSH is in the 1- to 2-μM range in human blood plasma and cysteine is 10- to 20-μM range. Thus, there is less thiol to reduce DHA than in the cytoplasm. In addition, there is little or no NADH or NADPH in the extracellular medium. Thus, ASC, which is present in relatively high concentrations in extracellular fluids, may not be maintained in its reduced state by the same mechanisms as found intracellularly. This issue is particularly important because ASC has been found to be among the quantitatively most important extracellular antioxidants (8).

Studies of antioxidants present in human blood plasma which inhibit lipid peroxidation in lipoproteins showed that ASC is the primary antioxidant (8). Similarly, studies of antioxidants in bronchoalveolar lavage fluid of different species (9) show that ASC is one of the major antioxidants in the pulmonary epithelial lining fluid (Table 1). Thus, one must address the mechanisms of how ASC can be effectively recycled after oxidation. This issue is important in any extracellular fluid where reactive O_2 species are generated, such as occurs during the respiratory burst by activated neutrophils, but is especially important in the lungs, where high concentrations of oxidants can be inspired or generated as a result of high ambient O_2 concentrations.

At least three mechanisms may be operative in maintaining extracellular ASC. Most cells have rapid DHA uptake systems (10) so that direct release of ASC and uptake of DHA could serve to maintain extracellular ASC (Fig. 1a). In addition, all cells appear to release GSH, and some release CYS (11). These thiols could be part of a shuttle mechanism to maintain extracellular ASC (Fig. 1b), because oxidation of either GSH or CYS can result in increased cystine (CYS_2) which is actively taken up by many cell types (11). A third

Table 1 Effect of Smoking on Antioxidant Status

	Control		Smokers	Reference
Plasma (μmol/L)[a]				
Ascorbate	46.9 ± 14.3		37.0 ± 17.5	72
Glutathione	3.0 ± 0.6		2.8 ± 0.8	101
α-Tocopherol	1.2 ± 0.4		1.2 ± 0.5	67
Bronchoalveolar lavage (μmol/L)				
Ascorbate	1.7 ± 1.5	(160 μM)	3.4 ± 1.4	67
Glutathione	1.7 ± 0.3	(165 μM)	9.1 ± 2.2	61,102
α-Tocopherol	0.02 ± 0.002	(2.5 μM)	0.003 ± 0.001	103

mechanism involves reduction of SDA via intracellular NADH (Fig. 1c), which is catalyzed by a plasma membrane oxidoreductase (12). The activity of this latter system is variable in different cell types and has also been implicated in regulation of cell growth. Thus, although it remains unclear which of these systems is quantitatively most important, it is clear that the extracellular redox state and antioxidant capacity are intimately linked to the extracellular ASC pool and that this pool is ultimately controlled by cellular redox status and plasma membrane systems.

Intracellular Pools of Ascorbate

Charged polar compounds such as ASC are not readily permeable to cellular membranes, and therefore ASC transfer between compartments probably occurs mostly by transport systems. ASC is not extensively bound to cellular proteins and detectable amounts are found in membrane-bound compartments such as secretory vesicles, mitochondria, and microsomes (endoplasmic reticulum) (13). Such distribution is in accordance with functions known to occur in subcellular compartments (e.g., dopamine β-hydroxylase in secretory vesicles and ε-N-trimethyllysine hydroxylase in the mitochondria). Because the

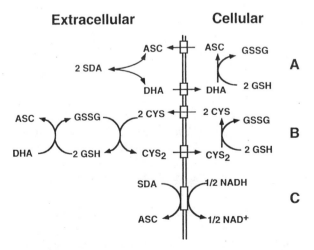

Figure 1 Potential mechanisms for control of extracellular redox status.

redox states of different compartments differ, e.g., the mitochondrial $NADH/NAD^+$ is more reduced than the cytosolic pool (4) and the cytosolic GSH/GSSG is more reduced than the cisternae of the endoplasmic reticulum (14), it appears likely that the concentration and redox state of ASC may differ in various compartments. Moreover, since ASC is sequestered into vesicles where catecholamines, peptide hormones, and collagen are synthesized or processed by ASC-dependent reactions, it appears possible that a large fraction of intracellular ASC may be in organelles rather than in the aqueous cytoplasm in some cells. Indeed, the distribution of ASC in tissues shows that it is highest in secretory cells (13,15). Thus, it appears possible that ASC may be secondary to thiols as an antioxidant in the aqueous cytoplasm of cells but is the most important redox-active component in specific subcellular compartments.

Studies by Meister and collaborators (16) showed that inhibition of GSH synthesis in vivo by administration of buthionine sulfoximine, an inhibitor of this pathway, resulted in decreased tissue ASC and increased lung injury by disruption of lamellar body structure. They found that this injury could be ameliorated by treatment with ASC. Thus, their results suggest that ASC, which is maintained in its reduced state by GSH, is a required component for formation and secretion of surfactant. These findings underscore the important relationship between GSH and ASC in which GSH is an essential component to reduce DHA back to ASC and ASC serves as a reductant for processes which are not kinetically favorable when GSH serves directly as a reductant.

Little is known about the transport systems which move ASC across intracellular membranes. However, secretory vesicles contain a specific cytochrome system which allows transfer of reducing equivalents from cytoplasmic ASC to vesicular semidehydro ascorbate (SDA) without transfer of the carbon skeleton (17). This system contains cytochrome b_{561}, a protein which spans the membrane and catalyzes this transmembranal electron transfer. Since transfer of reducing equivalents across the plasma membrane of some cells also occurs by an NADH-dependent system which reduces extracellular SDA to ASC (12), it appears that transmembranal electron transfer may provide an important and general mechanism for use of cytoplasmic reducing power to maintain ASC in other compartments.

FUNCTIONS OF ASCORBATE IN THE LUNG

The biological functions of ASC range from a rather specific reductant in hydroxylation reactions to an antioxidant which principally functions to prevent reaction inactivation of enzymes as a result of oxidation of an essential metal in a catalytic center of an enzyme and to terminate free radical reactions. The enzyme-catalyzed reactions have been frequently reviewed, as have the functions of ASC as an antioxidant (18,19). The activities are consistent with the generalization that ASC functions along with NADH, NADPH, and GSH as a water-soluble electron carrier which is essential to maintain cellular redox biochemical processes. In this function, ASC principally cycles between ASC and SDA so that it has a somewhat unique role as a le^- carrier in the aqueous environment. Other redox-active components can replace many of these activities to some extent, but this characteristic does not obscure the quantitatively important role of ASC in many le^- transfer reactions in cells.

In the lung, ASC has both extracellular and intracellular functions as an antioxidant, has a critical role in the synthesis and vesicular processing of collagen and surfactant apoproteins, and may have other roles in chemical detoxication, immune function, and redox control of transcription. In its role as an antioxidant, ASC cannot be viewed individually because it functions in concert with GSH, α-tocopherol, and other antioxidants to prevent oxidative damage in the highly oxygenated lung tissue (20). As described later, hyperoxia, asthma, and other conditions with elevated generation of reactive O_2 species result in decreased cellular and extracellular ASC. When oxidant generation exceeds the amount which the detoxication systems can control, extensive oxidation of cellular components results in necrotic cell death and loss of functional alveoli. Exposure to oxidants at concentrations which do not cause acute cell death can nonetheless cause loss of function as a consequence of enhanced utilization and depletion of ASC. Even under conditions where cells do not die, exposure to oxidants can impair hormone-stimulated surfactant secretion and thus limit lung function (21). This loss of function can be prevented by either ASC or GSH.

Ascorbate is used within the endoplasmic reticulum, Golgi apparatus, and related vesicles to support the processing of procollagen that is required for mature collagen secretion (22). Thus, excessive utilization of ASC as an antioxidant can result in loss of ASC and impaired collagen deposition. Because type II cells must reside on collagen type IV matrix to mature into type I cells, impaired deposition of collagen type IV can result in loss of differentiation of type II cells and thus preclude repair and replacement of the pulmonary epithelium.

An additional problem with ASC deficiency occurs as a consequence of failure of protein processing. Surfactant apoproteins A and D have collagen-like domains that require hydroxylation for proper folding and stability (23,24). Decreased ASC can therefore affect the production of these proteins, resulting in deficient surfactant production. Because surfactant turnover is much more rapid than collagen turnover, effects on surfactant production may occur much faster in response to oxidant-induced decreases in ASC or ASC deficiency.

Because ASC is a central redox-active molecule, it may also function in redox control of gene expression (25,26). Substantial changes in total messenger ribonucleic acid (mRNA) levels occur upon ASC repletion in scorbutic guinea pigs. In addition, changes in extracellular redox state affect cell proliferation (7), transcriptional regulation via transcription factors are at least partially under redox control (27,28), and apoptosis is stimulated by oxidants and inhibited by certain reductants and free radical trapping agents (29,30). Thus, variations in ASC or oxidation of ASC can potentially have effects not readily attributed to specific coenzymatic functions.

Finally, ASC may have a general coenzymatic activity in protecting enzymes which function through a free radical mechanism. Many enzymes undergo autooxidation upon purification and require thiols for maintenance of activity (31). Others, such as indoleamine dioxygenase, undergo reaction inactivation because of autooxidation during the reaction cycle (32). Still others, such as some cytochrome P450s, catalyze reactions which occur by a free radical mechanism (33). Ascorbate can function in each of these to preserve enzyme function. However, the latter is particularly important given the high activities of some cytochrome P450s in the lung.

Cytochrome P450 is well known as a family of detoxication enzymes which also have the capability of generating reactive, toxic, mutagenic, and carcinogenic products. One of the well characterized reactions is the formation of a radical product from the $1e^-$ reduction of *tert*-butylhydroperoxide (*t*-BuOOH):

$$tBuOOH + cytP450(Fe^{2+}) \rightarrow tBuO^{\cdot} + {}^{\cdot}OH + cytP450(Fe^{3+})$$

The *t*BuO· rearranges to acetone with the elimination of a methyl radical (34) which can initiate lipid peroxidation and cause extensive oxidative damage. In the presence of ASC, the *t*BuO· largely is reduced to *t*BuOH with generation of SDA (Fig. 2). The SDA is readily

$$\text{1/2 NADPH + ROOH} \xrightarrow{\text{P450}} \text{1/2 NADP}^+ + \text{RO} \cdot + {}^-\text{OH}$$

$$\text{RO} \cdot + \text{ASC} \longrightarrow \text{ROH} + \text{SDA} \cdot$$

$$\text{SDA} \cdot + \text{1/2 NADH} \xrightarrow{\text{SDA R}} \text{ASC} + \text{1/2 NAD}^+$$

Figure 2 Ascorbate as a cofactor for coupled NADPH-, NADH-dependent reduction of peroxides to alcohols in the endoplasmic reticulum. P450, cytochrome P450; SDAR, Semidehydroascorbate reductase; NADPH, reduced nicotinamide-adenine dinucleotide phosphate; NADH, reduced nicotinamide-adenine dinucleotide.

reduced back to ASC by the NADH-dependent SDA reductase in the microsomes. Thus, ASC is a coenzyme for the overall reduction of tBuOOH to tBuOH, a process which effectively prevents release of significant amounts of the reactive t-BuO· radical from the enzyme. Because cytochromes P450 as well as flavoproteins and other enzymes can catalyze free radical formation, ASC can have an important function by preventing release of these radicals from the enzyme active site.

DISORDERS

Asthma

Numerous studies have focused on a link between ASC and vitamin C. In 1803, Reisseissen reported convulsive asthma in patients with scurvy (35). Asthma is defined as a hyper-responsiveness of the tracheobronchial tree resulting in a narrowing of the air passages. In response to extrinsic factors such as allergies, mast cells release mediators such as prostaglandins, leukotrienes, bradykinin, histamine, platelet activating factor, and chemotactic factors. These mediators then lead to bronchoconstriction followed by an inflammatory response. This inflammatory response is characterized by migration and degranulation of eosinophils, releasing major basic protein, eosinophilic cationic protein, and superoxide radicals into the airway. Further obstruction and bronchoconstriction are secondary to eosinophil degranulation.

Guinea pigs on low and ASC-deficient diets for 3–4 weeks developed significant airway hyperresponsiveness to aerosolized histamine (36). In guinea pigs with hyperreactive airways, ASC treatment reduced the airway sensitivity to aerosolized histamine (37). Coadministration of indomethacin, a cyclooxygenase inhibitor, abolished the protective effect of ASC and suggested that the ASC effects were mediated through alteration of prostaglandin metabolism (37). In contrast, another study using scorbutic guinea pigs demonstrated increased airway hyperreactivity but there were no concomitant changes in prostanoid generation or electrophysiological properties of airway smooth muscle (36). However, the possibility of other arachidonic acid metabolic products being generated could not be excluded.

Analysis of the data accumulated in the National Health and Nutrition Examination Survey (NHANES) revealed an association between ASC intake and asthma. Low dietary ASC level was associated with increased bronchitis and wheezing (38) and decreased pulmonary function (39). Reports of plasma ASC content in asthmatics are conflicting. Studies of blood leukocytes and plasma have shown significantly lower concentrations of ASC (40,41). However, there were no significant differences in ASC concentrations of red blood cells from asthmatics (42).

Oral ASC has been reported to reduce the number and severity of attacks in subjects with asthma (43). In human subjects, the intensity and the duration of acute bronchoconstriction induced by methacholine, histamine, or exercise are diminished if subjects receive an oral dose of ASC 1 h before the challenge (44–47). The protective effect of ASC could be blocked by indomethacin treatment (45,46). In human lung parenchymal slices, ASC increased prostaglandin E_2 (PGE$_2$), PGF$_{2\alpha}$, thromboxane B_2, and 6-keto-PGF$_{1\alpha}$ and the accumulation was inhibited by indomethacin (48). These studies support the hypothesis that ASC modulates bronchoconstrictor activity through alteration of prostanoid generation to stimulate synthesis of bronchodilators. This may be particularly important in asthmatic subjects where the ratio of prostaglandin E to F is abnormal (49) and where there is increased sensitivity to aspirin (50).

Other clinical studies have been unable to demonstrate a role for ASC in modulating airway hyperreactivity (51–53). A review of the 20 clinical studies and their outcomes has been presented by Bielory and Gandhi (54) with 11 studies suggesting that 1–2 g of ASC supplements may provide modest protection against airway hyperreactivity. However, the majority of these studies gave ASC for 1 h to 4 days before the airway challenge and studied a small patient pool. Studies of the effects of ASC on polymorphonuclear leukocyte motility demonstrated significant improvement (52,55). This suggests that long-term ASC supplements may be beneficial to asthmatics by reducing infections through increased leukocyte chemotaxis and activation of the C1q complement factor. Additional studies of the effects of short-term and long-term ASC supplements on the antioxidant status of the epithelial lining fluid, the oxygen radical burden, or nitric oxide generation may provide fresh insight into these older studies.

Cigarette Smoke

Cigarette smoke is rich in free radicals and free radical generating compounds which cause pulmonary oxidative injury. This pulmonary injury is potentiated by the infiltration of activated polymorphonuclear leukocytes which release proteolytic enzymes (56) and additional radicals which inactivate important protective proteinase inhibitors (57). In addition to the free radical injury, the smoke can induce formation of multiple nonpolar/aromatic deoxyribonucleic acid (DNA) adducts (58,59). Long-lived free radicals are also present in the tar phase (60). Thus, antioxidants may be important in the prevention of cigarette smoke–induced lung injury. Since ASC is one of the most abundant antioxidants in the epithelial lining fluid (61), it may be particularly important as a modulator of lung injury caused by cigarette smoke.

When compared to those of nonsmokers, the serum ASC concentration (62) and dietary ASC intake (63) are lower in smokers and are proportional to cigarette consumption (64) (Table 1). Increased ASC requirements have been estimated to be 140 mg/d in smokers relative to nonsmokers (recommended dietary allowance [RDA] = 100 mg/day) (65). The plasma ASC concentration of nonsmokers regularly exposed to environmental cigarette smoke (passive smokers) was also significantly decreased when compared to that of nonexposed nonsmokers (66). Severe ASC deficiency (<23 μmol/L of plasma) was observed in 24% of active smokers and 12% of passive smokers compared to no deficiencies in nonexposed nonsmokers (66). This decrease in plasma ASC is in contrast to the increased ASC present in the epithelial lining fluid and alveolar macrophage of smokers when compared to those of nonsmokers (67) (Table 1). This increase suggests that upon exposure to cigarette smoke there is a more rapid metabolism of antioxidants and there is an adaptive defense mechanism to increase the content of ASC and other antioxidants such as GSH content on the alveolar surface to protect the alveolar cells from the radicals (68).

In patients with emphysema or chronic bronchiolitis, low ASC intake was associated with significant loss of pulmonary function (69). Both functional vital capacity and functional expiratory volume are related to smoking history (70). Increasing the ASC intake by one standard deviation was associated with a 25% increase in functional vital capacity and functional expiratory capacity (70). Alternatively, increasing the ASC intake by one standard deviation could prevent the adverse effects of 5–7 pack-years of smoking (70).

One potential mechanism for ASC protection may be through its effects on polymorphonuclear leukocytes. Smokers have significantly higher circulating polymorphonuclear leukocytes than nonsmokers (71). Using leukocytes isolated from human smokers or laboratory animals exposed to cigarette smoke, the effects include increased response to chemotactic stimuli (52), cytokine release (72), release of superoxide anions (73), increased release of elastase (74), and enhanced aggregability (75). In the epithelial lining fluid ASC would then detoxify the oxidant radicals present in cigarette smoke as well as those produced by the polymorphonuclear leukocytes. In addition, extracellular ASC in the range of that present in the epithelial lining fluid can inhibit the release of oxidant radicals by polymorphonuclear leukocytes (76).

The superoxide anion released by polymorphonuclear leukocytes is unstable and dismutes into hydrogen peroxide. Myeloperoxidase, which is released by activated polymorphonuclear leukocytes, utilizes hydrogen peroxide to oxidize chloride ions to hypochlorous acid (HOCl) (77). Oxidants, especially HOCl, can inactive α-1-proteinase inhibitor, a major inhibitor of the elastase released by activated neutrophils. Inactivation of this inhibitor results in degradation of elastin fibers resulting in emphysema. In vitro studies (78) and clinical studies (79) demonstrated that ASC protects α-1-protease inhibitor from this oxidative inactivation.

Cancer

Epidemiological studies have documented an association between cigarette smoke and cancer of the respiratory tract (International Agency for Research on Cancer, 1986). This may be related to the increased oxygen radical production discussed earlier or the formation of aromatic DNA adducts via oxygen radicals (58). In vitro studies demonstrated that preincubation of aqueous cigarette smoke condensate extracts with ASC decreased the extracts' capacity to generate DNA adduct formation (58). Given the role of ASC in decreasing radical formation and propagation in cigarette smoke and the decreased plasma ASC levels in smokers, it is not unreasonable to suggest that ASC may be protective in lung cancer mortality.

Nitric oxide is produced by inflammatory cells and other cells as a physiological response to infection. A variety of other cell types produce nitric oxide as an intercellular second messenger. In addition, nitric oxide is a significant component of many combustion processes such as cigarette smoke. Ubiquitous exposure of humans to endogenous and exogenous nitric oxide may play a significant role in the carcinogenic process through nitrosation of amines (80). Formation of nitration products depends on the presence of oxygen radicals such as superoxide radicals also found in cigarette smoke. Endogenous antioxidants such as that present in the epithelial lining fluid may be particularly important in attenuating some of the adverse effects of excess exposure to nitric oxide (81–83).

Determining the relationship between ASC and lung cancer has been difficult because most of the epidemiological studies have focused on vitamin A or carotenoids and the diet questionnaires were not designed to assess ASC (84,85). But a higher risk of lung cancer is associated with infrequent intake of fruits and vegetables (86). A cohort study of over one million Americans reported that infrequent fruit intake was associated with a higher risk of subsequent lung cancer mortality and this may relate to the ASC intake (87).

In a prospective study in 1960, men aged 40–59 years were followed for 25 years in the Netherlands (88). Ascorbate intake was strongly inversely related to 25-year lung cancer mortality. Vitamin preparation users had a significantly lower risk ratio for 25-year lung cancer mortality than nonsmokers. The survival curve was calculated at different levels of risk factors. A 55-year-old man who smoked one pack of cigarettes a day for 40 years was assessed to have a 25%, 12%, or 7% risk of lung cancer mortality if his ASC intake was in the lowest quartile, highest quartile, or highest quartile plus he took vitamin preparations respectively.

In the Louisiana area, a daily consumption of <90 mg of ASC was associated with a risk estimate of 1.5 ($p < 0.001$) when compared to those who daily consumed greater than 140 mg of ASC (89). The ASC results also suggested an association with squamous and small cell carcinomas but revealed no significant relationship with adenocarcinomas. The ASC effect became stronger after results were adjusted for carotene intake. This is in contrast to the apparent disappearance of the carotene protection when adjusted for ASC intake.

Other studies have suggested a protective effect by ASC but the effects were not statistically significant (90,91). Ascorbate was in the protective direction but was not statistically significant in studies that depended on ASC supplements in the preceding 3 months (92,93) or studies based on a 24-h recall (94). In a recent review of the most well designed and well conducted epidemiological studies, a strong inverse association with ASC was found in only two out of six dietary studies (95). There was only one serum ASC study and no protection was observed. Additional studies examining the relationship between plasma ASC and lung cancer would be useful because they would eliminate the ambiguities associated with assessment of ASC intake through dietary evaluations.

Acute Respiratory Distress Syndrome (ARDS)

In acute respiratory distress syndrome (ARDS), a variety of inflammatory mediators are released, and this acute diffuse inflammatory reaction is important in the lung injury and development of the disease. Polymorphonuclear leukocytes normally constitute approximately 2% of the cells obtained from a bronchoalveolar lavage. But in the first few days of ARDS, the alveoli fill with proteinaceous fluid containing red blood cells, polymorphonuclear leukocytes, macrophages, and cell fragments. The number of polymorphonuclear leukocytes sequestered in the capillaries is markedly increased, and the number of extravasated polymorphonuclear leukocytes in the interstitium and alveoli is increased (96).

As stated, the activated polymorphonuclear leukocyte releases highly reactive oxygen species as well as elastase. The increased oxidant burden in the patient with ARDS is supported by the increased exhalation of hydrogen peroxide when compared to that of the critically ill patient without ARDS (97). The presence of ASC in the epithelial lining fluid may then be particularly important in scavenging the oxidants released by polymorpho-nuclear leukocytes.

In the sheep model of *Escherichia coli* endotoxin–induced ARDS, ASC infusion prevented the expected early phase pulmonary hypertension and increase in pulmonary vascular resistance (98). In the late phase of injury, ASC improved the neutropenia, lung permeability damage, and pulmonary gas exchange associated with ARDS. This improvement may be through increased scavenging of the radicals released by the polymorphonuclear leukocytes (98) or inhibiting of the release of oxidant radicals by polymorphonuclear leukocytes (76). Other mechanisms of protection by ASC may be have been through protection of surfactant which is sensitive to inactivation by HOCl (99) or decreased polymorphonuclear leukocyte–endothelial adherence (100). These results suggest that ASC plays an important modulatory role in the development and severity of this disease process.

SUMMARY

The lung is one of the few organs consistently exposed to relatively high oxygen concentrations and must constantly maintain antioxidant defenses to balance oxidant radical production. An imbalance of oxidant radicals can result from inhaled toxic gases such as oxygen, ozone, nitric oxide, nitrogen dioxide, and cigarette smoke. Excess oxidant radicals can also be generated in disorders resulting in inflammatory cell invasion such as asthma or acute respiratory distress syndrome. Regardless of the cause, the excess generation of oxidant radicals results in pulmonary injury.

As discussed, ASC may be an important modulator of the disease process. Through its role as an antioxidant, it may scavenge free radicals and attenuate lipid peroxidation and thus maintain cellular integrity. This may be through direct scavenging of the radical or through its role in maintenance of other antioxidants such as vitamin E or glutathione in their active forms. Alternatively modulation of oxidant radicals may affect gene expression. Some protection may be through the effects of ASC on the immune system, including stimulation of interferon production and stimulation of complement C1q activity or modulation of polymorphonuclear leukocyte responses. Alternatively, protection may be through the role of ASC on collagen synthesis, basement membrane integrity, and the subsequent role of the basement membrane on cellular differentiation. The role of ASC in the epithelial lining fluid may be particularly important in direct detoxification of the radicals before they reach the cells, decreasing the initial generation of lipid peroxides, buffering the tissue, and buffering the inflammatory cells present in the airspace.

REFERENCES

1. Njus D, Jalukar V, Zu J, et al. Concerted proton-electron transfer between ascorbic acid and cytochrome b561. Am J Clin Nutr 1991; 54:1179S–1183S.
2. Buettner GR, Jurkiewicz BA. Chemistry and biochemistry of ascorbic acid. In: Cadenas E, Packer L, eds. Handbook of Antioxidants. New York: Marcel Dekker, 1996:91–115.
3. Schneider W, Staudinger H. Reduced nicotinamide-adenine dinucleotide-dependent reduction of semidehydroascorbic acid. Biochim Biophys Acta 1965; 96:157–159.
4. Sies H. Nicotinamide nucleotide compartmentation. In: Sies H, eds. Metabolic Compartmentation. New York: Academic Press, 1982:205–231.
5. Winkler BS. Unequivocal evidence in support of the nonenzymatic redox coupling between glutathione/glutathione disulfide and ascorbic acid/dehydroascorbic acid. Biochim Biophys Acta 1992; 1117:287–290.

6. Winkler BS, Orselli SM, Rex TS. The redox couple between glutathione and ascorbic acid: a chemical and physiological perspective. Free Radical Biol Med 1994; 17:333–349.

7. Hwang C, Sinskey AJ. The role of oxidation-reduction potential in monitoring growth of cultured mammalian cells. In: Spier RE, Griffiths JB, Meignier B, eds. Production of Biologicals from Animal Cells in Culture. Oxford: Halley Court, 1991:548–567.

8. Frei B. Ascorbic acid protects lipids in human plasma and low-density lipoprotein against oxidative damage. Am J Clin 1991; 54:1113S–1118S.

9. Slade R, Crissman K, Norwood J, et al. Comparison of antioxidant substances in bronchoalveolar lavage cells and fluid from humans, guinea pigs, and rats. Exp Lung Res 1993; 19:469–484.

10. Rose RC, Bode AM. Biology of free radical scavengers: an evaluation of ascorbate. FASEB J 1993; 7:1135–1142.

11. Dahm LJ, Jones DP. Clearance of glutathione disulfide from rat mesenteric vasculature. Toxicol Appl Pharmacol 1994; 129:272–282.

12. Navas P, Villalba JM, Córdoba F. ASC function at the plasma membrane. Biochim Biophys Acta 1994; 1197:1–13.

13. Moser U. Uptake of ascorbic acid by leukocytes. Ann NY Acad Sci 1987; 498:200–214.

14. Hwang C, Sinskey AJ, Lodish HF. Oxidized redox state of glutathione in the endoplasmic reticulum. Science 1992; 257:1496–1502.

15. Schorah CJ. The transport of vitamin C and effects of disease. Proc Nutr Soc 1992; 51:189–198.

16. Meister A. On the antioxidant effects of ascorbic acid and glutathione. Biochem Pharmacol 1992; 44:1905–1915.

17. Fleming PJ, Kent UM. Cytochrome b561, ascorbic acid, and transmembrane electron transfer. Am J Clin Nutr 1991; 54:1173S–1178S.

18. Sauberlich HE. Pharmacology of vitamin C. (Review). Annu Rev Nutr 1994; 14:371–391.

19. Niki E. Vitamin C as an antioxidant. In: Simopoulos AP, ed. Selected Vitamins, Minerals, and Functional Consequences of Maternal Malnutrition. World Rev Nutr Diet 1991; 64:1–30.

20. Buettner GR. The pecking order of free radicals and antioxidants: lipid peroxidation, a-tocopherol, and ASC. Arch Biochem Biophys 1993; 300:535–543.

21. Brown LA. Glutathione protects signal transduction in type II cells under oxidant stress. Am J Physiol 1994; 266:L172–L177.

22. Fessler JH, Doege KJ, Duncan KG, et al. Biosynthesis of collagen. J Cell Biochem 1985; 28:183–189.

23. Benson B, Hawgood S, Schilling, et al. Structure of canine pulmonary surfactant apoprotein: cDNA and complete amino acid sequence. Proc Natl Acad Sci USA 1985; 82:6379–6383.

24. Persson A, Chang D, Rust K, et al. Purification and biochemical characterization of CP4 (SP-D): a collagenous surfactant-associated protein. Biochemistry 1989; 27:6361–6367.

25. Senoo H, Hata R. Extracellular matrix regulates cell morphology, proliferation, and tissue formation. Kaibogaku Zasshi 1994; 69:719–733.

26. Alcain FJ, Buron MI. ASC on cell growth and differentiation. J Bioenerg Biomembr 1994; 26:393–398.

27. Meyer M, Schreck R, Baeuerle PA. H_2O_2 and antioxidants have opposite effects on activation of NF-kappa B and AP-1 in intact cells: AP-1 as secondary antioxidant-responsive factor. EMBO J 1993; 12:2005–2015.

28. Abate C, Patel L, Rauscher FJ, et al. Redox regulation of fos and jun DNA-binding activity in vitro. Science 1990; 249:1157–1161.

29. Malorni W, Rivabene R, Santini MT, et al. N-acetylcysteine inhibits apoptosis and decreases viral particles in HIV-chronically infected U937 cells. FEBS Lett 1993; 327:75–78.

30. Jones DP, Maellaro E, Jiang S, et al. Effects of N-acetyl-L-cysteine on T-cell apoptosis are not mediated by increased cellular glutathione. Immunol Lett 1995; 45:205–209.

31. Webb JL, ed. Enzyme and Metabolic Inhibitors. New York: Academic Press, 1996.

32. Hirata F, Hayaishi O. Studies on indoleamine 2,3-dioxygenase. I. Superoxide anion as substrate. J Biol Chem 1975; 250:5960–5966.

33. White RE, Coon MJ. Oxygen activation by cytochrome P-450. Annu Rev Biochem 1980; 49: 315–356.
34. Vaz ADN, Coon MJ. Hydrocarbon formation in the reductive cleavage of hydroperoxidase by cytochrome P-450. Proc Natl Acad Sci USA 1987; 84:1172–1176.
35. Spannhake EW, Menkis HA. Vitamin C: new tricks for an old dog (Editorial). Am Rev Respir Dis 1983; 127:139–140.
36. Mohsenin V, Tremmel PG, Rothberg KG, et al. Airway responsiveness and prostaglandin generation in scorbutic guinea pigs. Prostaglandins Leukocyt Essential Fatty Acids 1988; 33: 149–155.
37. Popa V, Douglas JS, Bouhuys A. Airway responses to histamine, acetylcholine, and propranolol in anaphylactic hypersensitivity in guinea pigs. J Allergy Clin Immunol 1973; 51: 344–356.
38. Schwartz J, Weiss ST. Dietary factors and their relationships to respiratory symptoms: NHANES II. Am J Epidemiol 1990; 132:67–76.
39. Schwartz J, Weiss ST. Relationship between dietary vitamin C intake and pulmonary function in the First National Health and Nutrition Examination Survey (NHANES I). Am J Clin Nutr 1994; 59:110–114.
40. Olusi SO, Ojutiku OO, Jessop WJE, Iboko MI. Plasma and white blood cell ascorbic acid concentrations in patients with bronchial asthma. Clin Chem Acta 1979; 92:161–166.
41. Aderele WR, Ette SI, Oduwoule O, Ikpeme SJ. Plasma, vitamin C (ascorbic acid) levels in asthmatic children. Afr J Med Sci 1985; 14:115–120.
42. Powell CVE, Nash AA, Powers HJ, Primhak RA. Antioxidant status in asthma. Pediatr Pulmonol 1994; 18:34–38.
43. Anah CC, Jarike LN, Baig HA. High dose of ascorbic acid in Nigerian asthmatics. Trop Geogr Med 1980; 32:132–137.
44. Zuskin E, Lewis AJ, Bouhuys A. Inhibition of histamine in airway constriction by ascorbic acid. J Allergy Clin Immunol 1973; 51:218–226.
45. Mohsenin V, DuBois AB, Douglas JS. Effect of ascorbic acid on response to methacholine challenge in asthmatic subjects. Am Rev Respir Dir 1983; 127:143–147.
46. Ogilvy CS, DuBois AB, Douglas JS. Effect of ascorbic acid and indomethacin on the airways of healthy male subjects with or without induced bronchoconstriction. J Allergy Clin Immunol 1981; 67:363–369.
47. Schachter EN, Schlesinger A. The attenuation of exercise-induced bronchospasm by ascorbic acid. Ann Allergy 1982; 49:146–151.
48. Fann Y-D, Rothberg KG, Tremmel PG, et al. Ascorbic acid promotes prostanoid release in human lung parenchyma. Prostaglandins 1986; 31:361–368.
49. Allegra J, Trautlein J, Demers L, et al. Peripheral plasma determinations of prostaglandin E in asthmatics. J Allergy Clin Immunol 1975; 58:546–550.
50. McDonald JR, Mathison DA, Stevenson DD. Aspirin intolerance in asthma. J Cell Clin Immunol 1972; 50:198–205.
51. Ting S, Mansfield LE, Varbrough J. Effect of ascorbic acid on pulmonary functions in mild asthma. J Asthma 1983; 20:39–42.
52. Anderson R, Hay I, VanWyk HA, Theron A. Ascorbic acid in bronchial asthma. S Afr Med J 1983; 63:649–652.
53. Kreisman H, Mitchell C, Bouhuys A. Inhibition of histamine-induced airway constriction-negative results with oxtriphylline and ascorbic acid. Lung 1977; 154:223–229.
54. Bielory L, Gandhi R. Asthma and vitamin C. Ann Allergy 1994; 73:89–96.
55. Boxer LA, Watanabe AM, Rister M. Correction of leukocyte function in Chediak-Higashi Syndrome by ascorbate. N Engl J Med 1976; 295:1041–1045.
56. McGowan SE, Hunninghake GW. Neutrophils and emphysema. N Engl J Med 1989; 321:968–970.
57. Johnson D, Travis J. The oxidative inactivation of human alpha-1-proteinase inhibitor. J Biol Chem 1979; 254:4022–4026.

58. Randerath E, Danna TF, Randerath K. DNA damage induced by cigarette smoke condensate in vitro as assayed by ^{32}P-postlabeling. comparison with cigarette smoke–associated DNA adduct profiles in vivo. Mutat Res 1992; 268:139–153.

59. Geneste O, Camus A-M, Castegnaro S, et al. Comparison of pulmonary DNA adduct levels measured by ^{32}P-postlabeling and aryl hydrocarbon hydroxylase activity in lung parenchyma of smokers and ex-smokers. Carcinogenesis 1991; 12:1301–1305.

60. Pryor WA. Biological effects of cigarette smoke, wood smoke and the smoke from plastics: the use of electron spin resonance. Free Radical Biol Med 1992; 13:659–676.

61. Slade R, Crissman K, Norwood J, Hatch G. Comparison of antioxidant substances in broncho-alveolar lavage cells and fluid from humans, guinea pigs and rats. Exp Lung Res 1993; 19: 469–484.

62. Mahalko JR, Johnson LK, Gallagher SK, Milne DB. Comparison of dietary histories and seven day food records in a nutritional assessment of older adults. Am J Clin Nutr 1985; 42:542–553.

63. Bolton-Smith C, Casey CE, Gey KF, et al. Antioxidant vitamin status intake assessed using a food frequency questionnaire: correlation of biochemical markers in smokers and nonsmokers. Br J Nutr 1991; 65:337–346.

64. Pelletier O. Vitamin C and tobacco. Int J Vitam Nutr Res Suppl 1977; 16:147–170.

65. Schechtman G, Byrd JC, Hoffman R. Ascorbic acid requirements for smokers: analysis of a population survey. Am J Clin Nutr 1991; 53:1466–1470.

66. Tribble DL, Giuliano LJ, Fortmann SP. Reduced plasma ascorbic acid concentrations in nonsmokers regularly exposed to environmental tobacco smoke. Am J Clin Nutr 1993; 58: 886–890.

67. Bui MH, Sauty A, Collet F, Leuenberger P. Dietary vitamin C intake and concentrations in the body fluids and cells of male smokers and nonsmokers. J Nutr 1992; 122:312–316.

68. Kallner AB, Hartmann D, Hornig DH. On the requirements of ascorbic acid in man and steady-state turnover and body pool in smokers. Am J Clin Nutr 1981; 34:1347–1355.

69. Stachan DP, Cox BD, Erzinclioglu SW, et al. Ventilatory function and winter fresh fruit consumption in a random sample of British adults. Thorax 1991; 46:624–629.

70. Britton JR, Pavord ID, Richards KA, et al. Dietary antioxidant vitamin intake and lung function in the general population. Am J Respir Crit Care Med 1995; 151:1383–1387.

71. Friedman GD, Siegelaub AB, Seltzer CC, et al. Smoking habits and the leukocyte count. Arch Environ Health 1971; 26:137–143.

72. Tappia PS, Troughton KL, Langley-Evans SC, Grimble RF. Cigarette smoking influences cytokine production and antioxidant defenses. Clin Sci 1995; 88:485–489.

73. Anderson R. Assessment of the roles of vitamin C, vitamin E and β-carotene in the modulation of oxidant stress mediated by cigarette smoke-activated phagocytes. Am J Clin Nutr 1991; 53:358S–361S.

74. Blue ML, Janoff A. Possible mechanisms of emphysema in cigarette smokers: release of elastase from human polymorphonuclear leukocytes by cigarette smoke condensate in vitro. Am Rev Respir Dis 1978; 117:317–325.

75. Lehr H-A. Adhesion-promoting effects of cigarette smoke on leukocytes and endothelial cells. Ann NY Acad Sci 1993; 686:112–118.

76. Anderson R, Theron AJ, Ras GJ. Regulation by the antioxidants ascorbate, cysteine, and dapsone of the increased extracellular and intracellular generation of reactive oxidants by activated phagocytes from cigarette smokers. Am Rev Respir Dis 1987; 135:1027–1032.

77. van Antwerpen L, Theron AJ, Myer MS, et al. Cigarette smoke-mediated oxidant stress, phagocytes, vitamin C, vitamin E and tissue injury. Ann NY Acad Sci 1993; 686:53–65.

78. Nowak D, Piasecka G, Antczak A, Pietras T. Effect of ascorbic acid on hydroxyl radical generation by chemical, enzymatic and cellular systems: importance for antioxidant prevention of pulmonary emphysema. Biomed Biochim Acta 1991; 50:265–272.

79. Theron AJ, Anderson R. Investigation of the effects of oral administration of ascorbate on the functional activity of serum α-1-protease inhibitor and oxidant release by blood phagocytes

from cigarette smokers in a placebo controlled, doubleblind, crossover trial. Int J Vitam Nutr Res 1988; 58:218–224.

80. Arroyo PL, Hatch-Pigott V, Mower NF, Cooney RV. Mutagenicity of nitric oxide and its inhibition by antioxidants. Mutat Res 1992; 281:193–202.

81. d'Ischia M, Costantini C. Nitric oxide-induced nitration of catecholamine neurotransmitters: a key to neuronal degeneration? Bioorg Med Chem 1995; 3:923–927.

82. Eiserich JP, van der Vliet A, Handelman GJ, et al. Dietary antioxidants and cigarette smoke-induced biomolecular damage: a complex interaction. Am J Clin Nutr 1995; 62:1490S–1500S.

83. Grisham MB, Ware K, Gilleland HE Jr, et al. Neutrophil-mediated nitrosoamine formation: a role of nitric oxide in rats. Gastroenterology 1992; 103:1260–1266.

84. Byers T, Perry G. Dietary carotenes, vitamin C, and vitamin E as protective antioxidants in human cancers. Annu Rev Nutr 1992; 12:139–159.

85. Block G. Vitamin C and cancer prevention: the epidemiologic evidence. Am J Clin Nutr 1991; 53:270S–282S.

86. Knekt P, Jarvinen R, Seppanen R, et al. Dietary antioxidants and the risk of lung cancer. Am J Epidemiol 1991; 134:471–479.

87. Long-de W, Hammond EC. Lung cancer, fruit, green salad and vitamin pills. Clin Med J 1985; 98:206–210.

88. Kromhout D. Essential micronutrients in relation to carcinogenesis. Am J Clin Nutr 1987; 45:1361–1367.

89. Fontham ETH, Pickle LW, Haenszel W, et al. Dietary vitamins A and C and lung cancer risk in Louisiana. Cancer 1988; 62:2267–2273.

90. Kvale G, Bjelke E, Gart JJ. Dietary habits and lung cancer risk. Int J Cancer 1983; 31:397–405.

91. Bjelke E. Dietary vitamin A and human lung cancer. Int J Cancer 1975; 15:561–565.

92. Hinds MW, Kolonel LN, Hankin JH, Lee J. Dietary vitamin A, carotene, vitamin C and risk of lung cancer in Hawaii. Am J Epidemiol 1984; 119:227–237.

93. Kolonel LN, Hinds, MW, Nomura AMY, et al. Relationship of dietary vitamin A and ascorbic acid intake to the risk for cancers of the lung, bladder and prostate in Hawaii. Natl Cancer Inst Monogr 1985; 69:137–142.

94. Shekelle RB, Lepper M, Liu S, et al. Dietary vitamin A and risk of cancer in the Western Electric study. Lancet 1981; 2:1185–1190.

95. Flagg EW, Coates RJ, Greenberg RS. Epidemiologic studies of antioxidants and cancer in humans. J Am College Nutr 1995; 14:419–427.

96. Weiland JE, David WB, Holter JF, et al. Lung neutrophils in the adult respiratory distress syndrome: clinical and pathophysiologic significance. Am Rev Respir Dis 1986; 133: 218–225.

97. Kietzmann D, Kahl R, Müller M, et al. Hydrogen peroxide in expired breath condensate of patients with acute respiratory failure and with ARDS. Intensive Care Med 1993; 19:78–81.

98. Dwenger A, Pape HC, Bantel C, et al. Ascorbic acid reduces the endotoxin-induced lung injury in awake sheep. Eur J Clin Invest 1994; 24:229–235.

99. Merritt TA, Amirkhanian JD, Helbock H, et al. Reduction of the surface-tension-lowering ability of surfactant after exposure to hypochlorous acid. Biochem J 1993; 295:19–22.

100. Jonas E, Dwenger A, Hager A. In vitro effect of ascorbic acid on endothelial cell interaction. J Biolumin Chemilumin 1993; 8:15–20.

101. Cantin AM, North SL, Hubbard RC, Crystal RG. Normal alveolar epithelial lining fluid contains high levels of glutathione. J Appl Physiol 1987; 63:152–157.

102. Linden M, Håkansson L, Ohlsson K, et al. Glutathione in bronchoalveolar lavage fluid from smokers is related to humoral markers of inflammatory cell activity. Inflammation 1989; 13: 651–658.

103. Pacht ER, Kaseki H, Mohammed JR, et al. Deficiency of vitamin E in the alveolar fluid of cigarette smokers: influence on alveolar macrophage cytotoxicity. J Clin Invest 1986; 77: 789–796.

15

Vitamin C and Asthma

GARY E. HATCH

U.S. Environmental Protection Agency, Durham, North Carolina

INTRODUCTION

In spite of general health improvements in the population, the prevalence of asthma appears to have risen in recent years. During the period of 1982 to 1992, physician-diagnosed asthma in the United States increased by 58% (from 40.1 to 63.4 cases/1000) in people under the age of 18 (1). For ages 18–44 (same period) asthma prevalence increased by 55%, and for ages 45–65, by 24%. The same trend of increasing asthma over time has been reported in the United Kingdom, New Zealand, Australia, Finland, and Sweden (2,2a). Migration from subsistence societies to economically developed countries appears to be associated with an increased prevalence of asthma (3,4). Increased asthma in youth appears to persist into adulthood. Only 15% of women and 28% of men appear to "outgrow" childhood asthma (5). Recent studies suggest that asthma begins in early childhood with a higher incidence and earlier onset in males (6).

Asthma has a broad definition and is a complex disease involving several subtypes. Clinical symptoms include wheezing, chest tightness, and recurrent cough. More definitive measures include changes in maximal expiratory flow or airway resistance after exposure to nebulized bronchoconstrictors, increased blood eosinophil counts and immunoglobulin E (IgE) concentrations, and airway inflammation and hypersecretion of mucus (7). Most asthma (especially in the young) has a definite allergic basis (extrinsic or allergic asthma), whereas some cases have no apparent cause. In allergic asthma, inhalation of an antigen and both acute and delayed phases of response are known to be important. Strategies for the prevention of asthma have been classed as "primary" (prevention of development) and "secondary" (decreasing severity of asthmatic episodes) (8). Most work to date has focused on secondary rather than primary prevention strategies.

As reasons for increased asthma prevalence are sought, it is natural to suspect diet and environmental pollutants. The realization that oxidants and mutagens are commonly encountered in food and air and are endogenously produced has led to an increased interest in antioxidants (9). This interest is enhanced by the realization that even in developed countries, there appear to be deficits in consumption of foods containing antioxidants (10). The increased appreciation for the role of antioxidants in lung defenses (11) provides a backdrop for the question, Could deficiencies in vitamin C and perhaps other dietary antioxidants contribute to asthma? This chapter will examine recent research relating asthma, inhaled oxidant pollutants, internally generated oxidants, and dietary vitamin C. We examined some aspects of this topic in another publication (12). A review of the therapeutic value of C supplements in ongoing asthmatics (13) and a short review paper examining possible contributions of environmental pollution, allergen challenge, genetics, and diet to asthma (2,2a) have been published.

Vitamin C is one of the most abundant antioxidant substances in the extracellular lining fluid of the human as well as animal lung (14), and it appears to function both as a water-soluble oxidant scavenger and as a regenerating agent for vitamin E (15). The underlying hypothesis being explored in this chapter is that oxidative stress is a contributor to asthma, that C can function as an antioxidant against both environmental and endogenously generated oxidants, and that C is sometimes rate-limiting in people at developmental stages of asthma or during asthma attacks. For reasons that will become apparent, it is difficult to dissociate the discussion of vitamin C and asthma from a discussion of inhaled oxidants including cigarette smoke and common outdoor and indoor air pollutants.

ENVIRONMENTAL OXIDANTS AND ASTHMA

Cigarette Smoke

Epidemiological links between passive smoke exposure and asthma provide some of the best evidence for an environmental oxidant component of asthma which could theoretically be reduced by C. For example, in children of smoking mothers asthma is 2.6 times as likely to develop in the first year of life (16). Active smoking probably constitutes the largest inhaled oxidant challenge from an environmental source that is commonly encountered in humans. Mainstream and sidestream cigarette smoke contains nitrogen oxides at concentrations as high as 300 ppm, and long-lived free radicals are also present in the tar phase (17). Cigarette smoke exposure of human blood plasma in vitro causes rapid oxidation of the C present and a slower oxidation of vitamin E (18). After the degradation of C by smoke, lipid peroxidation in the plasma is initiated and becomes greater with time of exposure. Evidence that smoking exerts an oxidative load in vivo in humans includes the finding of increased ethane in exhaled breath of smokers (19).

Smokers have higher airway reactivity when challenged with bronchoconstrictors than nonsmokers although this effect requires many years to develop (20–22). Airway hyper-responsiveness does not appear to be a problem in adult smokers or in healthy adult nonsmokers after smoking their first cigarette (23,24). A cumulative smoking history is usually necessary in adults for development of asthma symptoms (25).

In contrast to the relative insensitivity of adults to mainstream cigarette smoke, infants and children appear to be very sensitive to passive smoke. Out of 11 epidemiological studies performed between 1987 and 1993 comparing children of smokers with children of non-smokers, 8 showed significant increases in one or more of the following: prevalence of asthma, emergency room visits for asthma, bronchial responsiveness to cold air, asthma symptoms score, parental reports of asthma, and physician diagnoses of asthma (26,27). Numbers of children included in each study ranged from 191 to 3482, and ages ranged from

0 to 21 years. More recent studies report the significance of maternal smoking on wheezing in children (28,29). Some of these effects appear to arise from preexisting abnormalities of respiratory function associated with in utero exposure to tobacco smoke products (30). In one study, asthmatic children of smoking mothers were found to be four times more responsive to histamine aerosol than asthmatic children of nonsmoking mothers (31). In another, an association was found between maternal smoking and degree of broncho-constriction provoked by inhalation of subfreezing air (32). A study of 9-year-old Italian children (87 girls, 85 boys) showed a marked increase in carbachol responsiveness among boys of smoking parents (33). Girls were only slightly affected. Studies published since the review cited (26) seem to bear out the same conclusions. An investigation of 2765 children from rural regions of Australia showed an association among airway responsiveness to histamine, passive smoke exposure, and respiratory infection (34). A report from the United Kingdom showed that parental smoking increased the prevalence of asthma in children aged 3–10 (35). It has been suggested that exposure to smoke is not causal but may be a modifier of the severity of asthma in children with preexisting tendencies toward this disorder (27). For example, blood IgE levels in newborns appear to be associated with development of asthma and other atopic diseases by later childhood (36,37).

Immunoglobulin E–mediated reactions appear to be involved in a large proportion of asthma cases (38). Elevated eosinophil counts in blood may also indicate the presence of allergic reactions in asthmatics. Active smokers have higher serum IgE and blood eosino-phil counts than nonsmokers (26). Children of smoking parents have higher serum IgE levels and higher eosinophil counts than children of nonsmoking parents (39). Immediate skin sensitivity to respirable antigens also correlates with asthma. Children of smoking parents have elevated skin prick sensitivity to a battery of inhaled antigens, and this effect appears to be related to the total number of cigarettes smoked by the parents (33).

Possible reasons for the apparent association between asthma symptoms and passive cigarette smoke exposure are obscured by the high incidence of respiratory infections also reported in children of smoking parents. Fifteen studies published between 1969 and 1992 originating from several countries all link parental smoking with increased incidence and severity of respiratory infections in their children (26). An additional 15 studies link parental smoking to middle ear infections in children (26). Effects of smoke exposure on infections appear to be greatest in infants aged 3 months or less with a trend of decreasing susceptibility up to school age. Several studies published prior to 1983 as well as more recent reports show that lower respiratory tract illnesses occurring early in life are associ-ated with a significantly higher prevalence of asthma and other chronic respiratory diseases at later ages (40).

Environmental Air Pollutants

Controlled studies of school age children and adults exposed to low concentrations of the oxidant gases ozone and nitrogen dioxide (NO_2) have shown at least mildly increased asthmalike symptoms. Numerous studies show that ozone and NO_2 exposure of exercising normal or asthmatic adults causes a transient increase in both basal airway constriction and responsiveness to inhaled bronchoconstrictors (41,42). Although increases in responsive-ness due to oxidant exposures in asthmatics are modest, they add to a much higher than normal background and thus are more critical.

Associations between oxidant air pollutant exposure and asthma have been described (43). The frequency of severe asthma and allergy attacks is strongly associated with spikes in air pollutant levels (44,45). A recent study of nonsmoking men living in different locations in California found an increased risk of asthma that correlated with average concentrations of ozone in the different localities (46). Increases in childhood asthma have been particularly marked among black children from low-income families. A study of such children in a large U.S. city suggested that ozone pollution of indoor air in homes without air conditioning may be involved in asthma (47). In another study, people living close to a major highway (a source of NO_2 and other pollutants) suffered more frequent and severe allergic reactions than cohorts living 5 miles away from the highway, although they had comparable exposures to airborne pollen (48). A German study showed an association between decreased lung function and combined indoor and outdoor NO_2 exposure in asthmatic children (49). Australian children (aged 3–4 years) had an increased prevalence of asthma, wheezing, and other respiratory symptoms when living in homes where parents smoked or where unvented natural gas was used for cooking (50).

ENDOGENOUS OXIDANTS AND ASTHMA

The potential contribution of oxidants from activated leukocytes to the asthmatic state is receiving increased attention. Infection as well as inhaled pollutants can activate leukocytes to produce oxidants. Barnes (51) proposed a self-perpetuating interaction involving over-production of oxidants by leukocytes in asthma on the basis of the following evidence: Eosinophils appear to play a critical role in asthma because their presence in bronchoalveo-lar lavage and blood is associated with bronchial hyperresponsiveness (52). Eosinophils, alveolar macrophages, and neutrophils from asthmatics produce higher levels of reactive oxygen species (superoxide, hydrogen peroxide, hypohalides, etc.) than those from normal subjects (53–57). The significance of the oxidative challenge accompanying acute allergic reactions has recently been demonstrated in guinea pigs (58). The challenge exposure in sensitized guinea pigs induced a large increase in eosinophils and lipid peroxidation products in bronchoalveolar lavage fluid and a decrease in vitamins C and E in the same fluid. In another report, a challenge exposure to antigen in sensitized dogs caused increased production of oxygen radicals in bronchoalveolar lavage cells (59).

Reactive oxygen species directly contract airway smooth muscle preparations, and this effect is enhanced when the epithelium is injured or removed (51). These findings might provide a mechanistic link between epithelial injury arising from a variety of causes and airway hyperresponsiveness. Reactive oxygen species also appear to stimulate histamine release from mast cells and mucus secretion from airway epithelial cells directly (60,61). It has been suggested that airway epithelial cells may respond to oxidant pollutants by the activation of transcription factors, such as nuclear factor kappa B, resulting in increased transcription of genes for certain cytokines (interleukin 8, etc.) and inflammatory enzymes (inducible NO synthase and cyclooxygenase), which might contribute in ways as yet not clearly defined to asthmatic symptoms (62). The induction of NO synthase in asthma has received increased attention because asthmatics have been shown to exhale greater amounts of NO than normal individuals (63). In this respect, asthma may be similar to some infections and inflammatory conditions (64).

VITAMIN C AND ASTHMA: HUMAN STUDIES

Lung Function and Vitamin C Status

Although an association between scurvy and "convulsive" asthma was reported in 1803 (65) and a report on the effect of nutrition on asthma appeared in 1953 (66), it has been only recently that the possible association between intake of vitamin C and lung disease has been studied seriously. In a prospective study from the Netherlands, solid fruit in the diet was found to be inversely associated with the 25-year risk for contracting asthma, chronic bronchitis, or emphysema (67). Analysis of data from the U. S. National Health and Nutrition Examinations showed an association between low dietary C intake and pulmonary function impairments including bronchitis and wheezing (68,69). A diet low in C, assessed by 24-h recall of foods eaten, correlated with decreased pulmonary function, suggesting that choice of foods poor in C may predispose to asthma. Likewise, low serum C level was found to correlate with increased wheezing and bronchitis. The correlations observed appear to be independent of smoking status, age, and numerous other confounding variables. A recent study from the United Kingdom showed that a 40-mg/day higher dietary intake of C was associated with a 25-ml higher forced expiratory volume (per second) in 2633 subjects aged 18 to 70 (70). Ironically, a study of 78,000 nurses in the United States published at the same time showed increased asthma symptoms associated with the use of vitamin C and E supplements (71). The latter study might be unusual in that nurses are known to have a higher background C consumption than the general population, and that it was found that the nurses were treating themselves with vitamin supplements when respiratory symptoms appeared. A recent study of 96 British men and women aged 65–74 reported a positive correlation between serum C, serum levels of acute phase proteins and hemostatic factors, and forced expiratory volume in 1 s (71a).

Plasma C in Asthmatics

Asthmatics have been reported to have lower than normal concentrations of C in plasma and blood leukocytes. One study examining 62 asthmatic and 57 normal adults of both sexes showed 35% and 50% lower concentrations of C in blood leukocytes and plasma of asthmatics, respectively (72). Another study comparing 51 asthmatic children with matched controls showed significantly lower plasma C concentrations in asthmatics, although the C concentration did not correlate with severity of the asthma or with the diagnosis of atopy (73). The reason for the lower C in asthmatics is not known. It may be the result of increased oxidant generation or it may be a symptom of other complex factors that predispose to asthma.

Therapeutic Efficacy of C in Asthmatics

Supplementation of asthmatics with C has been examined in several studies and recently reviewed (13). Since 1973, 12 studies have reported giving vitamin C supplements to asthmatic and normal subjects and examining respiratory symptoms (74–85) (Table 1). Half of these studies showed significant improvements in respiratory measurements. The combined number of subjects in all of these studies is quite small: 158 total, 60% of which were in the positive studies. Supplementation usually amounted to 0.5 to 2 g of C/day, often administered within 3 h of bronchoconstrictor challenge and/or pulmonary function assessments. The results suggest the potential for a modest effect of high-level supplementation of C in reversing hyperresponsiveness and other symptoms of ongoing asthma. Reasons for differences between the studies could have been differences between the baseline C status of the subjects prior to supplementation or the existence of other nonoxidant factors in mediating the responses. Only two of the studies measured the plasma C levels before and after supplementation. The fact that the supplemented level of C is so high and given in spikes leaves questions as to whether the high C values in plasma actually reflect the C levels in the respiratory tissues. It is interesting to note that three of the studies showing

Table 1 Studies on Effects of Ascorbate Supplementation on Respiratory Measurements in Asthmatics

Study	Ascorbate effect	Ascorbate dose	Design	Type	Population	Respiratory measurement[a]	Results
Zuskin et al. 1973[74]	+	0.5 g oral 3–6 h before challenge	Longitudinal Prospective Interventional	Single-blinded Randomized	Healthy adults $n = 17$	Histamine bronchoprovocation PFTs (PEFV)	Ascorbic acid had a protective effect on histamine-induced bronchospasm
Kreisman et al. 1977[75]	0	0.5 g oral 4 per day 3 treatments over 2–6 months	Longitudinal Prospective Interventional	Double-blinded Randomized Controlled	Asthmatic adults $n = 7$	Histamine bronchoprovocation FVC; FEV_1; TLC	Ascorbic acid did not exert a protective effect against histamine-induced airway construction
Kordansky et al. 1979[76]	0	0.5 d/day for 1 week then 3 h before challenge	Longitudinal Prospective Interventional	Double-blinded Randomized Controlled	Ragweed sensitive asthmatics $n = 6$	Bronchial provocation (airway resistance and conductance); FEV_1; PD_{20}; FEV_1	Ascorbic acid ingestion did not affect FEV_1, and did not protect against ragweed antigen–induced bronchospasm
Anah et al. 1980[77]	+	1 g/day orally for up to 14 weeks	Longitudinal Prospective Interventional	Double-blinded Randomized Controlled	Asthmatics $n = 41$	Severity and frequency of asthma attacks; plasma ascorbic acid levels	Vitamin C ingestion led to a decrease in number of asthma attacks (possibly via a decrease in number of respiratory infections)
Ogilvy et al. 1981[78]	+	1 g C orally 3–4 h before challenge	Longitudinal Prospective Interventional	Single-blinded Cross-over	Healthy male adults $n = 6$	Airway tone Bronchoconstriction (intensity and duration)	Methacholine–induced bronchoconstriction decreased with prior ascorbic acid intake; Indomethacin blocked this effect
Anderson et al. 1982[79]	0	IV injection of 1 g C, 2.5 h before challenge	Longitudinal Prospective Interventional	Single-blinded Randomized Controlled	Asthmatic children $n = 16$	Flow volume curve; Immunoglobulins Complement levels	Ascorbic acid ingestion did not affect flow volume: intravenous ascorbic acid did not affect exercise-induced asthma in 10 subjects

Study	Effect	Design	Control/Blinding	Dose	Subjects	Measurements	Results
Schachter and Schlesinger 1982[80]	+	Observational Longitudinal Prospective Interventional	Double-blinded Randomized Controlled	0.5 g C, 1.5 h prior to exercise	Asthmatics $n = 12$	Exercise induced bronchospasm: PFT's (PEFR, MEFV, FVC, FEV$_1$)	Ascorbic acid exerted a partial antibronchospastic action
Fortner et al. 1982[81]	0	Longitudinal Prospective Interventional	Double-blinded Randomized Controlled	0.25 to 1.0 g, 4× per day, 3 days	Adults with seasonal allergic rhinitis $n = 8$	Cutaneous reactivity Nasal airway resistance; Urine ascorbic acid levels; Skin tests to antigen, histamine and morphone	Ascorbic acid had no significant effect on skin testing to antigen or on nasal airway resistance
Mohsenin et al. 1983[82]	+	Longitudinal Prospective Interventional	Single-blinded Controlled	1 g oral immediately prior to methacholine	Asthmatics $n = 14$	Methacholine challenge: Airway resistance and conductance; PFTs (FEV$_1$, VC, TLC, RV); PD$_{40}$ with methacholine	After oral ascorbic acid ingestion, 11 of 14 patients had a decreased response to methacholine challenge; indomethacin ingestion blocked this effect
Ting et al. 1983[83]	0	Longitudinal Prospective Interventional	Uncontrolled	0.5 g, 4 times/day 3 days plus 1 dose immediately before	Asthmatic adults $n = 20$	Pulmonary functions (PVC, FEV$_1$, FEF$_{25-75}$, PEFR)	Ascorbic acid ingestion did not effect pulmonary function measurements
Kawane et al. 1985[84]	+	Longitudinal Prospective Interventional	Unblinded Non-randomized	1 g oral 2 h prior	Healthy adults $n = 5$	Methacholine challenge; FEV MEFV, FVC, FEV$_1$; Ascorbic acid serum levels	Ascorbic acid exerted some effect against response to methacholine challenge in some of the subjects
Malo et al. 1986[85]	0	Longitudinal Prospective Interventional	Double-blinded Randomized Cross-over	1 g/day 1 h prior	Asthmatic adults $n = 16$	Histamine bronchoprovocation (FEV$_1$, FVC, PD$_{20}$ of histamine)	Ascorbic acid therapy did not reveal a significant change in FEV$_1$, or in histamine response

[a]Source: Adapted from Ref. 13.

PFT, pulmonary function test; FVC, forced vital capacity; TLC, total lung capacity; PEFV, partial expiratory flow volume; FEFR, forced expiratory flow resistance; RV, residual volume; FEV$_1$, forced expiratory volume in 1 s; PD$_{20}$, dose causing 20% increase in airway resistance; MEFV, mean expiratory flow volume.

positive effects of C involved methacholine-induced bronchoconstriction, and that the improvement due to C was abolished by indomethacin in two of these studies (78,82). The influence of C on cyclooxygenase pathways has been reviewed (82). Studies in guinea pigs suggest that higher levels of C might shift the metabolism of arachidonic acid away from the synthesis of bronchoconstrictors such as $PGF_{2\alpha}$ toward the synthesis of bronchodilators such as PGE_2 (86). The chemical basis for such a shift is not yet clear.

SMOKING AND VITAMIN C STATUS

Increased asthma could in part by caused by inadequate dietary C or other antioxidants, coupled with exposure to oxidant pollutants or inflammatory generation of endogenous oxidants. For example, increased asthma in smokers and their children could have some of its basis in low C status. Several studies have reported lower plasma C concentrations in smokers than nonsmokers (87). The most likely reason for this is that the oxidant burden of the smoke inhalation causes a mobilization of C to the lung from the plasma (15). There is also a net increase in the total body catabolism of C in smokers (88). In addition to this direct effect, there is an unexplained shift in dietary preferences induced by smoking (89). It is likely that lower plasma C in smoking mothers would be passed on to their children during pregnancy and lactation. Thereafter, altered food preferences of the parents might continue to influence the children's diet. Few investigators have addressed this problem. A study of 200 Austrian mothers and their newborns which measured umbilical cord blood and newborn plasma C concentrations suggested that smoking caused low C concentrations in both mothers and infants (90).

ESTABLISHING OPTIMAL VITAMIN C INTAKE

Vitamin C intake in the nonsmoking population may give less than optimal protection against environmental pollutants as a result of (1) inadequacy of recommended daily allowances (RDAs) and (2) low compliance with RDAs. The present U.S. RDA for C (60 mg for adults) was determined in 1980 with a later (1989) revision added to increase the RDA for smokers to 100 mg (91,92). A recent study has recommended that the RDA be increased to 200 mg/day (92a). The present RDA is based largely on incomplete or inadequate information on the rates of C catabolism with supplementary information from pharmacokinetic studies involving injections of radiolabeled C (88,93). These studies attempted to generate estimates of the total body pool of C and also of the rates of catabolism. One concern about the adequacy of the 60-mg/day RDA is that it is based on estimates of C catabolism in C-deficient subjects. Since C deficiency appears to lower the rate of C catabolism, the RDA appears to understate the requirement (94). The most recent study recommending the 200-mg/day RDA (92a) provides data from several doses in a broad dose range from subjects on a well controlled diet. Information remains incomplete for women, ill patients, smokers, and the elderly. There is also no consensus as to which biological function is most sensitive to less than optimal dietary levels of C (94). Whereas the previous studies have focused mostly on prevention of scurvy, a reevaluation based on protection from insults from environmental or endogenous oxidants is needed (2). None of the human subjects in any of the pharmacokinetic studies involving establishment of the RDA has been exposed to exogenous or endogenous oxidant stresses such as might be encountered in everyday life. Another point of confusion in the establishment of the RDA has been the total body pool size of C. The fact that increased excretion of C occurs at higher pool sizes has sometimes discouraged efforts to increase the pool size beyond a certain point. However, higher tissue concentrations of C and the greatest beneficial effect might only be achievable at pool sizes where considerable C excretion occurs. Indeed, the 200-mg/day RDA intake is associated with about a 50% fractional excretion (fraction of a single dose excreted) into the urine (92a).

Aside from the inadequacy of the RDA, an even more important issue is that of compliance with it. A recent analysis of NHANES II data (1976–1980) on >11,000 U.S. adults showed that the actual consumption of C did not meet the RDA in the case of 43% of nonsmokers and 72% of smokers (95).

Supplementation of heavy smokers may represent a unique case requiring special consideration because of the complex changes induced by smoking. The same study cited earlier (95) showed that when smokers consumed the RDA for C, their plasma levels of C remained below those of nonsmokers. In fact, the RDA appeared to provide less than half of the amount of C required to achieve the plasma levels found in nonsmokers. Another study showed that in active smokers, high C supplementation paradoxically caused greater airway responsiveness than was present before supplementation (96). Studies in guinea pigs suggest a biphasic response to histamine challenge, with mild deficiencies causing increased responsiveness and more severe deficiencies showing decreased responsiveness (97). Other issues of concern include the possibility of a prooxidant effect of C supplementation. Patients with sepsis syndrome are similar to patients with asthma in that they have low plasma C levels and increased NO exhalation. The fact that these patients also have increased plasma "free" iron levels (98) raises concern that asthmatics may as well. Cautions have been raised about excess C supplementation during iron overload stemming from prooxidant effects observed in vitro with this couplet as well as clinical data from intravenous (IV) infusion of C (99,100).

POSSIBLE INTERACTION BETWEEN VITAMIN C AND OXIDES OF NITROGEN

Interactions between endogenously produced or environmentally derived nitrogen oxides and vitamin C might explain some of the effects of cigarette smoke. For example, in addition to being present in smoke, NO is exhaled in increased amounts in asthma (63). NO_3^-, a transformation product of NO, is excreted during infection and inflammation (101). NO is a radical that is reported to be capable of reacting directly with deoxyribonucleic acid (DNA) and other biomolecules (102), and its oxidation in the body may involve formation of reactive intermediates such as NO_2, $ONOO^-$, N_2O_3, and N_2O_4 (103). Studies examining the protective effects of C on formation of nitrosamines in the gastrointestinal tract from nitrite added to meats suggest that C is a very effective protective agent against harmful nitrogen oxides (104). Studies of C reactivity with $ONOO-$ suggest that C levels normally present intracellularly would be effective in scavenging this molecule (105). C is one of the most abundant antioxidants present in the extracellular lining fluid of human and animal lungs (13). This fluid is probably an important site of release of endogenously produced oxidants, as well as being directly exposed to inhaled environmental oxidants. Further studies are needed to examine the role of C in modulating tissue responses to NO and its derivatives.

Studies of NO_2 inhalation toxicological mechanisms show a clear inhibitory effect of C supplementation. NO_2 exposure (2.0 ppm, 1 h) in nonasthmatic adults causes airway hyperresponsiveness to methacholine challenge which can be completely prevented by C pretreatment (106). That oxidative injury is involved in this effect of NO_2 is shown by increased oxidation of lipids and proteins in bronchoalveolar lavage of NO_2 exposed subjects and the reversal of this oxidation by C and E supplementation (106). Studies in guinea pigs show that NO_2 induced injury occurs more readily during C deficiency. In one study, guinea pigs with varying degrees of C deficiency were exposed to normally innocuous levels of NO_2 (5 ppm, 3 h). Lung injury (measured as permeability to plasma proteins) became detectable when the lung concentrations of C decreased more than 50%, and became increasingly severe as the C decreased further (107). NO_2 exposure appears to cause mobilization of C into the lungs of both normally fed and C-deficient animals. However, in C-deficient animals this mobilization results in only a partial return to normal lung C concentrations and it appears to occur at the expense of C in plasma and other tissues (107). NO_2 injury in C-deficient animals is associated with an increase in lung glutathione and a decrease in vitamin E (108), suggesting that interactions between C and other antioxidants may be important. The protection afforded by C (assessed by measuring susceptibility of mildly C-deficient guinea pigs) appears to depend upon the nature of the oxidant insult, with a different spectrum of protection by C depending on the inhaled toxicant gas. When guinea pigs are exposed to equally injurious concentrations of phosgene, ozone, or nitrogen dioxide (assessed by lung lavage protein increases), the highest level of protection by C is observed with NO_2 (109).

Direct effects of altered C status on allergy are not well understood, and relatively few studies have been carried out in this area. Studies in scorbutic guinea pigs suggest that C deficiency decreases sensitivity to antigen aerosols regardless of whether it is present during initial antigen challenge or whether the period of antigen sensitization corresponds with the period of C deficiency (97). The release of histamine from sensitized scorbutic guinea pig lungs exposed to antigen in vitro is less than that of similarly treated lungs from normally fed animals. Further studies of mildly C-deficient animals which may give different results are needed. The possibility that oxidant exposure can alter the development of allergic responses is receiving increased attention. Recent studies have shown that inhaled oxidants can exert a "priming effect" on allergen challenge, resulting in an increased response over that seen with allergen alone. NO_2 exposure of rats prior to antigen (dust mite) challenge increases IgE levels and indicators of inflammation upon subsequent challenge (110). Ozone, an oxidant similar to NO_2, has a priming effect on nasal inflammation (increased eosinophils, neutrophils, and chemotactic protein) induced by exposure to dust mite antigen in allergic human subjects (111).

Another possible mechanism for oxidant/antioxidant interactions is that oxidants may increase susceptibility to infections, which in turn causes lung injury, and eventually leads to asthma. A large number of animal studies have shown that susceptibility to inhaled bacterial aerosols, and to a lesser extent viral challenges, is enhanced by NO_2 and ozone (42). This effect of oxidant gases appears to involve inhibition of alveolar macrophage phagocytosis and other forms of antimicrobial defense (112). There is strong evidence that C enhances leukocyte phagocytosis, motility, and other functions. Anderson (113) reviewed several studies which suggest that a major mechanism by which C enhances leukocyte function is through protection from their own oxidant generation.

FUTURE STUDIES NEEDED

Evidence points to the hypothesis that suboptimal C nutrition in children, combined with other factors, such as environmental oxidant exposure and perhaps increased exposure to infectious agents, may be contributing to the development of asthma and the increased asthma incidence in recent years. Infants may be at a critical stage with regard to susceptibility to infection, unique response to antigen challenge, or altered response to injury from infection. Although a large number of studies have examined adult responses to inhaled oxidants and dietary deficiencies, few examine newborns, who in the epidemiological studies appear to be the important target population. Further studies that address the developmental causes of asthma are needed.

With regard to prevention of secondary effects or acute asthma attacks, several studies have been reported. The oxidant/antioxidant balance appears to have the potential to modulate symptoms of ongoing asthma in adults. Studies in which asthmatics have taken C supplements give conflicting results: only half of the studies show an improvement. However, these studies have not yet examined very large numbers of subjects, nor have they examined the influence of the supplementation regimens used on tissue or bronchoalveolar lavage levels of C. Although endogenously produced oxidants may contribute substantially to asthma, the supplementation regimens for C may be too short or too sudden to cause changes in C at the sites where oxidant injury is occurring. Methods are needed to evaluate the total oxidant burden resulting from the sum of environmental and internally generated oxidant sources and the contribution of that burden to the asthmatic response. The fact that oxidant burdens probably fluctuate over time suggests that the need for supplementation may also vary with time. Genetically determined factors, such as plasma IgE concentrations and cytokines, need to be determined in the same subjects undergoing airway hypersensitivity studies. Further studies of the absorption and mobilization of C and other antioxidants in asthmatics are also needed.

The question of whether vitamin C supplementation per se or consumption of fruits and vegetables is the important factor needs further investigation. Most studies to date have employed "pharmacological" supplementation at high doses for short periods rather than continuous low-level supplementation or simply altered eating styles. Attention needs to be given to measuring both tissue and plasma C concentrations. For example, the C concentrations in leukocytes in the lung or lung lining fluids may be critical determinants of their response to antigens and the production of mediators in asthma. Further studies are needed to interpret the significance of low levels of C in plasma of asthmatics and in people with other inflammatory conditions.

SUMMARY

Epidemiological studies suggest associations among cigarette smoke exposure, infection, and increased asthma, particularly in children. Decreased preference for foods containing vitamin C and decreased concentrations of vitamin C in blood plasma also appear to be associated with asthma. Both environmental and endogenously produced oxidants may contribute to injury and asthma. Nitrogen oxides are examples of oxidants which may arise from both endogenous and environmental sources and which are protected against by vitamin C. Future studies which focus on the developing lung and on interactions between deficiencies in vitamin C and other dietary antioxidants, and on exposure to environmental as well as endogenous oxidants, may provide clues to understanding and controlling asthma.

ACKNOWLEDGMENTS

The author thanks Drs. Daniel Costa, Linda Birnbaum, and Ian Gilmour for their critical review and helpful suggestions on this chapter.

REFERENCES

1. Lung Disease Data. New York: American Lung Association, 1995.
2. Seaton A, Godden DJ, Brown K. Increase in asthma: a more toxic environment or a more susceptible population? Thorax 1994; 49:171–174.
2a. Burr ML. Pollution: does it cause asthma? Arch Dis Child 1995; 72:377–387.
3. Van Niekerk CH, Weinberg EG, Shore SC, et al. Prevalence of asthma: a comparative study of urban and rural Xhosa children. Clin Allergy 1979; 9:319–324.
4. Woolcock AJ, Dowse G, Temple K, et al. Prevalence of asthma in the South Fore people of Papua New Guinea: a method for field studies of bronchial reactivity. Eur J Respir Dis 1983; 64:571–581.
5. Roorda RJ, Gerritsen J, van Aalderen WMC, et al. Risk factors for the persistence of respiratory symptoms in childhood asthma. Am Rev Respir Dis 1993; 148:1490–1495.
6. Yunginger JW, Reed CE, O'Connell EJ, et al. A community-based study of the epidemiology of asthma: incidence rates, 1964–1983. Am Rev Respir Dis 1992; 146:888–894.
7. US Department of Health and Human Services. Guidelines for the diagnosis and management of asthma. Bethesda, MD: National Institutes of Health, Publication No. 91–3042, 1991.
8. Etzel RA. Indoor air pollution and childhood asthma: effective environmental interventions. Environ Health Perspect 1995; 103(suppl 6):55–58.
9. Ames BN, Shigenaga MK, Hagen TM. Oxidants, antioxidants, and the degenerative diseases of aging. Proc Natl Acad Sci 1993; 90:7915–7922.
10. Patterson BH, Block G, Rosenberger WF, et al. Fruit and vegetables in the American diet: data from the NHANES II Survey. Am J Public Health 1990; 80:1443–1449.
11. Menzel DB. Antioxidants in lung disease. Toxicol Ind Health 1993; 9(1–2):323–336.
12. Hatch GE. Asthma, inhaled oxidants, and dietary antioxidants. Am J Clin Nutr 1995; 61 (suppl):625S–630S.
13. Bielory L, Gandhi R. Asthma and vitamin C. Ann Allergy 1994; 73:89–96.
14. Slade R, Crissman K, Norwood J, Hatch G. Comparison of antioxidant substances in broncho-alveolar lavage cells and fluid from humans, guinea pigs, and rats. Exp Lung Res 1993; 19: 469–484.
15. Bendich A, Machlin LJ, Scandurra O, et al. The antioxidant role of vitamin C. Adv Free Radical Biol Med 1986; 2:419–444.
16. Weitzman M, Gortmaker S, Walker DK, Sobol A. Maternal smoking and childhood asthma. Pediatrics 1990; 85:505–511.
17. Pryor WA. Biological effects of cigarette smoke, wood smoke, and the smoke from plastics: the use of electron spin resonance. Free Radical Biol Med 1992; 13:659–676.
18. Frei B, Forte M, Ames BN, Cross CE. Gas phase oxidants of cigarette smoke induce lipid peroxidation and changes in lipoprotein properties in human blood plasma: protective effects of ascorbic acid. Biochem J 1991; 277:133–138.
19. Habib MP, Clements NC, Garewal HS. Cigarette smoking and ethane exhalation in humans. Am J Respir Crit Care Med 1995; 151:1368–1372.
20. Malo JL, Filiatrault S, Martin RR. Bronchial responsiveness to inhaled methacholine in young asymptomatic smokers. J Appl Physiol 1982; 52:1464–1470.
21. Cockroft DW, Berscheid BA, Murdock KY. Bronchial response to inhaled histamine in asymptomatic young smokers. Eur J Respir Dis 1983; 64:207–211.
22. Buczko GB, Day A, Vanderdoelen JL, et al. Effects of cigarette smoking and short-term smoking cessation on airway responsiveness to inhaled methacholine. Am Rev Respir Dis 1984; 129:12–14.
23. McIntyre EL, Ruffin RE, Alpers JH. Lack of short-term effects of cigarette smoking on bronchial sensitivity to histamine and methacholine. Eur J Respir Dis 1982; 63:535–542.
24. Suauki S, Sano F, Suzuki J, et al. Lack of effect from a single cigarette challenge on bronchial responsiveness in healthy non-smoking subjects. Thorax 1988; 43:401–406.

25. Neijens HJ. Determinants and regulating processes in bronchial hyperreactivity. Lung 1990; 168(suppl):268–277.

26. US Environmental Protection Agency, Office of Research and Development, Office of Air and Radiation. Respiratory health effects of passive smoking: lung cancer and other disorders. Washington, DC: US Environmental Protection Agency, Publication No. EPA/600/6–90/006F, 1992.

27. Sherman CB, Tosteson TD, Tager IB, et al. Early childhood predictors of asthma. Am J Epidemiol 1990; 132:83–95.

28. Martinez FD, Wright AL, Taussig LM, et al. Asthma and wheezing in the first six years of life. N Engl J Med 1995; 323:133–138.

29. Stoddard JJ, Miller T. Impact of parental smoking on the prevalence on wheezing respiratory illness in children. Am J Epidemiol 1995; 141:96–102.

30. Tager IB, Hanrahan JP, Tosteson TD, et al. Lung function, pre- and post-natal smoke exposure, and wheezing in the first year of life. Am Rev Respir Dis 1993; 147:811–817.

31. Murray AB, Morrison BJ. The effect of cigarette smoke from the mother on bronchial responsiveness and severity of symptoms in children with asthma. J Allergy Clin Immunol 1986; 77:575–581.

32. O'Connor GT, Weiss ST, Tager IB, Speizer FE. The effect of passive smoking on pulmonary function and non-specific bronchial responsiveness in a population based sample of children and young adults. Am Rev Respir Dis 1987; 135:800–804.

33. Martinez FD, Antognoni G, Macri F, et al. Parental smoking enhances bronchial responsiveness in nine-year-old children. Am Rev Respir Dis 1988; 138:518–523.

34. Haby MM, Peat JK, Woolcock AJ. Effect of passive smoking, asthma, and respiratory infection on lung function in Australian children. Pediatr Pulmon 1994; 18:323–329.

35. Kay J, Mortimer MJ, Jaron AG. Do both paternal and maternal smoking influence the prevalence of childhood asthma? A study into the prevalence of asthma in children and the effects of parental smoking. J Asthma 1995; 32:47–55.

36. Kjellman NI. Predictive value of high IgE levels in children. Acta Paediatr Scand 1976; 65: 465–471.

37. Hjalte K, Croner S, Max Kjellman N-I. Cost-effectiveness of neonatal IgE-screening for atopic allergy before 7 years of age. Allergy 1987; 42:97–103.

38. Burrows B, Halonen M, Barbee RA, Lebowitz MD. The relationship of serum immunoglobulin E to cigarette smoking. Am Rev Respir Dis 1981; 124:523–525.

39. Ronchetti R, Macri F, Coifetta G, et al. Increased serum immunoglobulin E and increased prevalence of eosinophilia in 9-year-old children of smoking parents. J Allergy Clin Immunol 1990; 86:400–407.

40. Samet JK, Tager IB, Speizer FE. The relationship between respiratory illness in childhood and chronic air-flow obstruction in adulthood. Am Rev Respir Dis 1983; 127:508–523.

41. US Environmental Protection Agency, Office of Research and Development. Air Quality Criteria for Ozone and Related Photochemical Oxidants, Vol. III. Washington, DC: US Environmental Protection Agency, Publication No. EPA/600/AP-93/004c, 1993.

42. US Environmental Protection Agency, Office of Research and Development. Air Quality Criteria for Oxides of Nitrogen, Vol. III. Washington, DC: US Environmental Protection Agency, Publication No. EPA/600/8-91/049cF, 1993.

43. Pierson WE, Koenig JQ. Respiratory effects of air pollution on allergic disease. J Allergy Clin Immunol 1992; 90:557–565.

44. Bates DV, Sixto R. Hospital admissions and air pollutants in Southern Ontario: the acid summer haze effect. Environ Res 1987; 43:317–331.

45. Cody RP, Weisel CP, Birnbaum G, Lioy PJ. The effect of ozone associated with summertime photochemical smog and the frequency of asthma visits to hospital emergency departments. Environ Res 1992; 58:184–194.

46. Greer JR, Abbey DE, Burchette RJ. Asthma related to occupational and ambient air pollutants in nonsmokers. J Occup Med 1993; 35:909–915.

47. White MC, Etzel RA, Wilcox WD, Lloyd C. Exacerbations of childhood asthma and ozone pollution in Atlanta. Environ Res 1994; 65:56–68.

48. Ishizaki T, Koizumi K, Ikemori R, et al. Studies of prevalence of Japanese cedar pollinosis among the residents in a densely cultivated area. Ann Allergy 1987; 58:265–270.

49. Moseler M, Hendel-Kramer A, Karmaus W, et al. Effect of moderate NO_2 air pollution on the lung function of children with asthmatic symptoms. Environ Res 1994; 67:109–124.

50. Volkmer RE, Ruffin RE, Wigg NR, Davies N. The prevalence of respiratory symptoms in South Australian preschool children. II. Factors associated with indoor air quality. J Paediatr Child Health 1995; 31:115–120.

51. Barnes PJ. Reactive oxygen species and airway inflammation. Free Radical Biol Med 1990; 9:235–243.

52. Frigas E, Gleich GJ. The eosinophil and the pathology of asthma. J Allergy Clin Immunol 1986; 77:527–537.

53. Chanez P, Dent G, Yukawa T, et al. Increased eosinophil responsiveness to platelet-activating factor in asthma. Clin Sci 1988; 74:5.

54. Shult PA, Graziano FM, Busse WW. Enhanced eosinophil luminol-dependent chemiluminescence in allergic rhinitis. J Allergy Clin Immunol 1986; 77:702–708.

55. Cluzel M, Damon M, Chanez P, et al. Enhanced alveolar cell luminol-dependent chemiluminescence in asthma. J Allergy Clin Immunol 1987; 80:195–201.

56. Kelly CA, Ward C, Stenton SC, et al. Numbers and activity of cells obtained at bronchoalveolar lavage in asthma, and their relationship to airway responsiveness. Thorax 1988; 43:684–692.

57. Ward C, Kelly CA, Stenton SC, et al. The relative contribution of bronchoalveolar macrophages and neutrophils to lucigenin- and luminol-amplified chemiluminescence. Eur Respir J 1990; 3:1008–1014.

58. Shvedova AA, Kisin ER, Kagan VE, Karol MH. Increased lipid peroxidation and decreased antioxidants in lungs of guinea pigs following an allergic pulmonary response. Toxicol Appl Pharmacol 1995; 132:72–81.

59. Stevens WHM, Inman MD, Wattie J, O'Byrne PM. Allergen-induced oxygen radical release from bronchoalveolar lavage cells and airway hyperresponsiveness in dogs. Am J Respir Crit Care Med 1995; 151:1526–1531.

60. Mannaioni PF, Giannella E, Palmerani B, et al. Free radicals as endogenous histamine releases. Agents Actions 1988; 23:129–142.

61. Adler KB, Holden-Stauffer WJ, Repine JE. Oxygen metabolites stimulate release of high-molecular-weight glycoconjugates by cell and organ cultures of rodent respiratory epithelium via an arachidonic acid dependent mechanism. J Clin Invest 1990; 85:75–85.

62. Barnes PJ. Air pollution and asthma: molecular mechanisms. Mol Med Today 1995; 1:149–155.

63. Gaston B, Drazen J, Chee CBE, et al. Expired nitric oxide (NO) concentrations are elevated in patients with reactive airways disease. Endothelium 1993; 1:87.

64. Kharitonov SA, Yates D, Barnes PJ. Increased nitric oxide in exhaled air of normal human subjects with upper respiratory tract infections. Eur Respir J 1995; 8:295–297.

65. Reisseissen FD. De Pulmonis Structura. Strasborg, 1803.

66. McNally N. Preliminary report on the use of vitamin C in asthma. J Irish Med Assoc 1953; 33: 175–178.

67. Miedema IE, Feskens JM, Heederik D, Kromhout D. Dietary determinants of long-term incidence of chronic nonspecific lung disease: The Zutphen Study. Am J Epidemiol 1993; 138: 37–45.

68. Schwartz J, Weiss ST. Dietary factors and their relationship to respiratory symptoms: NHANES II. Am J Epidemiol 1990; 132:67–76.

69. Schwartz J, Weiss ST. Relationship between dietary vitamin C intake and pulmonary function in the First National Health and Nutrition Examination Survey (NHANES I). Am J Clin Nutr 1994; 59:110–114.

70. Britton JR, Pavord ID, Richards KA, et al. Dietary antioxidant vitamin intake and lung function in the general population. Am J Respir Crit Care Med 1995; 151:1383–1387.

71. Troisi RJ, Willett WC, Weiss ST, et al. A prospective study of diet and adult-onset asthma. Am J Respir Crit Care Med 1995; 151:1401–1408.

71a. Khaw K-T, Woodhouse P. Interrelation of vitamin C, infection, haemostatic factors, and cardiovascular disease. Br Med J 1995; 310:1559–1563.

72. Olusi SO, Ojutiku OO, Jessop WJE, Iboko MI. Plasma and white blood cell ascorbic acid concentrations in patients with bronchial asthma. Clin Chem Acta 1979; 92:161–166.

73. Aderele WR, Ette SI, Oduwoule O, Ikpeme SJ. Plasma, vitamin C (ascorbic acid) levels in asthmatic children. Afr J Med Sci 1985; 14:115–120.

74. Zuskin E, Lewis AJ, Bouhuys A. Inhibition of histamine induced airway constriction by ascorbic acid. J Allergy Clin Immunol 1973; 51:218–226.

75. Kreisman H, Mitchell C, Bouhuys A. Inhibition of histamine-induced airway constriction: negative results with oxtriphylline and ascorbic acid. Lung 1977; 154:223–229.

76. Kordansky DV, Rosenthal RR, Norman PS. The effects of vitamin C on antigen-induced bronchospasm. J Allergy Clin Immunol 1979; 63:61.

77. Anah CO, Jarike LM, Baig HA. High dose ascorbic acid in Nigerian asthmatics. Trop Geogr Med 1980; 32:132–137.

78. Ogilvy CS, DuBois AB, Douglas JS. Effect of ascorbic acid and indomethacin on the airways of healthy male subjects with and without induced bronchoconstriction. J Allergy Clin Immunol 1981; 67:363–369.

79. Anderson R, Hay I, Van Wyk HA, Theron A. Ascorbic acid in bronchial asthma. S Afr Med J 1983; 63:649–652.

80. Schachter EN, Schlesinger A. The attenuation of exercise induced bronchospasm by ascorbic acid. Ann Allergy 1982; 49:146–151.

81. Fortner BR, Danziger RE, Rabinowitz PS, Nelson HS. The effect of ascorbic acid on cutaneous and nasal response to histamine and allergen. J Allergy Clin Immunol 1982; 69:484.

82. Mohsenin V, Dubois AB, Douglas JS. Effect of ascorbic acid on response to methacholine challenge in asthmatic subjects. Am Rev Respir Dis 1983; 127:143–147.

83. Ting S, Mansfield LE, Yarborough J. The effects of ascorbic acid on pulmonary functions in mild asthma. J Asthma 1983; 20:39–42.

84. Kawane H, Soejima R, Matsushima T, et al. Effect of ascorbic acid on bronchoconstriction induced by methacholine inhalation challenge in healthy subjects. Kawasaki Med J 1985; 11:87–92.

85. Malo JL, Cartier A, Pinean L, et al. Lack of acute effects of ascorbic acid on spirometry and airway responsiveness to histamine in subjects with asthma. J Allergy Clin Immunol 1986; 78:1153–1158.

86. Puglisi L, Berti F, Bosisio E, et al. Ascorbic acid and $PGF_{2\alpha}$ antagonism on tracheal smooth muscle. In: Samuellson B, Paoletti R, eds. Advances in Prostaglandin and Thromboxane Research. Vol. 1. New York: Raven Press, 1976:503–506.

87. Schechtman G, Boyd JC, Gruchow HW. The influence of smoking on vitamin C status in adults. Am J Public Health 1989; 79:158–162.

88. Kallner AB, Hartmann D, Hornig DH. On the requirements of ascorbic acid in man: steady-state turnover and body pool in smokers. Am J Clin Nutr 1981; 34:1347–1355.

89. Subar AF, Harlan LC, Mattson ME. Food and nutrient intake differences between smokers and non-smokers in the US. Am J Public Health 1990; 80:1323–1329.

90. Heinz-Erian P, Achmuller M, Berger H, et al. Vitamin C concentrations in maternal plasma, amniotic fluid, umbilical cord blood, the plasma of newborn infants, colostrum and transitory and mature breast milk. Pediatr Paedol 1987; 22(2):163–178.

91. Food and Nutrition Board. Recommended Dietary Allowances, 9th ed. Washington, DC: National Academy Press, 1980:72–82.

92. National Research Council. Recommended Dietary Allowances, 10th ed. Washington, DC: National Academy Press, 1989.

92a. Levine M, Conray-Cantilena C, Wang Y, et al. Vitamin C pharmacokinetics in healthy volunteers: evidence for a recommended dietary allowance. Proc Natl Acad Sci USA 1996; 93:3704–3709.

93. Kallner A, Hartmann D, Hornig D. Steady-state turnover and body pool of ascorbic acid in man. Am J Clin Nutr 1979; 32:530–539.

94. Levine M. New concepts in the biology and biochemistry of ascorbic acid. N Engl J Med 1986; 314:892–902.

95. Schectman G, Byrd JC, Hoffmann R. Ascorbic acid requirements for smokers: analysis of a population survey. Am J Clin Nutr 1991; 53:1466–1470.

96. Bucca C, Rolla G, Caria E, et al. Effects of vitamin C on airway responsiveness to inhaled histamine in heavy smokers. Eur Respir J 1989; 2:229–233.

97. Mohsenin V, DuBois AB. Vitamin C and airways. Ann NY Acad Sci 1987; 498:259–268.

98. Galley HF, Davies MJ, Webster NR. Ascorbyl radical formation in patients with sepsis: Effect of ascorbate loading. Free Radical Biol Med 1996; 20:139–143.

99. Herbert V. Does mega-C do more good than harm, or more harm than good? Nutr Today 1993; 28:28–32.

100. Greene LS. Asthma and oxidant stress: nutritional, environmental, and genetic risk factors. J Am Coll Nutr 1995; 14:4.

101. Green LC, De Luzuriaga KR, Wagner DA, et al. Nitrate biosynthesis in man. Proc Natl Acad Sci USA 1981; 78:7764–7768.

102. Wink DA, Kasprzak KS, Maragos CM, et al. DNA deaminating ability and genotoxicity of nitric oxide and its progenitors. Science 1991; 254:1001–1003.

103. Gaston B, Drazen JM, Loscalzo J, Stamler JS. The biology of nitrogen oxides in the airways. Am J Respir Crit Care Med 1994; 149:538–551.

104. Tannenbaum SR, Wishnok JS, Leaf CD. Inhibition of nitrosamine formation by ascorbic acid. Am J Clin Nutr 1991; 53:247S–250S.

105. Squadrito GL, Jin X, Pryor WA. Stopped-flow kinetic study of the reaction of ascorbic acid with peroxynitrite. Arch Biochem Biophys 1995; 322:53–59.

106. Mohsenin V. Effect of vitamin C on NO_2-induced airway hyperresponsiveness in normal subjects: a randomized double-blind experiment. Am Rev Respir Dis 1987; 136:1408–1411.

107. Mohsenin V. Lipid peroxidation and antielastase activity in the lung under oxidant stress: role of antioxidant defenses. J Appl Physiol 1991; 70(4):1456–1462.

108. Hatch GE, Slade R, Selgrade MJK, Stead AG. Nitrogen dioxide exposure and lung antioxidants in ascorbic acid-deficient guinea pigs. Toxicol Appl Pharmacol 1986; 82:351–359.

109. Slade R, Highfill JW, Hatch GE. Effects of ascorbic acid or nonprotein sulfhydryl depletion on the acute inhalation toxicity of nitrogen dioxide, ozone, and phosgene. Inhal Toxicol 1989; 1: 261–271.

110. Gilmour MI, Park P, Selgrade MJK. Increased immune and inflammatory response to dust mite antigen in rats exposed to 5 ppm NO_2. Fundamentals Appl Toxicol 1996; 31:65–70.

111. Peden DB, Setzer RW, Devlin RB. Ozone exposure has both a priming effect on allergen-induced responses and an intrinsic inflammatory action in the nasal airways of perennially allergic asthmatics. Am J Respir Crit Care Med 1995; 151:1336–1345.

112. Gilmour MI, Park P, Selgrade MJK. Ozone-enhanced pulmonary infection with Streptococcus zooepidemicus in mice: the role of alveolar macrophage function and capsular virulence factors. Am Rev Respir Dis 1993; 147:753–760.

113. Anderson R. The immunostimulatory, anti-inflammatory and anti-allergic properties of ascorbate. Adv Nutr Res 1984; 6:19–45.

16

Effect of Vitamin C on Leukocyte Function and Adhesion to Endothelial Cells

HANS-ANTON LEHR
Johannes Gutenberg University, Mainz, Germany

RAINER K. SAETZLER
Temple University, Philadelphia, Pennsylvania

KARL E. ARFORS
Pharmacia AB, Uppsala, Sweden

Leukocytes are the most important players in the immune response against bacterial and fungal infections. Activation of circulating leukocytes, predominantly neutrophils, and their subsequent adhesion of the microvascular endothelium in response to various inflammatory mediators precede their emigration across the functionally and/or morphologically impaired endothelium (1). Through the respiratory burst and the release of reactive oxygen species, as well as through degranulation products, such as arachidonic acid metabolites, microbicidal peptides, and hydrolytic enzymes, activated leukocytes contribute to the host defense against microorganisms and to the elimination of foreign and necrotic material (1–3). Observations in patients with leukocyte adhesion deficiency, who suffer from recurrent bacterial infections, have demonstrated the importance of leukocyte adhesion and function in the mounting of an effective inflammatory reaction (4).

This review focuses on the effect of vitamin C on leukocyte function. These effects have to be separated into those that stimulate some leukocyte functions and those that counteract other leukocyte functions. As it becomes apparent, the net effect of vitamin C on leukocyte function is rather beneficial for the organism, resulting both in an improved cell-mediated immune response, and also in the protection from adverse effects of inadequately activated leukocytes.

VITAMIN C STIMULATES LEUKOCYTE FUNCTION

Vitamin C levels are pathologically reduced in the plasma and in leukocytes of preterm babies, of newborns, and of senescent people (5), as well as of human subjects who suffer from cancer (6), rheumatoid arthritis (7–9), tuberculosis (10), and acute phase reactions after surgery, stroke, or trauma (11–14). Furthermore, many studies have demonstrated that plasma and leukocyte vitamin C levels are significantly reduced in smokers (15–18). Many of these conditions are characterized by a depressed delayed-type hypersensitivity skin test, an inability of the organism to fight infections effectively, ultimately resulting in an increased risk of recurrent severe infections. Studies on vitamin C–deficient animals (20) and human subjects (10,21) have suggested that the inability to fight infections adequately may be due to impaired leukocyte function(s). On the basis of these studies, many researchers have investigated the effect of vitamin C on leukocyte function in vitro and in vivo.

In Vitro Studies

In 1974, Goetzl and coworkers observed that vitamin C stimulates the random mobility and chemotaxis of neutrophils and eosinophils, and to a lesser extent of monocytes in vitro, irrespective of the applied chemoattractant (22). These observations have later been confirmed in several reports (23–27). However, speculations concerning the possible mode of action of vitamin C vary extensively: whereas Goetzl ascribed the stimulatory effect of vitamin C to an enhancement of the hexose-monophosphate shunt activity in leukocytes (22), others suggested that the stimulation of neutrophil and monocyte chemotaxis by vitamin C could be due to increased levels of intracellular cyclic guanosine monophosphate (GMP) (26,28). The observation that the stimulatory effect of vitamin C was serum-dependent suggested that serum was necessary to maintain vitamin C in an unoxidized state (23,28). Therefore, Anderson speculated that the vitamin C–induced stimulation of neutrophil motility could be due to the ability of unoxidized (but not oxidized) vitamin C to scavenge reactive oxygen species (ROS), thus preventing the autooxidation of the neutrophil membrane by myeloperoxidase (MPO) and hydrogen peroxide (H_2O_2) released from neutrophils after exposure to chemoattractants and during phagocytosis (23). Anderson demonstrated that vitamin C concentrations that stimulate neutrophil motility in vitro and in vivo effectively inhibited the MPO/H_2O_2/halide system in leukocytes (23). Although MPO released into the extracellular space may contribute to microbicidal activity, it may also compromise leukocyte function by mediating the autooxidation of leukocyte membranes (29), resulting in membrane iodination and loss of sulfhydryl groups. Subsequently, Anderson could provide conclusive experimental evidence that vitamin C in vitro protects from leukocyte self-inactivation via inhibition of the MPO/H_2O_2/halide system (23). Support for this concept was later provided in studies which demonstrated that vitamin C exerts powerful antioxidant activities and has the ability to scavenge superoxide radicals and other ROS (30,31).

Independently of the effects of vitamin C on extracellular oxidants, it has been proposed that vitamin C may potentiate the intracellular antimicrobial activity of neutrophils (32,33). Proposed mechanisms of action include the stimulation of the hexose monophosphate shunt activity (32), the increased generation of ROS in a vitamin C/H_2O_2 system (34), and the potentiation of lysozyme activity (33). As alternative mechanisms, Orr (35) and Anderson (23) suggested that vitamin C may increase phagocytic antimicrobial activity by inactivating bacterial catalases, thus increasing the susceptibility of these microorganisms to the toxic effects of H_2O_2. Furthermore, Anderson suggested that vitamin C may increase phagocytic activity by preventing the degranulation of neutrophils (36), thus increasing that intracellular availability of more granules for the destruction of ingested organisms (37). The concept that vitamin C exerts different effects on the bactericidal phagocytes in the extracellular space (inhibition) than in the intracellular space (stimulation) was later supported in a study using luminol-enhanced chemiluminescence on human leukocytes ex vivo (38).

Vitamin C enhances the responsiveness of T-lymphocytes to diverse mitogens in vitro (39,40), and inhibits the inactivation of this lymphocyte responsiveness by the influenza virus (41). Others have described an improved migration of T-lymphocytes to serum-derived chemoattractants in the presence of vitamin C (42). By analogy with the mechanism of action of vitamin C on neutrophil motility, several modes of action of vitamin C on lymphocyte transformation have been suggested, including an increase in intracellular cyclic GMP (cGMP) levels (7), an inactivation of extracellular oxidants (23), and the preservation of energy-rich phosphates and glycerol-3-phosphate dehydrogenase activity (43).

In Vivo Studies

Because of the safety of ingesting large doses of vitamin C (see Chap. 21) and the ease of performing leukocyte function tests on samples obtained by venipuncture, most of the in vitro observations on the stimulatory effect of vitamin C on leukocyte function described have been repeated and mostly reproduced in studies on human volunteers (7,19,44,45). Intravenous injection of 1 g of vitamin C into human subjects resulted in increased neutrophil motility and increased lymphocyte transformation as early as 1 h after injection (23). Likewise, ingestion of 1–3 g of vitamin C/day for 1 week was associated with a significant increase in neutrophil migration and in lymphocyte responsiveness to different mitogens (phytohemagglutinin and concavalin A) (44). Similar findings have also been reported in diverse animal models using guinea pigs (46,47), mice (48), and calves (49). Experimentally to support the concept that vitamin C improves leukocyte function by preventing degranulation and extracellular release of bactericides while preserving the intracellular killing mechanisms directed toward ingested microorganisms, Anderson and coworkers demonstrated that vitamin C ingestion in human volunteers reduces the extracellular chemiluminescence response of leukocytes but leaves the intercellular chemiluminescence response intact (38).

Effect of Vitamin C on Leukocyte Function in Clinical Trials

Vitamin C has been used experimentally in patients having several different pathological conditions, all of which are characterized by a state of impaired leukocyte response, including chronic granulomatous disease, Chédiak–Higashi syndrome, disseminated neoplastic disease, and in patients with recurrent infections. Furthermore, vitamin C trials have been undertaken in otherwise healthy human subjects who suffer from impaired leukocyte function for other reasons such as very young or very old age or excessive physical activity.

    1.   Chronic granulomatous disease (CGD): The function of leukocytes is drastically compromised in children with CGD. These children suffer from recurrent bacterial infections caused by defective neutrophil motility and the inability of their neutrophils to fight the invading bacteria effectively. Anderson (23) treated three children with CGD with a vitamin C–supplemented diet for 2 years and assessed their leukocyte function before and at regular intervals after treatment. In all three children, dietary vitamin C supplementation resulted in a gradual improvement of neutrophil chemotaxis and staphylococcicidal activity. With the exception of one urinary tract infection, all three children remained free of infections over the entire 2-year treatment and observation period (23). A similar improvement by vitamin C ingestion was observed of neutrophil chemotaxis and phagocytosis, as well as lymphocyte response to various mitogens in a series of children suffering from asthma (44).

    2.   Chédiak-Higashi (CH) syndrome: Patients with CH syndrome suffer frequent and severe bacterial infections that are (as in CGD) due to a defective bactericidal function of neutrophils (50). In a much acclaimed case report, Boxer and coworkers could demonstrate that dietary supplementation with vitamin C normalized neutrophil chemotaxis and bacte-

ricidal activity, without affecting the neutrophil degranulation response (51). Similar results have been reported by Panush and coworkers (7), who administered vitamin C to two brothers suffering from CH syndrome and observed a normalization of natural killer cell function within 1 week after vitamin C administration; by Weening and coworkers (52), who observed a restoration of bactericidal activity of neutrophils in one patient with CH disease, who subsequently suffered from significantly less infectious complications; and by Yegin and coworkers (53), who observed improved neutrophil and monocyte motility in children with CH syndrome.

3. Disseminated neoplastic disease: Yonemoto (19) demonstrated that the abnormal lymphocyte transformation response to diverse mitogens in patients with advanced neoplastic disease is improved by vitamin C ingestion. Likewise, abnormal monocyte chemotaxis could be restored with vitamin C administration to patients with disseminated solid tumors (54).

4. Patients with recurrent infections, such as furunculosis or malignant external otitis, a severe and occasionally lethal infection of the external ear with *Pseudomonas* organisms, who have been found to have significantly depressed neutrophil and lymphocyte functions, have been found to profit markedly from vitamin C ingestion, in respect to both restoration of their leukocyte functions and resolution of the clinical picture (55,56).

5. Neonates: Vohra and coworkers reported that oral vitamin C improved neutrophil random (65%) and chemotactic migration (57%) within the first 24 to 48 h after birth in 20 neonates (57). They concluded that vitamin C should be included as an adjunct to the chemotherapy of neonatal sepsis.

6. Elderly people: Old people often have very low vitamin C levels (5). Dietary vitamin C significantly improves T-lymphocyte responsiveness to diverse mitogens in old people and enhances tuberculin skin hypersensitivity (5).

7. Marathon runners: The increased incidence of upper respiratory infections in marathon runners has been linked to an impaired neutrophil function secondary to the acute-phase response to the strenuous exercise (58). Vitamin C ingestion was found to reduce the incidence of upper respiratory tract infections in marathon runners significantly (59). However, since a direct effect on neutrophil function was not assessed in these subjects, it can only be speculated whether vitamin C exerted its protection from the respiratory tract infection through an improvement of neutrophil function.

Protective Effects of Vitamin C on Leukocyte-Directed Toxicity

Several in vitro and in vivo studies have shown that vitamin C has the capacity of protect leukocyte function against toxic injury. Most of these studies were focused on genotoxicity and deoxyribonucleic acid (DNA) strand breaks (60,61). However, some studies have demonstrated that vitamin C protects neutrophil motility and phagocytosis, and lymphocyte mitogen responsiveness, during attack by carcinogens (12), cadmium (63), and environmental toxins (64).

VITAMIN C INHIBITS LEUKOCYTE FUNCTION

Although leukocyte adhesion and emigration are involved in host defense and phagocytosis and thus serve a beneficial role during a well-contained inflammatory response, leukocytes can turn against the host and contribute to tissue damage (1–3). This damage is characterized in the acute stage by the loss of endothelial integrity, the extravasation of fluid and macromolecules into the interstitial space, and the uncontrolled recruitment of more leukocytes toward the focus of tissue damage. Leukocyte-mediated tissue damage was first postulated by Metchnikoff in 1887 (65) and has later been described in various physiological conditions, such as inflammatory bowel disease (66), endotoxemia (67), and localized (68–71) and systemic (72) ischemia and reperfusion. Chronic consequences of unwanted leukocyte activation and emigration are best seen in early atherosclerotic lesions, where emigrated leukocytes provide the basis for the formation of foam cells and complex atherosclerotic lesions (73–74). A central feature of leukocyte adhesion during these acute and chronic disease states is the excessive production of ROS, and the contribution of ROS to leukocyte adhesion has been well characterized (75,76). Consequently, the unwanted leukocyte adhesion and emigration, as well as leukocyte-mediated tissue damage may be counteracted effectively with antioxidants and ROS scavengers (71,75,77). Antioxidants have also been shown to inhibit experimental and clinical atherogenesis (15–17,78). Since vitamin C acts as a powerful scavenger of ROS (30,31), it is not surprising that efforts were undertaken to investigate whether it could affect the unwanted activation of leukocytes during the pathophysiological conditions described.

Inhibitory Effects of Vitamin C on Leukocyte Function In Vitro

Little information is available on the inhibitory effect of vitamin C on leukocyte function in vitro. Villa and coworkers (79) reported that vitamin C inhibits (in a dose-dependent fashion) the arachidonic acid–induced aggregation of human neutrophils and lymphocytes. On the basis of the finding that LTB_4-induced leukocyte aggregation was not affected by vitamin C, the authors speculated that vitamin C might function as a lipoxygenase inhibitor (79). This finding is consistent with the results obtained by others: in a different in vitro assay, using nylon fibers as the adhesion matrix, vitamin C did not affect LTB_4-induced leukocyte adhesion (80). These authors also observed no effect of vitamin C on the adhesion of resting neutrophils, suggesting that it does not act on the ability of neutrophils to adhere to matrix or endothelial cells per se, but rather on the stimuli of neutrophil adhesion (80). Consistently with this concept, Jonas et al. (81) showed that vitamin C, in a dose-dependent fashion, inhibited endotoxin-induced neutrophil adhesion to cultured endothelial cells, the production of ROS, and neutrophil-mediated endothelial cell injury, as assessed by ^{111}In-oxide release from labeled endothelial cells.

Inhibitory Effects of Vitamin C on Leukocyte Function In Vivo

With very few exceptions, the studies on the inhibitory effects of vitamin C on leukocyte function have been performed in established animal models of disease. The clinical corollaries to these studies are mostly of an epidemiological nature and thus contribute little to the understanding of the underlying mechanisms.

    1.   Adjuvant arthritis: On the basis of the observation that vitamin C can inhibit the migration of neutrophils into inflamed tissues (82), Davis and coworkers (83) showed that vitamin C inhibits leukocyte infiltration and tissue edema in a model of locally induced inflammation and arthritis in rat hind limbs. These findings are used as an explanation for the previous observation that vitamin C prevents and regresses adjuvant-induced arthritis (84). While no definite mode of action was identified in these studies, the authors speculate

that vitamin C might act by "mopping up" ROS, or by preventing the formation of other inflammatory mediators, such as prostaglandins, proteolytic enzymes, or leukotrienes (83).

2. Ischemia/Reperfusion: The contribution of ROS to leukocyte recruitment into postischemic tissue has been well documented (75). ROS are generated in endothelial cells by a mechanism that involves the conversion of xanthine dehydrogenase to xanthine oxidase (85), as well as by activated leukocytes within the reperfused tissue, resulting in the recruitment of more inflammatory cells into the lesion (75). In addition to exerting powerful chemotactic activities, ROS can directly upregulate adhesion molecules (86), and contribute to the breakdown of the endothelial cell barrier function. Consequently, several authors could demonstrate that inhibition of ROS formation and/or action significantly attenuates postischemic leukocyte adhesion and leukocyte-mediated tissue and organ damage (71,75, 77,87,88). On the basis of these findings Clavien and coworkers used a rat liver model of ischemia and reperfusion and demonstrated that vitamin C treatment significantly reduced the adhesion of leukocytes into the liver after a 45-min ischemia (89). To our knowledge, this is the only study published today which demonstrates the protective effect of vitamin C in experimental ischemia/reperfusion injury. However, there is one report on a clinical trial with vitamin C which is unfortunately published in a journal that is not listed by any of the major medical indexes. Eddy and coworkers (90) treated 28 patients with intravenous vitamin C or placebo control 1 h prior to cardiopulmonary bypass for open heart surgery. In addition to the intravenous treatment, vitamin C was also added to the cardioplegia solution. The release of lactic acid dehydrogenase and creatine phosphokinase (biochemical parameters of postischemic reperfusion injury) was almost entirely prevented by the vitamin C treatment. Unfortunately this study has received little attention and has not been followed up to date.

3. Cigarette Smoke–Induced Leukocyte Activation: Cigarette smoking is a major risk factor for the development of pulmonary and cardiovascular diseases. Features common to the pathomechanisms of most cigarette smoke–associated diseases are the activation and adhesion of circulating leukocytes to micro- and macrovascular endothelium (91,92), followed by acute and/or chronic leukocyte-mediated tissue damage (4,93). In agreement with earlier reports on the sequestration of leukocytes in the pulmonary microcirculation in animals (94–96) and humans (97), we have recently shown that cigarette smoke exposure of hamsters elicits the adhesion of leukocytes to micro- and macrovascular endothelium, as well as the aggregation of leukocytes with platelets in the blood stream. Both leukocyte adhesion and aggregate formation were prevented by pretreatment of the animals with dietary or intravenous vitamin C (98). These findings emphasize the contribution of ROS to cigarette smoke–related circulatory dysfunction and provide the explanation for protective effects of vitamin C in epidemiological surveys and in animal models of cigarette smoke–induced disease (15–17,99).

4. Leukocyte Adhesion with Relevance for Atherogenesis: The oxidation of low density lipoprotein (LDL) has been proposed to be a key event during early atherogenesis (100,101). One of the most prominent properties of oxidized LDL is its ability to stimulate the adhesion of leukocytes to endothelial cells (102,103). Vitamin C has been shown to prevent the oxidation of LDL effectively in vitro (104,105). Following up on observations that oxidized LDL-induced adhesion of leukocytes is dependent on the generation of a variety of inflammatory mediators, and also of ROS (103,106), we have studied the effect of dietary and intravenous vitamin C on oxidized LDL-induced adhesion of leukocytes to micro- and macrovascular endothelium. Both dietary and intravenous vitamin C inhibited

the stimulation of leukocyte adhesion to endothelial cells, and the formation in the blood stream of leukocyte/platelet aggregates (107). Vitamin C has been clearly associated with a reduced cardiovascular risk in large epidemiological surveys (15–17). The presumed threshold level for effective protection from cardiovascular disease in humans by vitamin C has been estimated at 40 to 50 μmol/L (16). This threshold level was surpassed by all the hamsters in our study (107), suggesting that the vitamin plasma levels measured in this study translate into levels found in humans, with low baseline vitamin levels in control hamsters corresponding to a predicted high risk of cardiovascular disease and high levels in vitamin-treated hamsters corresponding to a predictive low risk of cardiovascular disease (15–17). A comparable extent of protection from leukocyte adhesion and aggregation was obtained by acutely raising vitamin C plasma levels through a single bolus injection of vitamin C just 5 min prior to oxLDL injection, suggesting that vitamin C need not be incorporated into leukocytes but merely needs to be circulating in the blood stream (107). This finding is consistent with the notion that vitamin C acts by scavenging ROS in the blood stream (30,31), while not affecting the ability of leukocytes to adhere or aggregate per se (80). The exact mechanism by which vitamin C affects leukocyte function after challenge with oxLDL or with cigarette smoke remains a matter of speculation: vitamin C may interfere with the formation of platelet activating factor (PAF) or other lipid mediators. Recent in vitro evidence suggests that a ROS attack on membrane phospholipids results in the generation of fragmented phospholipids that activate leukocytes via the PAF receptor and have thus been called PAF-like lipids (108). Previous studies on the hamster skinfold chamber model have shown that pharmacological blockade of the PAF receptor significantly attenuates oxLDL-induced leukocyte adhesion and aggregation, demonstrating the role of the PAF receptor in this event (92). Alternatively, it is conceivable that oxLDL may act through ROS-mediated inhibition of nitric oxide synthase (109) and/or nitric oxide inactivation (110), steps that may well be prevented by the administration of vitamin C (111). Nitric oxide has been identified as a powerful antiadhesive and antiaggregatory mediator in vivo (112). Finally, vitamin C may act by preserving the endothelial cell production of antiadhesive and antiaggregatory prostacyclin, the formation of which may be suppressed by oxLDL or cigarette smoke exposure (113).

CONCLUSION

Reviewing the literature on the effects of vitamin C on leukocyte function has yielded two major results that may at first glance appear contradictory. A large body of evidence shows that vitamin C stimulates leukocyte functions (i.e., neutrophil chemotaxis, phagocytosis; lymphocyte mitogenic responsiveness), while a similarly prominent body of evidence demonstrates an inhibition of leukocyte functions by vitamin C (i.e., inhibition of stimulated leukocyte adhesion and aggregation). It is of interest that in the clinical use of vitamin C in the prophylaxis and treatment of diverse pathological conditions, its action is overwhelmingly positive. This apparent dilemma between basic and clinical science may be resolved when the differential effects of vitamin C on leukocyte function are integrated with the differential role of leukocytes in disease pathomechanisms. The Dr. Jekyll leukocyte attacks and kills microorganisms, removes necrotic and foreign material, and thus serves a beneficial role in the host defense. Vitamin C exerts several stimulatory actions on the ability of leukocytes to perform these tasks. The Mr. Hyde leukocyte is called to action during the body's response gone awry during inflammation, ischemia/reperfusion, cigarette smoke exposure, and early atherogenesis. These adverse leukocyte functions are ROS-mediated and are thus effectively counteracted by vitamin C.

REFERENCES

1. Granger DN, Kubes P. The microcirculation and inflammation: modulation of leukocyte-endothelial cell adhesion. J Leuk Biol 1994; 55:662–675.
2. Anderson BO, Brown JM, Harken AH. Mechanisms of neutrophil-mediated tissue injury. J Surg Res 1991; 51:170–179.
3. Lehr HA, Arfors KE. Mechanism of tissue damage by leukocytes. Curr Opin Hematol 1994; 1:92–99.
4. Anderson DC, Springer TA. Leukocyte adhesion deficiency: an inherited defect in the Mac-1, LFA-1, and p150,95 glycoproteins. Annu Rev Med 1987; 38:175–194.
5. Kennes B, Dumont I, Brohee D, et al. Effect of vitamin C supplements on cell-mediated immunity in old people. Gerontology 1983; 29:305–310.
6. Anthony HM, Schorah CJ. Severe hypovitaminosis C in lung-cancer patients: the utilization of vitamin C in surgical repair and lymphocyte-related host resistance. Br J Cancer 1982; 46:354–367.
7. Panush RS, Delafuente JC, Katz P, Johnson J. Modulation of certain immunologic responses by vitamin C. III. Potentiation of in vitro and in vivo lymphocyte responses. Int J Vitam Nutr Res Suppl 1981; 23:35–47.
8. Roberts P, Hemilä H, Wikström M. Vitamin C and inflammation. Med Biol 1984; 62:88.
9. Lunec J, Blake DR. The determination of dehydroascorbic acid and ascorbic acid in the serum and synovial fluid of patients with rheumatic arthritis. Free Radic Res Commun 1985; 1:31–39.
10. Gatner EM, Anderson R. An in vitro assessment of cellular and humoral immune function in pulmonary tuberculosis: correction of defective neutrophil motility by ascorbate, levamisole, metoprolol and propranolol. Clin Exp Immunol 1980; 40:327–336.
11. Hume R, Vallance BD, Muir MM. Ascorbate status and fibrinogen concentrations after cerebrovascular accident. J Clin Pathol 1982; 35:195–199.
12. Irvin TT. Vitamin C requirements in postoperative patients. Int J Vitam Nutr Res Suppl 1982; 23:277–286.
13. Louw JA, Werbeck A, Louw ME, et al. Blood vitamin concentrations during the acute-phase response. Crit Care Med 1992; 20:934–941.
14. Vallance S. Changes in plasma and buffy layer vitamin C following surgery. Br J Surg 1988; 75:366–370.
15. Enstrom JE, Kanim LE, Klein MA. Vitamin C intake and mortality among a sample of the United States population. Epidemiology 1992; 3:194–202.
16. Gey KF, Moser UK, Jordan P, et al. Increased risk of cardiovascular disease at suboptimal plasma concentrations of essential antioxidants: an epidemiological update with special attention to carotene and vitamin C. Am J Clin Nutr Suppl 1993; 57:787S–797S.
17. Riemersma RA, Wood DA, Macintyre CC, et al. Risk of angina pectoris and plasma concentrations of vitamins A, C, and E and carotene. Lancet 1991; 337:1–5.
18. Schectman G, Byrd JC, Gruchow HW. The influence of smoking on the vitamin C status in adults. Am J Public Health 1989; 79:158–162.
19. Yonemoto RH. Vitamin C and the immune response in normal controls and cancer patients. Int J Vitam Nutr Res Suppl 1979; 19:143–148.
20. Goldschmidt MC, Masin WJ, Brown LR, Wyde PR. The effect of ascorbic acid deficiency on leukocyte phagocytosis and killing of actinomyces viscosus. Int J Vitam Nutr Res 1988; 58:326–334.

21. Dowd PS, Kelleher J, Walker BE, Guillou PJ. Nutrition and cellular immunity in hospital patients. Br J Nutr 1986; 55:515–527.

22. Goetzl EJ, Wasserman SI, Gigli I, Austen KF. Enhancement of random migration and chemotactic response of human leukocytes by ascorbic acid. J Clin Invest 1974; 53:813–818.

23. Anderson R. Assessment of oral ascorbate in three children with chronic granulomatous disease and defective neutrophil motility over a 2-year period. Clin Exp Immunol 1981; 43:180–188.

24. Dallegri F, Lanzi G, Patrone F. Effects of ascorbic acid on neutrophil locomotion. Int Arch Allergy Appl Immunol 1980; 61:40–45.

25. Greendyke RM, Brierty RE, Swisher SN. In vitro studies on erythrophagocytosis. II. Effects of incubating leukocytes with selected cell metabolites. J Lab Clin Med 1964; 63:1016–1026.

26. Sandler JA, Gallin JI, Vaughan M. Effects of serotonin, carbamylcholine, and ascorbic acid on leukocyte cyclic GMP and chemotaxis. J Cell Biol 1975; 67:480–484.

27. Smith MJ, Walker JR. The effects of some antirheumatic drugs on an in vitro model of human polymorphonuclear leukocyte chemokinesis. Br J Pharmacol 1980; 69:473–478.

28. Anderson R, Theron A. Effects of ascorbate on leukocytes. Part I. Effects of ascorbate on neutrophil motility and intracellular cyclic nucleotide levels in vitro. S Afr Med J 1979; 56:394–399.

29. Anderson R, Grabow G. In vitro stimulation of neutrophil motility by metoprolol and sotalol related to inhibition of both H_2O_2 production and peroxidase mediated iodination of the cell and leukoattractant. Int J Immunopharmacol 1980; 2:321–326.

30. Hemilä H, Roberts P, Wikström M. Activated polymorphonuclear leukocytes consume vitamin C. FEBS Lett 1984; 178:25–30.

31. Halliwell B, Wasil M, Grootveld M. Biologically significant scavenging of the myeloperoxidase-derived oxidant hypochlorous acid by ascorbic acid. FEBS Lett 1987; 213:15–17.

32. De Chatelet LR, Cooper MR, McCall CE. Stimulation of the hexose monophosphate shunt in human neutrophils by ascorbic acid. Mechanism of action. Antimicrob Agents Chemother 1972; 1:12–16.

33. Miller TE. Killing and lysis of gram-negative bacteria through the synergistic effect of hydrogen peroxide, ascorbic acid and lysozyme. J Bacteriol 1969; 98:949–955.

34. Ericsson Y, Lundbeck H. Antimicrobial effect in vitro of the ascorbic acid oxidation. II. Influence of various chemical and physical factors. Acta Pathol Microbiol Scand 1955; 37:507–512.

35. Orr CWM. Studies on ascorbic acid. I. Factors influencing the ascorbate-mediated inhibition of catalase. Biochemistry 1967; 6:2995–3000.

36. Anderson R, Jones PT. Increased leukoattractant binding and reversible inhibition of neutrophil motility mediated by the peroxidase/H_2O_2/halide system: effects of ascorbate, cysteine, dithiothreitol, levamisole and thiamine. Clin Exp Immunol 1982; 47:487–492.

37. Anderson R. The immunostimulatory, anti-inflammatory and anti-allergic properties of ascorbate. Adv Nutr Res 1984; 6:19–45.

38. Anderson R, Lukey PT, Theron AJ, Dippenaar U. Ascorbate and cystine-mediated selective neutralization of extracellular oxidants during N-formyl-peptide activation of human phagocytes. Agents Actions 1987; 20:77–86.

39. Munster AM, Loadholdt CB, Leary AG, Barnes MA. The effect of antibiotics on cell-mediated immunity. Surgery 1977; 81:692–695.

40. Panush RS, Delafuente JC. Modulation of certain immunologic responses by vitamin C. II. Enhancement of concanavalin A-stimulated lymphocyte responses. Int J Vitam Nutr Res Suppl 1979; 19:179–185.

41. Manzella JP, Roberts NJ. Human macrophage and lymphocyte responses to mitogen stimulation after exposure to influenza virus, ascorbic acid and hyperthermia. J Immunol 1979; 123:1940–1944.

42. Smogorzewska EM, Layward L, Soothill JF. T-lymphocyte mobility: defects and effects of ascorbic acid, histamine and complexed IgG. Clin Exp Immunol 1981; 43:174–179.

43. Smit MJ, Anderson R. Biochemical mechanisms of hydrogen peroxide- and hypochlorous acid-mediated inhibition of human mononuclear leukocyte functions in vitro: protection and reversal by anti-oxidants. Agent Actions 1992; 36:58–65.

44. Anderson R, Hay I, van Wyk H, et al. The effect of ascorbate on cellular humoral immunity in asthmatic children. S Afr Med J 1980; 58:974–977.

45. Johnston CS, Martin LJ, Cai X. Antihistamine effect of supplemental ascorbic acid and neutrophil chemotaxis. J Am Coll Nutr 1992; 11:172–176.

46. Fraser RC, Pavlovi'c S, Kurahara CG, et al. The effect of variations in vitamin C intake on the cellular immune response of guinea pigs. Am J Clin Nutr 1980; 33:839–947.

47. Johnston CS, Huang SN. Effect of ascorbic acid nutriture on blood histamine and neutrophil chemotaxis in guinea pigs. J Nutr 1991; 121:126–130.

48. Siegel BV, Morton JI. Vitamin C and the immune response. Experientia 1977; 33:393–395.

49. Eicher-Pruiett SD, Morrill JL, Blecha F, et al. Neutrophil and lymphocyte response to supplementation with vitamins C and E in young calves. J Dairy Sci 1992; 75:1635–1642.

50. Stossel TP, Root RK, Vaughan M. Phagocytosis in chronic granulomatous disease and the Chédiak–Higashi syndrome. N Engl J Med 1972; 286:120–123.

51. Boxer LA, Watanabe AM, Rister M, et al. Correction of leukocyte function in Chédiak–Higashi syndrome by ascorbate. N Engl J Med 1976; 295:1041–1045.

52. Weening RS, Schoorel EP, Roos D, et al. Effect of ascorbate on abnormal neutrophil, platelet and lymphocyte function in a patient with the Chédiak–Higashi syndrome. Blood 1981; 57:856–865.

53. Yegin O, Sanal O, Yeralan O, et al. Defective lymphocyte locomotion in Chediak-Higasji Syndrome. Am J Dis Child 1983; 137:771–773.

54. Scheinberg MA. The effect of vitamin C on certain monocyte cell functions: an in vitro and in vivo approach. Int J Vitam Nutr Res Suppl 1983; 24:119–120.

55. Corberand J, Nguyen F, Fraysse B, Enjalbert L. Malignant external otitis and polymorphonuclear leukocyte migration impairment: improvement with ascorbic acid. Arch Otolaryngol 1982; 108:122–124.

56. Levy R, Schlaeffer F. Successful treatment of a patient with recurrent furunculosis by vitamin C: improvement of clinical course and of impaired neutrophil functions. Int J Dermatol 1993; 32:832–834.

57. Vohra K, Khan AJ, Telang V, et al. Improvement of neutrophil migration by systemic vitamin C in neonates. J Perinatol 1990; 10:134–136.

58. Newsholme EA, Parry-Billings M, McAndrew N, Budgett R. A biochemical mechanism to explain some characteristics of overtraining. In: Brouns F, ed. Advances in Nutrition and Top Sport. New York: Karger, 1991:79–93.

59. Peters EM, Goetzsche JM, Grobbelaar B, Noakes TD. Vitamin C supplementation reduces the incidence of postrace symptoms of upper respiratory tract infection in ultramarathon runners. Am J Clin Nutr 1993; 57:170–174.

60. Birnboim HC. Factors which affect DNA strand breakage in human leukocytes exposed to a tumor promotor, phorbol myristate acetate. Can J Physiol Pharmacol 1982; 60:1359–1366.

61. Andersen D, Basaren N, Blowers SD, Edwards AJ. The effect of antioxidants on bleomycin treatment in in vitro and in vivo genotoxicity assays. Mutat Res 1995; 329:37–47.

62. Medhat AM, el Din-Abdelwahab KS, er Aaser AA, et al. Soybean and ascorbate feeding in experimental carcinogenesis: immunologic studies. Tumori 1991; 77:372–378.

63. Kubov'a J, Tulinsk'a J, Stolcov'a E, et al. The influence of ascorbic acid on selected parameters of cell immunity in guinea pigs exposed to cadmium. Z Ernaehrungswiss 1993; 32:113–120.

64. Dunier M, Vergnet C, Siwicki AK, Verlhac V. Effect of Lindane exposure on rainbow trout immunity. IV. Prevention of nonspecific and specific immunosuppression by dietary vitamin C (ascorbate-2-polyphosphate). Ecotoxicol Environ Safety 1995; 30:259–268.

65. Metchnikoff E. Sur la lutte des cellules de l'organisms contre l'invasion des microbes. Ann Inst Pasteur 1887; 1:321–336.

66. Chester JF, Ross JS, Malt RA, Weitzman SA. Acute colitis produced by chemotactic peptides in rats and mice. Am J Pathol 1985; 121:284–290.

67. Dal Nogare AR. Septic shock. Am J Med Sci 1991; 302:50–65.

68. Hernandez LA, Grisham MB, Twohig B, et al. Role of neutrophils in ischemia-reperfusion-induced microvascular injury. Am J Physiol 1987; 253:H699–H703.

69. Korthuis RJ, Grisham MB, Granger DN. Leukocyte depletion attenuates vascular injury in post-ischemic skeletal muscle Am J Physiol 1988; 254:H823–H827.

70. Lehr HA, Guhlmann A, Nolte D, et al. Leukotrienes as mediators in positischemic leukocyte/endothelium interaction in a microcirculation model in the hamster. J Clin Invest 1991; 87:206–2041.

71. Menger MD, Pelikan S, Steiner D, Messmer K. Microvascular ischemia-reperfusion injury in striated muscle: significance of "reflow paradox." Am J Physiol 1992; 263:H1901–H1906.

72. Vedder NB, Winn RK, Rice CL, et al. A monoclonal antibody to the adherence-promoting leukocyte glycoprotein, CD18, reduces organ injury and improves survival from hemorrhagic shock and resuscitation in rabbits. J Clin Invest 1988; 81:939–944.

73. Ross R. Atherosclerosis: a defense mechanism gone awry. Am J Pathol 1993; 143:987–1002.

74. Lehr HA, Hübner C, Menger MD, Messmer K. Mechanisms and mediators of leukocyte/endothelium interaction during atherogenesis. Atheroscler Rev 1993; 25:49–57.

75. Granger DN. Role of xanthine oxidase and granulocytes in ischemia/reperfusion injury. Am J Physiol 1988; 255:H1269–H1275.

76. McIntyre TM, Patel KD, Zimmerman GA, Prescott SM. Oxygen radical-induced leukocyte adherence. In Granger DN, Schmid-Schoenbein GW, eds. Physiology and Pathophysiology of Leukocyte Adhesion. New York: Oxford University Press, 1995:261–277.

77. Suzuki M, Inauen W, Kvietys PR, et al. Superoxide mediates reperfusion-induced leukocyte-endothelial cell interactions. Am J Physiol 1989; 257:H1740–H1745.

78. Carew TE, Schwenke DC, Steinberg D. Antiatherogenic effect of probucol unrelated to its hypocholesterolemic effect: evidence that antioxidants in vivo can selectively inhibit low density lipoprotein degradation in macrophage-rich fatty streaks and slow the progression of atherosclerosis in the Watanabe heritable hyperlipidemic rabbit. Proc Natl Acad Sci USA 1987; 84:7725–7729.

79. Villa S, Lorico A, Morazzoni G, et al. Vitamin E and vitamin C inhibit arachidonate-induced aggregation of human peripheral blood leukocytes in vitro. Agents Actions 1986; 19:127–131.

80. Pfister RR, Haddox JL, Snyder TL. The effects of citrate on the adherence of neutrophils to nylon fibers in vitro. Invest Ophthalmol Vis Sci 1988; 29:869–875.

81. Jonas E, Dwenger A, Hager A. In vitro effect of ascorbic acid on neutrophil–endothelial cell interaction. J Biolumin Chemilumin 1993; 8:15–20.

82. Wilson CW. Clinical pharmacological aspects of ascorbic acid. Ann NY Acad Sci 1975; 258:355–376.

83. Davis RH, Rosenthal KY, Cesario LR, Rouw GR. Vitamin C influence on localized adjuvant arthritis. J Am Podiatr Med Assoc 1990; 80:414–418.

84. Hanley DC, Solomon WA, Saffran B, Davis RH. The evaluation of natural substances in the treatment of adjuvant arthritis. J Am Podiatr Med Assoc 72:275–284.

85. Parks DA, Bulkley GB, Granger DN, et al. Ischemic injury in the cat small intestine: role of superoxide radicals. Gastroenterology 1982; 82:9–15.

86. Lewis MS, Whatley RE, Cain P, et al. Hydrogen peroxide stimulates the synthesis of platelet-activating factor by endothelium and induces endothelial cell-dependent neutrophil adhesion. J Clin Invest 1988; 82:2045–2055.

87. Becker EL, Sigman M, Oliver JM. Superoxide production induced in rabbit polymorphonuclear leukocytes by synthetic chemotactic peptides and A23187. Am J Pathol 1979; 95:81–97.

88. Willy C, Thiery J, Menger MD, et al. Impact of vitamin E supplement in standard laboratory animal diet on microvascular manifestation of ischemia/reperfusion injury. Free Radical Biol Med 1995; 19:919–926.

89. Clavien PA, Harvey PR, Sanabria JR, et al. Lymphocyte adherence in the reperfused rat liver: mechanisms and effects. Hepatology 1993; 17:131–142.

90. Eddy L, Hurvitz R, Hochstein P. A protective role for ascorbate in induced ischemic arrest associated with cardiopulmonary bypass. J Appl Cardiol 1990; 5:409–414.

91. Janoff A. Elastases and emphysema: current assessment of the protease-antiprotease hypothesis. Am Rev Respir Dis 1985; 132:417–433.

92. Lehr HA, Seemüller J, Hübner C, et al. Oxidized LDL-induced leukocyte/endothelium interaction in vivo involves the receptor for platelet-activating factor. Arterioscler Thromb 1993; 13:1013–1018.

93. Janoff A, Carp H, Lee DK, Drew RT. Cigarette smoke inhalation decreases alpha 1-antitrypsin activity in rat lung. Science 1979; 206:1313–1314.

94. Kilburn KH, McKenzie W. Leukocyte recruitment to airways cigarette smoke and particle phase in contrast to cytotoxicity by vapor. Science 1975; 189:634–637.

95. Ludwig PW, Schwartz BA, Hoidal JR, Niewoehner DE. Cigarette smoking causes accumulation of polymorphonuclear leukocytes in alveolar septum. Am Rev Respir Dis 1985; 131:828–830.

96. Bosken CH, Doerschuk CM, English D, Hogg JC. Neutrophil kinetics during active cigarette smoking in rabbits. J Appl Physiol 1991; 71:630–637.

97. MacNee W, Wiggs B, Belzberg AS, Hogg JC. The effect of cigarette smoking on neutrophil kinetics in human lungs. N Engl J Med 1989; 321:924–928.

98. Lehr HA, Frei B, Arfors KE. Vitamin C prevents cigarette smoke-induced leukocyte aggregation and adhesion to endothelium in vivo. Proc Natl Acad Sci USA 1994; 91:7688–7692.

99. Kuhn C, Senior JA, Pierce JA. In: Witschi H, Nettesheim P, eds. Mechanisms of Respiratory Toxicology, Vol. 2. Boca Raton, FL: CRC Press, 1982; fl55–172.

100. Steinberg D, Parthasarathy S, Carew TE, et al. Beyond cholesterol: modifications of low-density lipoprotein that increase its atherogenicity. N Engl J Med 1989; 320:915–924.

101. Penn MS, Chisolm GM. Oxidized lipoproteins, altered cell function and atherosclerosis. Atherosclerosis 1994; 108:S21–S29.

102. Frostegard J, Nilsson J, Haegerrstrand A, et al. Oxidized low-density lipoprotein induces differentiation and adhesion of human monocytes and monocytic cell line U937. Proc Natl Acad Sci USA 1990; 87:904–908.

103. Lehr HA, Hübner C, Finckh B, et al. Role of leukotrienes in leukocyte adhesion following systemic administration of oxidatively modified human low-density lipoprotein in hamsters. J Clin Invest 1991; 88:9–14.

104. Frei B, Stocker R, Ames BN. Antioxidant defenses and lipid peroxidation in human blood plasma. Proc Natl Acad Sci USA 1988; 85:9748–9752.

105. Lehr HA, Becker M, Marklund SL, et al. Superoxide-dependent stimulation of leukocyte adhesion by oxidatively modified LDL in vivo. Atheroscler Thromb 1992; 12:824–829.

106. Niki E. Action of ascorbic acid as a scavenger of active and stable oxygen radicals. Am J Clin Nutr 1991; 54:1119S–1124S.

107. Lehr HA, Frei B, Olofsson AM, et al. Protection from oxidized LDL-induced leukocyte adhesion to microvascular and macrovascular endothelium in vivo by vitamin C, but not by vitamin E. Circulation 1995; 91:1525–1532.

108. Smiley PL, Stremler KE, Prescott SM, et al. Oxidatively fragmented phosphatidylcholines activate human neutrophils through the receptor for platelet activating factor. J Biol Chem 1991; 266:11104–11110.

109. Yang X, Cai B, Sciacca RR, Cannon PJ. Inhibition of inducible nitric oxide synthase in macrophages by oxidized low-density lipoproteins. Circ Res 1994; 74:318–328.

110. Gryglewski RJ, Palmer RM, Moncada S. Superoxide anion is involved in the breakdown of endothelium-derived vascular relaxing factor. Nature 1986; 320:454–456.

111. Keaney JF, Gaziano JM, Xu A, et al. Dietary antioxidants preserve endothelium-dependent vessel relaxation in cholesterol-fed rabbits. Proc Natl Acad Sci USA 1993; 90:11880–11884.

112. Kubes P, Suzuki M, Granger DN. Nitric oxide: an endogenous modulator of leukocyte adhesion. Proc Natl Acad Sci USA 1991; 88:4651–4655.

113. Eldor A, Vlodavsky I, Riklis E, Fuks Z. Revicery of prostacyclin capacity of irradiated endothelial cells and the protective effect of vitamin C. Prostaglandins 1987; 34:241–255.

17

Mechanisms Underlying the Action of Vitamin C in Viral and Immunodeficiency Disease

RAXIT J. JARIWALLA and STEVE HARAKEH
Linus Pauling Institute, Palo Alto, California

INTRODUCTION

The Essentiality of Vitamin C

In 1928 Albert Szent-Györgyi isolated L-ascorbic acid from vegetables and adrenal glands of animals. In 1932 this compound was given the name vitamin C, or ascorbic acid. It was discovered that primates, unlike most animals, are unable to synthesize vitamin C because they possess a mutated form of the gene encoding the enzyme L-gulono-gamma-lactone oxidase, required for the final step in L-ascorbic acid synthesis (1).

Vitamin C therefore is an essential nutrient in human physiological processes. Since people cannot make it endogenously, they depend on ingesting a sufficient supply wholly from exogenous sources. Ascorbic acid (AA) is particularly abundant in many fruits as well as in vegetables, such as the various *Capsicum* peppers, the crucifers (e.g., broccoli, cabbage, kale), and certain nightshade-family food plants (e.g., potatoes, tomatoes). A serious deficiency in this vitamin results in scurvy, notable symptoms of which are gum disease, fatigue, joint and muscle pain, skin lesions, and capillary bleeding (2). Ascorbate deficiency may also cause decline in mental function and contribute to depression (3).

Effects of Vitamin C on Viral and Immunodeficiency Diseases

A large body of evidence by now has shown that vitamin C can inactivate or inhibit a wide spectrum of viruses in vitro as well as protect against viral infections in vivo. Additionally, vitamin C has been demonstrated to restore immune function in both viral and nonviral conditions linked to immunodeficiency.

Early reports from in vitro studies showed that ascorbate mediated the inactivation of several different viruses, which included poliomyelitis, herpes simplex (fever blisters or cold-sores), foot and mouth, rabies, vaccinia, and bacterial viruses (1). In vivo, ascorbate was reported to control a wide spectrum of viral infections, including poliomyelitis, hepatitis, herpes simplex, herpes zoster (shingles), virus pneumonia, measles, virus encephalitis, rabies, and influenza (1,3).

. More recently, ascorbate was demonstrated to suppress the replication of rhinoviruses and retroviruses in infected host cells (4,5). A large number of studies have assessed vitamin C efficacy in the common cold. The overall weight of the evidence shows that although vitamin C may not affect incidence of colds (at low to moderate concentrations tested), it reduces the course of disease and severity of symptoms (3,6,7).

Immunodeficiency states in which supplementation with vitamin C has been said to have restored immune function include (1) Chédiak–Higashi disease, a condition characterized by impaired phagocytic function; (2) measles in children exhibiting abnormal helper/suppressor T-cell ratios; (3) human immunodeficiency virus (HIV) infection, associated with helper T-cell depletion and B-cell dysregulation; and (4) age-related weakening of immune systems in elderly persons (4).

In our work as virologists during the past decade in investigating the biochemical and cellular effects of HIV and acquired immunodeficiency syndrome (AIDS) on the immune system, we have learned a great deal about the potential or actual value of vitamin C and other micronutrients in addressing health problems of those suffering in this epidemic. We consider researchers' and clinicians' findings in studying or treating HIV infection to have important relevance to immune-deficient conditions generally.

Infection with (HIV) is commonly associated with weight loss, defined as a reduction of 10% or greater of the usual body weight, associated, in the absence of any illness, with chronic diarrhea and/or weakness and fever. As a result, "wasting syndrome," one of the most notable manifestations of AIDS, develops. Infection with HIV leads to an overall reduction in immunity, making the body more susceptible to secondary opportunistic infections and neoplasms.

A correlation has been found between survival and involuntary reduction of body weight. In a study of HIV-infected homosexuals, a greater loss of body weight was noted in HIV-seropositive patients than in those tested HIV-seronegative. The HIV-seropositive individuals had a lighter weight and thinner build. The most noticeable decrease in body weight and lean body mass occurred as patients approached the end stage of the disease (8).

The causes for this dramatic decline in body weight are known to be declining food intake (due to lack of appetite), improper attention to optimal nutrition designed for the condition, and chronic diarrhea, which moves nutrients through the gastrointestinal tract too rapidly for absorption. It is therefore believed by nutrition-oriented HIV researchers and physicians that effective dietary information and support can help the body better maintain normal weight as well as give it more strength to ward off secondary infections. These positive effects in turn can provide affected individuals with longer life spans and a better overall quality of life. Society itself can benefit from HIV-infected persons' overall increased productivity and lower health-care costs.

Primarily HIV attacks the immune system, and HIV infection is associated with a steady depletion of nutrients and vitamins in patients. Even asymptomatic patients have shown lower levels of vitamin C and other micronutrients and endogenous antioxidants in their plasma, as compared to uninfected individuals (9). A number of other immunodeficient conditions display similar deficiencies in key vitamins, minerals, and other beneficial biochemical compounds. For this reason, an agent that boosts the function of the immune system should help to bolster the body's mechanisms against HIV and other infections, as well as deter other immune dysfunctions.

It is highly probable that vitamin C, because of its numerous immune-stimulating, virus-suppressing, and protective properties, is just such a candidate for nutritional therapy in immunodeficiency diseases. The specific biological effects of vitamin C on viruses and the immune system and the strategic function of ascorbate in AIDS have been recently reviewed (4,5). This chapter will focus on the biochemical mechanisms that underlie ascorbate's beneficial effects in viral and immunodeficiency diseases. Specifically, we will present ascorbate's immunosupportive mechanisms involved in (1) protection from oxidative damage, (2) strengthening of connective tissues, (3) bolstering of the immune responses, (4) direct antiviral action and selective killing of virus-infected cells.

POTENTIATION OF PROTECTIVE HOST MECHANISMS THROUGH DIFFERENT FUNCTIONS

Ascorbic acid is a multifunctional physiological modulator. Aside from its well-documented role in hydroxylation reactions linked to collagen synthesis, ascorbate is a powerful reducing agent (antioxidant) and can exert a prooxidant effect under certain conditions (e.g., in the presence of transition metals). Additionally, it can stimulate both cell-mediated and humoral (antibody) responses and exert a direct antiviral action on virus activity and infected cells.

Accordingly, the mechanistic basis for the protective effect of ascorbate in viral and immune-related disorders is likely to derive from multiple functions rather than a single property. What follows will cover the known functions of ascorbate that are relevant to its beneficial effects in viral and immune diseases.

Cell Protection from Oxidative Damage

Protection against viral diseases depends in part on ascorbate's effectiveness as a reducing agent. Ascorbate ($C_6H_6O_6H_2$) acts as a reducing agent by virtue of its ability to donate electrons associated with two redox-active hydrogens. Depending on the concentration in the body, ascorbate can function as either a carrier or a source of high-energy electrons. At ordinary concentrations normally present in the diet, ascorbate serves as an electron carrier, neutralizing free radicals and undergoing oxidation in the process, only to be regenerated to its reduced form by glutathione. In contrast, at high concentrations supplied through supplementation, ascorbate can serve as a direct source of electrons, capable of reducing both free radicals and their scavengers without requiring regeneration to ascorbic acid for continued function (10). The latter property is essential under conditions of glutathione deficiency (see later discussion).

Ascorbate contributes up to 24% of the total antioxidant capacity for trapping peroxy radicals in human blood plasma (11). In a plasma in vitro system, ascorbate was demonstrated to function as an outstanding antioxidant, displaying more effectiveness than protein thiols, bilirubin, urate, or tocopherol in protecting against peroxidation of fatty acids (12). By trapping reactive radicals in plasma, ascorbate may lower the rate of oxidation of vital components of plasma, thereby conferring protection against damage by extracellular oxidants.

Additionally, vitamin C can function in concert with vitamin E to protect cell membranes against oxidative damage (13). Since protected cells are more resistant to viral entry than damaged cells, this property of ascorbate may in part contribute to resistance against viral invasion of target tissues.

Neutralization of Cytoplasmic/Extracellular Antioxidants Generated from Activated Neutrophils/Macrophages

On the basis of the reaction of vitamin C with oxidizing substances, Hemilä (6) suggested that the biochemical explanation for its beneficial effect in the common cold may be related to its antioxidant function. The amounts of vitamin C that confer protection from the common cold were also higher than those required to prevent scurvy associated with decreased collagen synthesis. Several experimental observations support the suggested mechanism. Oxidant production has been linked with viruses responsible for causing the common cold. Thus, activated neutrophils are consistently found in nasal passages of subjects infected with rhinovirus strains, and neutrophil invasion into the lung has been associated with infection by respiratory syncytial virus (14,15).

Neutrophil activation involves a process of respiratory burst in which activation of a membrane-associated oxidase leads to the formation of superoxide radical within a phagosome (16). Hydrogen peroxide generated from the action of superoxide dismutase then diffuses out into the extracellular space or gets converted to the highly reactive hypochlorous acid via the action of myeloperoxidase. Neutrophil activation is also associated with production of proteolytic enzymes which can leak out of the phagosome into the extracelluar space. One such protease is elastase, whose activity in plasma is kept in check by the alpha-1 proteinase inhibitor. However, inactivation of the latter by reactive free radicals can promote proteolytic activity (17,18).

There is evidence for utilization (oxidation) of endogenous vitamin C during phagocyte activation (17,19,20). Some is oxidized during respiratory burst and some in neutralizing cytoplasmic and extracelluar antioxidants generated during the activation process. Vitamin C was also shown to protect alpha-1 proteinase inhibitor from inactivation by myeloperoxidase-generated hypochlorite in vitro (21). Thus, as suggested by Hemilä and Herman (7), supplemental vitamin C may provide protection from viral infection in the common cold by neutralizing oxidizing substances generated during virus-mediated neutrophil activation.

A growing body of evidence links oxidative stress to other viral infections. Except for those of certain diseases such as poliomyelitis, the symptoms of most viral infections do not primarily result from direct cytopathic effects on infected cells, but rather from abnormal host response through activation of host effector functions (22). The latter are associated not only with oxidant production, but also with inflammatory cytokines and other biological-response mediators.

In this category, viruses such as Sendai virus (parainfluenza 1 virus), influenza virus of mice, and rabbit poxvirus can activate respiratory burst in phagocytic cells (macrophages/ neutrophils) to generate reactive oxygen species (ROS) in the absence of host antiviral components. Other viruses included in the herpesvirus, lentivirus, and togavirus families require antiviral antibodies to activate phagocytic cells. Recently, experimentally induced viral encephalitis was linked to nitric oxide generation (23,24). Nitric oxide and superoxide were also shown to mediate neurotoxicity induced by the surface glycoprotein (gp120) of human immunodeficiency virus (25).

Human immunodeficiency virus infection has been associated with a state of chronic immune-cell activation and inflammation consistent with increased oxidative stress and a high rate of selective apoptosis of disease-fighting lymphocytic cells (9,26,27). Consumption of specific micronutrients (including vitamin C) by HIV-seropositive persons was found to reduce the hazard of AIDS development (9). Administration of the antioxidant enzyme superoxide dismutase (SOD) was shown to protect against the symptoms induced by influenza virus in mice (28,29). Since vitamin C can react efficiently with superoxide radical and other oxidants, it may provide protection against toxic effects of viruses, in part by neutralizing ROS generated from host-cell activation.

Sparing of Glutathione and Cell Protection from Glutathione Deficiency

Aside from oxidant production, viral/immunodeficiency states are often associated with antioxidant imbalance. Specific abnormalities in antioxidant micronutrients can be detected early in HIV infection. These include decreased levels in blood serum of physiologically important vitamins (A, B-complex, C, E, and carotenes), trace elements (selenium and zinc), and endogenous sulfur-containing amino acids (cysteine, methionine) or peptide thiols such as glutathione (9).

Deficiency in acid-soluble thiols (cysteine) and glutathione (GSH) is widespread in HIV-infected persons (30,31). Glutathione deficiency occurs in both peripheral blood mononuclear cells and lung epithelial-lining fluid (31). Since micronutrient abnormalities are prevalent early in infection, they may contribute to progression of disease. Specifically, GSH deficiency may play a significant role in HIV pathogenesis. Loss of high GSH-containing CD8 T-cells has been linked to weakening of the cell-mediated cytotoxic response against viruses (26,32); GSH lung deficiency may predispose to pulmonary cell abnormality (31). Experimental animals with drug-induced GSH deficiency exhibit widespread organ damage, including cataract formation and a high rate of mortality (33). Administration of a diet containing large doses of another water-soluble antioxidant (ascorbic acid) was shown to spare GSH, confer protection from organ damage, and reduce the rate of mortality in a dose-dependent fashion (33,34).

The effect of both ascorbate and N-acetylcysteine (NAC) on a patient with hereditary deficiency of glutathione synthetase was recently studied by Jain et al. (35). They reported that the continous administration of high doses of ascorbic acid and N-acetylcysteine led to a decrease in erythrocyte turnover in patients with deficiency of glutathione. They attributed this to enhancement by NAC and AA of glutathione levels in both plasma and lymphocytes.

Thus, under conditions of GSH deficiency, ascorbate can serve as an essential antioxidant and provide protection from cellular damage and death due to multiple organ failure.

Increased Viral Resistance from Strengthening of Connective Tissues

It is well established that ascorbic acid can influence the activity of enzymes involved in hydroxylation reactions (36). Vitamin C deficiency has been associated with defective formation of collagen and connective tissue (37). Collagen synthesis and structure depend on the proper functioning of several hydroxylases, which include prolyl-4-hydroxylase, prolyl-3-hydroxylase, and lysyl hydroxylase. These enzymes require a reducing agent to maintain their activity, which is lowered in the tissues of ascorbate-deficient animals. There is evidence that ascorbate reactivates oxidatively inactivated enzymes by reducing the bound metal ion Fe^{3+} to Fe^{2+}, thereby facilitating the formation of hydroxyproline and hydroxylysine residues. The latter are required for stabilization of the triple helical structure of collagen. Thus by stimulating collagen synthesis, ascorbate can strengthen tissues and intercellular cement substance, resulting in resistance to viral infection. Early studies on the role of ascorbate in collagen formation and involvement of possible mechanisms have been reviewed (4). More recent studies supporting this role are summarized here.

Recently, Yeowell et al. (38) showed that ascorbate addition to dermal fibroblasts from patients with a connective tissue disorder (Ehlers-Danlos syndrome type VI) resulted in upregulation of lysyl hydroxylase and a twofold increase in collagen synthesis. Stimulation of collagen synthesis in dermal fibroblasts was independent of age (39).

In other studies, ascorbate enhanced collagen synthesis in (1) native collagen fibers used as a dermal substitute (40), (2) human dermal fibroblasts grown on a collagen matrix (41), (3) cultured endothelial cells (about sixfold), resulting in stimulation of barrier functions (42).

Extracellular matrix gene expression was also modulated by ascorbate in bovine chondrocyte cultures (43). Growth of ligament/skin fibroblasts and vascular smooth muscle cells in the presence of ascorbate resulted in an increased proportion of newly synthesized fibrillin within cell layers (44). Addition of moderately high doses (50–200 μg/ml) of ascorbate to the culture medium of trabecular meshwork cells of the human eye was shown to result in dose-dependent stimulation of hyaluronic acid synthesis and secretion. By strengthening the fibrillar network that surrounds and connects tissues, ascorbate provides a physical barrier against viral invasion.

Bolstering of Immunity

Stimulation and Protection of Lymphocyte Production and Function

Ascorbate plays an important role in lymphocyte physiological processes. Like neutrophils, lymphocytes concentrate ascorbate to high levels (45,46). Both lymphocyte function and production are influenced by ascorbate concentrations. This was reviewed earlier by us (5). Ascorbate can also protect lymphocytes against oxidative damage. Here we focus on the most recent findings pertaining to the immunoprotective effects of vitamin C on lymphocytic cells in culture, animals, and humans.

Bergsten et al. (47) studied the transport of ascorbic acid and its distribution in B-lymphocytes in humans. They reported that the activity or high-affinity transport component was dependent on both temperature and concentration. Carbonylcyanide-P-trifluoromethoxyphenylhydricone and ouabain inhibited the transport of AA and generated AA accumulation against a concentration gradient. Intracellularly, AA in human lymphocytes was predominantly bound to the cytosol and not to protein.

Chakrabarti et al. (48) reported that mice fed a diet supplemented with ascorbic acid showed potentiation of their immune system that was claimed to be due to stimulation and activation of large granular lymphocytes.

Aidoo et al. (49) studied the antimutagenic effects of vitamin C on the frequency of T-lymphocytes produced in rats dosed with the mutagenic agent N-ethyl-N-nitrosourea (ENu). In 344 Fischer rats, ascorbic acid significantly reduced the ENu-mediated mutagenic responses, suggesting an explanation for the effect of vitamin C intake on decreasing abnormal cell proliferation.

Both in vitro and in vivo studies conducted by Anderson et al. (5O) found that vitamin C, but not vitamin E, abolished chromosome-damaging responses induced by bleomycin in human peripheral lymphocytes and reduced responses in micronuclei from peripheral blood cells in mice. These effects were attributed to a protective role of vitamin C and a null effect of vitamin E against chromosome-mediated immune cell damage.

Anderson et al. (51) also studied the effects of antioxidants and other agents on deoxyribonucleic acid (DNA) damage generated by oxygen radical in human lymphocytes. They found that vitamin C had a clear dose-related protective effect when tested alone. In the presence of H_2O_2, vitamin C provided small protection at low concentrations but exacerbated effects of H_2O_2 at high doses; the latter were within the interexperimental variability range. In a different study, Umegaki et al. (52) found that beta-carotene but not ascorbic acid protected human lymphocytes from x-ray-induced genetic damage. In a study on workers in contact with molybdenum salts, ascorbic acid administration resulted in a decrease of the chromosomal structural rearrangements as measured by chromosomal aberrations and sister chromatid exchange (53).

Protection of Phagocytic Function

Vitamin C also plays an important role in the proper functioning of phagocytes (5). In addition to conferring protection against tissue damage linked to neutrophil activation (see the section, Neutralization of Cytoplasmic/Extracellular Antioxidants Generated from Activated Neutrophils/Macrophages), ascorbate also protects phagocytes against adverse oxidation effects.

Autooxidation of neutrophils can occur as a result of oxidants such as hydrogen peroxide produced endogenously during phagocytic activation. Such autooxidation can cause loss of neutrophil functions vital to phagocytosis (54). Vitamin C has been shown to reduce the autooxidative effects of hypochloride (17). Recent studies provide further support for the inhibitory effect of ascorbate against oxidative reactions linked to macrophage activity.

Stait and Leake (55) reported that whereas ascorbate inhibited low-density lipoprotein (LDL) oxidation by macrophages in freshly prepared LDL, it did not inhibit LDL modification in the presence of macrophages in autooxidized LDL left in the refrigerator for 10 weeks or longer after isolation. Rengstrom et al. (56) also reported that the formation of dienes from exposure of LDL to copper was inhibited by the addition of ascorbic acid.

In a study on the mechanism of LDL protection, Retsky et al. (57) found that ascorbic acid scavenged free radicals, thus preventing them from attacking and oxidizing LDL. Second, LDL was stably modified by dehydroascorbate or other decomposition products, thus making it more resistant to metal ion–dependent oxidation.

Kubova et al. (58) investigated the effect of different concentrations of ascorbic acid in guinea pigs exposed to cadmium (Cd). They found that Cd had a negative effect on the immune system, which was potentiated by suboptimal intake of ascorbic acid. However, the toxic effects of Cd were lowered by high intake of vitamin C, as evaluated by measurement of phagocytic activity (of polymorphonuclear leukocytes and monocytes) and total T-lymphocytes in peripheral blood.

Herbacznska-Cedro et al. (59) studied the effects of supplemental vitamins C and E in 13 healthy volunteers on reactive oxygen production in polymorphonuclear leukocytes stimulated with arachidonic acid. They found that supplementation caused a significant increase in serum content of vitamins C and E, which was correlated with a significant decrease in leukocytes' ability to produce oxygen free radicals and with a lowering of serum peroxides. This may contribute to the vascular protective effect of ascorbate and tocopherol.

Improvement in the clinical course of a patient with impaired neutrophil functions after vitamin C supplementation was reported recently by Levy and Schlaeffer (60). Also, Papatheofanis and Barmada (61) reported that pretreatment of human polymorphonuclear leucocytes with ascorbic acid before exposure to isobutyl-2-cyanoacrylate resulted in (1) significant reduction in superoxide production; (2) lowering of lactate dehydrogenase release; and (3) increase in glutathione levels. Their data showed that ascorbic acid reduced the cytotoxic properties of toxic chemicals associated with the abnormal formation of reactive oxygen intermediates.

Effect of Vitamin C on Antibody Production

It has been discussed earlier (4) that ascorbic acid and its derivatives function as effective immunostimulators of antibody production in humans and animals. More recently, Dunier et al. (62) showed that the specific and nonspecific immunosuppressive effect of the insecticide Lindane in rainbow trout can be prevented by vitamin C. They found that immunoglobulin (Ig) production and B-lymphocyte proliferation in response to mitogen were significantly reduced as a result of exposure to Lindane. This effect was reversed as a result of high levels of ascorbic acid in the fish diet. Lindane did not modify the humoral response to *Yersinia ruckeri*, but it was significantly increased by vitamin C for 1 month after injection with *Yersinia* antigen.

Tanaka et al. (63) investigated the effects of ascorbic acid or the frequent addition of ascorbate on antibody production by human peripheral blood lymphocytes (PBLs) after stimulation with *Staphylococcus aureus Cowan 1* or pokeweed mitogen. Ascorbate functioned as a potent immunostimulator for antibody production, as demonstrated in the increased numbers of IgM and IgG; intracellular levels of ascorbic acid were important in maintaining a good immune response to PBLs.

DIRECT ANTIVIRAL ACTION

In addition to conferring cellular protection from oxidative damage and enhancing immune functions, ascorbate can directly inactivate virus infectivity and/or its enzymatic activity. This effect of ascorbate on viruses appears to be mediated, paradoxically, via its prooxidant function. As a prooxidant, ascorbate can reduce redox-active transition metal ions by a one-electron transfer mechanism to their lower valency state: e.g., ferric to ferrous ($Fe^{3+} \rightarrow Fe^{2+}$), cupric to cuprous ($Cu^{2+} \rightarrow Cu^{+}$). By a two-electron mechanism, ascorbate can also reduce molecular O_2 to hydrogen peroxide (H_2O_2). The reduced products can react in the presence of oxygen to generate superoxide (O_2^{1-}) and hydroxyl ($^{\cdot}OH$) radicals by the following reactions (64):

$$Fe^{2+} \text{ or } Cu^{+} \rightarrow O_2^{1-} + Fe^{3+} \text{ or } Cu^{2+}$$
$$Fe^{2+} \text{ or } Cu^{+} + H_2O_2 \rightarrow OH^{-} + {}^{\cdot}OH + Fe^{+3} \text{ or } Cu^{2+}$$

The metal-ion catalyzed oxidation mediated by ascorbate can modify macromolecular structure, including that of lipids, proteins, and nucleic acids (65). A large number of enzymes have been shown to undergo oxidative inactivation by ascorbate and O_2 (64). Unlike free radical generation by oxidizing substances which cause random modification of target molecules, oxidative modification of proteins by ascorbate was found to affect only one or a few amino acid residues, indicating a site-specific mechanism of action (64,65). Similarly, cleavage of nucleic acid by ascorbate in the presence of oxygen was shown to be a site-specific event, resulting in formation of discrete breakdown products (66). These observations are consistent with a mechanism of action in which metal ions bound to specific sites on proteins or nucleic acid react with H_2O_2, leading to the localized production of ·OH radicals. Catalytic sites, or those important for biological activity, located in the vicinity of ·OH generation, undergo structural damage, resulting in specific loss of biological activity.

Virus Inhibition by Oxidative Inactivation of Specific Components

A number of observations suggest that inactivation of cell-free virus and suppression of virus replication by ascorbate may be mediated via its prooxidant action. Thus, Murata and coworkers (67,68) studied the susceptibility of bacterial viruses in vitro and found that both ribonucleic acid (RNA)- and DNA-containing phages were inactivated by exposure to ascorbate. Virus inactivation was dependent on the presence of O_2 and accelerated by trace quantities of transition-metal ions. Addition of free-radical scavengers inhibited virus inactivation, suggesting involvement of oxidative radicals. Fractionation of virion components showed that scission of phage nucleic acid had occurred after exposure to ascorbate—consistent with loss of viral infectivity. Damage to genomic RNA was also suggested as a probable mechanism for reduction in the infectivity and replication of Rous sarcoma virus (RSV) after ascorbate exposure of infected cells (69).

Although viral nucleic acid appeared to be the target in phage inactivation and RSV inhibition, other components appear to be involved in ascorbate-mediated suppression of HIV. Thus, studies conducted in our laboratory have shown that ascorbate suppresses HIV replication in unstimulated chronically and acutely infected cells (70,71) and inhibits viral expression in a latently infected line upon cell stimulation by cytokine or tumor promoter (72). Analysis of total RNA and proteins from an ascorbate-treated chronically infected line showed that the patterns of virus-specific RNAs and polypeptides were similar to the corresponding viral components in virus-specific RNAs in untreated cells (73). Ascorbate also did not affect regulatory *Tat* protein-mediated transactivation of reporter gene linked to HIV long-terminal repeat (LTR) in mixed cultures of infected and uninfected indicator cell lines (73).

More recent analysis by gel shift assays has shown that ascorbate does not affect activation of the nuclear transcription factor, NF-KB, a key step targeted for HIV inhibition by thiol-containing and liphophilic antioxidants (unpublished observations). In contrast to the preceding findings, ascorbate consistently lowered the enzymatic activity of virion-associated reverse transcriptase in culture supernatants harvested from ascorbate-treated infected cell lines. These results are consistent with a mechanism of action in which ascorbate suppresses HIV at least in part by impairing virus-specific enzymatic activity, possibly via oxidative modification.

Virus Inhibition Through Selective Killing of Infected Cells

Yet other mechanisms may operate in ascorbate-mediated virus inhibition. One such mechanism involves apoptosis, or programmed cell death. It has been well documented that ascorbate can cause selective killing of specific types of tumor cells. Certain populations of leukemic cells and tumor cells of neuroectodermal origin (melanoma, neuroblastoma) are highly susceptible to ascorbate-mediated cytotoxicity (74,75). Cell lines from neuroectodermal tumors display increased sensitivity to oxidative stress because of an abnormal pattern of antioxidant enzymes. They also contain high levels of ascorbate recycling (semidehydroascorbate and dehydroascorbate reducing activities) (75). Oxidative stress, including glutathione depletion, has been shown to promote cell death (76). Higher levels of ascorbate via increased regeneration may potentiate oxidation in tumor cells, leading to selective cell killing.

Virus-infected cells, particularly HIV-infected cells, are good candidates for oxidant-mediated cell death. As discussed in the section, Cell Protection from Oxidative Damage, both generalized antioxidant loss and glutathione deficiency are prevalent in HIV infection. Intracellular GSH depletion and loss of antioxidant enzymes occur in infected cells. Oxidant production associated with immune-cell activation is also prevalent in infected subjects. Peripheral blood mononuclear cells from HIV-infected subjects display a high rate of both spontaneous and activation-induced cell death, as compared to those from HIV-negative subjects. Consistent with the involvement of oxidative stress in apoptosis, the glutathione precursor and thiol antioxidants NAC was shown to increase cell survival in HIV-infected cells after cytokine exposure (77). In contrast, ascorbate was found to increase cellular toxicity in a cytokine-stimulated promonocytic cell line (78), supporting a prooxidative mechanism.

Although the mechanism of decreased cell survival in ascorbate-treated HIV-infected cells remains to be established, the data suggest that ascorbate may mediate selective killing of virus-infected cells.

SUMMARY

Vitamin C is an essential multifunctional nutrient with strong antioxidant and prooxidant activities. It inhibits a wide spectrum of viruses in vitro and provides protection against viral infection/invasion and immune dysfunction in vitro. The beneficial effects of ascorbate in viral and immunodeficiency disease appear to result from involvement of multiple mechanisms rather than a singular property or function of the vitamin. Important mechanisms involved include (1) protection of both virus-susceptible cellular targets and immune cells from oxidative/proteolytic damage, (2) potentiation of cell-mediated and humoral immune responses, and (3) direct antiviral action.

Ascorbate confers host cell protection from viral invasion by strengthening connective tissues, by neutralizing extracellular oxidizing substances liberated from activated infection-fighting phagocytes (macrophages/neutrophils), and by serving as an essential antioxidant in sparing glutathione and withstanding oxidative tissue damage associated with GSH deficiency. Ascorbate potentiates the immune response by stimulating lymphocyte production/function (including antibody synthesis), by enhancing neutrophil function (phagocytic activity), and by preventing autooxidation of activated cells involved in host defense. The vitamin appears to exert its direct antiviral action through its prooxidant function, which may mediate inactivation of cell-free virus, suppression of viral replication in infected cells, and selective killing (via apoptosis) of virally infected cells. These multiple actions of ascorbate combined with its low toxicity at high doses (against normal cells) distinguish it from other antioxidants and set it apart from conventional antiviral and immunodeficiency drugs.

ACKNOWLEDGMENT

We are grateful to Barbara Marinacci and Jola Walichiewicz for their help in processing this manuscript

REFERENCES

1. Stone I. The Healing Factor: Vitamin C Against Disease. New York: Grosset & Dunlap, 1972.
2. Lind J. Treatise on the Scurvy. 3d ed. Birmingham, AL: Classics of Medicine Library, 1980.
3. Pauling L. How to Live Longer and Feel Better. New York: WH Freeman, 1986.
4. Jariwalla RJ, Harakeh S. Ascorbic acid and AIDS: strategic functions and therapeutic possibilities. In: Watson R, ed. Nutrition and AIDS. Boca Raton, FL: CRC Press, 1994: 117–139.
5. Jariwalla RJ, Harakeh S. Antiviral and immunomodulatory activities of ascorbic acid. In: JR Harris, ed. Subcellular Biochemistry. Vol 25. Ascorbic Acid: Biochemistry and Biomedical Cell Biology. New York: Plenum Press, 1995:215–231.
6. Hemilä H. Vitamin C and the common cold. Br J Nutri 1992; 67:3–16.
7. Hemilä H, Herman ZS. Vitamin C and the common cold: a retrospective analysis of Chalmers' review. J Am Coll Nutr 1995; 14:116–123.
8. Kotler D. Malnutrition and HIV infection and AIDS. AIDS 1989; 3 (suppl):189, S175–180.
9. Jariwalla RJ. Micro-nutrient imbalance in HIV infection and AIDS: relevance to pathogenesis and therapy. J Nutr Environ Med 1995; 5:297–306.
10. Lewin S. Vitamin C: Its Biology and Medical Potential. New York, Academic Press, 1976.
11. Wayner DDM, Burton GW, Ingold KU, et al. The relative contributions of vitamin E, urate, ascorbate and proteins to the total peroxy radical-trapping antioxidant activity of human blood plasma. Biochim Biophys Acta 1987; 924:408–419.
12. Frei B, England L, Ames BN. Ascorbate is an outstanding antioxidant in human blood plasma. Proc Natl Acad Sci USA 1989; 86:6377–6381.
13. Jacob RA. The integrated antioxidant system. Nutr Res 1995; 15:755–766.
14. Faden H, Kaul TN, Ogra PL. Activation of oxidative and arachidonic acid metabolism in neutrophils by respiratory syncytial virus antibody complexes: possible role in disease. J Infect Dis 1983; 148:110–116.
15. Winther B, Farr B, Turner RB, et al. Histopathologic examination and enumeration of polymorphonuclear leukocytes in the nasal mucosa during experimental rhinovirus colds. Acta Otolaryngol Suppl 1984; 413:19–24.
16. Muggli R. Vitamin C and phagocytes. In: Cunningham-Rundles, ed. Nutrient Modulation of the Immune Response. New York: Marcel Dekker, 1993:75–90.
17. Anderson R, Lukey PT. A biological role for ascorbate in the selective neutralization of extracellular phagocyte-derived oxidants. Ann NY Acad Sci 1987; 498:229–247.
18. Jackson JH, Cochrane CG. Leukocyte-induced tissue injury. Hematol Oncol Clin North Am 1988; 2:317–334.
19. Winterbourn CC, Vissers MCM. Changes in ascorbate levels on stimulation of human neutrophils. Biochim Biophys Acta 1983; 763:175–179.
20. Frei B, Stocker R, Ames BN. Antioxidant defenses and lipid peroxidation in human blood plasma. Proc Natl Acad Sci USA 1988; 85:9748–9752.
21. Halliwell B, Wasil M, Grootveld M. Biologically significant scavenging of the myeloperoxidase-derived oxidant hypochlorous acid by ascorbic acid. FEBS Lett 1987; 213:15–18.
22. Peterhans E. Reactive oxygen, antioxidants, and autotoxicity in viral diseases. In: Pasquier et al., eds. Oxidative Stress, Cell Activation and Viral Infection. Basel, Switzerland: Birkhauser Verlag, 1994.
23. Koprowski H, Zheng YM, Katz H, et al. In vivo expression of inducible nitric oxide synthase in experimentally induced neurologic diseases. Proc Natl Acad Sci USA 1993; 90:3024–3027.

24. Hayman M, Arbuthnott G, Harkiss G, et al. Neurotoxicity of peptide analogues on the transactivating protein tat from Maedi-Visna virus and human immunodeficiency virus. Neuroscience 1993; 53:1–6.

25. Dawson VL, Dawson TM, Uhl GR, Snyder SH. Human immunodeficiency virus type-1 coat protein neurotoxicity mediated by nitric acid in primary cortical cultures. Proc Natl Acad Sci USA 1993; 90:3256–3259.

26. Staal FJT, Ela SW, Roederer M, et al. Glutathione deficiency and human immunodeficiency virus infection. Lancet 1992; 339:909.

27. Fauci AS. Multifactorial nature of human immunodeficiency virus disease: implications for therapy. Science 1993; 2:1011–1018.

28. Oda T, Akaike T, Hamamoto T, et al. Oxygen radicals in influenza-induced pathogenesis and treatment with pyran polymer-conjugated SOD. Science 1989; 244:974–976.

29. Sharonov BP, Dolganova AV, Kiselev OI. Effective application of superoxide dismutase on later stages of influenza. Vopr Virusol 1991; 36:477–481.

30. Eck HP, Gmunder H, Hartmann M, et al. Low concentrations of acid-soluble thiol (cysteine) in the blood plasma of HIV-1-infected patients. Biol Chem Hoppe Seyler 1989; 370: 101–108.

31. Buhl R, Holroyd KJ, Mastrangeli A, et al. Systematic glutathione deficiency in symptom-free seropositive individuals. Lancet 1989; 2:1294–1298.

32. Eck HP, Stahl-Henning C, Hunsmann G, Droge, W. Metabolic disorder as early consequence of simian immunodeficiency virus infection in rhesus macaques. Lancet 1991; 338:346.

33. Meister A. On the antioxidant effects of ascorbic acid and glutathione. Biochem Pharmacol 1992; 44:1905–1915.

34. Martensson J, Meister A. Glutathione deficiency decreases tissue ascorbate levels in newborn rats: ascorbate spares glutathione and protects. Proc Natl Acad Sci USA 1991; 88:4656.

35. Jain A, Buist NR, Kennaway NG, et al. Effect of ascorbate or N-acetylcysteine treatment in a patient with hereditary glutathione synthetase deficiency. J Pediatr 1994; 124(2):229–233.

36. Englard S, Seifter S. The biochemical functions of ascorbic acid. Annu Rev Nutr 1986; 6:365.

37. Ross R, Benditt EP. Wound healing and collagen formation II: Fine structure in experimental structure. J Cell Biol 1962; 12:533–551.

38. Yeowell HN, Walker LC, Marshall MK, et al. The mRNA and the activity of lysyl hydroxylase are up-regulated by the administration of ascorbate and hydralazine to human skin fibroblasts from a patient with Ehlers–Danlos syndrome type VI. Arch Biochem Biophys 1995; 321(2): 510–516.

39. Philips CL. Effects of ascorbic acid on proliferation and collagen synthesis in relation to the donor age of human dermal fibroblasts. J Invest Dermatol 1994; 103(2):228–232.

40. Middelkoop E, deVries HJ, Ruuls L, et al. Adherence, proliferation and collagen turnover by human fibroblasts seeded into different types of collagen sponges. Cell Tissue Res 1995; 280(2):447–453.

41. Gessin JC, Brown LJ, Gordon JS, Berg RA. Regulation of collagen synthesis in human dermal fibroblasts in contracted collagen gels by ascorbic acid, growth factors, and inhibitors of lipid peroxidation. Exp Cell Res 1993; 206(2):283–290.

42. Utoguchi N, Ikeda K, Saeki K, et al. Ascorbic acid stimulates barrier function of cultured endothelial cell monolayer. J Cell Physiol 1995; 163(2):393–399.

43. Hering TM, Kollar J, Huynh TD, et al. Modulation of extracellular matrix gene expression in bovine high-density chondrocyte cultures by ascorbic acid and enzymatic resuspension. Arch Biochem Biophys 1994; 314(1):90–98.

44. Kielty CM. Synthesis and assembly of fibrillin by fibroblasts and smooth muscle cells. J Cell Sci 1993; 106(1):167–173.

45. Evans RM, Currie L, Campbell A. The distribution of ascorbic acid between various cellular components of blood, in normal individuals, and its relation to the plasma concentration. Br J Nutr 1982; 47:473.

46. Bergsten P, Amitai G, Kehrl J, et al. Millimolar concentrations of vitamin C in purified mononuclear leukocytes: depletion and reaccumulation. J Biol Chem 1990; 265:2584.

47. Bergsten P, Yu R, Kehrl J, Levin M. Ascorbic acid transport and distribution in human B lymphocytes. Arch Biochem Biophys 1995 317(1):208–214.

48. Chakrabarti RN, Kayal A, Saha R, Panja P. Quantitative evaluation of large granular lymphocytes in mice on ascorbic acid supplement diet. Indian J Pathol Microbiol 1994; 37(2):153–158.

49. Aidoo A, Lyn-Cook LE, Lensing S, Warner W. Ascorbic acid (vitamin C) modulates the mutagenic effects produced by an alkylating agent in vivo. Environ Mol Mutagenesis 1994; 24(3):220–228.

50. Anderson D, Basaran N, Blowers SD, Edwards AJ. The effect of antioxidants on bleomycin treatment in in vitro and in vivo genotoxicity assays. Mutat Res 1995; 329(1):37–47.

51. Anderson D, Yu TW, Phillips BJ, Schmezer P. The effect of various antioxidants and other modifying agents on oxygen-radical-generated DNA damage in human lymphocytes in the COMET assay. Mutat Res 1994; 307(1):261–271.

52. Umegaki K, Ikegami S, Inoue IK, et al. Beta-carotene prevents x-ray induction of micronuclei in human lymphocytes. Am J Clin Nutri 1994; 59(2):409–412.

53. Bobyleva LA, Chopikashvili LV, Alekhina NI, Zasukhina GD. Modification with ascorbic acid of the level of spontaneous and induced chromosome aberrations and sister chromatid exchanges in lymphocytes of workers in contact with molybdenum salts. Genetika 1993: 29(3): 430–434.

54. Baehner RL, Boxer LA, Allen JM, Davis J. Autooxidation as a basis for altered function by polymorphonuclear leukocytes. Blood 1977; 50:327–335.

55. Stait SE, Leake DS. Ascorbic acid can either increase or decrease low density lipoprotein modification. FEBS Lett 1994; 341(2–3):263–267.

56. Regnstrom J, Strom K, Moldeus P, Nilsson J. Analysis of lipoprotein diene formation in human serum exposed to copper. Free Radical Res Commun 1993; 19(4):267–278.

57. Retsky KL, Freeman MW, Frei BJ. Ascorbic acid oxidation product(s) protect human low density lipoprotein against atherogenic modification: anti- rather than prooxidant activity of vitamin C in the presence of transition metal ions. J Biol Chem 1993; 268(2):1304–1309.

58. Kubova J, Tulinska J, Stolcova E, et al. The influence of ascorbic acid on selected parameters of cell immunity in guinea pigs exposed to cadmium. Z Ernaehrungswiss 1993; 32(2):113–120.

59. Herbaczynska-Cedro K, Wartanowicz M, Panczenko-Kresowska B, et al. Inhibitory effect of vitamins C and E on the oxygen free radical production in human polymorphonuclear leucocytes. Eur J Clin Invest 1994; 24(5):316–319.

60. Levy R, Schlaeffer F. Successful treatment of a patient with recurrent furunculosis by vitamin C: improvement of clinical course and of impaired neutrophil functions. Int J Dermatol 1993; 32(11):832–834.

61. Papatheofanis FJ, Barmada R. Increased superoxide anion production in polymorphonuclear leucocytes on exposure to isobutyl-2-cyanoacrylate. Biomaterials 1992; 13(6):403–407.

62. Dunier M, Vergnet C, Siwicki AK, Verlhac V. Effect of lindane exposure on rainbow trout (Oncorhynchus mykiss) immunity. IV. Prevention of nonspecific and specific immunosuppression by dietary vitamin C (ascorbate-2-polyphosphate). Ecotoxicology Environ Safety 1995: 30(3):259–268.

63. Tanaka M, Muto N, Gohda E, Yamamoto I. Enhancement by ascorbic acid 2-glucoside or repeated additions of ascorbate of mitogen-induced IgM and IgG productions by human peripheral blood lymphocytes. Jpn J Pharmacol 1994; 66(4):451–456.

64. Stadtman ER. Ascorbic acid and oxidative inactivation of proteins. Am J Clin Nutr 1991; 54: 11255–11285.

65. Chevion M. A site-specific mechanism for free radical induced biological damage: the essential role of redox-active transition metals. Free Radical Biol Med 1988; 5:27–37.

66. Kazakov SA, Astashkina TG, Mamsev SV, Vlassov VV. Site-specific cleavage of single-stranded DNA at unique sites by a copper-dependent redox reaction. Nature 1988; 335:186–188.

67. Murata A, Uike M. Mechanism of inactivation of bacteriophage M52 containing single-stranded RNA by ascorbic acid. J Nutr Sci Vitaminol 1976; 22:347.
68. Murata A, Kitagawa K. Mechanism of inactivation of bacteriophage J1 by ascorbic acid. Agric Biol Chem 1973; 37:1145–1151.
69. Bissell MJ, Hatie C, Farson DA, et al. Ascorbic acid inhibits replication and infectivity of avian RNA tumor virus. Proc Natl Acad Sci USA 1980; 77:2711.
70. Harakeh S, Jariwalla RJ, Pauling L. Suppression of human immunodeficiency virus replication by ascorbate in chronically and acutely infected cells. Proc Natl Acad Sci USA 1990; 87:7245.
71. Harakeh S, Jariwalla RJ. Comparative study of the anti-HIV activities of ascorbate and thiol-containing reducing agents in chronically HIV infected cells. Am J Clin Nutr 1991; 54:1231S.
72. Harakeh S, Jariwalla RJ. Ascorbate effect on cytokine stimulation of HIV production. Nutrition 1995; 11:684–687.
73. Harakeh S, Niedzwiecki, Jariwalla RJ. Mechanistic analysis of ascorbate inhibition of human immunodeficiency virus. Chem Biol Interact 1994; 91:207–215.
74. Park CH, Kimler BF. Growth modulation of human leukemic, preleukemic and myeloma progenitor cells by L-ascorbic acid. Am J Clin Nutr 1991; 54:1241S–1246S.
75. DeLaurenzi V, Melino G, Savini I, et al. Cell death by oxidative stress and ascorbic acid regeneration in human neuroectodermal cell lines. Eur J Cancer 1995; 31A(4):463–466.
76. Powis G, Briehl M, Oblong J. Redox signalling and the control of cell growth and death. Pharmacol Ther 1995; 68(1):149–173.
77. Malorni W, Rivabene R, Santini MT, Donelli G. N-Acetylcysteine inhibits apoptosis and decreases viral particles in HIV-chronically infected U937 cells. FEBS Lett 1993; 327(1): 75–78.
78. Aoki K, Nakashima H, Hattori T, et al. Sodium benzylideneascorbate induces apoptosis in HIV-replicating U1 cells. FEBS Lett 1994; 351:105–108.

18

Blood Vitamin C in Human Glucose-6-Phosphate Dehydrogenase Deficiency

DANIEL TSUN-YEE CHIU and MEI-LING CHENG
Chang Gung Medical College, Kwei-san, Tao-yuan, Taiwan

INTRODUCTION

Glucose-6-phosphate dehydrogenase (G6PD) is a key enzyme in the hexose-monophosphate shunt (pentose phosphate pathway). One of the major functions of this pathway is to generate NADPH, an important reducing equivalent in all cells. The deficiency of G6PD is one of the most common enzymopathies, affecting over 200 million people worldwide (1–3). Such deficiency predisposes subjects to neonatal jaundice, drug- or infection-mediated hemolytic crisis, favism, and, less commonly, chronic nonspherocytic hemolytic anemia (1–3). This disease was first discovered in the 1950s as an outgrowth of investigations of the hemolytic anemia induced in susceptible subjects by the antimalarial drug primaquine (3). Since its discovery, many advances have been made in the field of G6PD research, but the advances have been rather unbalanced. The molecular biological features associated with G6PD deficiency have largely been elucidated and related studies indicate that G6PD deficiency is largely due to diverse point mutations in the G6PD gene (4–18). In contrast, the pathophysiological characteristics of G6PD deficiency are far from completely understood.

One poorly understood aspect of the pathophysiological characteristics of G6PD deficiency is the precise sequence of events in drug- or fava bean–induced damage to red cells (RBCs) leading to eventual hemolytic crises, although an oxidative mechanism has been proposed (19). Frequently encountered environmental factors that are known to be associated with hemolytic episodes in G6PD deficiency include fava bean ingestion (2,3,19–22), infection (22), and use of certain drugs such as primaquine (2,3,19,21,22). The ability to generate free radical intermediate(s) is a common feature among these environmental factors (2,19,21,22). Our laboratory (23) has clearly demonstrated that a free radical generating system such as alloxan/glutathione (GSH) can drastically decrease the deformability of G6PD-deficient RBCs. In contrast, under identical conditions, normal RBCs, probably because of their intact antioxidant system, are far less susceptible to oxidant-induced decrease in deformability. Thus, our study (23) clearly demonstrates that G6PD-deficient RBCs are more susceptible to oxidative attack than normal RBCs.

In addition to our study, a preponderance of evidence has indicated that G6PD-deficient RBCs are more susceptible to oxidative damage (19,21–24). Since G6PD is a housekeeping enzyme, individuals with G6PD deficiency should have little or no G6PD activity in all their cells. However, very little is known about the oxidative susceptibility of G6PD-deficient cells other than RBCs. Unfortunately, there is no G6PD-deficient animal model to obtain information on the oxidative susceptibility of G6PD-deficient cells other than RBCs. Since plasma antioxidant status may in some way reflect the oxidative stress encountered by each individual, we evaluate plasma levels of vitamin C and other antioxidants in blood of subjects with G6PD deficiency.

MATERIALS AND METHODS

Reagents

All reagents are of analytical grade. Unless otherwise stated, most of the reagents, including trichloroacetic acid (TCA), L-ascorbic acid, uric acid, tricine, sodium hydroxide, and 2,4,6-tris(2-pyridyl)-s-triazine (TZPZ), were purchased from Sigma (St. Louis, Missouri). Ascorbic acid oxidase was obtained from Boehringer Mannheim (Indianapolis, Indiana).

Procurement of Blood Samples

After obtaining of informed consent from blood donors, blood samples were collected in: ethylenediaminetetracetic acid (EDTA)-anticoagulated tubes from G6PD-deficient individuals and matching controls. All blood donors were asked to fast overnight prior to blood collection. Leukocytes were removed by aspiration after low spin centrifugation at 4°C for 10 min. Plasma and RBCs were separated and RBCs were washed three times with phosphate-buffered saline (PBS) solution containing glucose (10 mM phosphate/150 mM NaCl/5 mM D-glucose, pH 7.4).

Glucose-6-Phosphate Dehydrogenase Activity

The G6PD activity in fresh RBC was quantitatively measured by using kit No. 345-B (Sigma), as previously described (12). The chemicals in the reagent kit included oxidized nicotinamide-adenine dinucleotide phosphate (NADP$^+$), maleimide (to inhibit 6-phosphogluconate dehydrogenase), and lysing buffer. The activity of G6PD was quantitated spectrophotometrically by following the change in absorbance at 340 nm.

Determination of Plasma Vitamin C by the Ascorbate Oxidase Method

Plasma vitamin C level was determined by the method of Liu et al. (25) by using ascorbate oxidase. In this method, samples were analyzed indirectly by measuring the formation of a complex of ferrous ion and 2,4,6-tris(2-pyridyl)-s-triazine (Fe^{+2}–TPTZ), which could be followed spectrophotometrically at 593 nm by a spectophotometer (Beckman Du-70).

Determination of Plasma Vitamin A and E

A modified method of Russell et al. (26) was used for the determination of plasma levels of vitamins A and E. In brief, an equal volume of absolute alcohol containing 1 μg/ml of retinyl palmitate and 0.25% butylated hydroxytoluene (BHT) was added to 0.5 ml of plasma sample while vortexing. After a further 10-s vortexing, 2.5 ml of hexane containing 0.0125% BHT was added and the mixture was vortexed for another 30 s. Then the mixture was centrifuged at $1000 \times g$ for 5 min and part of the hexane layer (approximately 2.0 ml) was transferred to a vial. The hexane was evaporated by blowing nitrogen into the vial at room temperature. The residue was redissolved in 1.0 ml of absolute alcohol and the resultant sample was ready for HPLC analysis of vitamins A and E. If the samples were not analyzed immediately after extraction, the sample vials were capped and stored at $-20°C$. The HPLC conditions for the analysis of vitamins A and E were as follows: A μBondpak C_{18} column was used. The mobile phase was acetonitrile and CH_2Cl_2 (80 : 20 volume/ volume [v/v]) and the flow rate was set at 1.6 ml/min. Vitamin A was detected by an ultraviolet (UV) detector at 325 nm and vitamin E was detected at 292 nm.

Biochemical Characterization of Normal and Glucose-6-Phosphate Dehydrogenase Deficient Red Blood Cells

The adenosine triphosphate (ATP) content of RBCs was measured by the method of Beutler (27). The NADPH and $NADP^+$ ratio was determined according to the method of Zerez et al. (28). The intracellular GSH level of RBCs was determined by following the method described by Beutler (27).

Analysis of Results

The pair T test was used to evaluate statistically the difference between the data obtained from G6PD-deficient subjects and those from the matching controls.

RESULTS

The biochemical data, including ATP, GSH, and $NADPH/NADP^+$ ratio in normal and G6PD-deficient RBCs, were just as expected (Table 1). Glucose-6-phosphate dehydro-

Table 1   Biochemical Data of RBCs from Normal and G6PD-Deficient Individuals[a]

Sample	ATP (nmol/g Hb)	$\dfrac{NADPH}{NADPH + NADP^+}$	GSH (mmol/g Hb)
Control ($n = 35$)	3976 ± 372	0.58 ± 0.15	4.93 ± 0.82
G6PD-deficient ($n = 35$)	3894 ± 388	0.19 ± 0.21	3.26 ± 1.37

[a]RBC, red blood cell; G6PD, glucose-6-phosphate dehydrogenase; ATP, adenosine triphosphate; NADPH, reduced nicotinamide-adenine dinucleotide phosphate; NADP, nicotinamide-adenine dinucleotide phosphate; GSH, glutathione.

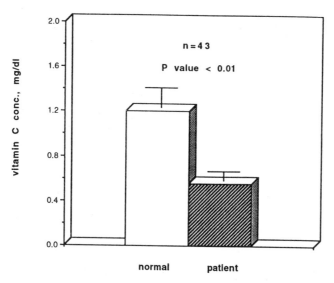

Figure 1 Plasma vitamin C level of G6PD-deficient patients and matching controls: Hatched bar, averaged plasma vitamin C level of 43 G6PD-deficient subjects, open bar, averaged plasma vitamin C level of 43 matching controls. Each value is expressed as mean ± standard error. G6PD, glucose-6-phosphate dehydrogenase.

genase–deficient RBCs have a low NADPH/NADP$^+$ ratio that is due to impairment of the hexose monophosphate shunt, which is the only biochemical pathway in RBCs to generate NADPH. The G6PD-deficient RBCs also had low GSH content. However, low levels of reducing equivalents in G6PD-deficient RBCs did not affect the ATP content.

The mean plasma vitamin C levels of G6PD-deficient subjects and matching controls are shown in Figure 1. In general, G6PD-deficient subjects had a much lower plasma vitamin C level (0.56 ± 0.08 mg/dl, mean ± standard error [SE]) than that of matching controls (1.20 ± 0.18 mg/dl, mean ± SE). On average, the plasma vitamin C level of G6PD-deficient subjects was less than 50% of that of the matching controls and this difference is statistically significant at $p < 0.01$.

In addition, G6PD-deficient subjects had a significantly ($p < 0.01$) lower plasma vitamin E level (0.57 ± 0.03 mg/dl, mean ± SE) than that of matching controls (0.69 ± 0.02 mg/dl, mean ± SE), as shown in Figure 2. The averaged plasma vitamin E level of G6PD-deficient subjects was only 82% of that of the matching controls. Besides having lower plasma levels of vitamin C and vitamin E, G6PD-deficient subjects, on average, had 30% less plasma vitamin A (32.09 + 2.14 μg/dl, mean ± SE) than matching controls (45.59 ± 2.50 μg/dl, mean ± SE) as shown in Figure 3. This difference was statistically significant at $p < 0.01$.

DISCUSSION

The data obtained from our current study clearly demonstrate that G6PD-deficient subjects have lower plasma levels of vitamin C (Fig. 1), vitamin E (Fig. 2), and vitamin A (Fig. 3) than matching controls. The averaged levels of plasma vitamins in G6PD-deficient subjects

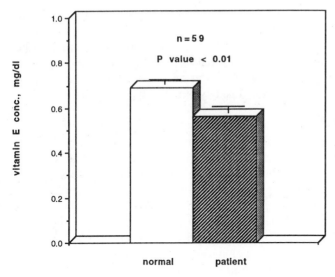

Figure 2   Plasma vitamin E level of G6PD-deficient patients and matching controls: Hatched bar, averaged plasma vitamin E level of 59 G6PD-deficient subjects, open bar, averaged plasma vitamin E level of 59 matching controls. Each value is expressed as mean ± standard error. G6PD, glucose-6-phosphate dehydrogenase.

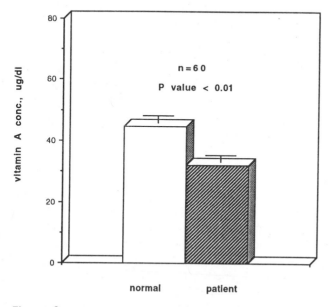

Figure 3   Plasma vitamin A level of G6PD-deficient patients and matching controls: Hatched bar, averaged plasma vitamin A level of 60 G6PD-deficient subjects, open bar, averaged plasma vitamin A level of 60 matching controls. Each value is expressed as mean ± standard error. G6PD, glucose-6-phosphate dehydrogense.

are only 46.7%, 70.3%, and 82.6% for vitamins C, A, and E, respectively, of those of matching controls. These decreases in plasma levels of vitamins with an antioxidant property may be attributed to an increase in oxidative stress due to G6PD deficiency. On the other hand, such a decrease in antioxidants can render G6PD-deficient subjects more susceptible to oxidative attack, initiating a vicious cycle. In any event, we feel that it is of paramount importance to evaluate the antioxidant systems in subjects with G6PD deficiency systematically.

As stated, the pathophysiological characteristics of G6PD deficiency are far from being completely understood. Oxidative damage to cells has long been proposed as a major cause of many diseases (21,22,29–31), particularly degenerative disorders such as cancer, cataracts, brain dysfunction, immune-system decline, and cardiovascular diseases (30,31). Since G6PD is a housekeeping enzyme for every cell of the body against oxidative insults, its deficiency can render cells more susceptible to oxidative attack (19,21–24) and hence, a propensity of deficient individuals to certain disorders. In addition to the classical presentation of hemolytic anemia, G6PD deficiency has recently been reported to be correlated positively with cholelithiasis (32), diabetes mellitus (33), and tuberculosis (34). Whether individuals with G6PD deficiency are more prone to certain degenerative diseases should be carefully evaluated. Moreover, oxidative stress has recently been reported to affect many cellular processes such as signal transduction (35–37), gene expression (38–40), cell proliferation (41), and cellular differentiation (42). Together with the fact that G6PD-deficient cells are more susceptible to oxidative attack, these new findings provide a basic rationale for the speculation that G6PD-deficient subjects would be more prone to certain degenerative disorders.

Preliminary studies from our laboratory suggest that G6PD-deficient individuals are more susceptible to certain types of viral infection. For example, the incidence of G6PD deficiency in the general male population of Taiwan is about 3% (43), whereas the incidence in males with hepatitis B infection in Taiwan is about 6.1% (unpublished observation). In addition, G6PD-deficient individuals seem to be more susceptible to contracting the common cold (unpublished observation). Vitamin C has long been proposed to affect susceptibility to infection by influenza virus (44). It has also been proposed to inhibit human immunodeficiency virus (45). Evidence is emerging to suggest that oxidants promote the proliferation of certain types of virus (46–48) whereas reducing agents suppress viral proliferation (49–51). Whether G6PD-deficient individuals are indeed more susceptible to certain types of viral infection and whether such increased susceptibility to viral infection is related to a decrease in the vitamin C level in these individuals remain to be clarified.

Perhaps most important of all from a medical point of view is how to design or at least recommend a health promotion program for the nearly 2 million people affected by G6PD deficiency worldwide. What has happened in sickle cell anemia may help to illustrate this point. Sickle RBCs are more susceptible to oxidative damage (52–55) in part because of the presence of unstable hemoglobin S. Such enhanced susceptibility to oxidative damage has led to a decrease in vitamin E (56) and vitamin C (57). Vitamin E supplementation of patients with sickle cell anemia has been reported to have beneficial effects on these patients (58). Since recent studies have shown that high doses of vitamin E supplementation can reduce the incidence of cardiovascular disease (59,60), dietary antioxidant supplementation may have beneficial effects for G6PD-deficient patients and such a potential remedy to prevent or, at least to minimize, oxidative damage in these patients should be explored.

ACKNOWLEDGMENTS

This project is supported by grants from Chang Gung College of Medicine & Technology (CMRP389 and NMRP366) and from the National Science Council of Taiwan (NSC83-0412-B182-034, NSC83-0412-B182-054-M02, and NSC84-2331-B182-034-MO2).

REFERENCES

1. Luzzatto L, Battistuzzi G. Glucose-6-phosphate dehydrogenase. Adv Hum Genet 1985; 14: 217–329.
2. Beutler E. Glucose-6-phosphate dehydrogenase deficiency. N Engl J Med 1991; 324:169–174.
3. Beutler E. Study of glucose-6-phosphate dehydrogenase: history and molecular biology. Am J Hematol 1993; 42:53–58.
4. Chiu DTY. Molecular basis of G6PD deficiency. J Biomed Lab Sci 1993; 5:1–9.
5. Vulliam TJ, D'Urso M, Battostuzzi G, et al. Diverse point mutations in the human glucose-6-phosphate dehydrogenase gene cause enzyme deficiency and mild or severe hemolytic anemia. Proc Natl Acad Sci (USA) 1988; 85:5171–5151.
6. Hirono A, Beutler E: Molecular cloning and nucleotide sequence of cDNA for human glucose-6-phosphate dehydrogenase variant A(-). Proc Natl Acad Sci USA 1988; 85:3951–3954.
7. Vulliamy T, Beutler E, Luzzatto L. Variants of glucose-6-phosphate dehydrogenase are due to missense mutations spread throughout the coding region of the gene. Hum Mutat 1993; 2: 159–167.
8. Chiu DTY, Zuo L, Chen E, et al. Two commonly occurring nucleotide base substitutions in Chinese G6PD variants. Biochem Biophys Res Comm 1991; 180:988–993.
9. Chao L, Du CS, Louie E, et al. A to G substitution identified in exon 2 of the G6PD gene among G6PD deficient Chinese. Nucleic Acids Res 1991; 19:6056.
10. Tang TK, Huang CS, Huang MJ, et al. Diverse mutations result in glucose-6-phosphate dehydrogenase (G6PD) polymorphism in Taiwan. Blood 1992; 79:2135–2140.
11. Chang JG, Chiou SS, Perng LI, et al. Molecular characterization of glucose-6-phosphate dehydrogenase (G6PD) deficiency by natural and amplification created restriction sites: five mutations account for most G6PD deficiency in Taiwan. Blood 1992; 80:1079–1082.
12. Chiu DTY, Zuo L, Chao L, et al. Molecular characterization of glucose-6-phosphate dehydrogenase deficiency in patients of Chinese descent and identification of new base substitutions in the human G6PD gene. Blood 1993; 81:2150–2154.
13. Lo YS, Lu CC, Chiou SS, et al. Molecular characterization of glucose-6-phosphate dehydrogenase deficiency in Chinese infants with or without severe neonatal hyperbilirubinaemia. Br J Haematol 1994; 86:858–862.
14. Tang TK, Yeh CH, Huang CS, Hunag MJ. Expression and biochemical characterization of human glucose-6-phosphate dehydrogenase in *Escherichia coli*: a system to analyze normal and mutant enzymes. Blood 1994; 83:1436–1441.
15. Takizawa T, Yoneyama Y, Miwa S, Yoshida A. A single nucleotide base transition is the basis of the common human glucose-6-phosphate dehydrogenase variant A(+). Genomics 1987; 1: 228–231.
16. Stevens DJ, Wanachiwanawin W, Mason PJ, et al. G6PD Canton a common deficient variant in South East Asia is caused by a 459 Arg to Leu mutation. Nucleic Acids Res 1990; 18:7190.
17. MacDonald D, Town M, Mason P, et al. Deficiency in red blood cells. Nature 1991; 350:115.
18. Hirono A, Fujii H, Shima M, Miwa S: G6PD Nara. A new class 1 glucose-6-phosphate dehydrogenase variant with an eight amino acid deletion. Blood 1993; 82:3250–3252.
19. Arese P, Deflora A. Pathophysiology of hemolysis in glucose-6-phosphate dehydrogenase deficiency. Semin Hematol 1990; 27:1–40.

20. Lin JY, Ling K-H. Studies on favism. 3. Studies on the physiological activities of vicine in vivo. J Formosan Med Assoc 1962; 61:490–494

21. Chiu D, Lubin B, Shohet SB. Peroxidative reactions in red cell biology. In Pryor W, ed. Free Radicals in Biology. New York: Academic Press, 1982:115–160.

22. Chiu D, Kuypers FA, Lubin B. Lipid peroxidation in human red cells. Semin Hematol 1989; 26(4):257–276.

23. Liu TZ, Lin TF, Hung IJ, et al. Enhanced susceptibility of erythrocytes deficient in glucose-6-phosphate dehydrogenase to alloxan/GSH-induced decrease in red cell deformability. Life Sci 1994; 55:PL55–60.

24. Scott MD, Zuo L, Lubin BH, Chiu DTY: NADPH, not glutathione, status modulates oxidant sensitivity in normal and glucose-6-phosphate dehydrogenase-erythrocytes. Blood 1991; 77:2059–2064.

25. Liu TZ, Chin N, Kiser MD, Bigler WN. Specific spectrophotometry of ascorbic acid in serum or plasma by use of ascorbate oxidase. Clin Chem 1982; 28(11):2225–2228.

26. Russel MJ, Thomas BS, Wellok E. Simultaneous assay of serum vitamin A and vitamin E by high performance liquid chromatography using time-switched UV and fluorimetric detectors. J High Resolut Chromatogr Chromatogr Commu 1986; 9:281–284.

27. Beutler E. Red Cell Metabolism: A Manual of Biochemical Methods. 3d ed. Orlando, FL: Grune & Stratton, 1984.

28. Zerez CR, Lee SJ, Tanaka KR. Spectrophotometric determination of oxidized and reduced pyridine nucleotides in erythrocytes using a single extraction procedure. Anal Biochem 1987; 164:367–373.

29. Halliwell B, Gutteridge JMC, Cross CE. Free radicals, antioxidants and human disease: where are we now? J Lab Clin Med 1992; 119:598–620.

30. Rice-Evans C, Burdon R. Free radical–lipid interactions and their pathological consequences. Prog Lipid Res 1993; 32:71–110.

31. Ames BN, Shigenaga MK, Hagen TM. Oxidants, antioxidants and the degenerative diseases of aging. Proc Natl Acad Sci USA 1993; 90:7915–7922

32. Meloni T, Forteleoni G, Noga G. Increased prevalence of glucose-6-phosphate dehydrogenase deficiency in patients with cholelithiasis. Folia Haematologica-Internationales Magozine für Klinische und Morphologische Blutforschung 1989; 116:745–752.

33. Niazi GA. Glucose-6-phosphate dehydrogenase deficiency and diabetes mellitus. Int J Hematol 1991; 54:295–298.

34. Insanov AB, Alleve NA, Adbullaev FM, Umniashkin AA. Clinico-immunologic characteristics of patients with pulmonary tuberculosis, psychic disease and congenital glucose-6-phosphate dehydrogenase deficiency. Probl Tuberk 1989; 6:10–15.

35. Heffetz D, Zick Y. H_2O_2 potentiates phosphorylation of novel putative substrates for the insulin receptor kinase in intact Fao cells. J Biol Chem 1989; 264:10126–10132.

36. Garcia-Morales P, Minami Y, Luong E, Klausner RD. Tyrosine phosphorylation in T cells is regulated by phosphatase activity: studies with phenylarsine oxide. Proc Natl Acad Sci USA 1990; 87:9255–9259.

37. Sullivan SG, Chiu DTY, Errasfa M, et al. Effects of H_2O_2 on protein tyrosine phosphatase activity in HER14 cells. Free Radical Biol Med 1994; 16:399–403.

38. Storz G, Tartaglia LA, Ames BN. Transcriptional regulator of oxidative stress-inducible genes: direct activation by oxidation. Science 1990; 248:189–194.

39. Keyse SM, Emslie EA. Oxidative stress and heat shock induce a human gene encoding a protein-tyrosine phosphatase. Nature 1992; 359:644–647.

40. Toledano MB, Kullik I, Trinh F, et al. Redox-dependent shift of OxyR-DNA contacts along an extended DNA-binding site: a mechanism for differential promoter selection. Cell 1994; 78: 897–909.

41. Murrel GAC, Francis MJO, Bromley L. Modulation of fibroblast proliferation by oxygen free radicals. Biochem J 1990; 265:659–665.

42. Yang KD, Shaio MF. Hydroxyl radicals as an early signal involved in phorbol ester-induced monocytic differentiation of HL60 cells. Biochem Biophys Res Commun 1994; 200:1650–1657.

43. Hsiao KJ. Genetic disorders and neonatal screening. In: Miyai K, Kanno T, Ishikawa E, eds. Clinical Biochemistry. Amsterdam: Elsevier 1992:289–292.

44. Pauling L. Ascorbic acid and the common cold. Scott Med J 1973; 18:1–2

45. Harakeh S, Niedzwiecki A, Jariwalla RJ. Mechanistic aspects of ascorbate inhibition of human immunodeficiency virus. Chem Biol Interact 1994; 91:207–215.

46. Kameoka M, Kimura T, Ikuta K. Superoxide enhances the spread of HIV-1 infection by cell to cell transmission. FEBS Lett 1993; 331:182–186.

47. Piette J, Legrand-Poels S. HIV-1 reactivation after an oxidative stress mediated by different reactive oxygen species. Chem Biol Interact 1994; 91:19–89.

48. Yao Y, Hoffer A, Chang CY, Puga A. Dioxin activates HIV-1 gene expression by an oxidative stress pathway requiring a functional cytochrome P450 CYP1A1 enzyme. Environ Health Perspect 1995; 103:366–371.

49. Garaci E, Palamara AT, Di Francesco P, et al. Glutathione inhibits replication and expression of viral proteins in cultured cells infected with Sandai virus. Biochem Biophys Res Comm 1992; 188:1090–1096.

50. Sappreg C, Legrand-Poels S, Best-Belpomme M, et al. Stimulation of glutathione peroxidase activity decrease HIV type 1 activation after oxidative stress. AIDS Res Hum Retroviruses 1994; 10:1451–1461.

51. Simon G, Moog C, Obert G. Effects of glutathione precursors on human immunodeficiency virus replication. Chem Biol Interact 1994; 91:217–224.

52. Chiu D, Lubin B, Shohet SB. Erythrocyte membrane lipid reorganization during the sickling process. Br J Haematol 1979; 41:223–234.

53. Marva E, Hebbel RP. Denaturing interaction between sickle hemoglobin and phosphatidylserine liposomes. Blood 1994; 83:242–249.

54. Kuross SA, Rank BH, Hebbel RP. Excess heme in sickle erythrocyte inside-out membranes: possible role in thioloxidation. Blood 1988; 71:876–882.

55. Hebbel RP, Morgan WT, Eaton JW, Hedlund BE. Accelerated autoxidation and heme loss due to instability of sickle hemoglobin. Proc Natl Acad Sci USA 1988; 85:237–241.

56. Chiu D, Lubin B. Abnormal vitamin E and glutathione peroxidase levels in sickle cell anemia. J Lab Clin Med 1979; 94:542–548.

57. Chiu DTY, Vinchinsky E, Ho SL, et al. Vitamin C deficiency in patients with sickle cell anemia. Am J Pediatr Hematol 1990; 12:262–267.

58. Natta CL, Machlin LJ, Brin M. A decrease in irreversibly sickled erythrocytes in sickle cell anemia patients given vitamin E. Am J Clin Nutr 1980; 33:968–971.

59. Stampfer MJ, Hennekens CH, Manson JE, et al. Vitamin E consumption and the risk of coronary heart disease in women. N Engl J Med 1993; 328:1444–1449

60. Rimm EB, Stampfer MJ, Ascherio A, et al. Vitamin E consumption and the risk of coronary heart disease in men. N Engl J Med 1993; 328:1450–1456

19

Vitamin C in Cutaneous Biology

JÜRGEN FUCHS and MAURIZIO PODDA

Johann Wolfgang Goethe University, Frankfurt, Germany

INTRODUCTION

Vitamin C is an essential nutrient that is receiving growing attention for its antioxidant function in human biological systems including the skin. In clinical dermatology vitamin C has been tried with varying success rates in treatment of several skin disorders. However, today ascorbate plays no significant role in clinical dermatological therapy. Cutaneous signs of vitamin C hypovitaminosis are characteristic and often lead to the diagnosis. On the contrary, excessive vitamin C intake is not associated with any skin symptoms. In experimental dermatological practice topical vitamin C is used in photoprotection and may also be effective as an antiinflammatory agent under certain conditions. The endogenous semioxidation product of vitamin C, the ascorbyl radical, may be useful as a marker of oxidative stress in skin.

SCURVY

The most important observation that has been made about ascorbic acid is that its absence in the diet causes scurvy. Scurvy as a consequence of a deficiency was described in the ancient writings of the Egyptians, Greeks, and Romans. The disease, a scourge of early sea voyagers, was first encountered on the voyages of Vasco da Gamma in 1489. In 1753 the Scottish physician Lind described scurvy and its dietary control (1). The identification of the dietary factor as ascorbate was reported in 1932 (2,3). Reports of vitamin deficiencies have become relatively rare in Western and other developed countries. Vitamin deficiencies are usually due to neglect, error, addictions, mental disorders, or malabsorption syndrome. In developed countries, persons most at risk for the development of scurvy are single elderly men who for reasons of chronic alcoholism, small budget, or mental incapacity have an inadequate diet (4–9). Aberrant eating behavior (food faddim), e.g., for philosophical reasons, may play a role in certain cases (10).

Skin Signs of Scurvy

It is essential for the clinician to recognize the symptoms of scurvy since untreated scurvy ultimately has a fatal outcome, caused by cachexia, infection, or hypotension. Skin appears to be especially vulnerable to ascorbate deficiency. The first symptoms of scurvy appear after 30–90 days of insufficient intake. When Crandon, a Harvard surgeon, placed himself on an ascorbate-free diet for 6 months, hyperkeratotic papules with ingrown hairs developed, followed by petechiae on the lower limbs (11). Recognition of the characteristic cutaneous manifestations of this entity is often the first step in making the correct diagnosis. In humans, experimental scurvy may differ from acquired scurvy, because patients with acquired scurvy usually have multiple dietary deficiencies. However, in both the acquired and the experimental conditions, patients have similar symptoms such as weakness, fatigue, follicular hyperkeratosis, perifollicular hemorrhage, ecchymoses, and bleeding gums. In experimental scurvy edema, arthralgia, ocular hemorrhage, Sjögren's syndrome, and poor wound healing are frequently observed. The skin manifestations of scurvy are follicular hyperkeratosis with fragmented corkscrewlike hairs that result from a decreased number of reduced disulfide bonds. On the posterior side of the thighs, the anterior side of the forearms, and the abdomen perifollicular hemorrhages are often found within the hyperkeratotic areas. Petechiae may develop on all the hair-bearing areas. On the site of trauma, ecchymosis can occur. Intracutaneous hemorrhage ranges from petechiae to ecchymoses. Hemorrhage also may be subungual, subconjunctival, subcutaneous, intramuscular, intra- or perineural, as well as intraarticular. Symmetrical edema, hyperpigmentation, and pseudoschlerema followed by ulceration may develop on the lower limbs. Ungual alterations such as koilonychia are described. Uncommon findings of ascorbate deficiency are xerostomia, keratoconjunctivitis sicca, and enlargement of submandibular, salivary, or parotid glands, a Sjögren-like syndrome (12).

Gums become edematous and friable, with bluish shiny masses in the regions of interdental papillae. Ascorbate is required for proper osteodentin formation, and in its absence, teeth soften and are predisposed to infection. Changes are most evident in persons with prior gingivitis (12); with good oral hygiene they may not occur. The tongue and the lips are usually not affected.

Noncutaneous Symptoms of Scurvy

Noncutaneous findings include generalized weakness, fatigue, weight loss, depression, and hemorrhages into joints and viscera followed by joint swelling, arthralgias, dyspnea, neuralgia, edema of the legs, epistaxis, and diarrhea (6,7). Normochromic and normocytic anemia is common and may be due to tissue hemorrhage or intravascular hemolysis (5,7,8). Sometimes a megaloblastic anemia, which is not observed in experimental ascorbate deficiency and is possibly due to aberrant folate metabolism (7,13), is found.

Scurvy of the Infant

Scurvy of the infant (Morbus Moeller-Barlow disease) has similar symptoms to adult scurvy; however, subperiosteal bleeding, particularly in the region of long bone epiphyses, is frequently observed. In this case, epiphyseal thickening and development of pseudo-paralysis are seen; gums are only affected if teeth are present (5).

Pathophysiological Characteristics of Scurvy

The characteristic capillary and tissue fragility in scurvy patients has been attributed to a defect in collagen biosynthesis. Ascorbate is a cofactor for several hydroxylating enzymes in the body (14,15), including proline hydroxylase and lysyl hydroxylase. It is also required for hydroxylation reactions in carnitine and catechol biosynthesis, conversion of folic acid to folinic acid, and metabolism of cyclic nucleotids, prostaglandins, and histamine (16). Although ascorbate is involved in the production of norepinephrine from dopamine, a clinical decrease in norepinephrine levels does not occur in scurvy patients (12). Most cutaneous manifestations of vitamin C deficiency are related to the role of vitamin C as a cofactor for proline hydroxylation in collagen synthesis. Ascorbate is a reducing agent in hydroxylation reactions. For proline, the enzyme prolyl hydroxylase, which has iron at its active site, is involved in the transformation. By reducing the iron atom to its ferrous state, ascorbate maintains the enzyme in its active form. Collagen synthesized in the absence of ascorbate is insufficiently hydroxylated and hence cannot properly form fibers. The compromised vessel patency in scurvy patients results from impaired synthesis of basal lamina, media adventitia, and surrounding connective tissue structures. Hydroxyproline is essential for maximal stability of the triple helix and consequently for secretion of procollagen from the cell. Hydroxylysine, on the other hand, participates in cross-link formation and serves as a site for covalent attachment of galactosyl or glucosylgalactosyl residues during collagen biosynthesis. In addition, ascorbate increases the synthesis of procollagen, apparently independently of hydroxylation. The mechanism for stimulation of gene transcription is unclear but may be related to the prooxidant properties of ascorbate (17).

Diagnosis and Therapy of Scurvy

The most reliable test for laboratory diagnosis of ascorbate deficiency is the analysis of leukocyte or thrombocyte ascorbate concentration, because blood and urinary levels reflect only oral intake. At the beginning of scurvy the intracellular level of ascorbate may be inside normal limits, however (18). Radioactive labeled ascorbate studies show that 90% depletion occurs within the first 90 days of deprivation and that clinical signs of scurvy begin to appear when the daily rate of ascorbate ingestion falls substantially below 7.5 mg (12). Replacement therapy with 100–300 mg ascorbate/day leads within 24 h to resolution of hypotension and spontaneous bleeding, gum changes in 2-3 days, ecchymoses in 10–20 days, and anemia in 2–3 weeks (13).

ASCORBATE AS A DRUG IN DERMATOLOGY

It is rational to use vitamin supplementation in clinical conditions where deficiencies are likely to occur. In addition, high-dose vitamin intake has been advocated in the treatment and prevention of several nondeficiency disorders. A beneficial effect of ascorbate has been claimed for an extraordinary number of clinical conditions in nondeficiency states, including the common cold (19,20), and allergic and toxic states of almost every kind; it is also claimed to influence certain aspects of the immune system (21,22), modulate cholesterol metabolism (23), and improve several kinds of cancer (24). The enormous literature on which these claims are based consists mainly of uncontrolled clinical trials or anecdotal reports. Only a few studies have made use of the techniques of randomization and double blinding (25). Evidence is conflicting or inconclusive as to the use of vitamin C in the common cold, asthma, and enhancement of athletic capacity, and the use of vitamin C in advanced stages of cancer has been rejected.

A literature review of clinical trials with vitamin C in dermatology indicates a broad spectrum of skin diseases in which clinical improvement has been reached with varying success rates (26). The disease states include furunculosis, pyoderma, erythema induratum, erythema nodosum, erythema exsudativum multiforme, glossitis rhomboidae mediana, stomatitis, glossititis, aphthosis, chloasma, acne vulgaris, psoriasis arthropatica, radiation dermatitis, cutaneous burns, purpura, pruritus, allergic contact dermatitis, and impaired wound healing. Most of these claims, however, are not supported by valid scientific data. The evaluation of the clinical case studies and reports of treatment of various dermatoses with ascorbate does not discover convincing evidence of its clinical efficiency in most cases. Today ascorbate plays no significant role in clinical dermatological therapy. Prospecto demonstrate unequivocally the clinical efficacy of the vitamin in distinct skin diseases. Such studies are presently not available. Evidence from clinical studies reveals only a beneficial therapeutic effect of vitamin C in pressure sores (27,28) and chronic ulcera cruris; patients suffering from thalassaemia major also seem to benefit from supplemental ascorbate (29).

Wound Healing

It is clearly established that in scorbutic humans wound healing is poor. Furthermore, it is recognized that in postoperative patients ascorbic acid tissue concentrations are decreased (30,31), probably by increased utilization by wound tissue or intraoperative/postoperative stress. In healing surgical wounds it becomes concentrated (32,33), and its circulating levels are acutely diminished after skin injury (30). In patients with low plasma ascorbate levels an increased rate of wound dehiscence is observed (30). This has led surgeons to administer large doses of ascorbate to improve wound healing. However, there is no clinical evidence that wound healing can be accelerated by administration of more ascorbate than is required to maintain normal tissue levels (34). However, patients with severe illnesses or injuries can rapidly become ascorbate depleted because the water-soluble vitamin cannot be stored in large amounts in the body. In these cases supplemental ascorbate (1–2 g/day) is recommended until recovery.

Ascorbate as an Antioxidant Supplement

Ascorbic acid is probably one of the most effective and least toxic antioxidants identified in mammalian systems. It is a water-soluble chain-breaking antioxidant that reacts directly with several reactive oxidants and may also regenerate other antioxidants. A few clinical conditions are caused by oxidative stress, but more often the stress results from the disease. Sometimes it then makes a significant contribution to the disease, and sometimes it is just an epiphenomenon and antioxidants are unlikely to be of therapeutic benefit (35).

Ascorbate deficiency in epidermal or dermal microcompartments may be a consequence of endogenously or exogenously induced oxidative injury in skin. Dermatoses with significant involvement of reactive oxygen species in their pathogenesis include skin conditions mediated by electromagnetic radiation, inflammatory cells, prooxidant xenobiotics, and lipid peroxidation products. Dermatological disorders with significant involvement of oxidative damage may benefit from local and systemic ascorbate therapy. Hence, ascorbate may be of potential use in treatment of distinct dermatoses, e.g., those which are associated with inflammatory cells and which are aggravated or induced by ultraviolet (UV) light. There is evidence that reactive oxidants are generated in vivo in skin by ultraviolet irradiation, and products of lipid and nucleic acid oxidation, lipid radicals, and antioxidant consumption have all been noted in ultraviolet irradiated skin (36,37). Molecular and morphological ultraviolet damage can be moderated by antioxidants. Photoaging, photocancer, and certain kinds of photodermatoses may be mediated in some way by reactive oxidant generation in skin. This assumption has led to several clinical trials, investigating the effects of antioxidant therapy on these clinical manifestations of solar damage. Ascorbate acts locally in the skin as an antioxidant and is depleted by UV irradiation. Irradiation of mice with solar simulated light at a dose of 5 J/cm^2 significantly decreased epidermal ascorbate and dehydroascorbate levels (38). Topical ascorbate has been shown to protect porcine skin from ultraviolet B (UVB)- and UVA-induced phototoxic reactions (39).

CUTANEOUS SIDE EFFECTS OF ASCORBATE

Megadose vitamin C intake is not associated with skin symptoms. In anecdotal reports allergic and/or intolerance reactions to vitamin C were reported (40,41). The clinical significance, however, is presumably not relevant. Ascorbate has extremely low acute, subacute, and chronic toxicity and lacks mutagenic, cancerogenic, and embryotoxic effects. Administration of very high doses (up to 20 g daily in some cases) of ascorbate to healthy young humans appears to do no significant harm and no cutaneous side effects are reported (42).

SKIN CONCENTRATION OF ASCORBATE

Although many methods exist for monitoring vitamin C in biological specimens, high-performance liquid chromatography (HPLC) with electrochemical or ultraviolet detection is, because of its simplicity and high sensitivity, the method of choice for routine analysis. In humans the physiological pool of ascorbate approaches about 1500 mg per average body weight (20 mg/kg) and the pool turns over with a half-life of 10–20 days (43). In human serum and plasma, ascorbate concentrations were found to vary from 7 to 15 µg/ml (44) or 1–15 µg/ml (45). Symptoms of scurvy occur when the body pool drops below 300 mg ascorbate. It has been pointed out that the physiological pool size of about 1500 mg ascorbate may not be sufficient for optimal human health. Human studies have shown that the body pool can be expanded to 2300–2800 mg by daily ingestion of 200 mg ascorbate (46). At this point the plasma concentration reaches a plateau of about 1.4 mg %. However, it has been suggested that a larger ascorbate pool is to be obtained at the expense of decreased gastrointestinal absorption and increased excretion of unmetabolized ascorbate. These data may have no bearing on optimal ascorbate requirements, since there may be no relation between the threshold of ascorbate excretion and optimal tissue concentrations. Any intake in excess of the daily rate of metabolism (5–20 mg/day) is absorbed but immediately excreted unchanged through the kidneys.

Tissue concentration of ascorbate in human tissue has been analyzed: adrenal gland 550 mg/kg, skleletal muscle 35 mg/kg, brain 140 mg/kg, liver 125 mg/kg, skin 30 mg/kg, adipose tissue 10 mg/kg, lungs 70 mg/kg, blood 9 mg/kg, kidneys 55 mg/kg, heart 55 mg/kg

(47). In most of these tissues, common functions of ascorbate will entail maintaining structural integrity through collagen synthesis. The higher levels in some of the organs may reflect some more specialized roles, e.g., in hormone synthesis, immune response, and antioxidant protection. Human skin fibroblasts rapidly accumulate extracellular ascorbate. A high-affinity active transport mechanism, which is concentration- and temperature-dependent, saturable, and sodium-dependent must be differentiated from a low-affinity transport mechanism (48). Confluent fibroblasts contain an undetectable amount of ascorbate; after incubation with micromolar ascorbate concentrations they accumulate a 15-fold excess in a few hours, leading to picomole ascorbate concentration per microgram cell protein (49), equivalent to several hundred micromolar (48). Ascorbate/dehydroascorbate content in mouse epidermis and dermis determined by HPLC with electrochemical detection was found to be 1.3 μmol (229 μg) ascorbate/g epidermis, 1.3 μmol dehydroascorbate/g dermis, 1.0 μmol (176 μg) ascorbate/g dermis, and 0.9 μmol dehydroascorbate/g dermis (50). Dehydroascorbate concentration is typically much lower in cells than that of ascorbate but is increased under conditions of oxidative stress. No significant amounts of dehydroascorbate were found in human plasma using HPLC and electrochemical or fluorimetric detection (44,45). Presumably dehydroascorbate content may be found to be increased in biological samples when the sample is mishandled or subject to oxidative stress.

ASCORBYL RADICAL AS A MARKER OF OXIDATIVE STRESS IN SKIN

The ascorbyl free radical is readily detectable by electron paramagnetic resonance (EPR) spectroscopy at low steady-state levels in rodent skin (51,52). The ascorbyl radical is usually detectable by EPR as a doublet signal with $a^H = 1.8$ G, $dH_{pp} = 0.6$ G, and $g = 2.0052$. However, each line of the ascorbate doublet is actually a triplet of doublets. As oxidative stress increases in a biological system, the steady-state concentration of the ascorbyl radical increases. Since the first EPR observations of ascorbyl radicals, it has been used as an indicator of oxidative events. It was proposed that the ascorbyl radical, which is naturally present in biological systems, can be used as a noninvasive indicator of oxidative stress, because it is relatively stable, is nontoxic, and is easily detectable (53,54), particularly when free radical production is low and other methods are insensitive. The ascorbyl radical as a marker of oxidative stress has been demonstrated to be useful in the study of free radical reactions in mouse skin (51–53). Electron paramagnetic resonance spectroscopy and imaging techniques are currently being explored for biological in vivo investigations (55,56). Skin is a target organ of the in vivo EPR technique, because microwave penetration is not a limiting factor in this tissue. In vivo EPR spectroscopy was successfully performed in human skin using surface coils at S-band frequency (57). This technique may prove useful in the future for noninvasive in vivo measurement of ascorbyl radicals in human skin under physiological and pathophysiological conditions.

REFERENCES

1. Stewart CP, Guthrie DA, eds. A Treatise on the Scurvy. Edinburgh: Edinburgh University Press, 1953.
2. Svirbely JL, Szent-Györgi A. The chemical nature of vitamin C. Biochem J 1932; 26:865–870.
3. Waugh WA, King CG. Isolation and identification of vitamin C. J Biol Chem 1932; 97:325–331.

4.   Walker A. Chronic scurvy. Br J Dermatol 1968; 80:625–630.
5.   Wallerstein RO, Wallerstein RO Jr. Scurvy. Semin Hematol 1976; 13:211–218.
6.   Leung FW, Guze PA. Adult scurvy. Ann Emerg Med 1981; 10:652–655.
7.   Chazan JA, Mistilis SP. The pathophysiology of scurvy. Am J Med 1963; 34:350–358.
8.   Vilter RW, Woolford RM, Spies TD. The pathophysiology of scurvy: a clinical and hematologic study. J Lab Clin Med 1946; 31:609–630.
9.   Mc Keanna KE, Dawson JF. Scurvy occurring in a teenager. Clin Exp Dermatol 1993; 18:75–77.
10. Sherlock P, Rothschild EO. Scurvy produced by a Zen macrobiotic diet. JAMA 1967; 199: 794–798.
11. Crandon JH, Lund CC, Dill DB. Experimental human scurvy. N Engl J Med 1940:223:353–369.
12. Hodges RE, Hood J, Canham JE. Clinical manifestations of ascorbic acid deficiency in man. Am J Clin Nutr 1971; 24:432–443.
13. Ellis CN, Vanderveen EE, Rasmussen JE. Scurvy: a case caused by peculiar dietary habits. Arch Dermatol 1984; 120:1212–1214.
14. Englard S, Seifer S. The biochemical functions of ascorbic acid. Annu Rev Nutr 1986; 6:365–406.
15. Levine M. New concepts in the biology and biochemistry of ascorbic acid. N Engl J Med 1986; 314:892–902.
16. Bates CJ. The function and the metabolism of vitamin C in man. In: Counsell, Hornig, eds. Vitamin C (Ascorbic Acid). London: Applied Science, 1981:1–22.
17. Chojkier M, Houglum K, Solis-Herruzo J, Brenner DA. Stimulation of collagen gene expression by ascorbic acid in cultured human fibroblasts: a role for lipid peroxidation. J Biol Chem 1989; 264:16957–16962.
18. Price NM. Vitamin C deficiency. Cutis 1980; 26:375–377.
19. Coulehan JL, Reisinger KS, Rogers KD, Bradley DW. Vitamin C prophylaxis in a boarding school. N Engl J Med 1974; 290:6–10.
20. Pauling L. Vitamin C and the Common Cold. San Francisco: Freeman, 1970.
21. Prinz W, Bortz R, Bregin B, Hersch M. The effect of ascorbic acid supplementation on some parameters of the human immunological defense system. Int J Vitam Nutr Res 1977; 47: 248–257.
22. Cathcart RF. The vitamin C treatment of allergy and the normally unprimed state of antibodies. Med Hypotheses 1986, 21:307–321.
23. Ginter E, Cerna O, Budlovsky J. Effect of ascorbice acid on plasma cholesterol in humans in a long term experiment. Int J Vitam Nutr Res 1977; 47:123–134.
24. Cameron E, Pauling L. Supplemental ascorbate in the supportive treatment of cancer: prolongation of survival times in terminal human cancer. Proc Natl Acad Sci USA 1976; 73:3685–3689.
25. Ovesen L. Vitamin therapy in the absence of obvious deficiency. What is the evidence? Drugs 1984; 27:148–170.
26. Wulf K. Vitamine. In Marchionini A, ed. Handbuch der Haut- und Geschlechtskrankheiten. Ergänzungswerk. Berlin, Göttingen, Heidelberg: Springer Verlag, 1962; Fünfter Band, Erster Teil; 382–469.
27. Burr RG, Rajan KT. Leukocyte ascorbic acid and pressure sores in paraplegia. Br J Nutr 1972; 28:275–281.
28. Taylor TV, Rimmer S, Day B, et al: Ascorbic acid supplementation in the treatment of pressure sores. Lancet 1974; 2:544–546.
29. Afifi AM, Ellis L, Huntsman RG, Said MI. High dose ascorbic acid in the management of thalassemia leg ulcers: a pilot study. Br J Dermatol 1975; 92:339–341.
30. Crandon JH, Lennihan R Jr, Mikhal S. Ascorbic acid economy in surgical patients. Ann NY Acad Sci 1961; 246–267.
31. Irvin TT, Chattopadhyay DK, Smythe A. Ascorbic acid and requirements in postoperative patients. Surg Gynecol Obstet 1978; 147:49–55.
32. Barlett MK, Jones CM, Ryan AE. Vitamin C and wound healing II. ascorbic acid content and tensile strength of healing wounds in human beings. N Engl J Med 1942; 226:474–481.

33. Abt AF, von Schuching S. Catabolism of L-ascorbic-1-C^{14} acid as a measure of its utilization in the intact and wounded guinea pig on scorbutic maintenance and saturation diets. Ann NY Acad Sci 1961; 92:148–158.

34. Levenson SM, Demetriou AA. Metabolic factors. In: Cohen IK, Diegelmann RF, Lindblad WJ, eds. Wound Healing: Biochemical and Clinical Aspects. 1992:248–273.

35. Halliwell B. Drug antioxidant effects: A basis for drug selection? Drugs 1991; 42:569–605.

36. Fuchs J, ed. Oxidative injury in dermatopathology. Heidelberg: Springer Verlag, 1992.

37. Fuchs J, Packer L, eds. Oxidative Stress in Dermatology. New York: Marcel Dekker, 1993.

38. Shindo Y, Witt E, Han Derick, Packer L. Dose response effects of acute ultraviolet irradiation on antioxidants and molecular markers of oxidation in murine epidermis and dermis. J Invest Dermatol 1994; 102:470–475.

39. Darr D, Combs S, Dunston S. Topical vitamin C protects porcine skin from ultraviolet radiation induced damage. Br J Dermatol 1992; 127:247–253.

40. Rust S. Über allergische Reaktionen bei Vitamintherapie. Z Haut Geschl Kr 1954; 17:317–321.

41. Rust S. Hypervitaminosen. Z Haut Geschl Kr 1954; 16:350–355.

42. Bendich A, Machlin LJ, Scandurra O, et al. The antioxidant role of vitamin C. Adv Free Radical Biol Med 1986; 2:419–444.

43. Hornig D. Metabolism and requirements of ascorbic acidin man. S Afr Med J 1981; 60:818–823.

44. Dhariwal K, Hartzell W, Levine M. Ascorbic acid and dehydroascorbic acid measurements in human plasma and serum. Am J Clin Nutr 1991; 54:712–716.

45. Capellmann M, Becka M, Bolt. A note on distribution of human plasma levels of ascorbic acid and dehydroascorbic acid. J Physiol Pharmacol 1994, 45:183–187.

46. Baker EM, Saari JC, Tolbert BM. Ascorbic acid metabolism in man. Am J Clin Nutr 1966; 19:371–378.

47. Brown LAS, Jones DP. The biology of ascorbic acid. In: Cadenas E, Packer L, eds. Handbook of Antioxidants. New York: Marcel Dekker, 1996:117–154.

48. Welch RW, Bergsten P, Butler JD, Levine M. Ascorbic acid accumulation and transport in human fibroblasts. Biochem J 1993: 294:505–510.

49. Butler JD, Bergsten P, Welch RW, Levine M. Ascorbic acid accumulation in human skin fibroblasts. Am J Clin Nutr 1991; 54:1144S–1146S.

50. Shindo Witt E, Packer L. Antioxidant defense mechanisms in murine epidermis and dermis and their response to ultraviolet light. J Invest Dermatol 1993; 100:260–265.

51. Buettner GR, Motten AG, Hall RD, Chignell CF. ESR detection of endogenous ascorbate free radical in mouse skin: enhancement of radical production during UV irradiation following topical application of chlorpromazine. Photochem Photobiol 1987; 46:161–164.

52. Jurkiewicz VA, Buettner GR. Ultraviolet light induced free radical formation in skin: an electron paramagnetic resonance study. Photochem Photobiol 1994; 59:1–4.

53. Buettner GR, Jurkiewicz BA. Ascorbate free radical as a marker of oxidative stress: an EPR study. Free Radical Biol Med 1993; 14:49–55.

54. Roginsky VA, Stegmann HB. Ascorbyl radical as natural indicator of oxidative stress: quantitative regularities. Free Radical Biol Med 1994; 17:93–103.

55. Berliner LJ. The development and future of ESR imaging and related techniques. Phys Med 1989; 5:63–75

56. Swartz HM, and Walczak T. In-vivo EPR: prospects for the 90s. Phys Med 1993; 9:41–50

57. Fuchs J, Groth N, Herrling. In vivo electron paramagnetic resonance in human skin. Second International Workshop on In Vivo ESR and ESR Imaging. L'Aquila, Italy, September 10–14, 1995.

20

Human Metabolism and the Requirement for Vitamin C

BETTY JANE BURRI and ROBERT A. JACOB

Western Human Nutrition Research Center, USDA, San Francisco, California

INTRODUCTION

Vitamin C is an umbrella term for ascorbic acid and dehydroascorbic acid, organic acids. They are simple organic molecules with the formulas shown in Fig. 1.

Most animals synthesize vitamin C from either glucose or galactose (two abundant nutrients) through the glucuronic acid pathway (1). Humans need vitamin C because somewhere in evolution they lost the enzyme L-gulonolactone oxidase. In most species, L-gulonolactone oxidase oxidizes L-gulonolactone to 2-keto-gulonolactone, which then is isomerized to ascorbic acid. Only a few species (including humans, monkeys, guinea pigs, and fruit bats) lost this enzyme (1). Only these species need vitamin C in their diet.

Scientists have proposed many functions for vitamin C. Vitamin C may be an important antioxidant (2–4); it may promote normal teeth and gums (5,6); it may stave off colds (7–9), heart disease (10), cancers (11,12), cataracts (13,14), and mortality (15). However, scientists have identified only one nutritional syndrome that vitamin C, and only vitamin C, can prevent. Vitamin C prevents scurvy, a fatal nutritional disease.

Scurvy is characterized by joint pains, tooth loss, lethargy, bone and connective tissue disorders, poor wound healing, and death. Scurvy is of great historical importance (16). It devastated many ocean voyages, such as Anson's circumnavigation of 1740 to 1744. Almost half of the crew from that fleet died of scurvy. How do the symptoms of scurvy relate to the biochemical characteristics of vitamin C?

VITAMIN C METABOLISM

Biochemical Functions

Vitamin C (both ascorbic acid [AA] and dehydroascorbic acid [DHAA]) is a cofactor for a variety of biochemical reactions (Table 1). It functions in oxidation–reduction (redox)

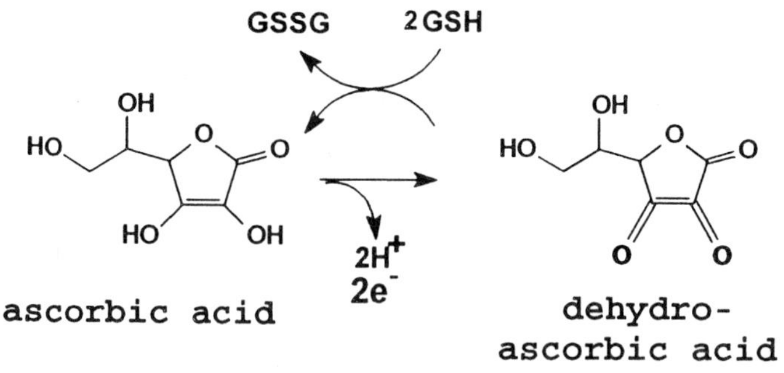

Figure 1 Ascorbic acid and dehydroascorbic acid. Ascorbic acid is the reduced form of vitamin C. The oxidized form, dehydroascorbic acid, can be reduced back to ascorbic acid by glutathione (GSH). (Adapted from Ref. 1.)

reactions; e.g., it provides electrons to reduce iron or copper at the catalytic sites of enzymes. It is only a moderately strong reducing agent. For example, equimolar concentrations of vitamin C will reduce copper and iron ions in the test tube. However, the oxidized form of vitamin C (DHAA) will itself be reduced by glutathione or reduced nicotinamide-adenine dinucleotide (NADH) (1). It is unclear whether vitamin C is really essential for most of these enzyme reactions. Theoretically, and in the test tube, vitamin C can be replaced with other redox reagents (1). Practically, it appears to be essential for the normal functions of these enzymes in healthy humans and animals (1).

Vitamin C also participates in less specific redox reactions, typically as an antioxidant. It joins vitamin E, the carotenoids, selenium, and other antioxidant nutrients that function to protect the body from oxidative damage. It may be the most important water soluble antioxidant. Finally, there is some evidence that vitamin C may influence iron, vitamin, and cholesterol metabolism.

Table 1   Biochemical Functions of Ascorbic Acid

Enzyme	Function
Enzymes that require ascorbic acid	
Proline hydrolase	Collagen synthesis
Procollagen-proline-2-oxoglutarate-3-dioxygenase (prolyl hydroxylase)	Collagen synthesis
Lysine hydrolase	Collagen synthesis
Trimethyllysine-2-oxoglutarate dioxygenase	Carnitine synthesis
Gamma-butyrobetaine,2-oxoglutarate-4-dioxygenase	Carnitine synthesis
Dopamine-beta-hydroxylase	Catecholamine synthesis
Peptidyl-glycine-alpha-amidating-monooxygenase	Peptide amidation
4-Hydroxyphenylpyruvate dioxygenase	Tyrosine metabolism
Antioxidant	Mixed function oxidase
Possible functions	
Promoting nonheme iron metabolism	
Influencing cholesterol metabolism	
Influencing folate, tocopherol, and B vitamin metabolism	

Source: Adapted from Refs. 1 and 17.

Functions Related to Scurvy

Most of the enzyme reactions listed in Table 1 require iron or copper. The metal ions used by these enzymes are oxidized during their hydroxylation reactions. Vitamin C typically acts as a cofactor in these reactions, by reducing the metal ions back to their original state.

Vitamin C is required for the posttranslational hydroxylation of the peptide-bound proline residues of procollagen (Fig. 2) (18,19). Enzyme-bound iron is oxidized during the hydroxylation reaction. Vitamin C reactivates the enzyme by reducing the iron to the ferrous state. Vitamin C is also required for lysine hydroxylation, which is a copper-dependent reaction (1,20). Vitamin C reactivates the enzyme by reducing copper at the active site of the enzyme. These hydroxylation reactions stabilize the triple-helical structure of the collagen molecule. Collagen stabilization strengthens connective tissues (18–20). Vitamin C depletion produces weak, defective connective tissue (18–20). Defective connective tissue is probably responsible for the gum and bone changes, as well as the poor wound healing, seen in scurvy.

Vitamin C also appears to be essential for the synthesis of muscle carnitine (20,21), which is required for transferring fatty acids into mitochondria (1). Carnitine biosynthesis involves lysine methylation, which requires ascorbic acid as well as iron. Carnitine biosynthesis is essential for optimal energy production. Vitamin C depletion results in low carnitine production, weakness, and lassitude (1,21–24). Many anecdotal reports from trained observers suggest that weakness and lassitude are early signs of scurvy (25,26). Carnitine depletion may be responsible for the weakness and lassitude in scurvy.

Vitamin C is used for the hydroxylation of dopamine to norepinephrine (noradrenaline) in the brain (1,27–29). Ascorbic acid is a cofactor for the copper-containing enzyme dopamine-beta-monooxygenase. Vitamin C is concentrated actively by the brain. These

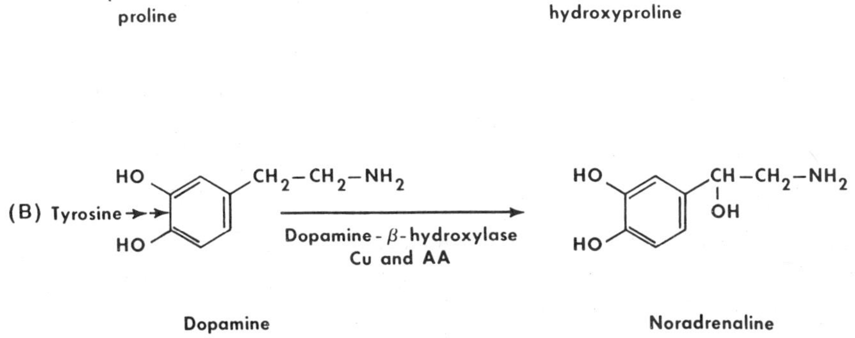

Figure 2 Vitamin C reactions: A, Hydroxylation of proline. Ascorbic acid (AA) is a cofactor involved in regenerating ferrous iron. α-KG, α-ketoglutaric acid; B, hydroxylation of dopamine. (From Ref. 1.)

concentrations are maintained in animal brain tissue even after prolonged depletion (1). Scientists know little about vitamin C metabolism in the human brain. However, depression, hypochondria, and mood changes frequently occur during scurvy (25,26,30). Malfunctions of dopamine hydroxylation may cause these symptoms.

Functions with Unknown Connections to Scurvy (Extrascorbutic Functions)

Scurvy is very rare today, even in famine. Scurvy was not reported as a major problem during the 900-day siege of Stalingrad (Kenneth Carpenter, personal communication). Doctors still do report scurvy occasionally (31), but it does not appear to be a common nutritional disease anywhere in the world. Protein-calorie malnutrition has always been much more common. So are anemia, goiter, xerophthalmia (nutritional blindness), and rickets (caused by deficiencies of iron, iodine, vitamin A, and vitamin D, respectively) (32). Thus, the global importance of vitamin C to human health does not depend on scurvy prevention. It depends on the extrascorbutic functions of vitamin C: whether these extrascorbutic functions are essential, or at least very useful, for human health, and whether vitamin C can be replaced in these extrascorbutic functions.

Does marginal vitamin C status cause other, more subtle, health problems? Some evidence suggests that it does. First, vitamin C is required for reactions in tyrosine metabolism and peptide amidation (17). Scientists have not observed changes in tyrosine metabolism during vitamin C depletion in humans (30). Simple relationships between the functions of these enzymes and the symptoms of scurvy have not been ascertained. Second, scurvy is an end-stage vitamin C deficiency, a lethal disease. It is identified by well-defined, easily recognized symptoms such as tooth loss. It would be surprising if the first and only symptom of vitamin C deficiency in the human body were these characteristic scurvy symptoms. Many studies of experimentally induced scurvy suggest that characteristic symptoms are preceded by other symptoms such as lassitude, hypochondria, anxiety, and muscle pain or weakness (25,26). These symptoms are nonspecific, difficult to quantify accurately, and difficult to correlate to indices of vitamin C status. They probably depend on individual health and behavioral characteristics. Third, vitamin C may have beneficial functions that are not related to scurvy prevention. These extrascorbutic functions may require more vitamin C than scurvy prevention does.

There are experimental studies suggesting that vitamin C may be useful for preventing gingivitis (5,6). Others show that vitamin C lowers the level of serum cholesterol (33,34). Vitamin C may facilitate intestinal absorption of nonheme iron (35,36), which is useful in counteracting low iron intake. Similarly, vitamin C appears to influence copper transport (37). Moderately high vitamin C intakes may benefit people with schizophrenia (38), Parkinson's disease (39), or diabetes (40,41). Higher vitamin C intake has been associated with improved pulmonary function (42). Other results suggest that vitamin C may improve fertility in males (43–46). Some human studies show that it can affect a variety of immune response functions (47,48), though these results are contradicted by results of other studies (49). It may prevent or ameliorate colds (7–9).

Conversely, vitamin C may have extrascorbutic functions that are harmful. Increased nonheme iron absorption may be bad, if it contributes to iron overload (50). Pharmacological doses of vitamin C might increase hemolysis in people with sickle cell trait (51). It may produce "rebound scurvy" (52,53), scurvylike symptoms that sometimes appear in people who have stopped taking high vitamin C supplements. It may increase oxalate and kidney stone formation, especially in renal patients (54). It might lead to loss of tooth enamel (55,56).

Vitamin C is an antioxidant (2–4). Its extrascorbutic role in the antioxidant defense system is described elsewhere in this book. Briefly, vitamin C may protect lipoproteins from oxidation. Vitamin C is an antioxidant because of its structure (several conjugated double bonds and a ring structure). Its shares this antioxidant function with many other molecules that have similar structural features. These include other essential nutrients (selenium, vitamin E), food constituents (beta-carotene and lycopene), and organic molecules such as bilirubin and uric acid. Many epidemiological studies suggest that vitamin C is an important nutrient. The large majority of these studies show inverse relationships between vitamin C and disease endpoints. People with low vitamin C status or intake have a greater tendency to have a variety of cancers (11,12), coronary heart disease (10), and cataracts (13,14,57). A far smaller number of epidemiological studies have shown no effect, or even possible vitamin C action as a prooxidant, potentially accelerating cancer formation (58). Unfortunately, these epidemiological studies cannot prove that vitamin C is useful or necessary for cancer or coronary heart disease prevention. Epidemiological studies can only show associations. They do not prove cause and effect.

Actually, one of the more remarkable characteristics of vitamin C is that large variations in vitamin C intake appear to have little influence on human health. Millions of people consume 25 mg of vitamin C (or less) per day with no apparent ill effects. Millions of people eat 2 or 3 g or more of vitamin C per day, also with no apparent ill effects. Imagine the calamitous results that would occur if people ate an 100-fold range of calories! Harmful effects from extreme ranges of consumption of protein, fats, iodine, selenium, vitamin D, vitamin A, and many other nutrients would be obvious. The reason that massive changes in vitamin C consumption have so little effect must also be related to its metabolism.

Humans would not need vitamin C if they did not have a rare deleterious mutation. If humans did not have this mutation, vitamin C might not seem so important to us. Many other molecules (such as glucose, citric acid, or fructose) also perform multiple functions in the human body. Would scientists study vitamin C any more than they study these other molecules if humans did not have this mutation? Would scientists have identified all of the functions ascribed to vitamin C, if humans biosynthesized it? Probably not. The anecdotal evidence linking vitamin C to cold prevention was probably no stronger than the anecdotal evidence linking chicken soup or chocolate candy to cold prevention. However, humans who do not eat enough vitamin C contract scurvy. There is no nutrient deficiency associated with a lack of chicken soup or chocolate in the diet. As we discuss the role of vitamin C in human nutrition and metabolism, it is well to remember that if we synthesized vitamin C we might not write books about it.

HUMAN STUDIES

We know surprisingly little about vitamin C metabolism in humans. The reason for our lack of knowledge is that human studies are expensive, time-consuming, and labor-intensive. Human beings are not guinea pigs. We live long, active lives. We are exposed to different diseases, environments, and stresses. We eat many things. In short, humans are difficult research subjects. There are two major types of human nutrition studies: controlled and free-living. Both types have unique drawbacks. It is necessary to understand these drawbacks in order to evaluate nutrition research findings.

A controlled study takes place in a metabolic unit or in a hospital. In a classic strict controlled nutrition study, the people who participate in the study live in a metabolic unit or hospital under supervision for months or years. Cooks prepare all of their food to uniform specifications. Medicines and medical conditions that might interfere with results are prohibited.

There are great advantages of all this control. Scientists can be confident that changes in biochemical or physiological status are caused by differences in diet. Another advantage is that complete collections of urine and feces can be obtained, preventing sampling errors. Finally, blood can be collected at the most critical times for metabolic studies. The drawbacks of these controlled studies are also great. First, scientists must limit the number of people studied to the number who can sleep in the metabolic unit. This number may be too small to allow researchers to see the subtler effects of nutrient depletion or effects that occur only in small groups of genetically or environmentally predisposed people. Second, the living conditions in the unit are unusual. Third, the studies are very expensive.

Free-living studies are much more common. Subjects in free-living nutritional studies typically go about their usual lives, with small differences. They either eat a special diet or record what they eat. Scientists then compare what the subjects say they ate to changes in health status, biochemical, or physiological changes. Free-living studies have several advantages over controlled studies. Only imagination (or, more often, funding), limits the number and types of subjects in the study. The study can run for years or even decades. The disadvantage is that free-living subjects in the same study eat different diets, have different life-styles, and experience different exposures to disease than other subjects participating in the same study. Furthermore, only a relatively small number of fruits and vegetables are good sources of vitamin C. Thus, day-to-day consumption of vitamin C is probably more variable than consumption of other nutrients (such as riboflavin or folate) that are more evenly distributed in foods. Differences in daily consumption may impact the results of free-living studies, even if the subjects eventually eat similar amounts of the nutrient. Intervention trials are a special example of a free-living study. Scientists developed clinical intervention trials to measure the effectiveness of new drugs and treatments. Ideally, the subjects have never been exposed to the drug before. The scientist compares one group of people who have the drug to another group who do not. Nutrient intervention trials work less well. The scientist must compare one group of people who ate the nutrient, are eating the nutrient, and will continue to eat the nutrient to another group, who have eaten, do eat, and will eat the nutrient. This is a special problem for vitamin C intervention trials, because vitamin C has been available as a self-prescribed intervention in the U.S. population for years.

METABOLISM AND TURNOVER STUDIES

Depletion Studies

Modern studies of vitamin C deficiency in humans are rare. They have also been relatively short-term and have typically focused on specific vitamin C interactions. Unfortunately, very few have measured antioxidant or iron status. Few have attempted to estimate psychological status, fatigue, or stress. Long-term, more severe depletion studies were more common between 1930 and 1970 (25,26,30,59–66). These older studies provide most of our information on the amount of vitamin C that protects against severe symptoms of scurvy. These studies are important. They were conducted with care, and they probably cannot be repeated. These scurvy studies were limited, of course, by methodological problems. Scientists conducted these studies by using small numbers of relatively similar people. They provide almost no information on vitamin C requirements of infants, children, adolescents, and the elderly. They provide little information about psychological status or stress, none on antioxidant status, and none on individual enzyme reactions. They typically used methods for estimating serum vitamin C concentrations that had artifacts and have been replaced by modern chromatography methods (67). Despite these drawbacks, the scurvy studies provide most of our information about vitamin C metabolism during periods of low vitamin C intake and about the amount of vitamin C needed to prevent scurvy. Much of this information is remarkably consistent.

Several scurvy studies still have major impact on the recommended dietary intake of vitamin C (26,60–64). These studies include the Scorby Research Institute study of vitamin C depletion (60) in healthy young adults and the U.S. Army/Iowa State University Scurvy studies 1 and 2, of vitamin C metabolism and depletion in adult males (26,61–64).

Scorby Research Institute Study

The longest study of scurvy was conducted in Sheffield, England, during 1944 and 1945 (60). Twenty conscientious objectors (19 men and 1 woman) were housed at the Scorby Institute for up to 18 months. It was a free-living study but had more control than is typical for these types of studies. Some subjects held outside jobs, and subjects could choose their diet from a restricted list of foods. However, opportunities for unapproved foods and activities were restricted by wartime conditions. Three subjects served as controls, eating the low vitamin C diet plus 70 mg per day vitamin C. An additional 7 subjects received a supplement of 10 mg per day vitamin C. Ten subjects (9 men and the woman) received the restricted diet alone. Scurvy developed in at least 8 of the 10 depleted subjects. Scurvy symptoms developed later than in other controlled depletion studies (61–64), probably because the diet contained small amounts of vitamin C. (Scorby Institute scientists estimated that the diet contained approximately 1 mg per day vitamin C. However, reanalysis of the dietary data provided (60) by Food Processor 2 software (68) suggests that the diet contained 2 to 3 mg per day of vitamin C.)

In the subjects who received the vitamin C supplement of 10 mg per day consistent symptoms of scurvy did not develop. All symptoms reported for the depleted group were cleared up with a supplement of 10 mg per day vitamin C (except possibly one case of acne, which needed 20 mg per day). However, physical fatigue tests (which were poorly described and reported) left doubt as to whether 10 mg per day of vitamin C was enough to maintain health.

Half of the subjects (four in the depletion group) had also participated in a lengthy vitamin A (and carotenoid) depletion study conducted previously at the same institute. These subjects had been fed a low vitamin A/carotenoid diet, containing 50 mg per day vitamin C, for up to 2 years. There was no significant difference between the time of onset of the first reported symptoms (100 ± 45 days versus 119 ± 67 days) or of the diagnosis of scurvy (207 ± 11 days versus 216 ± 50 days) in the group that had participated in the vitamin A depletion study compared to the group who had not. However, the 2 subjects in whom life-threatening illnesses developed during this study had participated in both depletion studies. This may be noteworthy, since vitamin C and beta-carotene both are antioxidants that have been implicated in disease prevention.

Scurvy Studies 1 and 2

U.S. Army and Iowa State University scientists conducted two controlled nutrition studies on vitamin C depletion in the 1960s. The subjects in the studies were nine healthy male adult prisoners (26,61–64). The subjects on these studies ate a controlled formula diet that was devoid of vitamin C for most of the experiments. The diet was adequate in most other nutrients, although it was also devoid of carotenoids. In the first study 4 men, 33 to 44 years old, consumed a liquid diet for 113 days, followed by a controlled solid diet for 97 days. Subjects were repleted with variable amounts of vitamin C from day 100. On the second study 5 men aged 26 to 52 years ate a solid diet containing 77.5 mg ascorbic acid for 13 days to stabilize their vitamin C concentrations before depletion, followed by a low vitamin C liquid diet for 84 to 97 days (62). The liquid diet was so unpalatable that the subjects administered their diets to themselves by stomach tube. (This may result in overestimates of normal dietary absorption from these studies, because food was administered directly into the stomach instead of eaten orally.) Staff supervised and controlled activities, which were strenuous. The subjects walked 10 miles per day. Scientists estimated the vitamin C absorption and metabolism of these subjects by radioisotope dilution. In all subjects classic signs of scurvy, including petechia, follicular hyperkeratosis, joint pains, and increased gingivitis, developed. In five of nine ocular lesions, which are not among the classic scurvy symptoms (62), also developed. Scientists included psychological tests in the second scurvy study only.

Most of the metabolic information from the Army studies was remarkably constant, even for a small group of people. The average pool size at the beginning of the experiment was 1500 mg, with a range from 1486 to 1549 mg (Table 2) (62). This difference is likely to be similar to the range produced by experimental error alone. The utilization rate for each person varied from 2.6% to 4.1% per day (62), depending on lean body mass. However, clinical changes occurred over a very wide range of pool sizes of vitamin C. For example, ecchymoses occurred at pool sizes ranging from 19 to 438 mg (Table 2) (62). Gum changes occurred at pool sizes ranging from 63 to 360 mg (62). Furthermore, scurvy symptoms developed at markedly different times, and in different orders of appearance. Perhaps the first symptoms that developed were psychological, subjects manifested the classic neurotic

Table 2   Estimates of the Body Pool Size of Vitamin C

n	Sex	Body pool (grams)	Reference
1	M	4.0–6.0	25
3	M	1.2–1.7	69
1	M	1.7–3.2	70
1	M	2.8	71
9	M	1.5	62
4	F	2.2–2.8	72
		Pool size estimate for onset of clinical symptoms	
9	M	0.02–0.44 For ecchymoses	62
9	M	0.03–0.32 For congested follicles	62
9	M	0.06–0.34 For hyperkeratosis	62
9	M	0.06–0.36 For gum changes	62
9	M	0.10–0.49 For petechiae	62

triad (hypochondria, depression, and hysteria) (26). Hypochondria occurred first; the critical value changes in this symptom occurred at a mean body pool size of 761 mg vitamin C (26). These psychological changes did not occur in the vitamin A depletion studies done by the same scientists under similar conditions, so they were probably caused by vitamin C depletion. Additional support for an interaction between vitamin C metabolism and clinical factors comes from their previous study. One subject during that study showed triple his normal ascorbic acid excretion during a brief period of great psychological stress. (Two subjects escaped from prison during this study.)

Both the Scorby Research Institute and U.S. Army depletion–repletion studies suggested that 6 to 12 mg per day of vitamin C prevented the onset of scurvy. Both suggested 6 to 12 mg per day of vitamin C was all that was necessary to clear up the symptoms of scurvy in most people, at least if the dose were fed for prolonged periods. Both suggested that a somewhat higher intake of vitamin C (perhaps 20 to 30 mg) might be necessary to correct some of the milder symptoms of scurvy (such as fatigue, acne, or the neurotic syndrome) in a few of the people tested. Both also showed that 6 to 12 mg per day of vitamin C did not raise blood vitamin C concentration to that found in normal healthy individuals.

Other Depletion Studies

Other depletion studies were conducted for shorter times. These studies typically suggest that somewhat higher concentrations of vitamin C (7 to 130 mg per day) are necessary to maintain vitamin C concentrations in blood at a normal (or even measurable) level (30,65, 66,73–75). The results from several suggested that somewhat higher concentrations (7 to over 130 mg per day) are necessary to treat or prevent mild deleterious health problems (such as fatigue, acne, bleeding gums, or petechia) from occurring in some people (5,6, 30,73,74).

For example, 150 Royal Canadian Airforce workers who had been treated for gingivitis were fed diets containing 10, 25, 75, and 80 mg of vitamin C per day (6). Gingivitis recurred more frequently at the lowest vitamin C intakes. Recurrence was 33% with 10 mg per day, 23% with 25 mg per day, 13% at 80 mg per day, and 8% with 75 mg per day. A second study of 11 men in a metabolic unit (5) showed that gingival bleeding sites (an early indication of gingivitis) increased when the subjects were fed a controlled diet containing 5 mg per day of ascorbic acid (Fig. 3). Gingival bleeding sites decreased during both a 65 and a 605 mg/ day repletion period, but the 605 mg per day supplement may have been a slight improvement over the 65-mg supplement.

Results from one metabolic unit study suggest that some individuals may need at least 60 mg per day of vitamin C to ameliorate some of the milder symptoms of scurvy (74). Eleven women were fed a formula diet devoid of vitamin C for 54 days. After the first 12 days, five women received the diet plus 600 mg per day of erythorbic acid (d-isoascorbic acid, a food additive); six received the formula diet alone. All were supplemented with 30 mg vitamin C per day from study days 25 to 34; 60 mg per day from days 35 to 44; and 90 mg per day from days 45 to 54. Scorbutic signs (inflamed, bleeding gums) unexpectedly developed in five of the six women fed the formula diet alone (unsupplemented with erythorbic acid). In nine subjects acne, which improved during the 90 mg per day ascorbic acid supplement, developed. This study appears anomalous, because symptoms of scurvy developed faster than expected, and subjects retained symptoms at higher vitamin C supplements than typical. The reason for this anomaly may be the study design. First, the study did not have a stabilization period. Subjects were fed the vitamin C depleted diet immediately, whereas previous studies stabilized vitamin C intake (e.g., subjects were fed

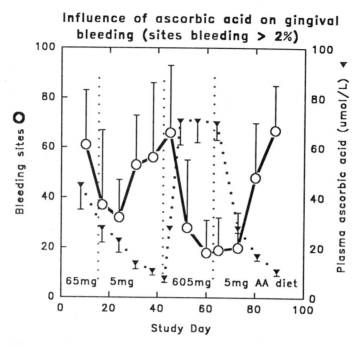

Figure 3 The influence of vitamin C on gingival bleeding sites. The number of gingival bleeding sites is an early measure of gingivitis. (Adapted from Ref. 5.)

77 mg per day for 13 days for the U.S. Army studies, and up to 2 years at 50 mg per day for the Scorby study). Initial marginal status may have resulted in the rapid appearance of symptoms. Second, the symptoms were obvious, but milder than observed in prior studies (H. Sauberlich, M. Kretsch, personal communication), so the criteria for reporting were different.

Depletion studies also show that vitamin C does not influence many physiological parameters, at least for the short term. Anemia did not increase (62). Hemoglobin and hematocrit values did not change (5,60). The immune response to typhoid vaccine was normal (62). Major psychiatric illness did not occur, although milder symptoms [depression and anxiety (25), introspection and anxiety (26,60), fatigue and listlessness (30)] were frequent. There were no significant interactions with oxalate, B vitamins, vitamin E or A, or iron (5). There were no significant increases in the incidence of infection (60,62). However, there may have been a marginally significant increase in cold severity and length (mean duration 3.3 nondeprived versus 6.4 days deprived, $p < 0.1$) (60).

Kinetic Studies

Recently, more metabolic information has been collected from people who are on controlled (but not deficient) dietary intakes of vitamin C. Important metabolic studies have been conducted by Kallner (76–78), Blanchard et al. (79–82), and Melethil et al. (83).

Kallner measured vitamin C status and turnover by radioisotope dilution in 15 healthy male nonsmokers (76) and 15 healthy male smokers (77). These were free-living studies; the men were asked to eat a low vitamin C diet based on rice and spaghetti. They were fed the diet plus 30, 60, 90, or 180 mg vitamin C per day for 2 weeks. Kinetic constants were calculated on the basis of a three compartment model. It was assumed that the subjects had attained equilibrium during these relatively brief supplementation periods. The half-life of vitamin C varied from 7 to 40 days (Table 3). Kinetics were complex: the half-life was inversely related to dosage. Smokers had a shorter half-life and appeared to need 30–40 mg per day more ascorbic acid than nonsmokers (76–78).

Blanchard (79) fed 14 young adult women (aged 20 to 29 years), 14 elderly women (65 to 72 years), 15 young adult men (21 to 28 years), and 15 elderly men (66 to 74 years) 10 mg per day vitamin C for 5 weeks, then 500 mg per day for 2 1/2 weeks in a free-living study. All were healthy Caucasian nonsmokers who were not on medications. The subjects' dietary intake of vitamin C was estimated with food records. Kinetics appeared to be a first-order process, with the half-life inversely related to entry ascorbic acid concentrations below 85 μmol/L. Above 85 μmol/L the half-life was constant and averaged 14.2 days. Elimination of vitamin C was slower when the concentration was below 85 μmol/L. These results suggested that vitamin C was conserved at low concentrations. Kinetic constants did not vary with age, but they did vary with sex. The reaction rate was smaller, and the half-life longer in men. Entry and depleted ascorbic acid concentrations did not differ between the sexes, but repleted plasma concentrations were higher in women. The depletion process occurred faster in women. Plasma levels after supplementation were higher in women than in men. Fat-free mass (the best predictor measured) was inversely related to vitamin C concentrations during repletion.

Melethil (83) fed pharmacological doses of vitamin C to four nonsmoking subjects (three men and one woman, aged 22 to 29 years). The subjects were fed 500, 1000, and 2000 mg vitamin C per day for 1 week each. Vitamin C kinetics were complex. The recovery of dose in the urine was 73%, 47%, and 36% of dose, respectively, for 500, 1000, and 2000 mg intakes. Both gastrointestinal absorption and reabsorption appeared to be saturable. This suggested that the systemic effects of pharmacological doses of vitamin C are open to question, because it is uncertain how much may be absorbed, retained, and excreted.

Several other studies have attempted to calculate body pool sizes or kinetic constants,

Table 3   Estimates of Apparent Half-Life of Vitamin C Metabolism

n	Sex	Diet intake (mg per day)	Mean days	Range days	Reference
9	M	0	17.3	12.2–22.7	62
1	M	10	13.7		71,85
58	30 M	10	19.9	12.2–44.7	79
58	28 F	10	16.0	9.3–53.7	79
4	M	30	28.0	16.5–40.1	76
3	M	60	25.3	23.1–27.0	76
9	M	60	14.3	± 2.91 SEM	84
3	M	90	12.9	9.1–17.0	76
4	M	180	11.0	7.9–12.8	76
1	M	250	8.0		71,85
9	M	600	6.9	± 2.65 SEM	84

often on single individuals. For example, Baker et al. (71,85) estimated the pool size and kinetic constants for a single male subject using radioisotope dilution. He calculated that the initial pool size of this individual was 2.8 g. The rate of ascorbic acid turnover varied reciprocally with ascorbic acid intake (and pool size), from 13.7 days on an intake of 10 mg per day to 8 days at an intake of 250 mg per day. Additional studies and their results are listed in Tables 2 and 3.

Many other studies have attempted to calculate the amount of vitamin C required to saturate tissues (Table 4). These studies produce variable results, depending on their criteria for saturation, the methods used to measure vitamin C status and intake, and the population. For example, Morse (86) measured vitamin C status in 19 mentally handicapped women (27 to 64 years of age) for 5 months. The subjects ate a modified institutional diet. Vitamin C intake was estimated from weighed food consumption recorded for 16 days at the beginning and end of the study. The women were fed approximately 33 mg of vitamin C per day for 7 weeks, then an additional 25 mg per day supplement for 5 weeks, then an additional 50 mg per day for 5 more weeks, and finally an additional 100 mg per day for the last 5 weeks. Blood ascorbic acid concentrations dropped when the subjects were fed 33 mg per day. Plasma and white blood cell ascorbic acid concentrations were correlated at 33, 58, and 83 mg per day, but not at 133 mg per day intake. This suggests that vitamin C saturation may occur between 83 and 133 mg per day.

In summary, these studies suggest that vitamin C metabolism is complex. In healthy adults it appears to depend on the intake of vitamin C and the body stores of vitamin C. Vitamin C metabolism appears to be influenced by sex, body composition, smoking, and possibly to some degree age.

Furthermore, the amount of vitamin C calculated to meet estimated requirements or saturation depends on the test used and the tissue measured. Finally, the estimated requirement depends on the philosophical and political criteria used for the requirement: whether the "requirement" refers to the amount needed to prevent scurvy, to establish tissue saturation, or to promote "optimal health."

Table 4   Estimates of the Maintenance Requirement for Vitamin C[a]

Method	Estimated requirement (mg per day) for each age group					
	0–1	2–5	6–12	13–17	18–64	65+ years
Scurvy	20	—	—	—	6.5–45	—
Whole blood-A	20	—	—	—	55–70	50–80
Plasma-S	—	—	45–125	—	70–131	—
Plasma-A	—	—	52–72	70–97	38–100	—
Leukocytes-S	—	—	50–100	—	22–83	—
Leukocytes-A	—	—	—	62–100	60–100	—
Urine excretion-S	20–40	21–50	35–130	125	26–125	50–75
Urine excretion-A	—	—	50–100	60–65	15–25	—

[a]The total number of studies and the total number of people analyzed in this conspectus and summarized herein were: 21 studies of 368 adults; 5 studies of 178 infants; 5 studies of 16 children (2 to 5 years); 16 studies of 388 children (6 to 12 years); 4 studies of approximately 24 children (13 to 17 years); and 5 studies of 323 elderly people. S, estimated requirement for tissue saturation; A, estimated requirement for "acceptable" concentration.
Source: Ref. 73.

METABOLISM OF PHARMACOLOGICAL DOSES

Most scientists define pharmacological doses of vitamin C as intakes that are very difficult to obtain from food. For example, an intake of 1 g or more of vitamin C is a pharmacological dose. Many Americans consume these pharmacological (mega) doses of vitamin C routinely. In effect, they are participating in a nutritional experiment, with the goal of improving their health and quality of life. Why would millions of Americans use themselves as guinea pigs in a long-term nutritional experiment? And what have been the results of this experiment? Our first question has a deceptively simple answer.

Linus Pauling, winner of two Nobel Prizes (one for Chemistry, one for Peace), published *Vitamin C and the Common Cold* in 1970 (9). This book has arguably been the most influential book in the history of nutrition. Pauling collected anecdotal, circumstantial, evolutionary (87), and (minimal) experimental data to support his claim that gram doses of vitamin C helped ameliorate the common cold. He suggested that gram doses of vitamin C also promote health, well-being, and alertness (7,9). Surprisingly, the book became very popular. It appears to have elicited an almost emotional response among millions of people. Thousands have apparently consumed pharmacological doses of vitamin C for years, on the basis of his advice (15,42,88,89).

The response to this book by other scientists was swift and forceful. Opponents argued that the book was not the best science. (This was true; it contained few well-done experiments.) They argued that pharmacological doses of vitamin C might result in a multitude of serious health problems, such as rebound scurvy (52,53), iron overload (50), tooth enamel loss (55,56), B vitamin deficiency (90), and gallstones (54). These arguments were good in theory. Unfortunately, many were supported by anecdotal, circumstantial, or experimental evidence as minimal as Pauling's. Recent controlled experiments have not provided much supporting evidence for these deleterious actions of vitamin C. Vitamin C did influence nonheme iron uptake. However, most of this influence occurred at relatively low, recommended intakes of vitamin C (35,36). Vitamin C concentrations in serum and leukocytes did drop faster after large intakes of vitamin C (5,91), but this did not lead to signs of scurvy. The apparent effect of ascorbic acid on B_{12} and B_6 vitamins turned out to be an artifact of the measurement methods used (92). Several studies have shown no link between high intake of vitamin C and increased oxalate or kidney stone production in humans (93,94). Furthermore, many people in the United States eat pharmacological doses of vitamin C daily (15,88,89). Thousands, possibly millions, have taken pharmacological doses of vitamin C for 25 or 30 years! Reports of adverse effects should be common if they occurred regularly. That does not mean that toxicity symptoms and deleterious effects of pharmacological (mega) doses of vitamin C never occur. They probably do occur, especially in people predisposed to defects in iron or folic acid metabolism. However, reviews of the literature show that they appear to be rare (95,96).

Recent experiments also show few acute benefits of pharmacological doses of vitamin C. The duration of cold symptoms may be decreased by large doses of vitamin C (9,97). Vitamin C may act as an antihistamine (98). Its effect, if any, is controversial and small. The most promising experiments result in approximately 1 day less of bed rest (8,9,97). Pharmacological doses of vitamin C may attenuate bronchial reactivity, relieving some symptoms of bronchitis and asthma, but this effect may be transitory (99,100). Even if scientists establish these benefits beyond reasonable doubt, it is difficult to see why a patient with a cold or asthma would take megadoses of vitamin C. Many over-the-counter remedies work better.

Vitamin C has also sometimes appeared to be beneficial to men with fertility problems (44–46), but a controlled study showed no improvement in sperm motility or other indices of fertility in healthy adult males with normal sperm functions (75).

Some studies also suggest that people who eat large amounts of vitamin C may have lower rates of cancer (12) or heart disease (10). However, nutrient intervention trials using vitamin C show minimal effects (101,102). The Linxian trial found that 120 mg supplements of vitamin C provided no benefit in reducing cancer risk, even though the study population may have had borderline nutritional status (101,102). Of course, higher doses given over a longer period might have shown a benefit. However, a few studies have suggested that larger intakes of vitamin C may even be associated with higher risks of cancer (58), suggesting that vitamin C may sometimes act as a prooxidant.

Why do these large doses of vitamin C have such a minimal effect—good or bad—on human health? Part of the reason centers on vitamin C metabolism. First, vitamin C absorption is regulated. The larger the intake of vitamin C, the smaller the proportion that is absorbed into the blood. Second, there is also a threshold for renal tubular reabsorption (83). Again, the larger the dose, the smaller the proportion that is reabsorbed. Most vitamin C is excreted when large doses are eaten. The amount excreted is directly proportional to the blood ascorbate concentration. Since both absorption and excretion are dose dependent, vitamin C metabolism is complex. However, this typically means that the larger the intake of vitamin C, the smaller the percentage of vitamin C that is actually utilized.

Several scientists have attempted to calculate the amount of vitamin C that would be safe and adequate for humans from metabolic data. So far, these attempts are in their infancy, because of the uncertainties caused by the complex metabolism of vitamin C. Two recent attempts have been the "recommended dietary intakes" calculated by the 9th RDA committee (103), and "in situ kinetics," by Levine (17,104).

RECOMMENDED DAILY DIETARY ALLOWANCES

Recommended Dietary Intake

The recommended dietary intake (RDI) (103) was an attempt to base the minimum requirement of vitamin C on metabolic criteria. Vitamin C requirements were calculated from absorption data (showing that vitamin C absorption decreases with increased intake) and information from the U.S. Army (61–64) studies relating pool sizes of vitamin C to scurvy symptoms. The RDI was calculated from the amount of vitamin C that provides a body pool greater than has ever been related to scurvy (900 mg in adult males); was threefold higher than the one that prevents scurvy; and provided a 1 month reserve for low intakes. The RDI was estimated as 40 mg per day for adult men, and 30 mg per day for adult women. This estimate was lower than previous estimates, primarily because the RDI committee believed that no benefit had been proved for higher intakes and that higher intakes might result in harm to some susceptible people (such as those at risk for iron overload). The RDI committee made a praiseworthy attempt to estimate vitamin C requirements from scientific information. However, they can probably be faulted for minimizing or ignoring the effects of individual and group variability in their calculations. For one example, the coefficient of variation used in their calculations was just 20% (103,105). For another, the difference in RDI for men and women was based on the difference in body weight of a reference man to a reference woman. (It is unlikely that differences in body weight account for differences in vitamin C metabolism, since these differences persist at the highest intakes of vitamin C (106). Furthermore, if differences in body weight were a primary factor determining the requirement of vitamin C, it would have been appropriate to list the RDI for different body weights, instead of assigning different RDIs by sex or age.)

In Situ Kinetics

In situ kinetics attempts to relate ascorbic acid functions to concentrations in tissues (17,104). Vitamin C is a cofactor in several enzyme reactions (Table 1). The hypothesis behind in situ kinetics is that the dietary intake of vitamin C that gives these enzymes maximal activity (at their site of action) without causing toxicity symptoms is the optimal dietary intake for vitamin C. By deriving kinetic profiles for the enzymes that utilize vitamin C, scientists should be able to derive the recommended daily dietary allowance for vitamin C. This is an attractive hypothesis, since it can be used to derive requirements from experiments in healthy, adequately nourished subjects. Thus, the requirement could be estimated without having to account for adjustments in metabolism induced by deficiency or toxicity in the subjects. Unfortunately, scientists do not yet have enough experimental information to use in situ kinetics to calculate the requirement for vitamin C. A great deal of experimental work is needed. Some of the experiments will require the prolonged use of a metabolic unit, cell culture facilities, stable isotope measurements, or all of these. Even when this work is completed, we do not know whether it will be possible always to identify the critical tissues where in situ kinetics will be most relevant. Finally, there may be several optimal kinetic configurations. The concentrations that result in optimal in situ kinetics for one person may not be optimal for another. In fact, they may be marginally deficient or toxic. Preliminary estimates of the requirement for vitamin C derived from in situ kinetics are 7 to 750 mg per day (104).

Highlight: Current Controversies Surrounding Recommended Dietary Intakes for Vitamin C

Recommended dietary intakes for vitamin C change with time. For example, the current daily U.S. RDA for adults is 60 mg (107). It was 45 mg in 1974. It would have been 40 mg for men and 30 for women, if the National Research Council of the United States had approved the initial recommendations of the committee of the 10th edition of the RDA in 1985 (103). Recommended intakes also vary between countries. Adult daily recommended intakes have ranged from a low of 30 mg in Great Britain to a high of 75 mg in Germany (108). The same few experiments form the basis for these recommendations. They measured the same small number of subjects, so why are the recommendations so different?

There are several reasons for the controversy. First, most humans appear to need less than 10 mg per day of vitamin C to prevent scurvy. However, it is unlikely that the first undesirable symptom of vitamin C deficiency is scurvy, a life-threatening disease. Second, vitamin C depletion experiments show that many undesirable symptoms occur before the onset of scurvy. These symptoms may be important, but they are nonspecific and vague. Most (such as fatigue, hypochondria, acne, and gingivitis) are complex phenomena. They do not present themselves in all subjects. They do not correlate to vitamin C concentrations easily. They may require hereditary, health, or behavioral predisposition. Third, the benefits proposed for high intakes of vitamin C, such as reducing symptoms of the common cold (8,9), preventing degenerative diseases (10–14), and improving fertility (43–46), are also nonspecific and difficult to measure. Fourth, many of these suggested benefits would require most people to consume vitamin supplements (instead of foods). Vitamin C has not undergone the pharmacological studies done for new drugs. It is difficult to compare it to other drugs used for the same purposes. Fifth, acute vitamin C toxicity is very rare. Sixth, although chronic intakes of large amounts of vitamin C may cause harmful effects in some people (such as those at risk for iron overload) (50), there is little evidence that these effects are actually widespread (95,96). Thus, the benefits to various intakes of vitamin C have no clearly defined limits. Similarly, the risks of various intakes are also largely unknown. This has meant that the RDA for vitamin C has incorporated differing philosophies and health status goals on a base of scientific evidence.

The recommended dietary intake for Great Britain is relatively low (30 mg per day). It was derived from the Scorby (Sheffield, England) study (60) of vitamin C depletion in conscientious objectors in World War II. The British base their recommended intake on the minimum safe requirement for vitamin C, calculated during a time of hardship. This is the amount required to prevent scurvy, plus a safety factor. The current U.S. recommended dietary intake (60 mg per day) is based on a combination of factors (107), which include average dietary intake, average depletion and turnover rates of vitamin C calculated from radioisotope studies of inmates conducted by the U.S. Army, and safety factors for losses during food preparation and increased needs during special circumstances. The German recommended intake is relatively high (75 mg per day). It is consistent with the turnover data from the recent radioisotope studies of Kallner in healthy male Swiss smokers and nonsmokers (77,78). Scientists recognize the limits of these studies. They incorporate data from 42 healthy adult men (aged 19 to 52 years) and 1 adult woman. Children, adolescents, and elderly adults were not studied.

Recommended dietary intakes incorporate safety factors, as well as precise science. Therefore, they include ideas and visions of disease prevention and optimal health. It is unlikely that the controversy surrounding recommended dietary intakes for vitamin C will be solved by scientific means alone. Scientists should perform several experiments to improve the RDA for vitamin C, which we will discuss in another section. However, scientists must also have open discussions of our nutritional paradigms. Are we setting standards that will prevent scurvy, provide average stores, or promote "optimal" health? Should we set standards for all three? On what basis? And for whom? Scientists may help prevent confusion and distrust if we discuss our social, economic, and philosophical views of recommended dietary intakes openly. Then, we might be able to separate the science from the controversy.

FACTORS BELIEVED TO INFLUENCE VITAMIN C METABOLISM AND REQUIREMENTS

Vitamin C metabolism is not constant. It is correlated with fat-free body mass (62). It depends on the dose of vitamin C administered and the amount of vitamin C already stored in the tissues (76–79). It varies between individuals, and probably also in the same individual. These variations may be caused by a variety of factors, such as sex, age, health status, exposure to smoke or pollution, diet, and heredity. We know very little about hereditary factors influencing vitamin C metabolism and requirement. We know somewhat more about environmental factors, such as health status and smoking. The importance of these factors, with the possible exception of smoking, has not been established.

Individual Variation

Controlled vitamin C depletion and repletion studies suggest that vitamin C metabolism has an approximately threefold variation (Tabes 2 and 3). Calculated body stores of vitamin C in healthy people range from about 1.2 to 4 g (Table 2). Calculated half-lives at similar vitamin C intakes can also vary widely, depending on the study (Table 3). These are not large variations, but they do suggest that some individuals may need more vitamin C than others. Furthermore, these studies were done in small, homogeneous populations (mostly healthy adult nonsmoking males). The actual normal range of vitamin C body pools and vitamin C utilization is probably larger. The possibility that vitamin C metabolism differs markedly between some individuals is also suggested by studies of scurvy. Symptoms of scurvy develop at markedly different rates in different people, and over a wide range of body pools (Table 2). Finally, case reports suggest that at least a small percentage of individuals must metabolize vitamin C differently than most. These individuals show vitamin C toxicity symptoms (51–53), or appear to be more susceptible to scurvy than others. Scientists do not yet know the extent or importance of these individual variations.

Age

Many epidemiological studies show that elderly people sometimes have lower concentrations of vitamin C in their blood than younger adults (109,110). This is not always the case, however, Several studies have shown that healthy, active elderly people have relatively high serum vitamin C concentrations (106,109,111). Scientists have searched for a physiological basis for the low vitamin C status of elderly people with little success. For example, Blanchard found little or no difference in the kinetic behavior of vitamin C between young and elderly adult men and women (79–82). Young and elderly adults had similar decreases in plasma concentrations of vitamin C during vitamin C depletion, and similar increases during vitamin C supplementation. Absorption kinetics and peak absorption concentrations were also similar. A review of the literature shows that studies calculating the maintenance requirement for vitamin C do not suggest differences in metabolism with old age (Table 4). Low vitamin C status in elderly people tends to be associated with either social isolation (112), or institutionalization (113), social conditions that tend to increase poor dietary habits. Most studies suggest that elderly people with low vitamin C status simply have lower dietary intakes of vitamin C (109,110), though the difference may be due in part to differences in health status. Elderly people have more infectious conditions than younger adults. They are also subject to more chronic diseases (such as diabetes and Parkinson's disease). Both chronic (39–41) and acute diseases may influence vitamin C metabolism and turnover.

Infants and very young children appear to need less vitamin C than adults (Table 4), but few rigorous studies have been done on these age groups. The serum concentrations and estimated requirements for vitamin C derived from studies in adults encompass the ranges of all the other age groups, including infants. Thus, age itself is likely to have minimal influence on vitamin C metabolism.

Sex

Women generally have higher serum concentrations of vitamin C than men (106,109,114). This difference probably is not based on differences in diet. For one thing, many studies from all over the world have compared men and women and reported that women had higher serum vitamin C concentrations (106,109,114–116). Cultural differences between the diets of men and women sometimes exist, but they are not as large as differences between cultures and incomes. For another, this difference is seen consistently, e.g., among smokers and vitamin supplement users. It is also unlikely that differences in health status cause this difference. Most surveys reporting vitamin C concentrations in men and women were done on either healthy, noninstitutionalized populations or on persons at the same institution. Although many studies have not reported their criteria for "healthy," others have used careful and clear-cut guidelines to select their subjects. Figure 4 shows serum vitamin C concentrations from healthy elderly men and women from Boston. Women had higher serum vitamin C concentrations at every estimated dietary intake. Experimental studies comparing men and women showed that women, on average, had significantly shorter half-lives for vitamin C metabolism (79–82). Women also attained higher plasma vitamin C concentrations upon vitamin C supplementation (79). Women typically have plasma vitamin C concentrations that are 10 to 20 μmol/L higher than those of men at similar dietary intakes of vitamin C. The difference in plasma vitamin C concentrations appears during adolescence (117). Hence, it appears that the sex difference in vitamin C concentrations is based on hormonal or physiological differences. Information on the influence of hormones on vitamin C concentrations is limited and contradictory. Oral contraceptives appear to influence vitamin C concentrations in serum and leukocytes (73). Some studies have shown that vitamin C concentrations vary with the stage of the menstrual cycle, but others have not (73).

Smoking

Smoking affects vitamin C serum concentrations, metabolism, and requirements (76–78, 118, 119). Smokers have lower vitamin C concentrations in serum (118), plasma, and other tissues (119). Smoking appears to alter vitamin C metabolism by increasing the turnover of the body pool. Kallner compared vitamin C turnover rates in healthy male smokers (77) and nonsmokers (76) and found that smokers had a faster turnover rate. Kallner estimated that smokers would need to eat at least 40 mg more ascorbic acid per day to maintain equivalent

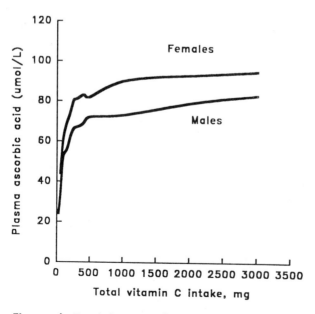

Figure 4 The influence of sex on serum concentrations of vitamin C in healthy elderly people in Boston. (From Ref. 106.)

serum vitamin C levels. Of course, smokers would benefit more by quitting smoking than by increasing their vitamin C intake. However, exposure to secondhand smoke may also affect the vitamin C status and requirement of nonsmokers. Wives of smokers, who presumably breathe in large amounts of secondhand smoke, had lower blood concentrations of vitamin C than matched controls (120). The lower vitamin C concentrations seen in wives of smokers may have been caused by exposure to secondhand smoke. However, wives of long-term smokers may be less health-conscious than nonsmoking wives of nonsmokers. They may eat fewer fruits and vegetables or take fewer vitamin supplements than wives of nonsmokers. However, if secondhand smoke does affect vitamin C status, it may be a significant influence on vitamin C metabolism in the general population. Secondhand smoke affects millions of people; more studies are needed to determine its influence on vitamin C metabolism.

Pregnancy and Lactation

Fetuses retain vitamin C (121). Vitamin C concentrations in cord blood and in newborn (term) infants is higher than that in the mother (122) (and presumably the father, since men tend to have lower concentrations of vitamin C than women). Therefore, vitamin C status in the mother must be influenced by the fetus, at least late in pregnancy. The 1989 RDA committee calculated that the total increment of vitamin C required by the mother over the length of the pregnancy would be approximately 3 to 4 mg per day (107). They suspected that this was an underestimate, and therefore proposed an increment of 10 mg vitamin C per day during the second and third trimesters of pregnancy (107). They also estimated that a lactating woman producing 750 ml of milk containing 30 to 100 µg/ml vitamin C would need approximately 35 mg more vitamin C per day during the first 6 months of lactation (107).

Stress

Many studies have suggested that various forms of stress may influence vitamin C metabolism (26,73,122). Hypothetically, stress could influence vitamin C metabolism by a number of mechanisms. For example, vitamin C is an antioxidant. Any stress that increases oxygen turnover or antioxidant requirements might increase vitamin C metabolism. Pollution or illness could easily increase antioxidant requirements (123–125). This might influence the requirement for vitamin C, especially if other antioxidants were in short supply. Vitamin C is used to convert dopamine to norepinephrine (27,29). Anything that increases the need for norepinephrine or the turnover of dopamine might increase vitamin C metabolism. Increased psychological stress might influence dopamine turnover directly. Heat, cold, trauma, and illness might all increase physical and psychological stress. Thus, all of these factors might influence the vitamin C requirement directly or indirectly.

Anecdotal evidence suggesting that stress increases the requirement for vitamin C has accumulated for centuries (16,25). Numerous experimental studies have also documented that stresses of various kinds sometimes appear to decrease vitamin C concentrations or increase utilization (26,73,122,126–128). Many types of stress are implicated. Specifically, heat stress (73), cold stress (73), trauma (73,126,127), illness (125,128), smog (123,124), and psychological stress (26,129) may all influence vitamin C metabolism. However, this evidence is contradicted by many other studies that did not find any effects of stress on vitamin C metabolism and requirement (60,73).

There are several reasons for controversies surrounding the effects (or lack thereof) of stress, illness, and trauma on vitamin C metabolism. The main reason is that other factors are more important determinants of vitamin C status and metabolism on a population basis; of these probably the most important determinant is diet. Vitamin C concentrations are highly correlated to dietary intake (and vitamin supplement usage) until intakes exceed approximately 75 to 150 mg per day (76–79,106,117) Other very important determinants are sex and smoking, either of which can influence vitamin C concentrations by 20% to 30% (106,117–119). The effects, if any, of stress can only be measured accurately if these other factors are minimized or accounted for accurately. Typically studies of the influence of stress on vitamin C status have not measured dietary intake accurately (73). The studies were conducted in small groups, with differing initial vitamin C status, antioxidant status, and exposure to stress. Second, there are many types of illness, trauma, and stress. Some are acute, some are chronic. The onset, duration, and degree of stress are often difficult to measure. Third, the influence of stress on vitamin C status and requirement is probably not universal. Different individuals react differently to stress. Some people appear to be unaffected by it; in others ulcers, high blood pressure, and psychological symptoms develop. Possibly we will understand the extent of the influence of stress on vitamin C only after we are able to measure it accurately and consistently.

GAPS IN SCIENTIFIC INFORMATION AND PRESENTATION

Normal, healthy people do have different requirements for vitamin C, although these differences may be very small. They also have different susceptibilities to the symptoms of scurvy and to cancer, heart disease, and colds. Scientists usually tend to minimize these individual differences; sometimes they present only averages of the data. Or they present averages and standard deviations. Unusual data points are not well represented by averages or by averages and standard deviations. The data may be unusual because they are wrong. On the other hand, they may represent accurate information about an individual who is not typical in some way. Comparing averaged data is usually more appropriate than comparing individual data. It gives a more accurate picture of the general population. However, averaging data can inadvertently exclude or ignore important differences. This has caused some conflicts in the scientific literature that might have been prevented. Many studies have shown that differences in vitamin C status influence a reaction or a measure of physiological status. Other studies have shown no change in these parameters. Two studies that show conflicting results for the influence of vitamin C on human health may both be correct—for the population studied.

Probably the worst gap in scientific presentation is the lack of information on adolescents. Very few studies on vitamin C metabolism, turnover, and requirement have ever been done on older children and adolescents (aged 6 to 18 years). These are ages of considerable interest, because many changes in metabolism are likely to occur during these years.

PROFITABLE AREAS FOR FUTURE RESEARCH

One important goal in human vitamin C research is to find a functional marker for marginal vitamin C status. Scientists have attempted to find this marker for years and have not been fully successful. However, they have neglected some potentially fruitful areas. For example, the activities of enzymes that are known to require vitamin C have seldom been measured. Developing simple, rapid, and cost-effective assays for these enzymes is necessary. Second, measuring these enzyme activities in the general population will be useful; for example, an enzyme that shows a wide range of activities in the general population probably warrants more investigation than an enzyme with a narrow range of activities. Third, testing the effect of smoking on these enzyme activities would be useful, since smoking may influence the kinetics of these enzymes. Work has begun in this area (17), but is in its infancy. Other areas that may provide functional markers for vitamin C status include studies of psychological changes (129); antioxidant status; adrenal, dopaminergic, and sex hormone functions; collagen metabolism; and gingival health. Preferably scientists should begin to compare these potential indices of vitamin C status to vitamin C body pool sizes estimated by stable isotopes or analogues of vitamin C. Then they can compare the indices to measures of vitamin C status and metabolism in the normal range of dietary intakes.

Another profitable area is to investigate why large variations in dietary intakes of vitamin C do not have more of an impact on human health. Why can one person consume hundreds of times more vitamin C than another without any acute health consequences? Small amounts of vitamin C prevent scurvy. Small amounts of vitamin C are essential for a number of enzyme activities. Small amounts of vitamin C influence bones, gums, and connective and ocular tissues. This is a highly active and important biological molecule, in small amounts. Larger intakes of vitamin C may or may not impact human health. However, the impact is not dramatic, rapid, or acute in most individuals. Can we really explain this entirely by an extremely efficient mechanism for vitamin C regulation? If so, why is this regulation so efficient? And what happens if, and when, this regulation breaks down? There are dozens of reports in the medical literature that suggest that high intakes of vitamin C may contribute to iron overload, B vitamin (thiamine, riboflavin, pantothenic acid) deficiency, gallstones, and intestinal trouble in some individuals. Many of the people in these reports are still alive. It would be interesting to measure their enzyme activities, nutritional status, and health status now. It would also be interesting to investigate whether these problems run in families, and therefore may be hereditary defects in vitamin C metabolism.

NOTE ADDED IN PROOF

The relationship among dose, plasma concentration, and bioavailability of vitamin C in healthy men (aged 20 to 26 years) eating a semicontrolled diet adequate in other nutrients has recently been determined by modern high-performance liquid chromatography (HPLC) methods (130). The men were nonsmokers, used no regular medications, and had normal blood chemical characteristics. They also had no history of genetic susceptibility to glucose-6-phosphate dehydrogenase deficiency or hemochromatosis, conditions thought to influence vitamin C status or metabolism. (The author's statement that recruitment of women in the study was encouraged, but none qualified, suggests additional unspecified recruiting criteria.) Volunteers were depleted of vitamin C, then supplemented sequentially with 30, 60, 100, 200, 400, 1000, and 2500 mg per day of ascorbic acid. Each supplement was given until plasma ascorbic acid concentrations stabilized. Seven men began the study, which ran for 4 to 6 months; three completed it. Plasma and intracellular ascorbic acid concentrations were saturated at about 200 mg per day supplementation, somewhat higher than estimates derived from earlier experiments (Table 4). Bioavailability estimates (from comparison of the response to identical intravenous and oral supplements) decreased at above 200 mg per day intake. The excretion of oxalate and urate, which are associated with kidney stone formation, increased at intakes of 1000 mg per day or above. These results support a relatively high RDA estimate of about 200 mg per day for healthy adult nonsmoking men.

REFERENCES

1. Basu TK, Schorah CJ. Vitamin C in Health and Disease. Westport, CT: AVI, 1982.
2. Hornig D, Strolz F. Recommended dietary allowance: support from recent research. J Nutr Sci Vitamnol 1992; Spec. No:173–176.
3. Retsky KL, Freeman MW, Frei B. Ascorbic acid oxidation product(s) protect human low density lipoprotein against atherogenic modification. Anti-rather than prooxidant activity of vitamin C in the presence of transition metal ions. J Biol Chem 1993; 268:1304–1309.
4. Sies H, Stahl W. Vitamins E and C, beta-carotene, and other carotenoids as antioxidants. Am J Clin Nutr 1995; 62:1315S–1321S.
5. Jacob RA, Omaye ST, Skala JH, et al. Experimental vitamin C depletion and supplementation in young men. Ann NY Acad Sci 1987; 498:333–346.
6. Linghorne WJ, McIntosh WG, Tice JW, et al. The relationship of ascorbic acid intake to gingivitis. Can Med Assoc J 1946; 54:106–119.
7. Pauling L. Are recommended daily allowances for vitamin C adequate? Proc Natl Acad Sci USA 1974; 71:4442–4446.
8. Hemila H, Herman ZS. Vitamin C and the common cold: a retrospective analysis of Chalmer's review. J Am Coll Nutr 1995; 14:116–123.
9. Pauling L. Vitamin C and the Common Cold. San Francisco: Freeman, 1970.
10. Gale CR, Martyn CN, Winter PD, Cooper C. Vitamin C and risk of death from stroke and coronary heart disease in cohort of elderly people. Br Med J 1995; 310:1563–1566.
11. Byers T, Guerrero N. Epidemiological evidence for vitamin C and vitamin E in cancer prevention. Am J Clin Nutr 1995; 62:1385S–1392S.
12. Block G. Vitamin C status and cancer: epidemiological evidence of reduced risk. Ann NY Acad Sci 1992; 669:280–290.
13. Robertson JM, Donner AP, Trevithick JR. A possible role for vitamins C and E in cataract prevention. Am J Clin Nutr 1991; 53:346S–351S.
14. Taylor A, Jacques P, Epstein EM. Relations among aging, antioxidant status, and cataract. Am J Clin Nutr 1995; 62:1439S–1447S.
15. Enstrom JE, Kanim LE, Klein MA. Vitamin C intake and mortality among a sample of the United States population. Epidemiology 1992; 3:194–202.
16. Carpenter KJ. The History of Scurvy and Vitamin C. New York: Cambridge University Press, 1987.
17. Levine M, Cantilena CC, Dhariwal KR. In situ kinetics and ascorbic acid requirements. World Rev Nutr Diet 1993; 72:114–127.
18. Peterkofsky B. Ascorbate requirement for hydroxylation and secretion of procollagen: relationship to inhibition of collagen synthesis in scurvy. Am J Clin Nutr 1991; 4:1135S–1140S.
19. Barnes MJ, Kodicek E. Biological hydroxylations and ascorbic acid with special regard to collagen metabolism. Vitam Hormon 1972; 30:1–43.
20. Rebouche CJ. Ascorbic acid and carnitine biosynthesis. Am J Clin Nutr 1991; 54:1147S–1152S.
21. Hulse JD, Ellis SR, Hendersen L. Carnitine biosynthesis: β-hydroxylation of trimethyllysine by an α-ketoglutarate-dependent mitochondrial dioxygenase. J Biol Chem 1978; 253:1654–1659.
22. Hughes RE. Recommended daily amounts and biochemical roles: the vitamin C, carnitine, fatigue relationship. In: Counsell JN, Hornig DH, eds. Vitamin C. London: Applied Science, 1981:75–85.
23. Feller AG, Rudman D. Role of carnitine in human nutrition. J Nutr 1988; 118:541–547.
24. Ciman M, Rizzoli V, Siliprandi N. Deficiency of carnitine induced by scurvy. IRCS Med Sci 1979; 7:253.
25. Crandon JH, Lund CC. Vitamin C deficiency in an otherwise normal adult. N Engl J Med 1940; 222:748–752.

26. Kinsman RA, Hood J. Some behavioral effects of ascorbic acid deficiency. Am J Clin Nutr 1971; 24:455–464.
27. Dilberto EJ Jr, Daniels AJ, Viveros OH. Multicompartmental secretion of ascorbate and its dual role in dopamine β-hydroxylation. Am J Clin Nutr 1991; 54:1163S–1172S.
28. Oke AF, May L, Adams R. Ascorbic acid distribution patterns in human brain. Ann NY Acad Sci 1987; 498:1–13.
29. Menniti FS, Knoth J, Dilberto EJ Jr. Role of ascorbic acid in dopamine beta-hydroxylation: the endogenous enzyme cofactor and putative electron donor for cofactor regeneration. J Biol Chem 1986; 261:16901–16908.
30. Steele BF, Hsu C, Pierce ZH, Williams HH. Ascorbic acid nutriture in the human. 1. Tyrosine metabolism and blood levels of ascorbic acid during ascorbic acid depletion and repletion. J Nutr 1952; 48:49–59.
31. Ramar S, Sivaramakrishnan V, Manoharan K. Scurvy: a forgotten disease. Arch Phys Med Rehab 1993; 74:92–95.
32. Faulkner F, ed. International Child Health: A Digest of Current Information. Vol. 6. No. 1. Rochester, NY: International Pediatric Association, 1995.
33. Ginter E, Zdichynec B, Holzerova O, et al. Hypocholesterolemic effect of ascorbic acid in maturity-onset diabetes mellitus. Int J Vitam Nutr Res 1978; 48:368–373.
34. Hemila H. Vitamin C and plasma cholesterol. Crit Rev Food Sci 1992; 32:33–57.
35. Hallberg L. Effect of vitamin C on bioavailability of iron from food. In: Counsell JN, Hornig DH, eds. Vitamin C. London: Applied Science, 1981:49–61.
36. Hoffman KE, Yanelli K, Bridges KR. Ascorbic acid and iron metabolism: alterations in lysosomal function. Am J Clin Nutr 1991; 54:1188S–1192S.
37. Harris ED, Percival SS. A role for ascorbic acid in copper transport. Am J Clin Nutr 1991; 54:1193S–1197S.
38. Suboticanec K, Folnegovic-Smalc V, Korbar M, et al. Vitamin C status in chronic schizophrenia. Biol Psychiatry 1990; 28:959–966.
39. Pardo B, Mena MA, Fahn S, Garcia de Yebenes J. Ascorbic acid protects against levadopa-induced neurotoxicity on a catecholamine-rich human neuroblastoma cell line. Movement Disord 1993; 8:278–284.
40. Cunningham JJ, Mearkle PL, Brown RG. Vitamin C: an aldolase reductase inhibitor that normalizes erythrocyte sorbitol in insulin-dependent diabetes mellitus. J Am Coll Nutr 1994; 13:344–350.
41. Clemetson CAB. Vitamin C. Vol 2. Boca Raton, FL: CRC Press, 1989:23–40.
42. Schwartz J, Weiss ST. Relationship between dietary vitamin C intake and pulmonary function in the First National Health and Nutrition Examination Survey. Am J Clin Nutr 1994; 59:110–114.
43. Millar J. Vitamin C: the primate fertility factor? Med Hypotheses 1992; 38:292–295.
44. Dawson EB, Harris WA, Rankin WE, et al. Effect of ascorbic acid on male fertility. Ann NY Acad Sci 1987; 498:312–323.
45. Dawson EB. Effect of ascorbic acid supplementation of the sperm quality of smokers. Fertil Steril 1992; 58:1034–1039.
46. Luck MR. Ascorbic acid and fertility. Biol Reprod 1995; 52:262–266.
47. Jacob RA, Kelley DS, Pianalto FS, et al. Immunocompetence and oxidant defense during ascorbate depletion of healthy men. Am J Clin Nutr 1991; 54:1302S–1309S.
48. Boxer LA, Watenabe AM, Rister M, et al. Correction of leukocyte function in Chediak-Higashi syndrome by ascorbate. N Engl J Med 76; 295:1041–1045.
49. Vogel RL, Lamster IB, Wechsler SA, et al. The effects of megadoses of ascorbic acid on PMN chemotaxis and experimental gingivitis. J Periodontol 1986; 57:472–479.
50. Herbert V, Shaw S, Jayatilleke E, Stopler-Kasdan T. Most free-radical injury is iron-related: it is promoted by iron, hemin, holoferritin and vitamin C, and inhibited by desferoxamine and apoferritin. Stem Cells 1994; 12:289–303.

51. Calabresis EJ. Does consumption of mega-doses of ascorbic acid pose a hemolytic risk to persons with sickle-cell trait and sickle-cell anemia? Med Hypotheses 1982; 9:647–649.

52. Schrauzer GN, Rhead WJ. Ascorbic acid abuse: effects of long-term ingestion of excessive amounts on blood levels and urinary excretion. Int J Vitam Nutr Res 1973; 43:201–211.

53. Tsao CS, Salimi SL. Evidence of rebound effect with ascorbic acid. Med Hypotheses 1984; 13:303–310.

54. Urivetzky M, Kessaris D, Smith AD. Ascorbic acid overdosing: a risk factor for calcium oxalate nephrolithiasis. J Urol 1992; 147:1215–1218.

55. Dannenberg JL. Vitamin C and enamel loss. J Am Dent Assoc 1982; 105:172–174.

56. Clark JW. Conditioned oral scurvy due to megavitamin C withdrawal. J Periodontol 1982; 54:182–183.

57. Gershoff SN. Vitamin C (ascorbic acid): new roles, new requirements? Nutr Rev 1993; 51: 313–326.

58. Alavanja MCR, Brown CC, Swanson C, Brownson RC. Saturated fat intake and lung cancer risk among nonsmoking women in Missouri. J Natl Cancer Inst 1993; 85:1906–1916.

59. Crandon JH, Lund CC, Dill DB. Experimental human scurvy. N Engl J Med 1940; 223: 353–369.

60. Peters R, Coward KH, Krebs HA, et al. Vitamin C Requirements of Human Adults: A Report by the Vitamin C Subcommittee of the Accessory Food Factors Committee. 280th ed. London: Her Majesty's Stationery Office, 1953.

61. Baker EM, Sauberlich HE, March SC, Hodges RE. Experimental scurvy in man: Army Science Conference Proceedings. Washington DC: Office, Chief of Research and Development, Department of the Army, 1968; 1:1–14.

62. Hodges RE, Hood J, Canham JE, et al. Clinical manifestations of ascorbic acid deficiency in man. Am J Clin Nutr 1971; 24:432–443.

63. Hodges RE, Canham JE. Vitamin deficiencies: studies of experimental vitamin C deficiency and experimental vitamin A deficiency in man. US Army Fitzimmons Reports 1971:115–128.

64. Hood J, Hodges RE. Ocular lesions in scurvy. Am J Clin Nutr 1969; 22:559–567.

65. Dodds ML, MacLeod FL. Blood plasma ascorbic acid levels on controlled intakes of ascorbic acid. Science 1947; 106:67.

66. Steele BF, Liner RL, Pierce ZH, Williams HH. Ascorbic acid nutriture in the human. II. Contents of ascorbic acid in the white cells and serums of subjects receiving controlled low intakes of the vitamin. J Nutr 1955; 57:361–368.

67. Jacob RA. Assessment of human vitamin C status. J Nutr 1990; 120:1480S–1485S.

68. ESHA Research. The Food Processor for Windows: Nutrition and Fitness Software. Salem, OR: ESHA Research, 1995.

69. Hellman L, Burns JJ. Metabolism of L-ascorbic acid-1-C14 in man. J Biol Chem 1958; 230:923–930.

70. Von Eekelen M. On the metabolism of ascorbic acid (vitamin C). Acta Brev Neerl Physiol 1935; 5:165–167.

71. Baker EM, Saari JC, Tolbert BM. Ascorbic acid metabolism in man. Am J Clin Nutr 1966; 19:371–378.

72. O'Hara PH, Hauck HM. Storage of vitamin C by normal adults following a period of low intake. J Nutr 1936; 12:413–427.

73. Irwin MI, Hutchins BK. A conspectus on vitamin C requirements of man. J Nutr 1976; 106:821–880.

74. Sauberlich HE, Kretsch MJ, Taylor PC, et al. Ascorbic acid and erythorbic acid metabolism in nonpregnant women. Am J Clin Nutr 1989; 50:1039–1049.

75. Jacob RA, Pianalto FS, Agee RE. Cellular ascorbate depletion in healthy men. J Nutr 1992; 122:1111–1118.

76. Kallner A, Hartmann D, Hornig D. Steady-state turnover and body pool of ascorbic acid in man. Am J Clin Nutr 1979; 32:530–539.

77. Kallner A, Hartmann D, Hornig D. On the requirements of ascorbic acid in man: steady-state turnover and body pool in smokers. Am J Clin Nutr 1981; 34:1347–1355.

78. Kallner A. Requirements for vitamin C based on human studies. Ann NY Acad Sci 1987; 498:418–423.

79. Blanchard J. Depletion and repletion kinetics of vitamin C in humans. J Nutr 1991; 121: 170–176.

80. Blanchard J, Conrad KA, Watson RR, et al. Comparison of plasma, mononuclear and polymorphonuclear leucocyte vitamin C levels in young and elderly women during depletion and supplementation. Eur J Clin Nutr 1989; 43:97–106.

81. Blanchard J, Conrad KA, Mead RA, Garry PJ. Vitamin C disposition in young and elderly men. Am J Clin Nutr 1990; 51:837–845.

82. Blanchard J, Conrad KA, Garry PJ. Effects of age and intake on vitamin C disposition in females. Eur J Clin Nutr 1990; 44:447–460.

83. Melethil S, Mason WD, Chang C. Dose-dependent absorption and excretion of vitamin C in humans. Int J Pharmaceut 1986; 31:83–89.

84. Omaye ST, Skala JH, Jacob RA. Plasma ascorbic acid in adult males: effects of depletion and supplementation. Am J Clin Nutr 1986; 44:257–264.

85. Tolbert BM, Chen AW, Bell EM, Baker EM. Metabolism of L-ascorbic-4-3H acid in man. Am J Clin Nutr 1967; 20:250–252.

86. Morse EH, Potgieter M, Walker GR. Ascorbic acid utilization by women: response of blood serum and white blood cells to increased levels of intake. J Nutr 1956; 58:291–298.

87. Pauling L. Evolution and the need for ascorbic acid. Proc Natl Acad Sci USA 1970; 67:1643–1648.

88. Dickinson VA, Block G, Russek-Cohen E. Supplement use, other dietary and demographic variables, and serum vitamin C in NHANES II. J Am Coll Nutr 1994; 13:22–32.

89. Schorah CJ. Vitamin C status in population groups. In: Counsell JN, Hornig DH, eds. Vitamin C. London: Applied Science, 1981:23–47.

90. Herbert V, Jacob E, Wong KTJ, et al. Low-serum vitamin B_{12} levels in patients receiving ascorbic acid in megadoses: studies concerning the effect of ascorbate on radioisotope B_{12} assays. Am J Clin Nutr 1978; 31:253–258.

91. Omaye ST, Skala JH, Jacob RA. Rebound effect with ascorbic acid in adult males. Am J Clin Nutr 1988; 48:379–381.

92. Marcus M, Prabhudesai M, Wassef S. Stability of vitamin B_{12} in the presence of ascorbic acid in food and serum: restoration by cyanide of apparent loss. Am J Clin Nutr 1980; 33:137–143.

93. Schmidt K-H, Hagmaier V, Hornig DH, et al. Urinary oxalate excretion after large intakes of ascorbic acid in man. Am J Clin Nutr 1981; 34:305–311.

94. Wandzilak TR, D-Andre SD, Davis PA, Williams HE. Effects of high dose vitamin C on urinary oxalate level. J Urol 1994; 151:834–837.

95. Diplock AT. Safety of antioxidant vitamins and beta-carotene. Am J Clin Nutr 1995; 62: 1510S–1516S.

96. Bendich A, Langseth L. The health effects of vitamin C supplementation: a review. J Am Coll Nutr 1995; 14:124–136.

97. Hemila H. Vitamin C and the common cold. Br J Nutr 1992; 67:3–16.

98. Clemetson CAB. Histamine and ascorbic acid in human blood. J Nutr 1980; 110:662–668.

99. Bielory L. Asthma and vitamin C. Ann Allergy 1994; 73:89–96.

100. Hatch GE. Asthma, inhaled oxidants, and dietary antioxidants. Am J Clin Nutr 1995; 61: 625S–630S.

101. Blot WJ, Li J, Taylor PR, et al. The Linxian trials: mortality rates by vitamin-mineral intervention group. Am J Clin Nutr 1995; 62:1424S–1426S.

102. Blot WJ, Li J, Taylor PR, et al. Nutrition intervention trials in Linxian, China: supplementation with specific vitamin/mineral combinations, cancer incidence, and disease-specific mortality in the general population. J Natl Cancer Inst 1993; 85:1483–1492.

103. Olson JA, Hodges RE. Recommended dietary intakes (RDI) of vitamin C in humans. Am J Clin Nutr 1987; 45:693–703.
104. Levine M, Dhariwal KR, Welch RW, et al. Determination of optimal vitamin C requirements in humans. Am J Clin Nutr 1995; 62:1347S–1356S.
105. Olson JA, Hodges RE, Press F, Isselbacher K. RDA Impasse. Nutr Notes 1985; 21:1–6.
106. Jacob RA, Otradovec CL, Russell RM, et al. Vitamin C status and nutritional interactions in a healthy elderly population. Am J Clin Nutr 1988; 48:1436–1442.
107. Subcommittee on the Tenth Edition of the RDAs. Recommended Dietary Allowances. 10th ed. Washington DC: National Academy Press, 1989:115–124.
108. Jacob RA. Vitamin C. In: Shils ME, Olson JA, Shike M, eds. Modern Nutrition in Health and Disease. Vol. 1. 8th ed. Philadelphia: Lea & Febiger, 1994:432–448.
109. Cohen M, Cheng L, Bhagavan HN. Vitamin C and the elderly: an update. In: Watson R, ed. Handbook of Nutrition in the Aged. 2d ed. Boca Raton, FL: CRC Press, 1994:204–262.
110. Cheraskin E. The prevalence of hypovitaminosis C. JAMA 1985; 254:2894.
111. Kemm JR, Allcock J. The distribution of supposed indicators of nutritional status in elderly patients. Age Ageing 1984; 13:2128.
112. Walker D, Beauchene RE. The relationship of loneliness, social isolation, and physical health to dietary inadequacy of independently living elderly. J Am Diet Assoc 1991; 91:300–304.
113. Marrazzi MC, Mancinelli S, Palombi L, et al. Vitamin C and nutritional status of institutionalized and noninstitutionalized elderly women in Rome. Int J Vitam Nutr Res 1990; 60:351–359.
114. Choi ES, McGandy RB, Dallal GE, et al. The prevalence of cardiovascular risk factors among elderly Chinese Americans. Arch Intern Med 1990; 150:413–418.
115. Fidanza A, Brubacher G, Simonetti MS, Cucchia LM. Nutritional status of the elderly. III. Vitamin nutriture in elderly pensioners in Perugia. Int J Vitam Nutr Res 1984; 54:355–359.
116. Dodds ML. Sex as a factor in blood levels of ascorbic acid. J Am Diet Assoc 1969; 54:32–33.
117. Garry PJ, Vaderjagdt DJ, Hunt WC. Ascorbic acid intakes and plasma levels in healthy elderly. Ann NY Acad Sci 1987; 498:90–99.
118. Smith JL, Hodges RE. Serum levels of vitamin C in relation to dietary and supplemental intake of vitamin C in smokers and nonsmokers. Ann NY Acad Sci 1987; 498:144–152.
119. Murata A. Smoking and vitamin C. World Rev Nutr Diet 1991; 64:31–57.
120. Tribble DL, Guiliano L, Fortmann SP. Reduced plasma ascorbic acid concentrations in nonsmokers regularly exposed to environmental tobacco smoke. Am J Clin Nutr 1993; 58:886–890.
121. Salmenpera L. Vitamin C nutrition during prolonged lactation: optimal in infants while marginal in some mothers. Am J Clin Nutr 1984; 40:1050–1056.
122. Baker EM. Vitamin C requirements in stress. Am J Clin Nutr 1967; 20:583–590.
123. Chatham MD, Eppler JH Jr, Sauder LR, et al. Evaluation of the effects of vitamin C on ozone-induced bronchoconstriction in normal subjects. Ann NY Acad Sci 1987; 498:269–279.
124. Bucca C, Rolla G, Farina JC. Effect of vitamin C on transient increase of bronchial responsiveness in conditions affecting the airways. Ann NY Acad Sci 1992; 669:175–187.
125. Pecoraro RE, Chen MS. Ascorbic acid metabolism in Diabetes Mellitus. Ann NY Acad Sci 1987; 498:248–258.
126. Lund CC. The effect of surgical operations on the level of cevitamic acid in the blood plasma. N Engl J Med 1939; 221:123–127.
127. Bartlett MK, Jones CM, Ryan AE. Vitamin C studies in surgical patients. Ann Surg 1940; 111:1–26.
128. Situnyake RD, Thurnham DI, Kootathep S, et al. Chain breaking antioxidant status in rheumatoid arthritis: clinical and laboratory correlates. Ann Rheum Dis 1991; 50:81–86.
129. Heseker H, Kubler W, Pudel V, Westenhoffer J. Psychological disorders as early symptoms of a mild-to-moderate vitamin deficiency. Ann NY Acad Sci 1992; 669:352–357.
130. Levine M, Conry-Catilena C, Wang Y, et al. Vitamin C pharmacokinetics in healthy volunteers: evidence for a recommended dietary allowance. Proc Natl Acad Sci USA 1996; 3704–3709.

21

Vitamin C Safety in Humans

ADRIANNE BENDICH
*Human Nutrition Research, Hoffmann-La Roche, Inc.,
Paramus, New Jersey*

INTRODUCTION

The most recently published paper on the safety of vitamin C (1) examined the literature up until 1993 and concluded that vitamin C was safe at levels 10 times or more than the current recommended dietary allowance (RDA) of 60 mg, even when taken for prolonged periods by healthy adults. The objectives of this review are to provide an update of the literature published mainly from 1993 to early 1996.

This chapter includes a discussion of the average and range of vitamin C intakes in the United States and a compilation of relevant epidemiological studies, which consistently report that individuals with the highest vitamin C intakes also have the lowest risk of morbidity and/or mortality from cancer and/or cardiovascular disease (CVD), the two major causes of death in U.S. adults. These data are presented to provide an indication of the lack of serious adverse effects associated with higher than average intakes of vitamin C.

This review also documents the safety of vitamin C seen in 30 recent intervention trials where known amounts of the vitamin are given to specific population groups for a defined period. The possible side effects of vitamin C supplementation in certain patient populations at risk for complications due to medical conditions are briefly discussed, as are the few studies which suggest that high intakes of vitamin C from foods and/or supplements may interfere with diagnostic testing.

It is hoped that the extensive tabulation of the clinical intervention studies provides further assurance of the safety of high doses of vitamin C for humans.

INTAKE LEVELS OF VITAMIN C

Vitamin C (ascorbic acid) has been described as the major water-soluble antioxidant in human serum (2) and has several other essential functions in the body (3). In the United

States, the foods that are the highest contributors of vitamin C are (in order of contribution) orange juice, grapefruit, tomatoes and tomato juice, and potatoes (4). Although the mean daily intake of vitamin C from foods is about 120 mg, about 25% of both men and women habitually consume less than 60 mg/day (the current RDA) and 10% of adults usually consume less than 30 mg/day (5). These data are corroborated in the recent NHANES III analysis for all ages (from 2 months to > 80 years) and sexes. The mean daily vitamin C intake from food was 105 mg; however, the median was only 78 mg, suggesting that a substantial proportion of Americans do not consume the RDA for vitamin C daily (6).

In addition to naturally occurring sources of vitamin C, fortified foods and vitamin supplements provide important sources of this vitamin for Americans. In fact, supplements containing vitamin C either as a component of multivitamins and/or as single-entity supplements are the chief source of the vitamin, providing 27.5% of total intake; fortified foods, the third major source, provide 7.8% of total intake (7). When all sources of vitamin C are included, data from NHANES II indicate that average vitamin C intake is approximately 160 mg/day (7).

The number of individuals who consume multivitamins routinely varies with age and sex but has been reported to be about 18% of U.S. adults; in contrast, 7.6% of the population use single supplements of vitamin C. The mean intake of vitamin C for users of multivitamins and single supplements was 395 mg/day, and in the 95th percentile, the average was 1069 mg/day. The 95th percentile of vitamin C intake for nonsupplement users was 500 mg/day (8). Thus, even for users of single supplements of vitamin C, the highest total vitamin C intake was about 1 g/day and was only twice the level seen in nonsupplement users. Moreover, Dickinson et al. (9) showed that regular supplement users also have higher intakes of vitamin C–rich fruits and vegetables than nonsupplement users. Therefore, the 95th percentile of total vitamin C intake for supplement users includes higher than average intakes from natural food sources as well as supplements. These data are provided to give the reader a prospective for examining the safety data from well-controlled intervention studies in which high doses of vitamin C were administered.

ABSORPTION, METABOLISM, EXCRETION, AND TISSUE CONCENTRATIONS

Human metabolism studies have shown that there is an inverse relationship between the dose of vitamin C ingested and the percentage absorbed. The renal threshold for vitamin C corresponds to a plasma concentration of approximately 0.8 mg/dl, which can be achieved at intakes of about 100 mg/day, although a recent study indicated that intakes of 250 mg/day did not result in increased urinary vitamin C (10). As intakes increase, a greater percentage of vitamin C is excreted in the urine; thus, there is a fairly consistent body pool of approximately 20 mg/kg body weight over a wide range of daily intakes (11). The kidney threshold thus provides a mechanism for the well-accepted safety of higher than RDA doses of vitamin C (1,3,12–19).

EPIDEMIOLOGICAL DATA OF REDUCED RISK OF CHRONIC DISEASE

Epidemiological studies have consistently reported a reduced risk of certain cancers and cardiovascular disease in populations with the highest intakes of vitamin C from food and/ or supplements (20–22).

Cancer

Correa and Fontham (23) tabulated 13 case-control studies in which cancer risk was significantly reduced in individuals with the highest intakes of fruits and vegetables. In another five studies, highest intakes of vegetables and fruits were specifically associated with lowered risk of lung cancer. In their own database, fruits as a group and dietary intake of vitamin C reduced the risk of gastric cancer by 50%. The mechanism of protection in this cancer may be prevention of *Helicobacter pylori* infection (a primary factor in gastric cancer development). *H. pylori* bacteria cannot replicate in the highly acidic environment of the stomach. Ascorbic acid, which is actively secreted into the stomach from the blood, helps to maintain the acidity of the stomach. Once *H. pylori* infection is present, ascorbic acid level is significantly decreased in the stomach (24). Several other mechanisms have been hypothesized for the lowered cancer risk: vitamin C blocks the formation of carcinogenic nitrosamines, reduces deoxyribonucleic acid (DNA) damage due to oxidative damage, and enhances immune responses (3).

Block (25) has specifically documented the association of high dietary intakes of vitamin C and lowered risk of several cancers seen in over 90 epidemiological studies. In the 50 epidemiological studies involving non-hormone-dependent cancers, all studies reported effects that were protective, "and not one was significantly harmful."

Cardiovascular Disease

Higher than average intakes of vitamin C (regardless of the exact amount associated with the "average intakes") are also linked to decreased risk of cardiovascular disease (CVD). Several mechanisms have been proposed for these findings.

Two studies (26,27) found that vitamin C reduced low-density lipoprotein (LDL) oxidation. There were also two reports (28,29) that vitamin C supplementation significantly reduced LDL triglyceride and cholesterol levels in type II diabetes. Moreover, a recent review (30) of 18 epidemiological and 21 interventional trials concluded that the cumulative data strongly suggest that higher vitamin C concentrations are linked with a decreased incidence of atherosclerosis.

High LDL levels and increased susceptibility of LDL to oxidation are considered risk factors for cardiovascular disease. In addition to the literature reviewed up until 1993 (1), which showed consistent reports of reduction in cardiovascular disease and stroke risk associated with the highest vitamin C intakes, there have been several other large epidemiological studies that found similar associations (22,31,32).

High-dose (2 g) ascorbic acid given to patients with documented coronary artery disease resulted in a rapid improvement in dilatation of brachial arteries compared to that of matched placebo responses (33). The authors hypothesize that vitamin C may reverse endothelial vasomotor dysfunction by facilitating the release of endothelium-derived relaxing factor (EDRF). Secretion of EDRF is blocked during oxidant stress; vitamin C, as a potent antioxidant (34), may reduce superoxide production, which has been found to inactivate EDRF.

In addition to preventing oxidative inactivation of EDRF, vitamin C supplementation (1000 mg/day) was shown to reduce the oxidative susceptibility of LDL from smokers (26). Oxidized LDLs are major components of the atherosclerotic plaques (35), and reduction in LDL oxidation is expected to lower cardiovascular disease risk.

Epidemiological data indicate that high intakes of fruits and vegetables are associated with a significant reduction in risk of stroke (36), although a direct relationship of this association with vitamin C could not be assessed in this study. However, in another epidemiological study, higher than average vitamin C intake (> 44 mg/day) and serum levels were significantly related to lower risk of stroke in an elderly population, but were not associated with lowered coronary heart disease (CHD) risk (31). There were two other studies that did find a lowered risk of CHD in women with the highest intakes of vitamin C (37,38).

In addition to reducing LDL susceptibility to oxidation and improving vasomotor activity, a third mechanism by which vitamin C may reduce CVD risk is suggested by the study of Khaw and Woodhouse (39), who reported an inverse relationship between vitamin C status (intake and serum levels) and serum fibrinogen and factor VII C concentrations. Higher than average serum levels of these hemostatic factors have been associated with increased CVD risk.

Vitamin C may reduce CVD risk in diabetics, who are at greater risk than nondiabetics by other mechanisms. In addition to reducing oxidative stress, vitamin C increased insulin action in type II diabetics and concurrently improved membrane microviscosity. Microviscosity affects the capability of blood components to move through the smallest blood vessels such as capillaries (40).

SAFETY OF HIGH DOSES OF VITAMIN C

Despite the epidemiological associations of highest vitamin C intakes and lowered risk of CVD and cancer, there continues to be misinformation in the scientific literature and lay press concerning vitamin C safety. It is therefore critical also to review the clinical studies in which doses of vitamin C were administered during double-blind, placebo-controlled, and other clinical intervention studies and contrast the data from these well-designed studies with anecdotal reports and hypotheses of potential adverse effects based upon little or no clinical data.

Double-Blind, Placebo-Controlled Intervention Studies

In 1995, Bendich and Langseth (1) reviewed the literature on vitamin C safety and efficacy and reported that 14 clinical trials published through 1993, using single supplements of vitamin C of dosages up to 10 g/day for up to 3 years, had not consistently reported any of the side effects mentioned in anecdotal reports or small case studies.

Since 1993, there have been several other intervention studies in which high doses of vitamin C have been examined for safety and efficacy (Tables 1 and 2). The 22 studies (26,28,41–47,48–58) reviewed in Table 1 included at least 20 participants, involved oral intake studies of vitamin C that were placebo-controlled and double-blind, and lasted a minimum of 14 days. Fourteen of the studies (28,41–52) examined the effects of 1000–6000 mg/day of vitamin C for up to 4 years. Many of the studies involved patients with diabetes or cancer; a number of them examined combinations of vitamins rather than single supplements of vitamin C.

There was no mention of side effects in 7/14 studies (41,46,48,50–52). Five studies directly stated that no side effects were seen (28,42–45,49). Of the 2 studies that do mention side effects (43,47), there was no consistent effect seen between studies and no effect specifically attributable to vitamin C in these reports.

Eight studies (27,29,53–58) examined the effects of 120–600 mg of vitamin C for up to 5 years in healthy as well as patient populations. In one study involving 1 year of supplementation of 600 mg of vitamin C and other micronutrients (53) a specific side effects questionnaire listing 21 possible symptoms was administered four times during the study. The one finding was an increase in nausea reported in the placebo group. In all other studies there was no indication of side effects.

Thus, in 22 well-controlled studies involving over 2200 participants, there were no consistent reports of vitamin C–related side effects. Moreover, in only one of them (47), two of five individuals who dropped out of the study were in the vitamin C group; the other three were in the placebo group.

In addition to the consistent finding of the safety of high doses of vitamin C, there were also findings which specifically addressed certain safety issues frequently raised in the literature. With regard to the potential for vitamin C to increase iron stores, there was a very modest effect of 1500 mg on iron status when taken for 35 days by healthy women with moderately low ferritin status (44). There was also no increase in body iron status seen when smokers with normal iron status were given 1000 mg of vitamin C for 28 days (26). There was, however, a beneficial increase in hemoglobin and other iron status parameters in vegetarians with initially low iron stores who were given 1000 mg of vitamin C for 60 days (63). These data agree with the analyses previously reported by Bendich and Cohen (66) that demonstrated the importance of vitamin C in enhancing nonheme iron absorption in individuals with low iron status, while not increasing iron status in iron-replete individuals.

Single-Blind and/or Non-Placebo-Controlled Intervention Studies

In addition to these 22 well-controlled studies, there were 8 other investigations involving dosages of 600 mg or more of vitamin C in single-blind or non-placebo-controlled studies (24,59–65). There was no mention of side effects in any of the studies, with the exception of a study involving supplementation with 10 g (10,000 mg) of vitamin C for 5 days (59). In this study, 2 of the 15 subjects experienced diarrhea; none of the 15 subjects had an increase in urinary oxalate during the study. Even though this was only a 5-day study it supports the lack of association of vitamin C supplementation with increased risk of kidney stones in nonstone formers (1). The potential for vitamin C to increase oxalate in nephrological disorders is discussed later.

Thus in 30 recent clinical studies involving males and females ranging in age from 10 to 88 years, there is no indication of any consistent, reproducible side effect associated with vitamin C intakes ranging from 120 mg to 10,000 mg/day taken for several days to several years.

Possible Side Effects in Risk Groups

Recent studies indicate that patients with severe kidney disease undergoing dialysis have an increase in urinary oxalate levels after supplementation with 100 mg/day of vitamin C. Thus, this supplementation is not usually recommended in this risk population group (67, 68). There may, however, be circumstances in which hemodialysis patients may benefit from vitamin C supplementation. Gastaldello et al. (69) administered 500 mg of vitamin C intravenously after hemodialysis to four patients with iron overload who were resistant to erythropoietin therapy. Vitamin C improved iron status and overcame erythropoietin resistance.

Table 1 Effect of Vitamin C Supplementation: Placebo-Controlled, Double-Blind Studies ($n > 20$)

Reference	Vit. C dose (mg/day)	Duration (day)	Population	Outcome	Reports of side effects
Klein et al., 1995 (41)	6000	28	$n = 24$ insulin-dependent diabetics, aged 35 ± 10 yrs	No effect on renal hemodynamics	No mention of side effects
Bostom et al., 1994 (42)	4500	84	$n = 44$ patients < 60 yr with coronary heart disease	No effect on Lp(a); no effect on plasma creatinine; no effect on plasma homocysteine	"High dose ascorbate was well tolerated"
Lamm et al., 1994 (43)	2000 + RDA multi and high doses of vitamins A, B$_6$, E, and zinc	1470	$n = 65$, aged 67 yr with bladder cancer	Significant reduction in bladder cancer recurrence	"No adverse reactions were noted with the exception of an occasional stomach upset"
Hunt et al., 1994 (44)	1500	35	$n = 25$ healthy nonpregnant women, 20–45 yr, with low serum ferritin level	Slight increase in serum ferritin	"The effect of ascorbic acid on body iron retention from whole diets seems to be considerably more modest and gradual than effects predicted from studies with single meals"
Abrahmsohn et al., 1993 (45)	1500	21	$n = 161$; aged 10–88 yr	Significant improvement in tooth extraction recovery	"No reports of side effects"
Weykemp et al., 1995 (46)	1500 or 750	84	$n = 30$ nondiabetic volunteers	No effect on hemoglobin glycation; no interference with assay	No mention of side effects
Greenberg et al., 1994 (47)	1000 + 400 IU Vitamin E ± 25 mg beta-carotene	1460	$n = 854$ patients, aged 59.2 yr with one colon polyp	No effect on polyp recurrence	Only 5 patients (out of 864) stopped taking the medication because of their presumed toxicity; 2 of the 5 were taking vitamin C

Paolisso et al., 1995 (28)	1000	120	$n = 40$ type II diabetics aged 72 ± 0.5 yr	Significant decrease in plasma free radicals; insulin; total and LDL cholesterol and triglycerides	"Compliance to vitamin C administration was 86 ± 0.9%. No patients dropped out of the study due to adverse effect of vitamin C administration. No significant differences in liver and renal function laboratory tests were found during vitamin C administration"
Jacques et al., 1995 (48)	1000	240	$n = 138$ aged 20–65 volunteers	No effect on HDL	No mention of side effects
ter Riet et al., 1995 (49)	1000	84	$n = 88$ patients with pressure ulcers	No improvement in ulcer healing	"No side effects were reported"
Dyke et al., 1994 (50)	1000	28	$n = 49$; adults	Significant reduction in gastric mucosal DNA damage	No mention of side effects
Fuller et al., 1996 (26)	1000	28	$n = 19$ smokers	Reduced LDL oxidative susceptibility; no increase in body iron stores	No mention of side effects
Vaxman et al., 1995 (51)	1000 + 200 mg pantothenic acid	21	$n = 49$ surgery patients	No effect of wound healing; intermediate endpoints improved	No mention of side effects
Kuhnz et al., 1995 (52)	1000 ± oral contraceptive	21	$n = 37$ healthy menstruating women	No effect of vitamin C on bioavailability of oral contraceptive	No mention of side effects
Benton et al., 1995 (53)	600 + vitamin A, B_1, B_2, B_6, B_{12}, folic acid, biotin, niacin, and vitamin E at 10 × RDA for England	365	$n = 129$ students aged 20.5 yr	Significant mood improvement	A side effects questionnaire listing 21 symptoms and an open question on spontaneous symptoms were administered 4× during the study. "On only one occasion was there a significant difference; on the third visit, those taking the placebo were more likely to report having felt nausea"

Table 1 Continued

Reference	Vit. C dose (mg/day)	Duration (day)	Population	Outcome	Reports of side effects
Herbaczynska-Cedro et al., 1995 (54)	600 + 600 mg vitamin E	14	n = 45 patients with acute myocardial infarction	Significantly decreased neutrophil oxygen free radical formation	No mention of side effects
Ghosh et al., 1994 (55)	500	42	n = 48 untreated hypertensive patients aged 74 yr	No significant effect on blood pressure; significant decrease in serum lipid peroxides	No mention of side effects
Nyyssonen et al., 1994 (27)	400 + 100 μg selenium, 200 mg vit. E, 30 mg beta-carotene	90	n = 40 men aged 30–58, smoking 15–40 cigarettes/day	Significantly increased LDL resistance to oxidation	"No clinical adverse events were observed during the trial in either the supplemented or placebo subjects"
Eriksson & Kohvakka, 1995 (29)	200 ± 600 mg/day of magnesium	90	n = 56 outpatient diabetics	Significantly improved glycemic control and HbA and lowered serum cholesterol and triglycerides	"During the 9 month study period 4 subjects dropped out, none due to side effects of the treatment"
Rokitzki et al., 1994 (56)	200 + 400 IU vitamin E	30	n = 24 trained long-distance runners aged 38.5 ± 8.5 yr	Decrease in muscle enzyme levels	No mention of side effects
Hunt et al., 1994 (57)	200	28	n = 57, aged 81 yr with acute bronchitis or bronchopneumonia	Reduction in major respiratory symptoms	No mention of side effects
Wang et al., 1994 (58)	120 + 30 μg molybdenum	1825	n = 201 aged 40–69 yr Linxian, China, residents	No effect on gastric cancer risk	No mention of side effects

RDA, recommended dietary allowance; Lp(a) LDL, low-density lipoprotein; HDL, high-density lipoprotein; DNA, deoxyribonucleic acid; RBC, red blood cell.

Table 2 Effect of Vitamin C Supplementation: Non-Placebo-Controlled and/or Single-Blind Studies

Reference	Vit. C dose (mg/day)	Duration (day)	Population	Outcome	Reports of side effects
Wandzilak et al., 1994 (59)	1000, 5000, and 10,000	5 days each dose	$n = 15$ men and women aged 28–30 ± 12 yr with no history of kidney stones	No increase in urinary oxalate	"Of 15 subjects, 13 tolerated all levels of vitamin C doses with no evidence of gastrointestinal disturbances. However, 2 of the 15 subjects experienced diarrhea while taking 10 g"
Lockwood et al., 1994 (60)	2850 + 2500 IU vitamin E, 32.5 IU beta-carotene, 387 µg selenium, other vitamins and minerals 1.2 g gamma-linolenic acid, 3.5 g n-3 fatty acids, 90 mg coenzyme Q_{10}	540	$n = 32$ women with breast cancer, aged 32–81 yr	No deaths vs. four expected; no weight loss, improved quality of life, reduced pain killer use	"None of the patients showed any sign of side effects, except for a tendency to yellowish palms due to the beta-carotene, and occasional fish oil taste for some patients"
Munoz et al., 1994 (61)	1000 or 2000	30	$n = 124$ healthy volunteers aged 17–74 yr	Significant decrease in Apo B	No mention of side effects
Kaugers et al., 1994 (62)	1000 + 800 IU vitamin E and 30 mg beta-carotene	270	$n = 79$ patients with oral leukoplakia	Clinical improvement	No mention of side effects
Sharma & Mathur, 1995 (63)	1000	60	$n = 28$ male or female vegetarians, 18–50 yr	Increased hemoglobin and other iron status parameters	"In contrast to iron preparations ascorbic acid is well tolerated, quite palatable and harmless"
Gilligan et al., 1994 (64)	1000 + 800 IU vitamin E and 30 mg betacarotene	30	$n = 19$, aged 52 ± 9 hypercholesterolemic patients	Reduced LDL oxidation susceptibility	No mention of side effects
Waring et al., 1996 (24)	1000	14	$n = 32$ gastritis patients	Increased gastric vitamin C	No mention of side effects
Cunningham et al., 1994 (65)	600 or 100	58	$n = 9$ insulin-dependent diabetics or 11 controls, 19–34 yr	Reduced sorbitol in RBC of diabetics	"Low toxicity"

Vitamin C Interference with Diagnostic Assays

High intakes of vitamin C from fruits and other foods as well as supplements has been shown to interfere with several urine-based diagnostic tests (70). Although newer diagnostic procedures, such as use of Rapimat, have been developed to override ascorbic acid interference, not all diagnostic tests have been reformulated.

High serum levels of vitamin C can also interfere with certain serum-based diagnostic assays (71,72). Thus, it is recommended that patients inform their physician of their use of vitamin C–containing supplements and/or higher than average intake of vitamin C–rich foods prior to their physician's use of vitamin C–sensitive diagnostic tests.

Conclusions

Several reviews have documented the safety of supplementation with levels of vitamin C that are 10 times or more than the current RDA of 60 mg. This review includes a discussion of intervention and epidemiological studies mainly published from 1993. The totality of the evidence indicates that vitamin C is safe for the majority of the population. There are, however, populations with health problems who should discuss the use of vitamin C supplements with their physicians prior to commencing supplementation. There may also be the possibility that the use of supplemental vitamin C and/or the consumption of diets rich in vitamin C–containing foods may result in interference with certain diagnostic procedures utilizing urine or serum samples. It is advised that physicians and patients discuss their use of vitamin C supplements prior to collection of urine and/or serum samples for diagnostic tests.

Finally, in addition to the cumulative data on the safety of vitamin C published since 1993, there has also been a growing literature documenting the reduction in risk of cancer and cardiovascular disease associated with higher than average intakes of vitamin C. These findings also add assurance of the safety as well as efficacy of higher than RDA intakes of vitamin C.

REFERENCES

1. Bendich A, Langseth L. The health effects of vitamin C supplementation: a review. J Am Coll Nutr 1995; 14:124–136.
2. Frei B. Ascorbic acid protects lipids in human plasma and low-density lipoprotein against oxidative damage. Am J Clin Nutr 1991; 54(suppl):1113S–1118S.
3. Moser U, Bendich A. Vitamin C. In: Machlin LJ, ed. Handbook of Vitamins. 2d ed. New York and Basel: Marcel Dekker, 1991.
4. Sinha R, Block G, Taylor PR. Problems with estimating vitamin C intakes. Am J Clin Nutr 1993; 57:547–550.
5. Block G, Subar AF. Estimates of nutrient intake from a food frequency questionnaire: The 1987 National Health Interview Survey. J Am Diet Assoc 1992; 92:969–977.
6. Alaimo K, McDowell MA, Briefel RR, et al. Advance data: dietary intake of vitamins, minerals, and fiber of persons ages 2 months and over in the United States: Third National Health and Nutrition Examination Survey, Phase 1, 1988–91. Advance data from vital and health statistics, no. 258. Hyattsville, MD: National Center for Health Statistics, 1994.
7. Block G, Sinha R, Gridley G. Collection of dietary sources by demographic characteristics. Am J Clin Nutr 1994; 59(suppl):232S–239S.
8. Subar AF, Block G. Use of vitamin and mineral supplements: demographics and amounts of

nutrients consumed: The 1987 Health Interview Survey. Am J Epidemiol 1990; 132:1091–1101.

9. Dickinson VA, Block G, Russek-Cohen E. Supplement use, other dietary and demographic variables, and serum vitamin C in NHANES II. J Am Coll Nutr 1994; 13:22–32.

10. King G, Beins M, Larkin J, et al. Rate of excretion of vitamin C in human urine. Age 1994; 17:87–92.

11. Kallner A, Hartmann D, Hornig D. Steady-state turnover and body pool of ascorbic acid in man. Am J Clin Nutr 1979; 32:530–539.

12. Rivers JM. Safety of high-level vitamin C ingestion. In: Burns JJ, Rivers JM, Machlin LJ, eds. Annals of the New York Academy of Sciences: Third Conference on Vitamin C, 498. New York: The New York Academy of Sciences, 1987.

13. National Research Council. Recommended Dietary Allowances, 10th ed. Washington, DC: National Academy Press, 1989.

14. Bendich A. Safety issues regarding the use of vitamin supplements. Ann NY Acad Sci 1992; 669:300–312.

15. Hemila H. The good and harm of vitamin C. Nutr Today 1994; 29:49–50.

16. Sauberlich HE. Pharmacology of vitamin C. In: Olson RE, Bier DM, McCormick DB, eds. Annual Review of Nutrition, 14. Palo Alto, CA: Annual Reviews, 1994.

17. Diplock AT. Safety of antioxidant vitamins and beta-carotene. Am J Clin Nutr 1995; 62:1510S–1516S.

18. Garewal HS, Diplock AT. How "safe" are antioxidant vitamins? Drug Safety 1995; 13:8–14.

19. Levine M, Dhariwal KR, Welch RW, et al. Determination of optimal vitamin C requirements in humans. Am J Clin Nutr 1995; 62:1347S–1356S.

20. Gridley G, McLaughlin JK, Block G, et al. Vitamin supplement use and reduced risk of oral and pharyngeal cancer. Am J Epidemiol 1992; 135:1083–1092.

21. Byers T, Guerrero N. Epidemiologic evidence for vitamin C and vitamin E in cancer prevention. Am J Clin Nutr 1995; 62:1385S–1392S.

22. Pandey DK, Shekelle R, Selwyn BJ, et al. Dietary vitamin C and beta-carotene and risk of death in middle-aged men: The Western Electric Study. Am J Epidemiol 1995; 142:1269–1278.

23. Correa P, Fontham ETH. Vitamins and cancer prevention: an epidemiologic overview. In: Bray GA, Ryan DH, eds. Vitamins and Cancer Prevention. Baton Rouge: Louisiana State University Press, 1992.

24. Waring AJ, Drake IM, Schorah CJ, et al. Ascorbic acid and total vitamin C concentrations in plasma, gastric juice, and gastrointestinal mucosa: effects of gastritis and oral supplementation. Gut 1996; 38:171–176.

25. Block G. Human data on vitamin C in cancer prevention. In: Gray GA, Ryan DH, eds. Vitamins and Cancer Prevention. 3d ed. Baton Rouge: Louisiana State University Press, 1993.

26. Fuller CJ, Grundy GM, Norkus EP, Jialal I. Effect of ascorbate supplementation on low density lipoprotein oxidation in smokers. Atherosclerosis 1996; 119:139–150.

27. Nyyssonen K, Porkkala E, Salonen R, et al. Increase in oxidation resistance of atherogenic serum lipoproteins following antioxidant supplementation: a randomized double-blind placebo-controlled clinical trial. Eur J Clin Nutr 1994; 48:633–642.

28. Paolisso G, Balbi V, Volpe C, et al. Metabolic benefits deriving from chronic vitamin C supplementation in aged non-insulin dependent diabetics. J Am Coll Nutr 1995; 14: 387–392.

29. Eriksson J, Kohvakka A. Magnesium and ascorbic acid supplementation in diabetes mellitus. Ann Nutr Metab 1995; 39:217–223.

30. Howard PA, Meyers DG. Effect of vitamin C on plasma lipids. Ann Pharmacother 1995; 29:1129–1136.

31. Gale CR, Martyn CN, Winter PD, Cooper C. Vitamin C and risk of death from stroke and coronary heart disease in cohort of elderly people. Br Med J 1995; 310:1563–1566.

32. Losonczy KG, Harris TB, Havlik RJ. Vitamin E with vitamin C use decreases nine year risk of all-cause and CHD mortality: the NIA EPESE studies (abstr). Gerontologist 1994; 34:207.

33. Levine GN, Frei B, Koulouris SN, et al. Ascorbic acid reverses endothelial vasomotor dysfunction in patients with coronary artery disease. Circulation 1996; 93:1107–1113.
34. Bendich A, Burton GW, Machlin LJ, et al. The antioxidant role of vitamin C. Adv Free Radical Biol Med 1986; 2:419–444.
35. Simon JA. Vitamin C and cardiovascular disease: a review. J Am Coll Nutr 1992; 11:107–125.
36. Gillman MW, Cupples LA, Gagnon D, et al. Protective effect of fruits and vegetables on development of stroke in men. JAMA 1995; 273:1113–1117.
37. Knekt P, Reunanen A, Jarvinen R, et al. Antioxidant vitamin intake and coronary mortality in a longitudinal population study. Am J Epidemiol 1994; 139:1180–1189.
38. Manson JE, Stampfer MJ, Willett WC, et al. A prospective study of vitamin C and incidence of coronary heart disease in women (abstr). Circulation 1992; 85:865.
39. Khaw KT, Woodhouse P. Interrelation of vitamin C, infection, haemostatic factors, and cardiovascular disease. Br Med J 1995; 310:1559–1563.
40. Paolisso G, D'Amore A, Balbi V, et al. Plasma vitamin C affects glucose homeostasis in healthy subjects and in non-insulin-dependent diabetics. Am J Physiol Endocrinol Metab 1994; 266:E261–E268.
41. Klein F, Juhl B, Christiansen JS. Unchanged renal haemodynamics following high dose ascorbic acid administration in normoalbuminuric IDDM patients. Scand J Clin Lab Invest 1995; 55:53–59.
42. Bostom AG, Yanek L, Hume AL, et al. High dose ascorbate supplementation fails to affect plasma homocyst(e)ine levels in patients with coronary heart disease. Atherosclerosis 1994; 111: 267–270.
43. Lamm DL, Riggs DR, Shriver JS, et al. Megadose vitamins in bladder cancer: a double-blind clinical trial. J Urol 1994; 151:21–26.
44. Hunt JR, Gallagher SK, Johnson LK. Effect of ascorbic acid on apparent iron absorption by women with low iron stores. Am J Clin Nutr 1994; 59:1381–1385.
45. Abrahmsohn GM, Halberstein RA, Fregeolle S. Vitamin C and dental healing: testing and placebo effect. General Dent 1993; 523–527.
46. Weykamp CW, Penders TJ, Baadenhuijsen H, et al. Vitamin C and glycohemoglobin. Clin Chem 1995; 41:713–716.
47. Greenberg ER, Baron JA, Tosteson TD, et al. A clinical trial of antioxidant vitamins to prevent colorectal adenoma: Polyp Prevention Study Group. N Engl J Med 1994; 331:141–147.
48. Jacques PF, Sulsky SI, Perrone GE, et al. Effect of vitamin C supplementation on lipoprotein cholesterol, apolipoprotein, and triglyceride concentrations. Ann Epidemiol 1995; 5:52–59.
49. ter Riet G, Kessels AG, Knipschild PG. Randomized clinical trial of ascorbic acid in the treatment of pressure ulcers. J Clin Epidemiol 1995; 48:1453–1460.
50. Dyke GW, Craven JL, Hall R, Garner RC. Effect of vitamin C supplementation on gastric mucosal DNA damage. Carcinogenesis 1994; 15:291–295.
51. Vaxman F, Olender S, Lambert A, et al. Effect of pantothenic acid and ascorbic acid supplementation on human skin wound healing process: a double-blind, prospective and randomized trial. Eur Surg Res 1995; 27:158–166.
52. Kuhnz W, Louton T, Humpel M, et al. Influence of high doses of vitamin C on the bioavailability and the serum protein binding of levonorgestrel in women using a combination oral contraceptive. Contraception 1995; 51:111–116.
53. Benton D, Haller J, Fordy J. Vitamin supplementation for 1 year improves mood. Neuropsychobiology 1995; 32:98–105.
54. Herbaczynska-Cedro K, Klosiewicz-Wasek B, Cedro K, et al. Supplementation with vitamins C and E suppresses leukocyte oxygen free radical production in patients with myocardial infarction. Eur Heart J 1995; 16:1044–1049.
55. Ghosh SK, Ekpo EB, Shah IU, et al. A double-blind, placebo-controlled parallel trial of vitamin C treatment in elderly patients with hypertension. Gerontology 1994; 40:268–272.
56. Rokitzki L, Logemann E, Sagredos AN, et al. Lipid peroxidation and antioxidative vitamins under extreme endurance stress. Acta Physiol Scand 1994; 151:149–158.

57. Hunt C, Chakravorty NK, Annan G, et al. The clinical effects of vitamin C supplementation in elderly hospitalised patients with acute respiratory infections. Int J Vitam Nutr Res 1994; 64: 212–219.

58. Wang GQ, Dawsey SM, Li JY, et al. Effects of vitamin/mineral supplementation on the prevalence of histological dysplasia and early cancer of the esophagus and stomach: results from the General Population Trial in Linxian, China. Cancer Epidemiol Biomarkers Prev 1994; 3:161–166.

59. Wandzilak TR, D'Andre SD, Davis PA, Williams HE. Effect of high dose vitamin C on urinary oxalate levels. J Urol 1994; 151:834–837.

60. Lockwood K, Moesgaard S, Hanioka T, Folkers K. Apparent partial remission of breast cancer in "high risk" patients supplemented with nutritional antioxidants, essential fatty acids and coenzyme Q10. Mol Aspects Med 1994; 15(suppl):s231–s240.

61. Munoz JA, Garcia C, Quilez JL, Andugar MA. Effect of vitamin C on lipoproteins in healthy adults. Ann Med Interne (Paris) 1994; 145:13–19.

62. Kaugars GE, Silverman S Jr, Lovas JG, et al. A clinical trial of antioxidant supplements in the treatment of oral leukoplakia. Oral Surg 1994; 78:462–468.

63. Sharma DC, Mathur R. Correction of anemia and iron deficiency in vegetarians by administration of ascorbic acid. Int J Physiol Pharmacol 1995; 39:403–406.

64. Gilligan DM, Sack MN, Guetta V, et al. Effect of antioxidant vitamins on low density lipoprotein oxidation and impaired endothelium-dependent vasodilation in patients with hypercholesterolemia. J Am Coll Cardiol 1994; 24:1611–1617.

65. Cunningham JJ, Mearkle PL, Brown RG. Vitamin C: an aldose reductase inhibitor that normalizes erythrocyte sorbitol in insulin-dependent diabetes mellitus. J Am Coll Nutr 1994; 13: 344–350.

66. Bendich A, Cohen M. Ascorbic acid safety: analysis of factors affecting iron absorption. Toxicol Lett 1990; 51:189–201.

67. Shah GM, Ross EA, Sabo A, et al. Effects of ascorbic acid and pyridoxine supplementation on oxalate metabolism in peritoneal dialysis patients. Am J Kidney Dis 1992; 20:42–49.

68. Urivetzky M, Kessaris D, Smith AD. Ascorbic acid overdosing: a risk factor for calcium oxalate nephrolithiasis. J Urol 1992; 147:1215–1218.

69. Gastaldello K, Vereerstraeten A, Nzame-Nze T, et al. Resistance to erythropoietin in iron-overloaded haemodialysis patients can be overcome by ascorbic acid administration. Nephrol Dial Transplant 1995; 10:44–47.

70. Brigden ML, Edgell D, McPherson M, et al. High incidence of significant urinary ascorbic acid concentration in a West Coast population: implications for routine urinalysis. Clin Chem 1992; 38:426–431.

71. Freemantle J, Freemantle MJ, Badrick T. Ascorbate interferences in common clinical assays performed on three analyzers (letter). Clin Chem 1994; 40:950–951.

72. Benzie IFF, Strain JJ. The effect of ascorbic acid on the measurement of total cholesterol and triglycerides: possible artefactual lowering in individuals with high plasma concentration of ascorbic acid. Clin Chim Acta 1995; 239:185–190.

22

Vitamin C in Prospective Epidemiological Studies

James E. Enstrom
School of Public Health, University of California, Los Angeles, California

INTRODUCTION

Vitamin C is an antioxidant that has received a great deal of attention in recent years with regard to prevention of cancer and cardiovascular disease (1,2). The human body is under constant attack by reactive oxygen molecules (free radicals and singlet oxygen) that are formed as a natural consequence of normal biochemical activity. Reactive oxygen can damage the body in many ways by altering membrane structure and function. Because this damage can be life threatening, the body has defense mechanisms to protect against oxidation. These defenses include small molecules like vitamin C that act as antioxidants or scavengers of reactive oxygen species. There are over 100 epidemiological studies that have examined some aspect of the relationship between vitamin C and disease. The majority of these are case-control studies of cancer patients. These case-control studies have been reviewed by Block (3) and are not discussed further here, except to say that the majority appear to show an inverse relation between vitamin C intake and risk of cancer when examined on a site by site basis.

The focus of this review is on prospective epidemiological studies that are generally methodologically superior to case-control studies because they obtain information about vitamin C intake and other characteristics before cancer or other diseases develop. There have been a number of review articles in recent years that focus on some aspects of this chapter (2–8). One of these articles lists all previous reviews on this subject (6). Included in this review are published papers, book chapters, abstracts, and dissertations. This chapter includes all known prospective epidemiological studies that involve vitamin C intake or an index of vitamin C intake. However, several prospective studies that have only fruit and/or vegetable intake as an independent variable are not included.

METHODS

This chapter presents the essential characteristics of 30 prospective studies that measured vitamin C intake in the diet (in the form of fruits, other foods containing vitamin C, and/or supplements containing vitamin C) or in blood samples (as plasma ascorbic acid and/or leukocyte ascorbic acid). The studies are described in chronological order. For some of these studies findings are reported for more than one follow-up period.

Table 1 describes the study population, geographic location, age, follow-up period, health status, and type of data collected for 24 population cohorts that were followed for mortality as an outcome variable (9–40). Table 1 also describes this same information for 6 population cohorts that were followed for incidence of cancer or cardiovascular disease (41–47).

Table 2 describes the results of those studies in Table 1 that give mortality from all causes for males and/or females. The number of years of follow-up observation, the high and low vitamin C intake groups, and the variables controlled for are presented along with the total number of subjects, total number of deaths, relative risk (RR) of high intake group versus low intake group, and 95% confidence interval (CI) or statistical significance level (p-value) for the relative risk.

Table 3 describes the results of these same studies dealing with all causes of death for both sexes combined. Table 4 describes the results of these same studies dealing with mortality from selected forms of cancer or cardiovascular disease for males, females, and/ or both sexes.

Table 5 describes the results of those studies in Table 1 that give incidence data for males and/or females. The number of years of follow-up observation, the high and low vitamin C intake groups, the disease outcome, and the variables controlled for are presented along with the sex and total number of subjects, total number of incident cases, relative risk of high intake group versus low intake group, and 95% confidence interval or statistical p-value.

Table 6 describes the study population, geographic location, age, follow-up period, health status, and type of data collected for eight intervention trials that involved vitamin C intake and control groups and mortality outcome (48–55).

Table 7 describes the results of those studies in Table 6 that are intervention trials. The placebo and intervention groups are described in terms of level of vitamin C supplementation, number of subjects, and number of deaths. Also presented are the characteristics controlled for, years of follow-up evaluation, relative risk of intervention versus placebo, and 95% confidence interval or statistical p-value.

RESULTS

Table 2 shows that the relative risks for all causes range between 0.52 and 1.00 for males and between 0.66 and 1.03 for females. The relative risks are based on comparing persons with the highest and lowest vitamin C intake, generally above and below the recommended dietary allowance (RDA) of 60 mg per day. Some comparisons are with serum or dietary vitamin C for survivors versus deceased persons. Particularly noteworthy are the National HANES Epidemiologic Followup Study (NHEFS) (27,30,32) and the Western Electric Study (34), which each showed an RR significantly less than 1.00 for males after controlling for numerous confounding variables. The relative risks for females are mostly less than 1.00 but not significantly so except for the NHEFS and early studies involving fairly small samples.

Table 3 shows that the relative risks for all causes range between 0.21 and 1.70 for both

Table 1 Description of Populations for Prospective Vitamin C Studies: Mortality and Incidence

Author (year)	Population description	Country	Ages at entry	Start	End	Initial health	Type of study
Mortality							
Chope (1954)	280 Males & 297 females; residents of San Mateo County, CA	USA	50–90	1948	1952	Healthy	Exam with food intake & clinical history
Chope (1956)	280 Males & 297 females; residents of San Mateo County, CA	USA	50–90	1948	1954	Healthy	Exam with food intake & clinical history
Wilson (1972)	50 Males & 109 females; random sample of patients at acute geriatric hospital	England	50–95	1968	1969	Seriously ill	Exam with venous blood sample
Burr (1975)	291 Males & 516 females; elderly people living in South Wales town	Wales	65–89	1971	1973	Low blood levels	Exam with blood samples
Gilmore (1975)	68 Males & 172 females; elderly people living at home in Glasgow	Scotland	65+	1969–71	1972–74	Living in own home	Exam with dietary intake
Hodkinson (1976)	343 Males & 322 females; random community sample from six areas	UK	65+	1967–68	1972	Average	Physical, medical, dietary, & biochemical exam
Mickelsen, Schlenker (1976)	100 Females; random sample of residents from Lansing, MI	USA	40–88	1948	1972	Average	Interview with dietary records & blood sample
Enstrom (1982)	223 Males & 256 females; white elderly PREVENTION questionnaire respondents from CA	USA	68+	1977	1980	Health conscious	Mailed dietary questionnaire
Burr (1982)	286 Males & 529 females; elderly people living in South Wales town	Wales	65–89	1971	1979	Low blood levels	Exam with blood samples
Hunt (1984)	98 Males & 101 females; patients at an acute geriatric ward in West Yorks	England	Elderly	~1982	~1983	Acute with severity score	Biochemical assessment in hospital
Long-de (1985)	136,281 White males from 25 states enrolled by ACS	USA	40–74	1960	1970	No history of cancer & not sick at entry	Mailed life-style & dietary questionnaire

Table 1   Continued

Author (year)	Population description	Country	Ages at entry	Start	End	Initial health	Type of study
Enstrom (1986)	1,369 Males & 1,654 females; representative sample of residents of Alameda County, CA	USA	16+	1974	1983	Noninstitutionalized	Life-style & dietary interview
Lapidus (1986)	1,462 Females; representative sample of residents in Gothenburg	Sweden	38–60	1968–69	1980–81	Average	Life-style & dietary interview & exam with blood samples
Gey (1987, 1993)	2,975 Male employees of the three major pharmaceutical companies in Basel	Switzerland	Ave. 51	1971–73	1980	Apparently healthy	Exam with blood samples
Kromhout (1987)	878 middle aged males randomly sampled from Zutphen	Netherlands	40–59	1960	1985	Average	Life-style & dietary interview
Stahelin (1991)	2,975 Male employees of the three major pharmaceutical companies in Basel	Switzerland	Ave. 51	1971–73	1985	Apparently healthy	Exam with blood samples
Chow (1992)	17,818 White males; Lutheran Brotherhood Insurance Society policy holders from 9 states	USA	35+	1966	1986	Already insured	Mailed life-style & dietary questionnaire
Enstrom (1992)	4,479 Males & 6,869 females; representative sample of civilian noninstitutionalized adults	USA	25–74	1971–74	1982–84	Average	Life-style & dietary interview & exam with blood samples
Volkert (1992)	73 Males & 227 females; elderly geriatric patients admitted to hospital in Heidelberg	Germany	75+	1987–88	1989	Moderately or severely ill	Clinical, anthropomorphic, & biochemical exam
Enstrom (1993, 1994)	4,479 Males & 6,869 females; representative sample of civilian noninstitutionalized adults	USA	25–74	1971–74	1987	Average	Life-style & dietary interview & exam with blood samples
Knekt (1994)	2,748 Males & 2,385 females; participants in multiphasic health exam in several regions	Finland	30–69	1966–72	1984	Free of known heart disease	Dietary history interview and health exam
Gale (1995)	359 Males & 307 females; stratified random sample from 8 areas	UK	65+	1973	1993	No history of CHD, stroke, or arteriosclerosis	Detailed dietary interview, health exam, blood sample

Reference	Sample	Country	Age	Years	End	Health status	Method
Pandey (1995)	1,556 Middle-aged male employees of Western Electric Company in Chicago, IL	USA	40–55	1958–59	1983	No history of CHD, cancer, or other serious illness	Life-style & dietary interview & numerous exams
Eichholzer (1996)	2,975 male employees of the three major pharmaceutical companies in Basel	Switzerland	Ave. 51	1971–73	1990	Apparently healthy	Exam with blood samples
Kushi (1996)	34,486 women recruited from a random DMV sample in Iowa	USA	55–69	1986	1993	No history of CHD	Mailed dietary questionnaire
Losonczy (1996)	~4,095 males & ~7,083 females; free-living persons from communities in MA, IA, CT & NC	USA	67–105	1984–86	1993	Average	Medical history, lifestyle & dietary interview
Sahyoun (1996)	254 males & 471 females; noninstitutionalized residents recruited from MA community groups	USA	60–101	1981–84	1992	Free of terminal disease and severe disorders	Physical, medical, dietary & biochemical exam
Enstrom (1996)	5,231 Males & 4,613 females; CA Mormon High Priest families	USA	25+	1980	1993	Mostly healthy	Mailed life-style & dietary questionnaire
Incidence							
Bjelke (1982)	13,785 Males & 2,928 females; random sample of men & their family members	Norway	≥35	1967	1978	Average	Mailed dietary questionnaire
Knekt (1991)	4,538 Males; participants in multiphasic health exam in several regions	Finland	20–69	1966–72	1986	Cancer-free	Dietary history interview and health exam
Shibata (1992)	~4,277 Males & ~7,300 females; elderly residents of Leisure World, Laguna Hills, CA	USA	>50 Ave. 74	1981–85	1989	Cancer-free, 1st year follow-up excluded	Mailed dietary questionnaire
Graham (1992)	18,586 women recruited from a mailing list of long-term New York State residents	USA	>50	1980	1987	Cancer-free	Mailed dietary questionnaire
Manson (1992, 93)	87,245 Female registered nurses in Nurses Health Study from 11 large states	USA	34–59	1980	1988	Healthy	Mailed dietary questionnaire
Hunter (1993)	87,494 Female registerd nurses in Nurses Health Study from 11 large states	USA	34–59	1980	1988	Cancer-free	Mailed dietary questionnaire
Rimm (1993)	39,910 Male non-MD health professionals from selected states after exclusions	USA	45–75	1986	1990	CHD-free, diabetes-free, hypercholesterolemia-free	Detailed dietary questionnaire

Table 2   Results for Prospective Vitamin C Studies: All Cause Mortality (Males and Females)

Author (year)	Low vitamin C group (L)	High vitamin C group (H)	Control variables	Years of FU	Males				Females			
					Total sample	Total deaths	RR (H vs L)	CI of RR	Total sample	Total deaths	RR (H vs L)	CI of RR
Wilson (1972)	LLA ≤ 25	LLA > 25		1	50	~35[a]	~80[a]	$p > .05$	109	61	0.73	$p < .01$
Burr (1975)	LLA < 15	LLA ≥ 15		2	291	63	0.52	$p < .01$	516	88	0.66	$p < .01$
Gilmore (1975)	VC < 30 mg/d	VC ≥ 30 mg/d	Age	3.34	68	24	~1.00[a]	$p > .05$	172	41	~1.00[a]	$p > .05$
Hodkinson (1976)	VC = low	VC = high		5	343	~200	~0.80[a]	$p < .02$	322	~200	~100[a]	$p > .05$
Mickelsen (1976)	mg/d For deceased	mg/d For survivors		24					100	60	0.70[b]	$p < .05$
Mickelsen (1976)	PAA For deceased	PAA For survivors		24					100	60	0.87[b]	$p < .05$
Schlenker (1976)	VC < 25 mg/d	VC > 25 mg/d		24					88	60	0.68[b]	$p < .05$
Burr (1982)	PAA For deceased	PAA For survivors		8	286	214	0.83[b]	$p < .05$	529	330	0.74[b]	$p < .05$
Burr (1982)	LAA for deceased	LAA for survivors		8	294	214	0.90[b]	$p > .05$	529	329	0.91[b]	$p > .05$
Enstrom (1986)	VC < 250 mg/d	VC ≥ 250 mg/d	Age	10	1,369	134	0.95	0.61–1.42	1,654	130	1.03	0.68–1.51
Lapidus (1986)	VC = low	VC = high	Age	12					1,424	75	~100[a]	$p > .05$

	PAA For deceased	PAA for survivors					0.92[b]	p < .01			0.77	0.53–1.06
Gey (1987)			Age, smoking	7	2,975	268	0.92[b]	p < .01				
Enstrom (1992)	VC < 50 mg/d	VC ≥ 50 mg/d & reg supps	Age	5	4,479	473	0.52	0.35–0.73	6,869	276	0.77	0.53–1.06
Enstrom (1992)	VC < 50 mg/d	VC ≥ 50 mg/d & reg supps	Age, 10 confounders	5	4,479	473	0.61	0.43–0.86				
Enstrom (1992)	VC ≥ 50 mg/d	VC < 50 mg/d & reg supps	Age	Ave. 10	4,479	1,069	0.59	0.47–0.72	6,869	740	0.90	0.74–1.09
Enstrom (1992)	VC < 50 mg/d	VC < 50 mg/d & reg supps	Age, 10 confounders	Ave. 10	4,479	1,069	0.78	0.62–0.97				
Enstrom (1993)	VC < 50 mg/d & ffv < 1/wk	VC < 50 mg/d & reg supps & ffv > 1/d	Age	Ave. 14	4,479	1,595	0.53	0.42–0.67	6,869	1,242	0.71	0.57–0.86
Enstrom (1994)	VC < 50 mg/d	VC < 50 mg/d & reg supps	Age	Ave. 14	4,479	1,595	0.63	0.53–0.74	6,869	1,242	0.86	0.73–1.00
Enstrom (1994)	VC < 50 mg/d	VC < 50 mg/d & reg supps	Age, 10 confounders	Ave. 14	4,479	1,595	0.80	0.67–0.96				
Pandey (1995)	VC = 21–82 mg/d	VC = 113–393 mg/d	Age, 11 confounders	Ave. 24	1,556	667	0.72	0.57–0.91				
Eichholzer (1996)	PAA for deceased	PAA for survivors	Age, smoking	17	2,974	801	0.92[b]	p < .01				
Enstrom (1996)	ff = 0 times/wk	ff > 7 times/wk	Age, health, smoking	14	5,231	815	0.96	0.90–1.02	4,613	386	0.98	0.90–1.07
Enstrom (1996)	No VC supps	Current VC supps	Age, health, smoking	14	5,231	815	0.85	0.73–0.99	4,613	386	0.94	0.75–1.18

[a]Calculated by extrapolating from published data.

[b]Ratio of mean for deceased divided by mean for survivors (for illustration, not for comparison to standard RR). VC, vitamin C intake in mg/day; LAA, leukocyte ascorbic acid in $\mu g/10^8$ cells); PAA, plasma ascorbic acid in mg/dl; ff, fresh fruits; ffv, fresh fruits and vegetables rich in vitamin C; VC supps, use of vitamin C supplements; reg supps, daily use of vitamin C and/or multivitamin supplements.

Table 3 Results for Prospective Vitamin C Studies: All Cause Mortality (Both Sexes)

Author (year)	Low vitamin C group (L)	High vitamin C group (H)	Control variables	Years of FU	Total sample	Total deaths	RR (H vs L)	CI of RR
Chope (1954)	VC < 50 mg/day	VC ≥ 50 mg/day		4	577	49	0.33	$p < .05$
Chope (1956)	VC < 50 mg/day	VC ≥ 50 mg/day		6	577	88	0.40	$P < .05$
Wilson (1972)	LAA < 12	LAA > 25		0.08	159	43	0.21	$p < .01$
Enstrom (1982)	VC = 100–999 mg/d	VC ≥ 2000 mg/d		3.25	479	34	1.70	$p > .05$
Enstrom (1982)	VC supps time = 1– 9 years	VC supps time ≥ 20 years		3.25	479	32	0.81	$p > .05$
Hunt (1984)	Low LAA	High LAA	Sex, severity of illness	1.33	199	59	0.61	$p < .05$
Enstrom (1986)	VC < 250 mg/d	VC ≥ 250 mg/d	Age, sex	10	3,023	264	0.97	0.67–1.38
Enstrom (1986)	VC < 250 mg/d	VC ≥ 250 mg/d	Age, sex, smoking	10	3,023	264	0.95	0.66–1.36
Enstrom (1992)	VC < 50 mg/d	VC ≥ 50 mg/d & reg supps	Age, sex	5	11,348	749	0.66	0.53–0.82
Enstrom (1992)	VC < 50 mg/d	VC ≥ 50 mg/d & reg supps	Age, sex, 10 confounders	5	11,348	749	0.68	0.52–0.89
Enstrom (1992)	VC < 50 mg/d	VC ≥ 50 mg/d & reg supps	Age, sex	Ave. 10	11,348	1,809	0.74	0.64–0.85
Enstrom (1992)	VC < 50 mg/d	VC ≥ 50 mg/d & reg supps	Age, sex, 10 confounders	Ave. 10	11,348	1,809	0.86	0.73–1.02
Volkert (1992)	PAA < 0.5 mg/dl	PAA ≥ 0.5 mg/dl		1.5	300	139	0.76	$p < .05$
Volkert (1992)	PAA for deceased	PAA for survivors		1.5	300	139	0.78[b]	$p < .05$
Enstrom (1993)	VC < 50 mg/d & ffv < 1/wk	VC ≥ 50 mg/d & reg supps & ffv > 1/d	Age, sex	Ave. 14	11,348	2,837	0.61	0.52–0.70
Enstrom (1994)	VC < 50 mg/d	VC ≥ 50 mg/d & reg supps	Age, sex	Ave. 14	11,348	2,837	0.76	0.68–0.85
Enstrom (1994)	VC < 50 mg/d	VC ≥ 50 mg/d & reg supps	Age, sex, 10 confounders	Ave. 14	11,348	2,837	0.88	0.82–0.99
Losonczy (1996)	No supps	Current VC supps	Age, sex	8	11,178	3,490	1.04	0.89–1.23
Losonczy (1996)	No supps	Current VC supps	Age, sex, 11 confounders	8	11,178	3,490	1.09	0.93–1.28
Losonczy (1996)	No supps	Current VC & VE supps	Age, sex.	8	11,178	3,490	0.58	0.42–0.79
Losonczy (1996)	No supps	Current VC & VE supps	Age, sex, 11 confounders	8	11,178	3,490	0.63	0.46–0.86
Sahyoun (1996)	VC < 90 mg/d	VC ≥ 388 mg/d	Age, sex	Ave. 10	725	217	0.53	0.33–0.84
Sahyoun (1996)	VC < 90 mg/d	VC ≥ 388 mg/d	Age, sex, 3 confounders	Ave. 10	725	217	0.55	0.34–0.88
Sahyoun (1996)	VC < 90 mg/d	VC ≥ 388 mg/d	Age, sex, 5 confounders	Ave. 10	725	217	0.55	0.32–0.93

[a]Calculated by extrapolating from published data.

[b]Ratio of mean for deceased divided by mean for survivors (for illustration; not for comparison to standard RR). VC, vitamin C intake in mg/day; LAA, leukocyte ascorbic acid in µg/10[8] cells; PAA, plasma ascorbic acid in mg/dl; ff, fresh fruits; ffv, fresh fruits ard vegetables rich in vitamin C; VC supps, use of vitamin C supplements; reg supps, daily use of vitamin C and/or multivitamin supplements; VE supps, use of vitamin E supplements.

Table 4 Results for Prospective Vitamin C Studies: Mortality from Selected Causes

Author (year)	Low vitamin C group (L)	High vitamin C group (H)	Control variables	Cause of death	Sex	Years of FU	Total sample	Total deaths	RR (H vs L)	CI of RR
Long-de (1985)	ff = 0–2 days/wk & no pills	ff = 5–7 days/wk	Age	Lung cancer	M	10	136,281	2,952	0.57	$p < .05$
Long-de (1985)	ff = 0–2 days/wk & no pills	ff = 5–7 days/wk & pills	Age	Lung cancer	M	10	136,281	2,952	0.61	$p < .05$
Lapidus (1986)	VC = low[a]	VC = high[a]	Age, smoking	MI	F	12	1,361	23	~1.00[a]	$p > .05$
Gey (1987)	PAA < 0.4	PAA > 0.4	Age, smoking	All cancer	M	7	2,975	102	0.72	$p > .05$
Gey (1987)	PAA < 0.4	PAA > 0.4	Age, smoking	GI cancer	M	7	2,975	26	0.42	$p < .05$
Kromhout (1987)	VC < 63 mg/d	VC = 83–103 mg/d	Age, smoking	Lung cancer	M	25	878	63	0.36	0.18–0.75
Kromhout (1987)	VC < 63 mg/d	VC = 83–103 mg/d	Age, smoking	All cancer	M	25	878	155	~1.00[a]	$p > .05$
Stahelin (1991)	PAA < 0.4	PAA > 0.4	Age, smoking, lipids	All cancer	M	12	2,975	204	0.83[a]	0.57–1.19
Stahelin (1991)	PAA < 0.4	PAA > 0.4	Age, smoking, lipids	GI cancer	M	12	2,975	37	~0.40[a]	0.2–0.7
Stahelin (1991)	PAA < 0.4	PAA > 0.4	Age, smoking, lipids	Stomach cancer	M	12	2,975	20	~0.30[a]	0.1–0.7
Stahelin (1991)	PAA < 0.4	PAA > 0.4	Age, smoking, lipids	Lung cancer	M	12	2,975	68	1.28[a]	0.7–2.5
Enstrom (1992)	VC > 50 mg/d	VC ≥ 50 mg/d & reg supps	Age	All cancer	M	Ave. 10	4,479	228	0.79	0.51–1.18
Enstrom (1992)	VC > 50 mg/d	VC ≥ 50 mg/d & reg supps	Age	All cancer	F	Ave. 10	6,869	169	0.93	0.60–1.40
Enstrom (1992)	VC > 50 mg/d	VC ≥ 50 mg/d & reg supps	Age	All CVD	M	Ave. 10	4,479	588	0.55	0.39–0.74
Enstrom (1992)	VC < 50 mg/d	VC ≥ 50 mg/d & reg supps	Age	All CVD	F	Ave. 10	6,869	371	0.75	0.55–0.99
Chow (1992)	VC = lowest quintile	VC = highest quintile	Age, smoking, industry	Lung cancer	M	20	17,818	219	0.80	0.5–1.2
Enstrom (1993)	VC < 50 mg/d & ffv < 1/wk	VC ≥ 50 mg/d & reg supps & ffv > 1/d	Age	All CVD	M	Ave. 14	4,479	815	0.52	0.37–0.71
Enstrom (1993)	VC < 50 mg/d & ffv < 1/wk	VC ≥ 50 mg/d & reg supps & ffv > 1/d	Age	All CVD	F	Ave. 14	6,869	636	0.58	0.42–0.78
Gey (1993)	PAA < 0.4	PAA > 0.4	Age, smoking	CHD	M	12	2,975	132	0.80	0.5–1.3
Enstrom (1994)	VC < 50 mg/d	VC ≥ 50 mg/d & reg supps	Age	All cancer	M	Ave. 14	4,479	346	0.69	0.47–0.97
Enstrom (1994)	VC < 50 mg/d	VC ≥ 50 mg/d & reg supps	Age	All cancer	F	Ave. 14	6,869	269	0.92	0.65–1.27

Table 4 Continued

Author (year)	Low vitamin C group (L)	High vitamin C group (H)	Control variables	Cause of death	Sex	Years of FU	Total sample	Total deaths	RR (H vs L)	CI of RR
Enstrom (1994)	VC < 50 mg/d	VC ≥ 50 mg/d & reg supps	Age	All CVD	M	Ave. 14	4,479	815	0.65	0.50–0.82
Enstrom (1994)	VC < 50 mg/d	VC ≥ 50 mg/d & reg supps	Age, 10 confounders	All CVD	F	Ave. 14	6,869	636	0.80	0.63–0.98
Knekt (1994)	VC < 61 mg/d	VC > 85 mg/d	Age, 5 confounders	CHD	M	Ave. 16	2,748	186	1.00	0.68–1.45
Knekt (1994)	VC < 62 mg/d	VC > 91 mg/d	Age, 5 confounders	CHD	F	Ave. 16	2,385	58	0.49	0.24–0.98
Gale (1995)	VC < 27.9 mg/d	VC ≥ 44.9 mg/d	Age, sex	Stroke	M/F	20	730	125	0.40	0.2–0.6
Gale (1995)	VC < 27.9 mg/d	VC ≥ 44.9 mg/d	Age, sex	CHD	M/F	•20	730	182	0.80	0.6–1.2
Eichholzer (1996)	PAA < 0.4	PAA > 0.4	Age, smoking, lipids	All cancer	M	17	2,974	290	0.81	0.59–1.12
Eichholzer (1996)	PAA < 0.4	PAA > 0.4	Age, smoking, lipids	Stomach cancer	M	17	2,974	28	1.41	0.31–6.25
Eichholzer (1996)	PAA < 0.4	PAA > 0.4	Age, smoking, lipids	Colon cancer	M	17	2,974	22	0.58	0.19–1.79
Eichholzer (1996)	PAA < 0.4	PAA > 0.4	Age, smoking, lipids	Lung cancer	M	17	2,974	87	0.55	0.26–1.16
Eichholzer (1996)	PAA < 0.4	PAA > 0.4	Age, smoking, lipids	Prostate cancer	M	17	2,974	30	1.08	0.36–3.23
Kushi (1996)	VC ≤ 87 mg/d (diet only)	VC ≥ 196 mg/d (diet only)	Age, 12 cofounders	CHD	F	7	17,107	122	1.43	0.75–2.70
Kushi (1996)	VC ≤ 112 mg/d (diet & supps)	VC ≥ 391 mg/d (diet & supps)	Age, 12 cofounders	CHD	F	7	34,486	242	1.49	0.96–2.30
Kushi (1996)	No supps	VC supps ≥ 1000 mg/d	Age, 12 cofounders	CHD	F	7	34,486	242	0.74	0.30–1.83
Losonczy (1996)	No supps	Current VC supps	Age, sex	All cancer	M/F	6	11,178	761	0.91	0.63–1.32
Losonczy (1996)	No supps	Current VC supps	Age, sex, 11 cofounders	All cancer	M/F	6	11,178	761	0.88	0.61–1.28
Losonczy (1996)	No supps	Current VC supps	Age, sex	CHD	M/F	6	11,178	1101	1.00	0.74–1.34
Losonczy (1996)	No supps	Current VC supps	Age, sex, 11 cofounders	CHD	M/F	6	11,178	1101	0.99	0.74–1.34
Sahyoun (1996)	VC < 90 mg/d	VC > 388 mg/d	Age, sex, 2 cofounders	All cancer	M/F	Ave. 10	<725	57	0.94	0.36–2.44
Sahyoun (1996)	VC < 90 mg/d	VC > 388 mg/d	Age, sex, 2 cofounders	All CVD	M/F	Ave. 10	<725	101	0.38	0.19–0.75
Sahyoun (1996)	PAA < 0.91 mg/dl	PAA > 1.56 mg/dl	Age, sex, 3 cofounders	All cancer	M/F	Ave. 10	<725	45	0.68	0.25–1.83
Sahyoun (1996)	PAA < 0.91 mg/dl	PAA > 1.56 mg/dl	Age, sex, 3 cofounders	All CVD	M/F	Ave. 10	<725	75	0.53	0.27–1.06

aCalculated by extrapolating from published data.

bRatio of mean for deceased divided by mean for survivors (for illustration; r of for comparison to standard RR). VC, vitamin C intake in mg/day; LAA, leukocyte ascorbic acid in µg/10^8 cells; PAA, plasma ascorbic acid in mg/dl; ff, fresh fruits; ffv, fresh fruits and vegetables rich in vitamin C; VC supps, daily use of vitamin C supplements; reg supps, daily use of vitamin C and/or multivitamin supplements.

Cause of death: GI cancer, gastrointestinal cancer; CHD, coronary heart disease or ischemic heart disease; MI, myocardial infarction; CVD, cardiovascular disease.

Table 5 Results for Prospective Vitamin C Studies: Incidence

Author (year)	Low vitamin C group (L)	High vitamin C group (H)	Control variables	Disease category	Sex	Years of FU	Total sample	Total cases	RR (H vs L)	CI of RR
Bjelke (1982)	VC index < 15	VC index > 22	Age, sex, region, urbanization	Stomach cancer	Both sexes	11.5	16,713	116	0.60	0.4–0.9[a]
Knekt (1991)	VC = lowest quintile	VC = highest quintile	Age (nonsmokers only)	Lung cancer	Males	Ave. 18	2,121	24	0.32	$p < .01$
Knekt (1991)	VC = lowest quintile	VC = highest quintile	Age (smokers only)	Lung cancer	Males	Ave. 18	2,417	93	1.23	$p = .36$
Shibata (1992)	VC < 145 mg/d	VC > 210 mg/d	Age, smoking	All cancer	Males	Ave. 7	~4,277	645	0.90	0.74–1.09
Shibata (1992)	VC supps = 0	VC supps = median 500 mg/d	Age, smoking	All cancer	Males	Ave. 7	~4,277	642	0.94	0.80–1.10
Shibata (1992)	VC < 155 mg/d	VC > 225 mg/d	Age, smoking	All cancer	Females	Ave. 7	~7,300	690	0.76	0.63–0.91
Shibata (1992)	VC supps = 0	VC supps = median 500 mg/d	Age, smoking	All cancer	Females	Ave. 7	~7,300	683	0.93	0.80–1.09
Graham (1992)	VC = 0–34 mg/d	VC = 79–498 mg/d	Age, education	Breast cancer	Females	7	18,586	344	0.81	0.59–1.12
Manson (1992,93)	VC < 93 mg/d	VC ≥ 359 mg/d[a]	Age	CHD	Females	8	87,245	552	0.58	0.44–0.77

Table 5 Continued

Author (year)	Low vitamin C group (L)	High vitamin C group (H)	Control variables	Disease category	Sex	Years of FU	Total sample	Total cases	RR (H vs L)	CI of RR
Manson (1992,93)	VC < 93 mg/d	VC ≥ 359 mg/d[a]	Age, CHD risk factors	CHD	Females	8	87,245	552	0.65	0.49–0.86
Manson (1992,93)	VC < 93 mg/d	VC ≥ 359 mg/d[a]	Age, CHD risk factors, multivitamins	CHD	Females	8	87,245	552	0.80	0.58–1.10
Hunter (1993)	VC < 93 mg/d	VC ≥ 359 mg/d	Age	Breast cancer	Females	8	89,494	1,439	1.05	0.9–1.2[a]
Hunter (1993)	VC < 93 mg/d	VC ≥ 359 mg/d	Age, 11 confounders	Breast cancer	Females	8	89,494	1,439	1.03	0.87–1.21
Hunter (1993)	VC supps = 0	VC supps ≥ 1,300 mg/d	Age, 11 confounders	Breast cancer	Females	8	89,494	1,439	1.12	0.75–1.69
Hunter (1993)	VC supps time = 0	VC supps time ≥ 10 years	Age, 11 confounders	Breast cancer	Females	8	89,494	1,439	1.12	0.87–1.43
Rimm (1993)	VC = median 92 mg/d	VC = median 1,162 mg/d	Age	CHD	Males	4	39,910	667	0.83	0.64–1.08
Rimm (1993)	VC = median 92 mg/d	VC = median 1,162 mg/d	Age, 10 confounders	CHD	Males	4	39,910	667	0.89	0.68–1.16
Rimm (1993)	VC = median 92 mg/d	VC = median 1,162 mg/d	Age, 10 confounders, antioxidants	CHD	Males	4	39,910	667	1.25	0.91–1.71

[a]Calculated by extrapolating from published data.
[b]Ratio of mean for deceased divided by mean for survivors (for illustration: not for comparison to standard RR). VC, vitamin C intake in mg/day; LAA, leukocyte ascorbic acid in μg/10[8] cells; PAA, plasma ascorbic acid in mg/dl; ff, fresh fruits; ffv, fresh fruits and vegetables rich in vitamin C; VC supps, use of vitamin C supplements; reg supps, daily use of vitamin C and/or multivitamin supplements.

Table 6 Description of Populations for Prospective Vitamin C Studies: Intervention Trials

Author (year)	Population description	Country	Ages at entry	Start	End	Initial health[a]	Type of trial
Wilson (1973)	194 Males & 344 females; patients admitted to acute geriatric hospital	England	52–97	1970	1971	Terminally ill	Randomized controlled trial
Burr (1975)	137 Males & 160 females; elderly people living in a South Wales town	Wales	65–89 Ave. 77	1971	1973	Elderly with low PAA & LAA	Randomized controlled trial
Cameron (1976)	52 Males & 48 females; terminal patients with cancer of 20 sites from Vale of Leven Hospital	Scotland	32–93	1971	1975	Terminal cancer	Trial with historical controls
Cameron (1978)	53 Males & 47 females; terminal patients with cancer of 16 sites from Vale of Leven Hospital	Scotland	38–93	1971	1978	Terminal cancer	Trial with historical controls (90 patients from 1976 study)
Creagan (1979)	76 Males & 47 females; terminal cancer patients from Mayo Clinic in Rochester, MN	USA	>40	1978	1978	Terminal cancer	Randomized controlled trial
Hunt (1984)	98 Males & 101 females; patients admitted to an acute geriatric ward in West Yorks	England	Elderly	~1982	~1983	Acutely ill	Double-blind randomized controlled trial
Moertel (1985)	57 Males & 43 females; terminal colorectal cancer patients from Mayo Clinic in Rochester, MN	USA		1982	1984	Terminal cancer	Randomized controlled trial
Blot (1993)	~6,600 Males & ~8,140 females out of 29,584 adults in trial from four Linxian communes	China	40–69	1986	1991	No debilitating diseases or prior cancer	Randomized community trial

[a]PAA, plasma ascorbic acid; LAA, leukocyte ascorbic acid.

Table 7 Results for Prospective Vitamin C Studies: Intervention Trials[a]

Author (year)	Placebo group (P)			Intervention group (I)			Control variables	Sex	Years of FU	RR (I vs P)	CI of RR
	Vitamin C supplement	Sample	Deaths	Vitamin C supplement	Sample	Deaths					
Wilson (1973)	0 mg	96	34	200 mg	98	37	Physical status	Males	0.08	1.07	$p > .05$
Wilson (1973)	0 mg	171	41	200 mg	173	41	Physical status	Females	0.08	0.99	$p > .05$
Wilson (1973)	0 mg	96	53	200 mg	98	62	Physical status	Males	0.50	1.15	$p > .05$
Wilson (1973)	0 mg	171	77	200 mg	173	75	Physical status	Females	0.50	0.96	$p > .05$
Burr (1975)	0 mg	59	20	50–150 mg	78	18	Age, blood levels of vitamin C	Males	2.00	0.68	$p > .05$
Burr (1975)	0 mg	93	15	50–150 mg	67	18	Age, blood levels of vitamin C	Females	2.00	1.67	$p > .05$
Cameron (1976)	0 mg	1000	880	10 g	100	47	Sex, age, site, tumor status	Both sexes	0.27	0.53	$p < .01$
Cameron (1978)	0 mg	1000	~900	10 g	100	~36	Sex, age, site, tumor status	Both sexes	0.27	~0.40	$p < .01$
Creagan (1979)	0 mg	63	56	10 g	60	54	Sex, age, site, tumor status	Both sexes	0.50	1.01	$p > .05$
Hunt (1984)	0 mg	105	28	200 mg	94	33	Sex, severity of illness	Both sexes	1.33	1.32	$p > .05$
Moertel (1985)	0 mg	49	24	10 g	51	25	Sex, age, prior radiation treatment	Both sexes	1.00	1.00	$p > .05$
Blot (1993)	0 mg	~3,700	280	120 mg – 30 µg Mo	~11,100	813	Sex, age, tobacco, cancer history	Both sexes	5.25	1.01	0.93–1.10
Blot (1995)	0 mg	~1,665	~126	120 mg + 30 µg Mo	~4,995	~366	Age, tobacco, cancer history	Males	5.25	0.93	$p \geq .05$
Blot (1995)	0 mg	~2,035	~154	120 mg + 30 µg Mo	~6,105	~447	Age, tobacco, cancer history	Females	5.25	1.12	$p \geq .05$

[a]FU, follow-up; CI, confidence interval; RR, relative risk; Mo, molybdenum.

sexes combined. Only two studies showed RRs that were greater than 1.00, although not significantly so. These two studies made companies based only on vitamin C supplement intake and one was based on small numbers. Most of the RRs involving high and low levels around the RDA are significantly less than 1.00, although several of these do not control for confounding variables. Some comparisons are with serum or dietary vitamin C for survivors versus deceased persons. Particularly consistent are the NHEFS results for three different follow-up periods and for two different sets of upper and lower intake limits (27,30,32). The RR differences remain significant after controlling for numerous confounding variables.

Table 4 shows that the relative risks for individual causes of death range between 0.30 and 1.41 for males, between 0.49 and 1.49 for females, and between 0.38 and 1.00 for both sexes combined. The relative risks are based on comparing persons with the highest and lowest vitamin C intake, generally above and below the RDA. Some comparisons are with serum or dietary vitamin C for survivors versus deceased persons. The NHEFS showed an RR for all cardiovascular disease (CVD) significantly less than 1.00 for males and females after controlling for numerous confounding variables (32). Several other RRs for males and females are also less than 1.00 but many do not control for confounding variables.

Table 5 shows that the relative risks for incidence from cancer and coronary heart disease (CHD) range between 0.32 and 1.25 for males and between 0.58 and 1.12 for females. The relative risks are based on comparing persons with the highest and lowest vitamin C intake, generally above the RDA. Particularly noteworthy is the Harvard Nurses Study, which showed an RR for CHD significantly less than 1.00 for females after controlling for CHD risk factors (7,46). Several other relative risks for males and females are also less than 1.00, but most do not control for confounding variables and most are not significantly less than 1.00.

Table 7 shows the results of intervention trials. Trials involving terminal geriatric patients given vitamin C supplements of about 200 mg/day showed no effect of supplementation. Two versions of a trial with terminal cancer patients given 10 g of vitamin C showed greatly improved survival rate compared with that of historical controls. However, two randomized controlled trials of terminal patients showed no benefit of supplements.

Correlation studies generally show an inverse relationship between vitamin C intake and selected causes of death such as stomach cancer and coronary heart disease (56–66). However, since these are not analytic studies they are not described further here.

CONCLUSIONS

The majority of studies show a decrease in mortality or a decrease in incidence with an increase in intake of vitamin C, particularly for levels of vitamin C intake above and below the U.S. RDA of 60 mg per day. The inverse relationship is strongest for males and both sexes combined and for all cause mortality. However, there are several studies that show no relationship and others in which the relationship is not significant after controlling for confounding variables. There does not appear to be a relationship at high levels of vitamin C supplement intake, but the number of studies addressing these high levels is small. The results of intervention trials show no effect of supplemental vitamin C.

ACKNOWLEDGMENTS

This research has been supported by the Wallace Genetic Foundation. The author thanks Richard J. Biermann, Linda E. Kanim, Cynthia A. Luppen, and Michael Succar for technical assistance.

REFERENCES

1. Gey KF. On the antioxidant hypothesis with regard to arteriosclerosis. Bibl Nutr Diet 1986; 37:53–91.
2. Committee on Diet and Health. Diet and Health: Implications for Reducing Chronic Disease Risks. Washington DC: National Research Council, National Academy Press, 1989.
3. Block G. Vitamin C and cancer prevention: the epidemiologic evidence. Am J Clin Nutr 1991; 53:270S–282S.
4. Dorgan JF, Schatzkin A. Antioxidant micronutrients in cancer prevention. Hematol/Oncol Clin North Am 1991; 5:43–68.
5. Simon JA. Vitamin C and cardiovascular disease: a review. J Am Coll Nutr 1992; 11:107–125.
6. Byers T, Perry G. Dietary carotenes, vitamin C, and vitamin E as protective antioxidants in human cancers. Annu Rev Nutr 1992; 12:139–159.
7. Manson JE, Gaziano JM, Jonas MA, Hennekens CH. Antioxidants and cardiovascular disease: a review. J Am Coll Nutr 1993; 12:426–432.
8. Bendich A, Langseth L. The health effects of vitamin C supplementation: a review. J Am Coll Nutr 1995; 14:124–136.
9. Chope HD. Relation of nutrition to health in aging persons. Calif Med 1954; 81:335–338.
10. Chope HD, Breslow L. Nutritional status of the aging. Am J Public Health 1956; 46:61–67.
11. Wilson TS, Weeks MM, Mukherjee SK, et al. A study of vitamin C levels in the aged and subsequent mortality. 1972; 14:17–24.
12. Burr ML, Hurley RJ, Sweetnam PM. Vitamin C supplementation of old people with low blood levels. Gerontol Clin 1975; 17:236–243.
13. Gilmore AJJ. Some characteristics of non-surviving subjects in a three-year longitudinal study of elderly people living at home. Gerontol Clin 1975; 17:72–79.
14. Hodkinson HM, Exton-Smith AN. Factors predicting mortality in the elderly in the community. Age Ageing 1976; 5:110–115.
15. Mickelsen O. The possible role of vitamins in the aging process. In: Rockstein M, Sussman ML, eds. Nutrition, Longevity, and Aging. New York: Academic Press, 1976:123–142.
16. Schlenker E. Nutritional status of older women. Dissertation, Michigan State University, 1976.
17. Enstrom JE, Pauling L. Mortality among health-conscious elderly Californians. Proc Natl Acad Sci 1982; 79:6023–6027.
18. Burr ML, Lennings CI, Milbank JE. The prognostic significance of weight and of vitamin C status in the elderly. Age Ageing 1982; 11:249–255.
19. Hunt C, Chakravorty NK, Annan G. The clinical and biochemical effects of vitamin C supplementation in short-stay hospitalized geriatric patients. Int J Vitamin Nutr Res 1984; 54:65–74.
20. Long-de W, Hammond EC. Lung cancer, fruit, green salad and vitamin pills. Chin Med J 1985; 98:206–210.
21. Lapidus L, Andersson H, Bengtsson C, Bosaeus I. Dietary habits in relation to incidence of cardiovascular disease and death in women: a 12-year follow-up of participants in the population study of women in Gothenburg, Sweden. Am J Clin Nutr 1986; 44:444–448.
22. Enstrom JE, Kanim LE, Breslow L. The relationship between vitamin C intake, general health practices, and mortality in Alameda County, California. Am J Public Health 1986; 76:1124–1130.
23. Kromhout D. Essential micronutrients in relation to carcinogenesis. Am J Clin Nutr 1987; 45:1361–1367.
24. Gey KF, Brubacher GB, Staehelin HB. Plasma levels of antioxidant vitamins in relation to ischemic heart disease and cancer. Am J Clin Nutr 1987; 45:1368–1377.
25. Kok FJ, de Bruijn AM, Vermeeren R, et al. Serum selenium, vitamin antioxidants, and cardiovascular mortality: a 9-year follow-up study in the Netherlands. Am J Clin Nutr 1987; 45:462–468.
26. Stahelin HB, Gey KF, Eichholzer M, et al. Plasma antioxidant vitamins and subsequent cancer

mortality in the 12-year follow-up of the prospective Basel Study. Am J Epidemiol 1991; 133: 766–775.

27. Enstrom JE, Kanim LE, Klein MA. Vitamin C intake and mortality among a sample of the United States population. Epidemiology 1992; 3:194–202.

28. Chow WH, Schuman LM, McLaughlin JK, et al. A cohort study of tobacco use, diet, occupation, and lung cancer mortality. Cancer Causes Control 1992; 3:247–254.

29. Volkert D, Kruse W, Oster P, Schlierf G. Malnutrition in geriatric patients: diagnostic and prognostic significance of nutritional parameters. Ann Nutr Metabol 1992; 36:97–112.

30. Enstrom JE. Vitamin C and mortality. Nutr Today 1993; 28:39–42.

31. Gey KF, Stahelin HB, Eichholzer M. Poor plasma status of carotene and vitamin C is associated with higher mortality from ischemic heart disease and stroke: Basel Prospective Study. Clin Invest 1993; 71:3–6.

32. Enstrom JE. Vitamin C intake and mortality among a sample of the United States population: new results. In: Packer L, Cadenas E, eds. Biological Oxidants and Antioxidants. Stuttgart, Germany: Hippokrates Verlag, 1994:229–241.

33. Knekt P, Reunanen A, Jarvinen R, et al. Antioxidant vitamin intake and coronary mortality in a longitudinal population study. Am J Epidemiol 1994; 139:1180–1189.

34. Pandey D, Shekelle R, Tangney C, Stamler J. Dietary vitamin C and beta carotene and risk of death in middle-aged men: The Western Electric Study. Am J Epidemiol 1995; 142:1269–1278.

35. Gale CR, Martyn CN, Winter PD, Cooper C. Vitamin C and risk of death from stroke and coronary heart disease in cohort of elderly people. Br Med J 1995; 310:1563–1566.

36. Eichholzer M, Stahelin HB, Gey KF, Ludin E, Bernasconi F. Prediction of male cancer mortality by plasma levels of interacting vitamins: 17 year follow-up of the prospective Basel study. Int J Cancer 1996; 66:145–150.

37. Kushi LH, Folsom AR, Prineas RJ, Mink PJ, Wu Y, Bostick RM. Dietary antioxidant vitamins and death from coronary heart disease in postmenopausal women. N Engl J Med 1996; 334:1156–1162.

38. Losonczy KG, Harris TB, Havlik RJ. Vitamin E and vitamin C supplement use and risk of all-cause and coronary heart disease mortality in older persons: the established populations for epidemiologic studies of the elderly. Am J Clin Nutr 1996; 64:190–196.

39. Sahyoun NR, Jacques PF, Russell RM. Carotenoids, vitamins C and E, and mortality in the elderly population. Am J Epidemiol 1996; 144:501–511.

40. Enstrom JE. Health practices and mortality among active California Mormons, 1980–93. In: JK Duke, ed. Latter-Day Saint Social Life. Provo, UT, 1996.

41. Bjelke E. The recession of stomach cancer: selected aspects. In: Magnus K, ed. Trends on Cancer Incidence. Washington, DC: Hemisphere, 1982:165–181.

42. Knekt P, Jarvinen R, Seppanen R, et al. Dietary antioxidants and the risk of lung cancer. Am J Epidemiol 1991; 134:471–479.

43. Shibata A, Paganini-Hill A, Ross RK, Henderson BE. Intake of vegetables, fruits, beta-carotene, vitamin C and vitamin supplements and cancer incidence among the elderly: a prospective study. Br J Cancer 1992; 66:673–679.

44. Graham S, Zielezny M, Marshall J, et al. Diet in the epidemiology of postmenopausal breast cancer in the New York State cohort. Am J Epidemiol 1992; 136:1327–1337.

45. Hunter DJ, Manson JE, Colditz GA, et al. A prospective study of the intake of vitamin C, E, and A and the risk of breast cancer. N Engl J Med 1993; 329:234–240.

46. Manson JE, Stampfer MJ, Willett WC, et al. A prospective study of vitamin C and incidence of coronary heart disease in women (abstr). Circulation 1992; 85:865.

47. Rimm EB, Stampfer MJ, Ascherio A, et al. Vitamin E consumption and the risk of coronary heart disease in men. N Engl J Med 1993; 328:1450–1456.

48. Wilson TS, Datta SB, Murrell JS, Andrews CT. Relation of vitamin C levels to mortality in a geriatric hospital: a study of the effect of vitamin C administration. Age Ageing 1973; 2: 163–171.

49. Burr ML, Hurley RJ, Sweetnam PM. Vitamin C supplementation of old people with low blood levels. Gerontol Clin 1975; 17:236–243.
50. Cameron E, Pauling L. Supplemental ascorbate in the supportive treatment of cancer: prolongation of survival time in terminal human cancer. Proc Natl Acad Sci USA 1976; 73:3685–3689.
51. Cameron E, Pauling L. Supplemental ascorbate in the supportive treatment of cancer: reevaluation of prolongation of survival time in terminal human cancer. Proc Natl Acad Sci 1978; 75: 4538–4542.
52. Creagan ET, Moertel CG, O'Fallon JR, et al. Failure of high-dose vitamin C (ascorbic acid) therapy to benefit patients with advanced cancer: a controlled trial. N Engl J Med 1979; 301: 687–690.
53. Hunt C, Chakravorty NK, Annan G. The clinical and biochemical effects of vitamin C supplementation in short-stay hospitalized geriatric patients. Int J Vitamin Nutr Res 1984; 54:65–74.
54. Moertel CG, Fleming TR, Creagan ET, et al. High-dose vitamin C versus placebo in the treatment of patients with advanced cancer who have had no prior chemotherapy: a randomized double-blind comparison. N Engl J Med 1985; 312:137–141.
55. Blot WJ, Li JY, Taylor PR, et al. Nutrition intervention trials in Linxian, China: supplementation with specific vitamin/mineral combinations, cancer incidence, and disease-specific mortality in the general population. J Natl Cancer Inst 1993; 85:1483–1492.
56. Knox EG. Ischaemic heart disease mortality and dietary intake of calcium. Lancet 1973; 1: 1465–1467.
57. Verlangieri AJ, Kapeghian JC, el-Dean S, Bush M. Fruit and vegetable consumption and cardiovascular mortality. Med Hypotheses 1985; 16:7–15.
58. Gey KF, Brubacher BG, Staehelin HB. Plasma levels of antioxidant vitamins in relation to ischemic heart disease and cancer. Am J Clin Nutr 1987; 45:1368–1377.
59. Gey KF, Stahelin HB, Puska P, Evans A. Relationship of plasma level of vitamin C to mortality from ischemic heart disease. Ann NY Acad Sci 1987; 498:110–123.
60. Guo WD, Li JY, Blot WJ, et al. Correlations of dietary intake and blood nutrient levels with esophageal cancer mortality in China. Nutr Cancer 1990; 13:121–127.
61. Riemersma RA, Oliver M, Elton RA, et al. Plasma antioxidants and coronary heart disease: vitamins C and E, and selenium. Eur J Clin Nutr 1990; 44:143–150.
62. Bolton-Smith C, Woodward M, Tunstall-Pedoe H. The Scottish Heart Health Study: Dietary intake by food frequency questionnaire and odds ratio for coronary heart disease risk. Eur J Clin Nutr 1992; 46.85–93.
63. Guo W, Zheng W, Li JY, et al. Correlations of colon cancer mortality with dietary factors, serum markers, and schistosomiasis in China. Nutr Cancer 1993; 20:13–20.
64. Bellizzi MC, Franklin MF, Duthie GG, James WP. Vitamin E and coronary heart disease: the European paradox. Eur J Clin Nutr 1994; 48:822–831.
65. Guo WD, Chow WH, Zheng W, et al. Diet, serum markers and breast cancer mortality in China. Jpn J Cancer Res 1994; 85:572–577.
66. Ocke MC, Kromhout D, Menotti A, et al. Average intake of anti-oxidant (pro)vitamins and subsequent cancer mortality in the 16 cohorts of the Seven Countries Study. Int J Cancer 1995; 61:480–484.

23

Nitrogen Oxides Are Important Contributors to Cigarette Smoke-Induced Ascorbate Oxidation

JASON P. EISERICH, CARROLL E. CROSS, and **ALBERT VAN DER VLIET**
University of California, Davis, California

INTRODUCTION

Cigarette smoking has been implicated as a major risk factor in chronic obstructive pulmonary diseases such as chronic bronchitis and emphysema (1,2), in carcinogenesis (3), and in cardiovascular disease (4). In fact, nearly 50% of the deaths in the industrialized world are a result of coronary artery disease, and it is becoming increasingly apparent that cigarette smoking contributes to much of this mortality (5). Although epidemiological relationships between a variety of diseases and cigarette smoking are reasonably well established, the precise chemical and biochemical mechanisms underlying the effects induced by cigarette smoking are incompletely understood.

There is a growing body of epidemiological evidence suggesting that free radical– and oxidant–mediated processes are involved in the pathobiology of chronic and degenerative diseases associated with cigarette smoking. Several reports have suggested that ascorbic acid levels are lower in plasma, leukocytes, and respiratory tract lining fluids (RTLFs) of cigarette smokers than in those of nonsmokers (6–11), possibly indicating the involvement of reactive oxidants. Tribble et al. (12) have also shown decreased levels of ascorbic acid in passive smokers, illustrating the potentially harmful effects of environmental tobacco smoke. Although reduced dietary intake of ascorbic acid can contribute to the deficiency of this vitamin observed in smokers (13), increased turnover resulting from the oxidative burden exerted by cigarette smoke, and from the ensuing inflammatory responses, cannot be excluded as a significant contributor to this apparent phenomenon. In fact, Kallner et al. (14) determined that cigarette smokers exhibited a 40% greater turnover rate of ascorbic acid as compared to nonsmokers with similar plasma levels of this antioxidant. Furthermore, the fact that increased levels of lipid peroxidation products (F_2-isoprostanes) are observed in the plasma of persons who smoke supports the hypothesis that smoking can cause oxidative modification of biomolecules in vivo (15). It is unclear, however, whether

Table 1 Calculated Concentrations of Some
Major Components in Gas-Phase Cigarette
Smoke and Their Levels When Deposited in
Respiratory Tract Lining Fluid

Component	In cigarette (μmol/cig)	In RTLF (μM)[a]
Nitrogen oxides[b]		
Nitric oxide (•NO)	12	1200
Nitrogen dioxide (•NO$_2$)	1.0	100
Organic radicals[c]		
(Alkyl, alkoxyl, peroxyl)	0.02	2.0
Aldehydes[d]		
Acetaldehyde	20	2000
Formaldehyde	1.5	150
Acrolein	0.8	80
Crotonaldehyde	0.2	20

[a]Assumes complete deposition of cigarette smoke components
into 10 ml of respiratory tract lining fluids (RTLFs).
[b]*Source*: Values adapted from Ref. 50.
[c]*Source*: Values adapted from Ref. 16.
[d]*Source*: Values are adapted from Ref. 46.

this oxidative stress placed on the smoker is a direct effect of the oxidative constituents in cigarette smoke, or whether the ensuing inflammatory response is primarily responsible.

Cigarette smoke consists of several thousands of compounds, many as yet unidentified. The complexity of the products found in cigarette smoke has made elucidating the mechanisms by which it induces its damaging effects on biological systems extremely difficult. An extensively studied group of compounds in cigarette smoke are the free radicals. Gas-phase cigarette smoke contains approximately 1×10^{15} radicals per puff, which are primarily of the alkyl, alkoxyl, and peroxyl types (16,17). Another important and highly abundant free radical in cigarette smoke is nitric oxide (•NO) and associated oxides of nitrogen. •NO is present in mainstream cigarette smoke in amounts of up to 500–1000 ppm and probably represents one of the greatest exogenous sources of •NO to which humans are normally and voluntarily exposed. •NO is a species of considerable recent interest, both because it is produced in vivo by nitric oxide synthase (NOS) and has multiple physiological roles and because of its potentially toxic effects when generated in excess (18). Although •NO is perhaps one of the most abundant chemical constituents in cigarette smoke (Table 1), its contribution to the overall toxicity associated with smoking is relatively unknown. The goal of this chapter is to address the possible chemical mechanisms by which •NO can oxidize ascorbate and other components in RTLFs and contribute to the pathogenesis of cigarette smoking.

ANTIOXIDANT COMPOSITION OF RESPIRATORY TRACT LINING FLUIDS

The respiratory tract lining fluids (RTLFs) form an interface between the underlying respiratory tract epithelial cells and the external environment and are the first biological

Table 2 Concentration of Various
Antioxidants in Human Respiratory Tract
Lining Fluid and Blood Plasma

Antioxidant (μM)	RTLF (μM)[a]	Plasma (μM)
Ascorbate	54 ± 15	63 ± 24
Urate	178 ± 9	379 ± 186
Glutathione	181 ± 79	1.0 ± 0.8

[a]Respiratory tract lining fluids (RTLFs) were obtained
from healthy human subjects ($n = 10$) by single-cycle
bronchoalveolar lavage procedure.
Source: Data are derived from van der Vliet et al. (unpublished observations).

fluids to interact with inhaled pollutants such as cigarette smoke (19). These fluids are endowed with a number of antioxidant molecules, including ascorbate, urate, and glutathione (Table 2), which are thought to provide an initial defense against inhaled oxidants. These components are thought to protect both functional constituents of the fluids themselves (antiproteinases and surfactant), as well as the underlying epithelial cells, against free radicals and oxidants that may be presented to the lung either from exogenous sources or from ensuing respiratory tract inflammatory/immune processes. Interest in RTLFs has stemmed partly from the observations that antioxidants such as glutathione (GSH) and ascorbate appear to be subnormal in a variety of disease states where oxidative stress is thought to be an operative factor (20). Since ascorbate and GSH provide the lung with a protective barrier to oxidative stress, an understanding of the reactions that may occur between RTLF antioxidants and nitrogen oxides, major components of cigarette smoke, is important to an understanding of their role in cigarette smoke–mediated toxicity.

FORMATION OF OXIDATIVE SPECIES BY REACTIONS OF NITRIC OXIDE

Although ˙NO is a free radical (possesses an unpaired electron), it displays highly selective reactivity (21). ˙NO does not react directly with many biological molecules; however, its reactions with other free radicals, either in cigarette smoke or with other free radicals present in the lung, are very rapid and are characteristic of typical radical–radical reactions. Thus, the oxidative conversion of ˙NO to more reactive species may be an essential factor associated with cigarette smoke–mediated oxidative reactions in the lung. The following sections demonstrate the chemical reactions which may facilitate the formation of reactive oxidants at the interface between inhaled cigarette smoke and the respiratory tract air-tissue surfaces and address the chemical species capable of oxidizing ascorbate in RTLFs.

Reactions of ˙NO with O_2 in Gas and Aqueous Phases

Since the lung has the highest oxygen tension of all the organs in the body, the oxidation of cigarette smoke–derived ˙NO may be an important pathway for its conversion to a more highly oxidant species. First, ˙NO can react with molecular oxygen (O_2), itself a diradical, in the gas phase to form the highly irritant and oxidizing species nitrogen dioxide (˙NO_2) (22).

$$2^\bullet NO + O_2 \rightarrow 2^\bullet NO_2 \tag{1}$$

Moreover, as $^\bullet NO$ is absorbed into oxygenated aqueous media, such as RTLFs, it reacts with O_2 to produce nitrite (NO_2^-) as the primary product (23) via a complex mechanism thought to involve a number of reactive intermediates (24,25). The individual reactions that are thought to be involved in this mechanism are shown in reactions 2–6.

$$^\bullet NO + O_2 \rightarrow ONOO^\bullet \tag{2}$$

$$ONOO^\bullet + {}^\bullet NO \rightarrow ONOONO \tag{3}$$

$$ONOONO \rightarrow 2^\bullet NO_2 \tag{4}$$

$$^\bullet NO_2 + {}^\bullet NO \rightleftharpoons N_2O_3 \tag{5}$$

$$N_2O_3 + H_2O \rightarrow 2NO_2^- + 2H^+ \tag{6}$$

The overall reaction, balanced stoichiometrically, is represented as follows:

$$4^\bullet NO + O_2 + 2H_2O \rightarrow 4NO_2^- + 4H^+ \tag{7}$$

Kinetic studies have revealed that the rate laws for the gas- and aqueous-phase reactions of $^\bullet NO$ with O_2 are $-d[^\bullet NO]/dt = 2k_g[^\bullet NO]^2[O_2]$ (22) and $-d[^\bullet NO]dt = 4k_{aq}[^\bullet NO]^2[O_2]$ (26–28), respectively, indicating that the reaction is second-order in $^\bullet NO$ and first-order in O_2 in both cases. Thus, at high concentrations of $^\bullet NO$, such as that found in mainstream cigarette smoke, oxidation of $^\bullet NO$ by O_2 would appear to be a significant reaction. These reactions involve the formation of reactive intermediates including $ONOO^\bullet$, $ONOONO$, $^\bullet NO_2$, and N_2O_3 (the latter has reaction characteristics of an "NO^+-like" species). The estimated one-electron reduction potentials of $^\bullet NO$ (Table 3) (29,30) suggest that it is not likely to oxidize substrates such as glutathione and ascorbate directly. However, the intermediates formed by $^\bullet NO$ oxidation possess reduction potentials that predict their ability to oxidize RTLF antioxidants such as ascorbate and GSH (Table 3) (31,32). Thus, it is likely that conversion of inhaled $^\bullet NO$ to more reactive intermediates could contribute to oxidation of RTLF

Table 3 Reduction Potentials for Pairs
of Nitric Oxide–Derived Species and
Extracellular Antioxidants

Redox pair	$E^{\circ\prime}(V)^a$	Reference
$ONOO^-, 2\,H^+/^\bullet NO_2$	+1.40	(30)
$NO^+/^\bullet NO$	+1.21	(29)
$ONOO^-, 2\,H^+/NO_2^-$	+1.20	(30)
$^\bullet NO_2/NO_2^-$	+1.04	(29)
$GS^\bullet/GS^-$	+0.90	(31)
$ONOO^\bullet/ONOO^-$	+0.43	(30)
$^\bullet NO/^3NO^-$	+0.39	(29)
$Asc^{\bullet-}, H^+/Asc^-$	+0.28	(32)
$DehydroAsc/Asc^{\bullet-}$	−0.17	(32)
$^\bullet NO/^1NO^-$	−0.35	(29)
$GSSG/GSSG^{\bullet-}$	−1.50	(32)

^{a}Values are for pH 7.0. $E^{\circ\prime}$, standard one-electron reduction potential (volts).

antioxidants, and this may represent an important mechanism to account for oxidative reactions associated with cigarette smoke.

Reactions of ·NO with Other Cigarette Smoke Components

Over the last several decades, Pryor and coworkers have extensively investigated the production of radical species derived from cigarette smoke (16,17). They have proposed a steady-state mechanism to explain radical production in cigarette smoke that is based on nitrogen oxide chemical characteristics. As discussed, the first step in this reaction mechanism involves the gas-phase oxidation of ·NO to form $·NO_2$, which subsequently reacts with unsaturated organic compounds (R) in cigarette smoke, such as isoprene, resulting in the formation of carbon-centered radicals (R·). Subsequent reactions of R·, O_2, and ·NO produce organic peroxyl (ROO·) and alkoxyl (RO·) radicals which combine further with ·NO, forming unstable organic nitrates (ROONO) and nitrites (RONO). These species may in fact contribute to oxidative reactions in the respiratory tract of a cigarette smoker, either by direct reactions with biological molecules (e.g., ascorbate) or by decomposition to more reactive free radical species. The significance of such reactions is underscored by the finding that organic nitrites rapidly oxidize ascorbate (33).

Other important species produced in cigarette smoke that may contribute to its oxidizing potential include semiquinone radials ($QH^{·-}$), which are thought to reside primarily in the cigarette tar matrix but likely also exist in both the gas and respirable particulate phases and would be inhaled into the lung, where they are deposited into the RTLFs. Semiquinone radicals exist in equilibrium with a number of quinones (Q) and hydroquinones (QH_2) (17) [(reaction 8)], species which are known to undergo redox cycling involving the reduction of O_2 to form superoxide ($O_2^{·-}$) [(reaction 9)] (34).

$$Q + QH_2 \rightleftharpoons 2H^+ + 2Q^{·-} \tag{8}$$

$$Q^{·-} + O_2 \rightarrow Q + O_2^{·-} \tag{9}$$

Since it is known that ·NO reacts with $O_2^{·-}$ at a near-diffusion-limited rate ($k = 6.7 \times 10^9$ $M^{-1}s^{-1}$) (35) to produce the cytotoxic and highly oxidant species peroxynitrite ($ONOO^-$) [(reaction 10)], this reaction may be important in regard to the oxidizing potential of cigarette smoke. Under physiological conditions $ONOO^-$ ($pK_a = 6.8$) is protonated to form peroxynitrous acid (ONOOH) [(reaction 11)], which is capable of oxidizing antioxidant substances such as ascorbate (36), urate (37), and glutathione (GSH) (38); inducing lipid peroxidation (39); and causing oxidation of amino acids in proteins (40).

$$·NO + O_2^{·-} \rightarrow ONOO^- \tag{10}$$

$$ONOO^- + H^+ \rightleftharpoons ONOOH \tag{11}$$

Although the mechanism by which ONOOH exerts its high reactivity is debated, it is thought to involve products arising from either homolytic fission to form free and solvent caged nitrogen dioxide ($·NO_2$) and hydroxyl radical (·OH) or a vibrationally excited species (*trans*-ONOOH*) (41). In any case, if formed in the lung, ONOOH is a highly reactive species capable of inflicting oxidative damage resulting from cigarette smoking.

In summary, because of their abundance in cigarette smoke and their high reactivity, nitrogen oxides are hypothesized to be significant contributors to oxidative lung injury associated with cigarette smoking.

CIGARETTE SMOKE AND ·NO-MEDIATED OXIDATION
OF ASCORBATE IN HUMAN PLASMA
Effects of Cigarette Smoke on Plasma Constituents

In order to study the interactions of inhaled cigarette smoke with constituents of RTLFs, experiments were designed in which human blood plasma was used as a model extracellular fluid and exposed to the gas phase of cigarette smoke. A 600 ml flask containing 10–20 ml of plasma, a rough estimate of the total volume of RTLFs, was evacuated and cigarette smoke was introduced into the flask, representing a "puff" of smoke. This smoke was then allowed to react with the plasma for various periods of time (1–20 min) and additional puffs were introduced subsequently (42).

Previous studies have demonstrated that exposure of plasma to cigarette smoke results in depletion of plasma antioxidants such as ascorbate, urate, protein thiols, α-tocopherol, carotenoids, and bilirubin (42–44). Ascorbate is the first antioxidant to be depleted in this system (complete depletion was observed after three puffs of cigarette smoke), and α-tocopherol and urate are found to be oxidized only after ascorbate is completely depleted, suggesting that ascorbate is perhaps the most easily oxidizable antioxidant in plasma. Alternatively, ascorbate may be indirectly oxidized by recycling initially oxidized urate and/or α-tocopherol. It was also demonstrated that gas-phase cigarette smoke can induce peroxidation of small amounts of plasma lipids, as indicated by formation of lipid hydroperoxides. Formation of lipid hydroperoxides could be detected only when ascorbate was completely depleted, implicating ascorbate as a critical extracellular antioxidant against cigarette smoke (42). Additionally, exposure of plasma to cigarette smoke was found to result in depletion of thiols (primarily associated with albumin) and formation of protein carbonyls, often used as a general measure of protein oxidation (45). These phenomena are, however, not related to the presence of ascorbate, and more likely reflect modification of thiols by the α,β-unsaturated aldehydes in cigarette smoke (Table 1) (46). Indeed, these effects of cigarette smoke could almost completely be mimicked by exposing plasma to a mixture of unsaturated aldehydes, at levels present in cigarette smoke (45). Also, exposure of plasma to these aldehydes did not result in depletion of ascorbate or peroxidation of plasma lipids. It appears, therefore, that cigarette smoke–induced thiol modification and oxidation of plasma antioxidants and lipids are mediated by independent mechanisms.

A Role for ·NO in Ascorbate Oxidation
by Cigarette Smoke

·NO and related nitrogen oxides are abundant species in cigarette smoke that are capable of inducing oxidation of important extracellular constituents. Indeed, nitrogen oxides such as ·NO$_2$ and ONOO$^-$ are capable of oxidizing critical extracellular antioxidants, lipids, and proteins (37,47), analogous to reactions of cigarette smoke. Moreover, these nitrogen oxides can oxidize and nitrate tyrosine residues in proteins by free radical–mediated mechanisms (48). These modifications were also demonstrated during exposure of tyrosine to cigarette smoke, and the extent of nitration was found to be dependent on the duration of exposure to cigarette smoke (49). Additionally, dityrosine, a product formed by the combination of tyrosyl radicals, is also formed under these reaction conditions and implicates a free radical–mediated mechanism. It is therefore feasible that the oxidation of ·NO may be an important cause of ascorbate oxidation by cigarette smoke.

In order to assess the extent to which ·NO (or oxidation products derived from ·NO) in cigarette smoke could contribute to oxidation of ascorbate in extracellular fluids, we exposed plasma to gas-phase cigarette smoke as described. Exposure of plasma to cigarette smoke resulted in depletion of ascorbate, and the extent of oxidation was found to increase in conjunction with exposure time, ranging from 1 to 10 min (Fig. 1). This suggests that the oxidation of plasma ascorbate by cigarette smoke depends on "aging" of the cigarette smoke. The oxidation of ascorbate was found to coincide with the accumulation of NO_2^- (the end-product of ·NO autoxidation) in the exposed plasma (Fig. 1), indicating that (auto)oxidation of ·NO in cigarette smoke is a causative factor in the oxidation of ascorbate.

The cigarette smoke from the mainstream smoke of one whole cigarette has been reported to contain about 300 μg of ·NO (50). In our experimental model, each puff of cigarette smoke burned approximately one-fourth of a cigarette, corresponding to 75 μg ·NO (2.5 μmol). This is introduced into a 600 ml volume of air (corresponding to 27 mmol, using a gas molar volume of 22.4 L/mol). Thus, the final concentration of ·NO in the

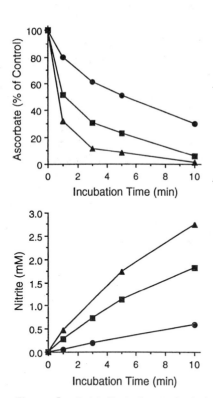

Figure 1 Oxidation of ascorbate by gas-phase cigarette smoke. Plasma (10 ml) was exposed to 1 (●), 2 (■), or 3 (▲) puffs of cigarette smoke in 600 ml flasks and allowed to react with each puff for the indicated period at 37°C: Above, remaining ascorbate was measured using HPLC with electrochemical detection (51) and expressed as a percentage of the initial ascorbate concentration (70.3 μM); below, accumulation of NO_2^- was measured using Griess reagent after exposure of plasma to cigarette smoke under similar conditions. HPLC, high-performance liquid chromatography.

exposure apparatus was approximately 100 ppm. In order to assess the contribution of ˙NO to cigarette smoke–mediated ascorbate oxidation, we exposed plasma to "puffs" of ˙NO by introducing 25 ml aliquots of ˙NO (3000 ppm in N_2) into the 600 ml flask, resulting in a final concentration of approximately 125 ppm ˙NO, similar to the estimated concentration of ˙NO in the cigarette smoke experiments. Exposure of plasma to this concentration of ˙NO was found to result in depletion of ascorbate. Figure 2 shows the chromatographic separation of plasma urate and ascorbate analyzed by high-performance liquid chromatography (HPLC) with electrochemical detection according to Frei et al. (51) and illustrates that exposure to ˙NO results in a time-dependent oxidation of ascorbate. Depletion of plasma ascorbate by ˙NO is quantitatively presented in Fig. 3, which demonstrates that ascorbate oxidation by ˙NO alone is considerably less extensive than that of cigarette smoke containing comparable levels of ˙NO (Fig. 1). Accumulation of NO_2^- during exposure of plasma to these levels of ˙NO was also substantially lower than that observed after exposure to cigarette smoke (Fig. 3), indicating that oxidation of ˙NO in air occurs at a much lower rate than in cigarette smoke. A significant difference between cigarette smoke and ˙NO alone is that the former is rich in organic materials and numerous other radicals which catalyze ˙NO oxidation, which may account for the differences in the accumulation of NO_2^- and extent of ascorbate oxidation in these two systems. Moreover, a number of other components in cigarette smoke including organic nitrates and nitrites may contribute to ascorbate oxidation, as these types of reactions have been shown to occur using model alkyl nitrites (33).

The extent of ascorbate oxidation by either cigarette smoke or ˙NO exposure was linearly related to the concentration of NO_2^- accumulated in the exposed plasma (Fig. 4). This suggests that (auto)oxidation of ˙NO is an important reaction leading to ascorbate oxidation, and that this accounts for a significant fraction of the ascorbate oxidized by cigarette smoke. The fact that the extent of ascorbate oxidation relative to NO_2^- accumulation is higher with cigarette smoke than with ˙NO alone (Fig. 4) indicates that additional

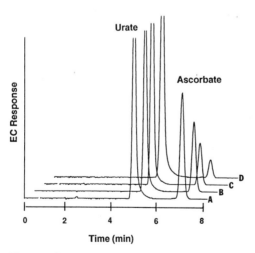

Figure 2 HPLC chromatograms representing oxidation of ascorbate by ˙NO. Plasma (before and after exposure to ˙NO) was analyzed by HPLC with EC detection: Trace A, untreated plasma; traces B, C, and D, plasma exposed to three "puffs" of ˙NO and incubated at 37°C for 1, 5, or 10 min, respectively. HPLC, high-performance liquid chromatography; EC, electrochemical.

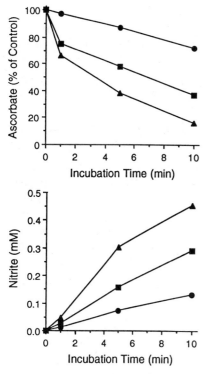

Figure 3 Oxidation of plasma ascorbate by exposure to ·NO. Plasma (10 ml) was exposed to 1 (●), 2 (■), or 3 (▲) 25 ml ''puffs'' of ·NO (3000 ppm in N_2) in 600 ml flasks (legend as in Fig. 1) for the incubated period: above, remaining ascorbate, or below, accumulated NO_2^- was measured as described in the legend to Fig. 1. Initial ascorbate concentration (control) was 67.7 μM.

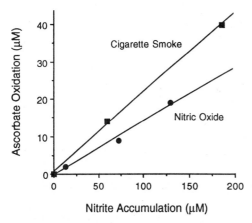

Figure 4 Correlation between ascorbate oxidation and NO_2^- accumulation by cigarette smoke or nitric oxide (·NO). Plasma was exposed to one puff of cigarette smoke or to 25 ml of 3000 ppm ·NO, and the decrease in ascorbate concentration was plotted against the accumulated concentration of NO_2^-.

mechanisms independent of ˙NO-mediated pathways contribute to ascorbate depletion by cigarette smoke. These may include other radical species in cigarette smoke (alkoxyl and peroxyl radicals) and compounds that may reduce oxygen to form superoxide, such as catechols.

Modulation of ˙NO-Induced Ascorbate Oxidation by Thiols

Since thiols, such as GSH, are important antioxidants in both the intra- and extracellular compartments, we hypothesized that these functionalities may modulate ascorbate oxidation by ˙NO. Our first approach was to deplete reduced thiols in plasma before exposure to ˙NO by alkylating the protein thiols with 1 mM N-ethylmaleimide (NEM). Subsequent exposure to ˙NO was found to cause increased depletion of ascorbate as compared to untreated plasma (Fig. 5). Thus, reduced protein thiols appear partly to attenuate the oxidation of ascorbate by ˙NO. Exposure of plasma to three "puffs" of ˙NO resulted in a modest, time-dependent oxidation of protein thiols. After 5 min incubation thiol levels were decreased by 16 μM, consistent with the enhanced ascorbate oxidation by ˙NO after pretreatment of plasma with NEM (Fig. 5).

A major difference between plasma and RTLFs is the concentration of GSH, which is much higher in RTLFs (Table 2). We investigated the possibility that GSH might modulate ascorbate oxidation by ˙NO under our conditions. Buffer solutions of ascorbate (100 μM in 100 mM phosphate, pH 7.4) were exposed to three "puffs" of ˙NO (5 min incubations each) in the absence or presence of various concentrations of GSH (200–1000 μM). The extent of ascorbate oxidation by ˙NO was not significantly affected by GSH at these concentrations (data not shown), a finding which appears inconsistent with the results in plasma containing protein thiols. A possible explanation is that oxidation of GSH by ˙NO (or nitrogen oxides formed during oxidation of ˙NO) results in formation of thiyl radicals. These radicals react rapidly with GS$-$ to form GSSG$^{˙-}$, which can then reduce O_2 to $O_2^{˙-}$. Thus, oxidation of GSH by radical mechanisms may indirectly result in ascorbate oxidation. Furthermore, $O_2^{˙-}$ may combine with ˙NO to form ONOO$^-$, which could also contribute to oxidation of

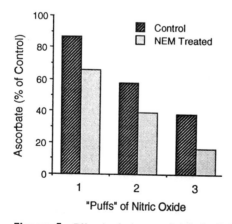

Figure 5 Effect of plasma thiol depletion on ascorbate oxidation by ˙NO. Plasma was exposed to ˙NO before and after depletion of reduced thiols, by preincubation with 1 mM N-ethylmaleimide (NEM), under conditions similar to those illustrated in Fig. 2. Remaining ascorbate was expressed in relation to initial levels (67.7 μM).

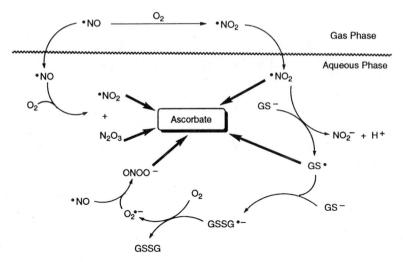

Figure 6 Proposed oxidation mechanisms of ascorbate in respiratory tract lining fluids during ˙NO inhalation.

ascorbate. The various events that may occur during ˙NO oxidation at the RTLF surface are schematically depicted in Fig. 6.

IN VIVO IMPLICATIONS

Since cigarette smoking is associated with recruitment and activation of phagocytes in the lung, which is associated with the production of inflammatory oxidants such as $O_2^{˙-}$, H_2O_2, and hypochlorous acid (HOCl), interactions between these oxidants and cigarette smoke-derived oxides of nitrogen should also be considered among the overall harmful prooxidant effects of smoking. Cigarette smoke–derived ˙NO could react with $O_2^{˙-}$ to form ONOO⁻, a highly oxidant species that could contribute to the oxidation of important biological molecules such as ascorbate and GSH in RTLFs. Moreover, our studies suggest that inhalation of cigarette smoke may cause substantial deposition of NO_2^- in RTLFs, which can also be involved in oxidative reactions. Acidic conditions may arise in the lung, either by intense inflammatory processes or by inhalation of acidifying gases (˙NO$_2$ or SO$_2$), and these conditions may catalyze oxidative reactions of nitrite by forming nitrous acid, a species which can decompose to a variety of reactive nitrogen species capable of oxidizing biomolecules including ascorbate (52). Moreover, we have recently shown that NO_2^- can be oxidized by HOCl at physiological pH to form reactive intermediates, one of which is thought to be nitryl chloride (NO_2Cl) (53). Previously unrecognized oxidant species such as NO_2Cl may thus contribute to cigarette smoke–induced toxicity in vivo.

SUMMARY AND CONCLUSIONS

Although ˙NO and associated nitrogen oxides are highly abundant chemical species in cigarette smoke, their role in oxidative stress associated with cigarette smoking is poorly defined and has received relatively little attention. Since these species are capable of oxidizing various biological constituents, we have hypothesized that nitrogen oxides can contribute importantly to the oxidative airway injury thought to be present in smokers. In fact, our results reported in this chapter indicate that oxidation of ˙NO to more reactive nitrogen oxides contributes significantly to depletion of ascorbate in extracellular fluids such as RTLFs. It is unclear whether this may have important implications in vivo regarding maintenance of ascorbate levels in RTLFs, as various mechanisms exist to recycle or restore extracellular ascorbate. However, these nitrogen oxides could represent a significant oxidant burden to the lung, especially in patients with inflammatory lung diseases, such as adult respiratory distress syndrome, cystic fibrosis, or asthma. Indeed, our findings are consistent with reports showing decreased airway and/or systemic levels of ascorbate in cigarette smokers.

Since ˙NO inhalation is now thought to be a useful therapeutic modality for the treatment of selected adults and preterm babies with respiratory distress syndromes and in selected cases of pulmonary hypertension and heart failure, our results may also have important implications for patients undergoing such treatment. Therapeutic doses of ˙NO used in these treatments may range from 5 to 80 ppm, and our studies demonstrate that similar levels could present an oxidative insult, as indicated by ascorbate depletion. The question may arise whether ascorbate levels in these patients should be monitored and/or whether these patients should be supplemented with ascorbate during treatment to maintain sufficient ascorbate levels in the respiratory tract. Further clinical studies seem warranted to address this important issue.

ACKNOWLEDGMENTS

The authors acknowledge a grant from the Cigarette and Tobacco Surtax Fund of the State of California (grant 1RT28) and NIH (grant HL 47628). JPE is a recipient of a research training fellowship from the California Affiliate of the American Lung Association. AvdV is a recipient of a postdoctoral fellowship from the California Affiliate of the American Heart Association, and is currently a Parker B. Francis Fellow in Pulmonary Research. We are grateful to Drs. William A. Pryor, Roland Stocker, and Balz Frei, and to our colleagues Drs. Lester Packer and Barry Halliwell for many helpful discussions concerning cigarette smoke bioreactivity.

REFERENCES

1. Evans MD, Pryor WA. Cigarette smoking, emphysema, and damage to α_1-proteinase inhibitor. Am J Physiol 1994; 266:L593–611.
2. Cantin A, Crystal RG. Oxidants, antioxidants and the pathogenesis of emphysema. Eur J Respir Dis 1985; 139(suppl):7–17.
3. Doll R, Peto R. Cigarette smoking and bronchial carcinoma: dose and time relationships among regular smokers and lifelong non-smokers. J Epidemiol Community Health 1978; 32: 303–313.
4. Kannel WB. Update on the role of cigarette smoking in coronary artery disease. Am Heart J 1981; 101:319–328.
5. Lakier JB. Smoking and cardiovascular disease. Am J Med 1992; 93:8S–12S.
6. Calder JH, Curtis RH, Fore H. Comparison of vitamin C in plasma and leukocytes of smokers and nonsmokers. Lancet 1963; 1:556–558.
7. Pelletier O. Vitamin C status of cigarette smokers and nonsmokers. Am J Clin Nutr 1970; 23:520–524.

8. Schectman G, Byrd JC, Gruchow HW. The influence of smoking on vitamin C status in adults. Am J Public Health 1989; 79:158–162.

9. Bui MH, Sauty A, Collet F, Leuenberger P. Dietary vitamin C intake and concentrations in the body fluids and cells of male smokers and nonsmokers. J Nutr 1992; 122:312–316.

10. Pamuk ER, Byers T, Coates RJ, et al. Effect of smoking on serum nutrient concentrations in African-American women. Am J Clin Nutr 1994; 59:891–895.

11. Mezzetti A, Lapenna D, Pierdomenico SD, et al. Vitamins E, C, and lipid peroxidation in plasma and arterial tissue of smokers and non-smokers. Atherosclerosis 1995; 112:91–99.

12. Tribble DL, Giuliano LJ, Fortmann SP. Reduced plasma ascorbic acid concentrations in non-smokers regularly exposed to environmental tobacco smoke. Am J Clin Nutr 1993; 58:886–890.

13. Smith JL, Hodges RE. Serum levels of vitamin C in relation to dietary and supplemental dietary intake of vitamin C in smokers and nonsmokers. Ann NY Acad Sci 1987; 498:144–151.

14. Kallner AB, Hartmann D, Hornig DH. On the requirements of ascorbic acid in man: steady-state turnover and body pools in smokers. Am J Clin Nutr 1981; 34:1347–1355.

15. Morrow JD, Frei B, Longmire AW, et al. Increase in circulating products of lipid peroxidation (F_2)-isoprostanes in smokers: smoking as a cause of oxidative damage. N Engl J Med 1995; 332:1198–1203.

16. Church DF, Pryor WA. Free-radical chemistry of cigarette smoke and its toxicological implications. Environ Health Perspect 1985; 64:111–126.

17. Pryor WA, Stone K. Oxidants in cigarette smoke: radicals, hydrogen peroxide, peroxynitrate and peroxynitrite. Ann NY Acad Sci 1993; 686:12–27.

18. Änggård E. Nitric oxide: mediator, murderer, and medicine. Lancet 1994; 343:1199–1206.

19. Hatch GE. Comparative biochemistry of the airway lining fluid. In: RA Parent, ed. Treatise on Pulmonary Toxicology. Vol. 1. Comparative Biology of the Normal Lung. Boca Raton, FL: CRC Press 1992:617–632.

20. Cross CE, van der Vliet A, O'Neill CA, et al. Oxidants, antioxidants, and respiratory tract lining fluids. Environ Health Perspect 1994; 102(suppl 10):185–191.

21. Stamler JS, Singel DJ, Loscalzo J. Biochemistry of nitric oxide and its redox-active forms. Science 1992; 258:1898–1902.

22. Huie RE. The reaction kinetics of NO_2. Toxicology 1994; 89:193–216.

23. Ignarro LJ, Fukuto JM, Griscavage JM, et al. Oxidation of nitric oxide in aqueous solution to nitrite but not nitrate: comparison with enzymatically formed nitric oxide from L-arginine. Proc Natl Acad Sci USA 1993; 90:8103–8107.

24. Wink DA, Darbyshire JF, Nims RW, et al. Reactions of the bioregulatory agent nitric oxide in oxygenated aqueous media: determination of the kinetics for oxidation and nitrosation by intermediates generated in the NO/O_2 reaction. Chem Res Toxicol 1993; 6:23–27.

25. Goldstein S, Czapski G. Kinetics of nitric oxide autoxidation in aqueous solution in the absence and presence of various reductants: the nature of the oxidizing intermediates. J Am Chem Soc 1995; 117:12078–12084.

26. Lewis RS, Deen WM. Kinetics of the reaction of nitric oxide with oxygen in aqueous solutions. Chem Res Toxicol 1994; 7:568–574.

27. Ford PC, Wink DA, Stanbury DM. Autoxidation kinetics of aqueous nitric oxide. FEBS Lett 1993; 326:1–3.

28. Kharitonov VG, Sundquist AR, Sharma VS. Kinetics of nitric oxide autoxidation in aqueous solution. J Biol Chem 1994; 269:5881–5883.

29. Stanbury DM. Reduction potentials involving inorganic free radicals in aqueous solution. Adv Inorg Chem 1989; 33:69–138.

30. Koppenol WH, Moreno JJ, Pryor WA, et al. Peroxynitrite, a cloaked oxidant formed by nitric oxide and superoxide. Chem Res Toxicol 1992; 5:834–842.

31. Surdhar PS, Armstrong DA. Reduction potentials and exchange reactions of thiyl radicals and disulfide anion radicals. J Phys Chem 1987; 91:6532–6537.

32. Buettner GR. The pecking order of free radicals and antioxidants: lipid peroxidation, α-tocopherol, and ascorbate. Arch Biochem Biophys 1993; 300:535–543.

33. Leis JR, Ríos A. Fast formation of NO in reactions of alkyl nitrites with ascorbic acid and analogues. J Chem Soc 1995: 169–170.

34. Nakayama T, Church DF, Pryor WA. Quantitative analysis of the hydrogen peroxide formed in aqueous cigarette tar extracts. Free Radical Biol Med 1989; 7:9–15.

35. Huie RE, Padmaja S. The reaction of NO with superoxide. Free Radical Res Commun 1993; 18:195–199.

36. Bartlett D, Church DF, Bounds PL, Koppenol WH. The kinetics of the oxidation of L-ascorbic acid by peroxynitrite. Free Radical Biol Med 1995; 18:85–92.

37. Van der Vliet A, Smith D, O'Neill CA, et al. Interactions of peroxynitrite with human plasma and its constituents: oxidative damage and antioxidant depletion. Biochem J 1994; 303: 295–301.

38. Radi R, Beckman JS, Bush KM, Freeman BA. Peroxynitrite oxidation of sulfhydryls: the cytotoxic potential of superoxide and nitric oxide. J Biol Chem 1991; 266:4244–4250.

39. Radi R, Beckman JS, Bush KM, Freeman BA. Peroxynitrite-induced membrane lipid peroxidation: the cytotoxic potential of superoxide and nitric oxide. Arch Biochem Biophys 1991; 288:481–487.

40. Ischiropoulos H, Al-Mehdi AB. Peroxynitrite-mediated oxidative protein modifications. FEBS Lett 1995; 364:279–282.

41. Pryor WA, Squadrito GL. The chemistry of peroxynitrite: a product from the reaction of nitric oxide with superoxide. Am J Physiol 1995; 268:L699–L722.

42. Frei B, Forte TM, Ames BN, Cross CE. Gas phase oxidants of cigarette smoke induce lipid peroxidation and changes in lipoprotein properties in human blood plasma: protective effects of ascorbic acid. Biochem J 1991; 277:133–138.

43. Eiserich JP, van der Vliet A, Handelman GJ, et al. Dietary antioxidants and cigarette smoke-induced biomolecular damage: a complex interaction. Am J Clin Nutr 1995; 62(suppl):1490S–1500S.

44. Handelman GJ, Packer L, Cross CE. Destruction of tocopherols, carotenoids, and retinol in human plasma by cigarette smoke. Am J Clin Nutr 1996; 63:559–565.

45. Reznick AZ, Cross CE, Hu M-L, et al. Modification of plasma proteins by cigarette smoke as measured by protein carbonyl formation. Biochem J 1992; 286:607–611.

46. Brenner JF, Proceedings of Tobacco and Health Conference, Report 2. Lexington, KY: University of Kentucky, Tobacco and Health Institute, 1970.

47. Halliwell B, Hu M-L, Louie S. Interaction of nitrogen dioxide with human plasma: antioxidant depletion and oxidative damage. FEBS Lett 1992; 313:62–66.

48. Van der Vliet A, Eiserich JP, O'Neill CA, et al. Tyrosine modification by reactive nitrogen species: a closer look. Arch Biochem Biophys 1995; 319:341–349.

49. Eiserich JP, Vossen V, O'Neill CA, et al. Molecular mechanisms of damage by excess nitrogen oxides: nitration of tyrosine by gas-phase cigarette smoke. FEBS Lett 1994; 353:53–56.

50. Cueto R, Pryor WA. Cigarette Smoke chemistry: conversion of nitric oxide to nitrogen dioxide and reactions of nitrogen oxides with other smoke components as studied by fourier transform infrared spectroscopy. Vibrational Spectroscopy 1994; 7:97–111.

51. Frei B, England L, Ames BN. Ascorbate is an outstanding antioxidant in human blood plasma. Proc Natl Acad Sci USA 1989; 86:6377–6381.

52. Tannenbaum SR, Mergens W. Reaction of nitrite with vitamins C and E. Ann NY Acad Sci 1980; 355:267–277.

53. Eiserich JP, Cross CE, Jones AD, et al. Formation of nitrating and chlorinating species by reaction of nitrite with hypochlorous acid: a novel mechanism for nitric oxide-mediated protein modification. J Biol Chem 1996; 271:19199–19208.

24

Vitamin C and Cigarette Smoke Exposure

CHING K. CHOW
University of Kentucky, Lexington, Kentucky

INTRODUCTION

Epidemiological and experimental evidence has implicated cigarette smoke exposure as a significant contributing factor in causing many degenerative diseases (1–7). Among them, increased risk of developing heart disease, lung cancer, pulmonary emphysema, and chronic bronchitis are the most serious diseases that have been attributed to smoke exposure. Smokers have a much higher mortality rate attributable to lung cancer, bronchitis, and emphysema in men than nonsmokers (2,3). Also, coronary thrombosis and myocardial infarction are more prevalent, and the death rate from coronary heart disease for both men and women is much higher in smokers than in nonsmokers (3,4). In addition, cigarette smoke exposure is associated with higher secretion of adrenal hormones, decreased birth weight of children, and higher death rate from peptic ulcer (3,5,8). While the mechanisms by which cigarette smoke exposure cause these increased risks are not yet understood, an imbalance of oxidative stress and antioxidant potential of smokers may account, in part, for the increased risk of these diseases among smokers (9,10).

If increased oxidative stress is a consequence of cigarette smoke exposure, the status of antioxidant nutrients may modulate the pathophysiological characteristics of cigarette smoking. On the other hand, the nutritional status and requirement for antioxidant nutrients may be altered after exposure to cigarette smoke. During the past decade, many studies dealing with the cellular effects of cigarette smoke exposure have been reported. This chapter deals primarily with the oxidative damage induced by cigarette smoke exposure and its interaction with vitamin C in human and animal studies.

CIGARETTE SMOKE EXPOSURE AND
OXIDATIVE DAMAGE

The chief reason that the underlying mechanisms by which cigarette smoke exposure is involved in the development of various disorders remain poorly understood is due to the complex nature of cigarette smoke. Cigarette smoke is a complex mixture containing numerous compounds. Over one thousand constituents of cigarette smoke, including nicotine, phenols, acetaldehyde, and cadmium, have been identified (11,12). Also, many free radicals, oxidants, or prooxidants are found in the smoke. Fresh cigarette smoke, for example, contains very high concentrations of oxides of nitrogen (9,13). Two different populations of free radicals, one in the tar and one in the gas phase, of cigarette smoke have been identified (13,14). The principal radical in the tar phase, a quinone/hydroquinone complex, is capable of reducing molecular oxygen to superoxide radicals, which may eventually lead to the generation of hydrogen peroxide as well as highly reactive peroxynitrite and hydroxyl radicals. The gas phase of cigarette smoke contains small oxygen- and carbon-centered radicals that are much more reactive than are the tar-phase radicals. Additionally, nitrogen dioxide formed in the flame may interact with other smoke components and generate more reactive species. Thus, cigarette smoke contains various oxidants, free radicals, and metastable products derived from radical reactions that may react with or inactivate essential cellular constituents.

Oxidative damage resulting from cigarette smoke exposure may also be mediated indirectly through inflammatory reactions. It has been well documented that cigarette smoke exposure induces an inflammatory response, as evidenced by the pulmonary accumulation of macrophages and neutrophils (15,16). In smokers, the cumulative smoking history is highly correlated with both leukocytosis and elevation of acute-phase reactants (16). In addition, cigarette smoke exposure causes an increase in oxidative metabolism of macrophages and neutrophils (17–20). Smokers have a greater number of lavageable cells than nonsmokers and exhibit significantly higher proportions of polymorphonuclear neutrophils and lymphocytes in their bronchoalveolar lavage cells (21–23). Alveolar macrophages, which account for most of the increase in lavageable cells from smokers, have the ability to release increased amounts of reactive oxygen species (17,18) and have higher levels of lysosomal enzymes (24,25). The increased oxidative metabolism of phagocytes is accompanied by increased generation of reactive oxygen species, such as hydrogen peroxide, nitric oxide, hydroxyl radicals, and superoxide radicals. Also, smokers have higher neutrophil myeloperoxidase activity than nonsmokers (26). Hydrogen peroxide and a myeloperoxidase product, hypochlorous acid, may be generated in biologically relevant quantities (27). These agents, if released extracellularly, can damage host tissue cells. Localized generation and extracellular release of superoxide, nitric oxide, hydrogen peroxide, and hypochlorous acid may overwhelm intrinsic antioxidant defenses and lead to oxidative injury to tissue cells. Hypochlorous acid, for example, may cause tissue damage indirectly by potentiating the extracellular proteolytic activity of neutrophil-derived protease, elastase, collagenase, and gelatinase, which attack key components of the extracellular matrix (26,27). Thus, smokers are subjected to not only oxidative stress resulting from oxidants and free radicals present in smoke but also reactive oxygen species generated by increased number of activated phagocytes. However, it should be noted that while activated phagocytes, mitochondria, and many other metabolic reactions are capable of generating reactive oxygen species, oxidative damage is usually self-limiting or prevented, under normal conditions, by various biological antioxidant mechanisms (28,29).

Results obtained from many in vitro studies support the view that exposure to the components of cigarette smoke can cause oxidative damage. For example, incubation of sonicated rabbit alveolar macrophages and pulmonary protective factor with an aqueous extract of cigarette smoke results in increased formation of lipid peroxidation products (30). An unidentified factor in cigarette smoke has been shown to oxidize thiols (31). Also, following activation with the synthetic chemotactic tripeptide N-formylmethionine-leucyl-phenylalanine, potentiated by cytochalasin B, blood neutrophils from smokers inflicted increased damage to the deoxyribonucleic acid (DNA) of cocultured mononuclear leukocytes and the damage to DNA was preventable by the inclusion of superoxide dismutase and catalase, individually or in combination (32). The latter report suggests that cigarette smoke exposure may prime phagocytes to generate increased amounts of potentially carcinogenic reactive oxidants.

Whether cigarette smoke induces free radical lipid peroxidation remains unclear, however. Bielicki et al. (33), for example, have shown that exposure of plasma to cigarette smoke for 6 h had no effect on the levels of lipid peroxidation products, determined as thiobarbituric acid reactants (TBARs), and ratio of arachidonic acid to palmitic acid, but treatment with 0.5 mM copper for 6 h caused a 3.0-, 4.0-, and 1.4-fold increase in TBARs, and a 17%, 25%, and 13% reduction in the ratio of arachidonic acid to palmitic acid in very low density lipoprotein (VLDL), LDL, and HDL fractions, respectively. The results obtained from this study suggest that unlike copper, cigarette smoke–induced inhibition of plasma enzyme activity is not resulting from free radical–induced lipid peroxidation.

An oxidative damage mechanism has been implicated to the development of lung cancer, emphysema, and other smoking-related disorders. For example, oxidative inactivation of alpha-1-antiprotease (antielastase or antitrypsin) is associated with the increased incidence of emphysema in smokers (9,13). However, whether increased oxidative damage is a consequence of cigarette smoke exposure in human subjects is not entirely clear. On the one hand, smokers have been shown to exhale significantly higher levels of breath pentane than nonsmokers, and supplement with vitamin E (800 mg/day for 2 weeks) decreases exhaled pentane in smokers (34). Also, smokers have higher levels of intracellular and extracellular chemiluminescence, an indicator for the release of reactive oxidants (20), and of plasma-conjugated dienes than nonsmokers. Furthermore, smokers have higher levels of 8-hydroxydeoxyguanosine, one of the oxidation products of DNA, in peripheral leukocytes (35), and supplementation of alpha-tocopherol and beta-carotene protect rats against ischemia/reperfusion injury to the heart caused by smoke exposure (36). Those studies support the oxidative damage mechanism of cigarette smoke. On the other hand, smokers have lower levels of lipid hydroperoxides in bronchoalveolar lavage fluid than nonsmokers (37), and the production of oxygen free radicals by neutrophils is decreased after exposure to nicotine and cotinine (38). Also, the levels of lipid peroxidation products, TBARs, in freshly isolated low-density lipoprotein (LDL) (39) or plasma (35) of smokers and nonsmokers are not different. The higher levels of TBARs found in the oxidized LDL of smokers than in nonsmokers appear to reflect lower levels of vitamin E in LDL of smokers, rather than the consequence of smoke exposure (39).

Several animal studies have been conducted to determine whether increased oxidative damage in the primary target lung tissue is a consequence of cigarette smoke exposure. The levels of lipid peroxidation products, TBARs, are found to be either decreased or unchanged, rather than increased, in the lungs of rats exposed to cigarette smoke as compared with those exposed to sham smoke (40,41). Thus, despite the possible attack by many free radicals and oxidants, increased formation of lipid peroxidation products did not seem to occur in the pulmonary tissue of animals exposed to cigarette smoke. The apparent lack of increased formation of lipid peroxidation products in the lung or bronchoalveolar lavage fluid of rats exposed to cigarette smoke has been attributed partly to the increased levels of antioxidant systems, including vitamin E, in the lungs (42–44).

The adaptive response of augmented antioxidant systems may serve to resist further damage or limit oxidant-mediated damage to alveolar structure. In addition to the levels of vitamin E (42,43) the activities of antioxidant enzymes have been shown to increase after cigarette smoke exposure. McCuster et al. (45), for example, have shown that the activities of superoxide dismutase and catalase from alveolar macrophages of smokers and smoke-exposed hamsters are twice that found in control subjects, but there is no change in the activity of GSH peroxidase. Also, smoke-exposed hamsters have prolonged survival in normobaric hyperoxia ($> 95\%$ O_2) than the controls (45). Additionally, smokers have higher pulmonary activity of DT-diaphorase, which catalyzes the two-electron reduction of quinones to less harmful hydroquinones, than nonsmokers (46).

VITAMIN C AND CIGARETTE SMOKE EXPOSURE

As mentioned, information obtained from many in vitro and cell culture studies generally supports the view that cigarette smoke is capable of inducing oxidative damage. The information available also suggests that vitamin C (ascorbic acid) can interact directly with the components of cigarette smoke, although it is not clear which component(s) in the smoke preferentially interacts with vitamin C. Exposure of human plasma to the gaseous phase of cigarette smoke, but not to whole smoke, causes lipid peroxidation and protein oxidation (47). Endogenous ascorbic acid has been shown to protect against oxidation of lipids, but not of protein (48). Also, aldehydes in cigarette smoke do not cause a depletion of plasma ascorbic acid or alpha-tocopherol and do not induce plasma lipid peroxidation (49). As aldehydes decrease plasma protein sulfhydryl concentrations and increase protein carbonyls, it is suggestive that thiols, GSH, and dihydrolipoic acid, but not vitamin C, may reduce aldehyde-induced protein modification.

Whether vitamin C and other antioxidants are capable of inhibiting cigarette-smoke–induced cytotoxicity has been examined. Exposure of tyrosine to cigarette smoke leads to the formation of 3-nitro- and di-tyrosine, and the conversion is partially inhibited by ascorbic acid, glutathione, and uric acid, suggesting oxides of nitrogen in cigarette smoke can oxidatively modify protein in the respiratory tract (50). Also, Bielicke et al. (33) have shown that exposure of plasma to cigarette smoke has no effect on the levels of TBARs and ratio of arachidonic acid to palmitic acid, while treatment with copper does, and that supplementation of plasma with vitamin C was unable to protect inhibition of lecithin/cholesterol acyltransferase (LCA) activity by cigarette smoke. The findings suggest that the cigarette smoke–induced inhibition of plasma LCA activity is unrelated to free radical–induced lipid peroxidation. Additionally, higher levels of 8-hydroxydeoxyguanosine found in the peripheral leukocytes of smokers suggest cigarette smoke may oxidize DNA. However, ascorbic acid has no effect on the mutagenic activity in *Salmonella typhimurium* TA98 or the clastogensis in mouse bone marrow induced by cigarette smoke (51).

Human Studies

If increased oxidative stress is a consequence of cigarette smoke exposure, the status of vitamin C may modulate the pathophysiological mechanism of cigarette smoke exposure. Also, the nutritional status and requirement for vitamin C may be altered after cigarette smoke exposure, and the nutritional status of vitamin C may mediate the development of smoke exposure–related disorders. Furthermore, increased utilization of vitamin C may be associated with cigarette smoke exposure. Many reports, indeed, have shown that the levels of vitamin C of smokers are lower in plasma and neutrophils while the urinary excretion of vitamin C is higher than in nonsmokers (16,52–57). Increased utilization and/or decreased intake/bioavailability of vitamin C in smokers may be responsible for the lower status of the vitamin.

Many studies have been conducted to determine whether lower intake is responsible for the lower status of plasma vitamin C in smokers. Tribble et al. (54), for example, have shown that hypovitaminosis C (< 23 μmol/L) is found in 24% of active smokers and 12% of passive smokers but none in nonexposed nonsmokers, and that reduced plasma ascorbic acid concentrations are associated with a lower vitamin C intake in smoke-exposed populations only. The findings suggest that chronic smoke exposure, particularly in association with lower vitamin C intake, may reduce ascorbic acid pools in both active and passive smokers. On the other hand, Tappia et al. (55) have shown that smokers have 21% lower plasma vitamin C concentration than nonsmokers despite a similar intake of ascorbic acid by the two groups and that plasma vitamins A and E concentrations are unaffected by the status of smoke exposure. Furthermore, Bui et al. (56) reported that the levels of ascorbic acid contents averaged 91 and 87 μmol/L in plasma, 2.1 and 2.1 μmol/L in mononuclear leukocytes, 3.2 and 1.7 μmol/L in bronchoalveolar lavage fluid, and 3.4 and 1.6 μmol/10^9 cells in alveolar macrophages from healthy male smokers and nonsmokers, respectively, and that the mean daily intake of vitamin C was 116 and 107 mg/day for smokers and nonsmokers, respectively. Those authors suggest that higher levels of ascorbic acid in alveolar macrophage and bronchoalveolar lavage of smokers than in nonsmokers observed may reflect a defensive change against free radicals derived from cigarette smoke.

Whether the nutritional status of vitamin C alters the generation of oxidation products of smokers has been studied. Male smokers have significantly lower arterial (internal mammary artery) and plasma levels of vitamins C and E and higher levels of fluorescent products of lipid peroxidation than nonsmokers (57). As lipid peroxidation products are significantly and inversely related to vitamin C in plasma, and to vitamin E in the tissue, it is suggested that vitamins C and E may be the primary antioxidant in the plasma and arterial tissue compartments, respectively.

If cigarette smoke–induced inflammation and cellular damage are oxidant-mediated, vitamin C may play a protective role. Decreased plasma and leukocyte concentrations of vitamin C have indeed been shown to be associated with increased numbers and activity of neutrophils (58–61). The findings suggest that there is an increased consumption of these micronutrients during neutralization of phagocyte-derived extracellular oxidants, that smokers have a faster rate of vitamin C utilization, and that cigarette smoke exposure might predispose them to enhanced oxidant attack on their lung parenchymal cells.

Efforts to correlate the status of vitamin C with the incidence of smoke exposure–related respiratory diseases have resulted in inconclusive findings. On the one hand, cigarette smoke exposure is associated with increased numbers and prooxidant activity of circulating neutrophils and monocytes, decreased plasma concentrations of vitamin C, and pulmonary dysfunction (62). Also, pulmonary dystrophy in smokers is highly correlated with the extent of generation of oxygen species by activated neutrophils (20). Additionally, Schwartz and Weiss (63) have shown that dietary vitamin C intake is positively and significantly associated with the level of FEV1. However, interaction between vitamin C intake and extent of smoke exposure and/or respiratory disease is not significant. Also, no significant correlation is found between plasma vitamin C levels and indices of smoking effects, such as pulmonary function abnormalities and cytogenetic changes. On the other hand, Richards et al. (20) have observed that pulmonary dystrophy in smokers was highly correlated with the extent of generation of oxygen species by activated neutrophils, but the plasma levels of vitamin C, vitamin E, and beta-carotene are not correlated with the release of reactive oxidants from circulating phagocyte or spirometric abnormalities in cigarette smokers (58).

Vitamin C status has been linked to the extent of oxidative damage in phagocytes. Van Antwerpen et al. (64), for example, have shown that smokers have higher levels of phorbol-12-myristate-13-acetate– (PMA-) activated luminol-enhanced chemiluminescence in whole blood, indicating cigarette smoke exposure sensitizes blood phagocytes to generate increased amount of reactive oxygen species. The levels of plasma vitamin C were significantly lower in smokers who work in mines, but not those associated with university work, than in nonsmokers. The discrepancy is likely due to differences in socioeconomic- and life-style-related vitamin C intake. Also, van Poppel et al. (65) have shown that smokers have higher sister chromatid exchanges (SCEs) levels in lymphocytes and lower levels of plasma beta-carotene and blood vitamin C. However, SCEs are weakly correlated with plasma cotinine, and micronuclei are not correlated with cotinine or antioxidants in smokers.

Animal Studies

The lung is vulnerable to injury from a variety of environmental agents, including cigarette smoke, because its airway and alveolar surface are directly exposed to the external environment. Animal studies allow for examining the cellular effect of cigarette smoke exposure on the pulmonary tissue, a process which is not feasible in human studies. However, no simple conclusion can be drawn even from a well-defined animal experiment. This is because there are a large number and variety of components present in cigarette smoke. Also, differences in species, age, sex, and nutritional status of experimental animals, as well as types of cigarette and exposure conditions employed, have made the task difficult to accomplish. For example, while an increase in free cell population in bronchoalveolar lavage has been found in experimental animals exposed to cigarette smoke, there is a species-dependent response to cigarette smoke. An onset of inflammatory cell response in mice exposed to cigarette smoke occurs within 6 weeks, compared to none in rats, suggesting a greater susceptibility of mice to cigarette smoke (66). Also, a more pronounced murine macrophage response to cigarette smoke has been demonstrated by morphometric analysis of lung tissue (67), and increased numbers of phagocytes are recovered in the lavage fluid of Syrian hamsters exposed to cigarette smoke (68).

Additionally, animals of different age and sex have been either maintained on a commercial chow diet or fed a synthetic diet for various lengths of time. For these animals the nutrition status of vitamin C differs unless they are maintained on the same chemically defined diet. To make the situation even more complicated, experimental animals have been exposed to whole smoke, the gaseous phase of the smoke, with or without sham smoke or unhandled room controls. Besides, animals have been exposed to different strengths (degree of dilution) of cigarette smoke generated from different types of smoke machines or exposed to mainstream (active) or sidestream (passive) smoke (69,70). Furthermore, animals have been exposed to a dose ranging from 1 to over 100 puffs of cigarette smoke in one or more sessions daily for only 1 day or up to 1 year or longer. Different types of cigarettes have very different levels of nicotine and other chemical constituents. It is, therefore, not surprising that varying results were obtained from a limited number of animal studies.

Partly because of the difficulty in deriving easily interpretable data only a few animal studies have aimed to determine the role of vitamin C in relation to the cellular effect of cigarette smoke exposure. The ability of rodents, the most commonly utilized experimental animals, to synthesize ascorbic acid further undercuts the usefulness of data obtained.

Similarly to the human studies, the plasma levels of ascorbic acid were lower in rats exposed acutely to cigarette smoke for 3–7 days than in the sham-exposed group, and the degree of decline was relatively greater in animals fed a vitamin E–deficient diet than in the supplemented group (40,71). Vitamin E supplement appears to aid in maintaining higher levels of plasma ascorbic acid in rats exposed to cigarette smoke. On the other hand, the levels of ascorbic acid were significantly increased in the lungs of animals on vitamin E–deficient diet, but not in supplemented animals, after exposure to acute cigarette smoke. It appears that increased amounts of ascorbic acid may be synthesized by cigarette-smoked rats to meet an increased need. A stimulation of hepatic ascorbic acid biosynthesis in rats and mice has been reported after exposure to various xenobiotics (72,73).

However, the levels of ascorbic acid in the plasma, liver, lungs, kidneys, or broncho-alveolar lavage fluid of rats exposed to cigarette smoke (mainstream, sidestream, or sham), 10 puffs daily for 16, 24, or 65 weeks, are not significantly different from those of room controls (42,44). As rodents are capable of synthesizing ascorbic acid, the lack of effect on ascorbic acid status after chronic cigarette smoke exposure suggests an adaptive change. Similarly, Bilimoria and Ecobichon (74) have shown that 0–6 h after acute exposure of adult rats to cigarette smoke (40–240 puffs), no reductions of ascorbic acid were observed in the blood, lung, liver, kidney, heart, and bladder at any exposure levels.

Several studies have shown that the nutritional status of vitamin C plays a role in attenuating the cellular effects of cigarette smoke exposure. For example, Sohn et al. (75) have shown that exposure of rats to cigarette smoke for 30 days resulted in mild histological changes in trachea and lungs. Also, the levels of TBARs and activities of super-oxide dismutase, catalase, and glutathione peroxidase were increased in the lung, while total sulfhydryl content was decreased in the exposed animals. Those changes were found to be attenuated by supplementing ascorbic acid (75). Using intravital fluorescent microscopy and scanning electron microscopy, Lehr et al. (76) have demonstrated in hamsters that cigarette smoke–induced leukocyte adhesion is not confined to the microcirculation, but that leukocytes also adhere singly and in clusters to the aortic endothelium; that cigarette smoke induces the formation in the bloodstream of aggregates between leukocytes and platelets; and that cigarette smoke–induced leukocyte adhesion to microvascular and macrovascular endothelium and leukocyte–platelet aggregate formation are preventable by dietary or intravenous pretreatment of vitamin C, but not by vitamin E or probucol. The findings suggest vitamin C contributes to protection from cigarette smoke–associated cardiovascular and pulmonary diseases in humans independently of its antioxidant function.

Guinea pigs, like humans, cannot synthesize ascorbic acid. In a study using guinea pigs as experimental animals, the levels of vitamin C in plasma, liver, kidneys, and lungs were found not to differ significantly among animal groups exposed to mainstream smoke, sidestream smoke, sham smoke, or room air twice (2 cigarettes per session at 10 puffs per person) daily for 17 or 20 weeks (43). Similarly, Bilimoria and Ecobichon (74) have shown that 0–6 h after acute exposure of adult Hartley guinea pigs to cigarette smoke (40–240 puffs), no reductions of ascorbic acid were observed in the blood, lung, liver, kidney, heart, and bladder at any exposure levels. The failure to demonstrate a decreased level of vitamin C in the lung of guinea pigs following cigarette smoke exposure is unexpected. However, the guinea pigs employed were fed a nutritionally adequate diet, and sufficient ascorbic acid from the diet may have been available to replenish the vitamin consumed. If those guinea pigs had been placed on a diet deficient or inadequate in vitamin C, the consequence of smoke exposure might have been different.

Since the respiratory system is the primary target of cigarette smoke, the vitamin C content of pulmonary tissue is likely to be adversely affected by exposure to it. The ability of guinea pigs to maintain normal levels of vitamin C observed in the lungs after chronic cigarette exposure (43,74) suggests an adaptive response that may protect pulmonary tissues against oxidative damage. As guinea pigs cannot synthesize vitamin C, a portion of vitamin C found in the lungs of smoke-exposed animals may result from mobilization of body stores. More studies, however, are needed to determine whether adaptive changes in vitamin C metabolism occur in guinea pigs after cigarette smoke exposure.

A functional interrelationship between vitamin C and other nutrients, notably vitamin E, selenium, iron, niacin, and sulfur-containing amino acids, has been recognized (28,29, 77,78). In addition to being an important water-soluble reducing agent and scavenger for free radicals and singlet oxygen (77), vitamin C has been shown to play a role in the regeneration of vitamin E (79–82) and to involve in modulation of iron status and metabolism (77,83). On the other hand, the reducing agents reduced nicotinamide-adenine dinucleotide (NADH) and reduced glutathione (GSH) seem to involve in the regeneration of vitamin C (29,84). Thus, to understand better the cellular function of vitamin C in cigarette smoke exposure, it is necessary to examine the status of those interacting compounds in smokers, too.

SUMMARY AND CONCLUSION

Cigarette smoke contains a large number of compounds, including many oxidants and free radicals that are capable of initiating and/or promoting oxidative damage. Also, oxidative damage may result from reactive oxygen species generated by increased and activated phagocytes after cigarette smoke exposure. The oxidative damage mechanism resulting from exposure to cigarette smoke has been implicated as playing a role in the pathogenesis of degenerative diseases. Results obtained from in vitro and cell culture studies generally support the hypothesis that increased oxidative damage, such as lipid peroxidation and oxidation of protein and DNA, is a consequence of cigarette smoke exposure.

As smoke exposure increases oxidative stress, vitamin C status may be adversely affected directly by smoke constituents, and indirectly by smoking-induced inflammation. Cigarette smoke exposure may also affect the intake, absorption, transport, utilization, turnover, and/or excretion of vitamin C. Also, the nutritional status of vitamin C may play a role in modulating the action and metabolism of smoke components. Data obtained from animal and human studies are generally supportive of the hypothesis that cigarette smoke interacts with vitamin C. However, whether increased lipid peroxidation or oxidative damage is a consequence of cigarette smoke exposure is not entirely clear. The adaptive responses, such as accumulation of vitamin E and increased activity of antioxidant enzymes in the lung and alveolar macrophages of smokers, may be responsible for the lack of clear evidence of lipid peroxidation or oxidative damage in in vivo studies. Because of the complexity of smoking exposure and lack of sensitive and specific methods for measuring lipid peroxidation products, the role of vitamin C and oxidative damage in causing smoking-related disorders remains to be elucidated. However, results obtained from many human and animal studies suggest that vitamin C plays a role in protecting cellular constituents from the deleterious effects of cigarette smoke exposure.

Future studies to determine the role of vitamin C in modulating the pulmonary effect of cigarette smoke exposure should employ guinea pigs as experimental animals. However, it is important that both the tissue and dietary content of vitamin C should be determined. Also, the status of its interacting nutrients, such as vitamin E, sulfur-containing amino acids, and Fe, needs to be monitored, and the possible metabolic adaptation of antioxidant systems needs to be examined. Furthermore, more sensitive and specific methods for assessing oxidative damage are needed.

REFERENCES

1. U.S. Department of Public Health Service. Smoking and Health: The Report of the Surgeon General. US DHEW Publication No. (PHS) 79-50066. Washington, DC: Government Printing Office, 1979.
2. Wynder EL. The epidemiology of cancer of the bronchus: facts and suppositions. Arch Otolaryngol Rhinol Laryngol 1967; 76:228–236.
3. Hammond EC. Smoking in relation to the death rates of one million men and women. Monograph 19, National Cancer Institute, January, 1966:127–204.
4. Doyle JT, Dawler TR, Kannel WB, Kinch SH, Kahn HA. The relationship of cigarette smoking to coronary heart disease. JAMA 1964; 190:886–890.
5. Diehl HS. Tobacco and Your Health: The Smoking Controversy. New York: McGraw-Hill, 1969.
6. US Department of Health and Human Service. Nicotine Action: A Report of the Surgeon General. DHEW Publication No. (CDC) 88-8406. Washington, DC: Government Printing Office, 1988.
7. US Department of Health and Human Service. The Health Consequences of Smoking: Chronic Obstructive Lung Disease. A Report of the Surgeon General. DHHS publication no. 84-50205. Washington, DC: Government Printing Office, 1984.
8. MacMahon B, Alpert M, Salber EJ. Infant weight and parental smoking habits. Am J Epidemiol 1965; 82:247–261.
9. Pryor WA. Oxidants in cigarette smoke: radical, hydrogen peroxide, peroxynitrite, and peroxynitrite. Ann NY Acad Sci 1993; 686:12–28.
10. Chow CK. Cigarette smoking and oxidative damage in the lung. Ann NY Acad Sci 1993; 686:289–298.
11. Schumacher JM, Green CR, Best FW, Newell MP. Smoke composition: an extensive investigation of the water-soluble portion of cigarette smoke. J Agric Food Chem 1977; 25:310–320.
12. Sakuma H, Ohsumi T, Sugawara S. Particular phase of cellulose cigarette smoke. Agric Biol Chem 1980; 44:555–561.
13. Church DF, Pryor WA. Free radical chemistry of cigarette smoke and its toxicological implications. Environ Health Perspect 1985; 64:111–126.
14. Pryor WA, Hales BJ, Premovic PI, Church DF. The radicals in cigarette tar: their nature and suggested physiological implications. Science 1983; 220:425–427.
15. Hunninghake CW, Crystal RG. Cigarette smoking and lung destruction: accumulation of neutrophils in the lungs of cigarette smokers. Am Rev Respir Dis 1983; 128:833–838.
16. Bridges RB, Chow CK, Rehm SR. Micronutrients and immune function in smokers. Ann NY Acad Sci 1990; 587:218–231.
17. Hoidal JR, Fox RB, LeMarbre PA, Perri R, Repine JE. Altered oxidative metabolic responses in vitro of alveolar macrophages from asymptomatic cigarette smokers. Am Rev Respir Dis 1981; 123: 85–89.

18. Hoidal JR, Niewoehner DE. Cigarette-smoke-induced phagocyte recruitment and metabolic alterations in human and hamsters. Am Rev Respir Dis 1982; 126:548–552.

19. Ludwig PW, Hoidal JR. Alterations in leukocyte oxidative metabolism in cigarette smokers. Am Rev Respir Dis 1982; 126:977–980.

20. Richards GA, Theron AJ, Van der Merwe CA, Anderson R. Spirometric abnormalities in young smokers correlate with increased chemiluminescence responses of activated blood phagocytes. Am Rev Respir Dis 1989; 139:181–187.

21. Hunninghake CW, Gadek JE, Kawanami O, Ferrans VJ, Crystal RG. Inflammatory and immune processes in the human lung in health and disease: evaluation by bronchoalveolar lavage. Am J Pathol 1979; 97:149–206.

22. Haslam PL, Turton CWG, Heard B, et al. Bronchoalveolar lavage in pulmonary fibrosis: comparison of cells obtained with lung biopsy and clinical features. Thorax 1980; 35:9–18.

23. Plowman PN. The pulmonary macrophage population of human smokers. Ann Occup Hyg 1982; 25:393–405.

24. Harris JO, Olssen GN, Castle JR, Maloney AS. Comparison of proteolytic enzyme activity in pulmonary alveolar macrophages and blood leukocytes in smokers and nonsmokers. Am Rev Respir Dis 1975; 111:579–580.

25. Martin RR. Altered morphology and increased acid hydrolase content of pulmonary alveolar macrophages from cigarette smokers. Am Rev Respir Dis 1973; 107:596–601.

26. Bridges RB, Fu MC, Rehm SR. Increased neutrophil myeloperoxidase activity associated with cigarette smoking. Eur J Respir Dis 1985; 67:84–93.

27. Wayner DD, Burton GW, Ingold KW, et al. The relative contributions of vitamin E, urate, ascorbate and protein to the total peroxy radical-trapping antioxidant activity of human blood plasma. Biochim Biophys Acta 1987; 924:408–419.

28. Chow CK. Interrelationship of cellular antioxidant defense systems. In: Chow CK, ed. Cellular Antioxidant Defense Mechanisms. Vol. 2. Boca Raton, FL: CRC Press, 1988:217–237.

29. Chow CK. Vitamin E and oxidative stress. Free Radical Biol Med 1991; 11:215–232.

30. Lentz PE, Di Luzio NRD. Peroxidation of lipids in alveolar macrophages: production by aqueous extracts of cigarette smoke. Arch Environ Health 1974; 28:279–282.

31. Fenner ML, Braven J. The mechanism of carcinogenesis by tobacco smoke: further experimental evidence and a prediction from the thio-defense hypothesis. Br J Cancer 1968; 22:474–479.

32. Schwalb G, Anderson R. Increased frequency of oxidant-mediated DNA strand breaks in mononuclear leukocytes exposed to activated neutrophils from cigarette smokers. Mutat Res 1989; 225:95–99.

33. Bielicki JK, McCall MR, van den Berg JJ, et al. Copper and gas-phase cigarette smoke inhibit plasma lecithin: cholesterol acyltransferase activity by different mechanisms. J Lipid Res 1995; 36:323–331.

34. Hoshino E, Shariff R, Van Gossum A, et al. Vitamin E suppresses increased lipid peroxidation in cigarette smokers. J Parent Enteral Nutr 1990; 14:300–305.

35. Duthie GG, Arthur JR, James WP, Vint HM. Antioxidant status of smokers and nonsmokers: effects of vitamin E supplementation. Ann NY Acad Sci 1989; 570:435–438.

36. Van Jaarsveld H, Kuyl JM, Albertz DW. Antioxidant vitamin supplementation of smoke-exposed rats partially protects against myocardial ischemia/reperfusion injury. Free Radical Res Commun 1992; 17:263–269.

37. Kawakami M, Kameyama S, Takizawa T. Lipid peroxidation in bronchoalveolar lavage fluid in interstitial lung diseases in relation to other components and smoking. Nippon Kyobu Shikkan Gakkai Zasshi 1989; 27:422–427.

38. Srivastava ED, Hallett MB, Rhodes J. Effect of nicotine and cotinine on the production of oxygen free radicals by neutrophils in smokers and non-smokers. Hum Toxicol 1989; 8:461–463.

39. Harats D, Naim M, Dabach Y, et al. Cigarette smoking renders LDL susceptible to peroxidative modification and enhanced metabolism by macrophages. Atherosclerosis 1989; 79:245–252.

40. Chow CK. Dietary vitamin E and cellular susceptibility to cigarette smoking. Ann NY Acad Sci 1982; 393:426–436.

41. Chow CK, Chen LH, Thacker RR, Griffith RB. Dietary vitamin E and pulmonary biochemical responses of rats to cigarette smoking. Environ Res 1984; 34:8–17.

42. Chow CK, Airriess GR, Changchit C. Increased vitamin E content in the lungs of chronic cigarette-smoked rats. Ann NY Acad Sci 1989; 570:425–427.

43. Airriess G, Changchit C, Chen LC Chow CK. Increased levels of vitamin E in the lungs of guinea pigs exposed to mainstream or sidestream smoke. Nutr Res 1988; 8:653–661.

44. Wurzel H, Yeh CC, Gairola C, Chow CK. Oxidative damage and antioxidant status in the lungs and bronchoalveolar lavage fluid of rats exposed chronically to cigarette smoke. J Biochem Toxicol 1995; 10:11–17.

45. McCuster K, Hoidal J. Selective increase of antioxidant enzyme activity in the alveolar macrophages from cigarette smokers and smoke-exposed hamsters. Am Rev Respir Dis 1990; 141:678–682.

46. Schlager JJ, Powis G, Cytosolic NAD(P)H: (quinone-acceptor) oxidoreductase in human normal and tumor tissue: effects of cigarette smoking and alcohol. Int J Cancer 1990; 45:403–409.

47. Renznik AZ, Cross CE, Hu ML, et al. Modification of plasma proteins by cigarette smoke as measured by protein carbonyl formation. Biochem J 1992; 286:607–611.

48. Cross CE, O'Neill CA, Rezenick AZ, et al. Cigarette smoke oxidation of human plasma constituents. Ann NY Acad Sci 1993; 686:72–89.

49. O'Neill CA, Halliwell B, van der Vliet A, et al. Aldehyde-induced protein modifications in human plasma: protection by glutathione and dihydrolipoic acid. J Lab Clin Med 1994; 124:359–370.

50. Eiserich LP, Vossen V, O'Neill CA, et al. Molecular mechanisms of damage by excess nitrogen oxides: nitration of tyrosine by gas-phase cigarette smoke. FEBS Lett 1994; 353:53–56.

51. Balansky R, Mircheva Z, Blagoeva P. Modulation of the mutagenic activity of cigarette smoke, cigarette smoke condensate and benzo(a)pyrene *in vitro* and *in vivo*. Mutagenesis 1994; 9: 107–112.

52. Pelletier O. Vitamin C status of cigarette smokers and nonsmokers. Am J Clin Nutr 1970; 23:520–528.

53. Pelletier O. Smoking and vitamin C levels in humans. Am J Clin Nutr 1969; 21:1259–1267.

54. Tribble DL, Giuliano LJ, Fortmann SP. Reduced plasma ascorbic acid concentrations in non-smokers regularly exposed to environmental tobacco smoke. Am J Clin Nutr 1993; 58:886–890.

55. Tappia PS, Troughton KL, Langley-Evans SC, Grimble RF. Cigarette smoking influences cytokine production and antioxidant defences. Clin Sci 1995; 88:485–489.

56. Bui MH, Sauty A, Collet F, Leuenberger P. Dietary vitamin C intake and concentrations in the body fluids and cells of male smokers and nonsmokers. J Nutr 1992; 122:312–316.

57. Mezzetti A, Lapenna D, Pierdomenico SD, et al. Vitamins E, C and lipid peroxidation in plasma and arterial tissue of smokers and non-smokers. Atherosclerosis 1995; 112:91–99.

58. Theron AJ, Richards GA, Van Rensburg AJ, et al. Investigation of the role of phagocytes and antioxidant nutrients in oxidant stress mediated by cigarette smoke. Int J Vitam Nutr Res 1990; 60:261–266.

59. Barton GM, Roath OS. Leukocyte ascorbic acid in abnormal leukocyte states. Int J Vitam Nutr Res 1976; 46:271–274.

60. Sakamoto W, Yoshikawa K, Shindoh M, et al. *In vivo* effects of vitamin E on peritoneal macrophages and T-kininogen level in rats. Int J Vitam Nutr Res 1989; 59:131–139.

61. Hemila H, Roberts P, Wikstrom M. Activated polymorphonuclear leukocytes consume vitamin C. FEBS Lett 1984; 178:25–30.

62. Theron AJ, Richards GA, Myer MS, et al. Investigation of the relative contributions of cigarette smoking and mineral dust exposure to activation of circulating phagocytes, alterations in plasma concentrations of vitamin C, vitamin E, and beta carotene, and pulmonary dysfunction in South African gold miners. Occup Environ Med 1994; 51:564–567.

63. Schwartz J, Weiss ST. Relationship between dietary vitamin C intake and pulmonary function in the First National Health and Nutrition examination Survey (NHANES I). Am J Clin Nutr 1994; 59:110–114.

64. van Antwerpen L, Theron AJ, Myer MS, et al. Cigarette smoke-mediated oxidant stress, phagocytes, vitamin C, vitamin E, and tissue injury. Ann NY Acad Sci 1993; 686:53–65.

65. van Poppel Verhagen H, van Veer P, van Bladeren PJ. Markers for cytogenetic damage in smokers: associations with plasma antioxidants and glutathione S-transferase mu. Cancer Epidemiol Biomarkers Prev 1993; 2:441–447.

66. Gairola CG. Free lung cell response of mice and rats to mainstream cigarette smoke exposure. Toxicol Appl Pharmacol 1986; 84:567–575.

67. Matulionis DH. Effects of cigarette smoke generated by different smoking machines on pulmonary macrophages in mice and rats. J Anal Toxicol 1984; 8:187–191.

68. Niewoehner DE, Peterson FJ, Hoidal JR. Selenium and vitamin E deficiencies do not enhance lung inflammation from cigarette smoke in the hamster. Am Rev Respir Dis 1983; 127: 227–230.

69. Griffith RB, Hancock R. Simultaneous mainstream- sidestream smoke exposure systems. 1. Equipment and procedure. Toxicology 1985; 34:123–138.

70. Griffith RB, Standafer S. Simultaneous mainstream- sidestream smoke exposure systems. II. The rat exposure system. Toxicology 1985; 35:13–24.

71. Chen LH, Chow CK. Effect of cigarette smoking and dietary vitamin E on plasma levels of vitamin C in rats. Nutr Rep Int 1980; 22:301–309.

72. Boyland E, Grove PL. Stimulation of ascorbic acid synthesis and excretion by carcinogenic and other foreign compounds. Biochem J 1961; 81:163–168.

73. Conney AH, Burns JJ. Stimulatory effects of foreign compounds on ascorbic acid biosynthesis and on drug-metabolizing enzymes. Nature 1959; 184:363–364.

74. Bilimoria MH, Ecobichon DJ. Protective antioxidant mechanisms in rat and guinea pig tissue challenged by acute exposure to cigarette smoke. Toxicology 1992; 72:131–144.

75. Sohn HO, Lim HM, Lee YG, et al. Effect of subchronic administration of antioxidants against cigarette smoke exposure in rats. Arch Toxicol 1993; 67:667–673.

76. Lehr HA, Frei B, Arfors KE. Vitamin C prevents cigarette smoke-induced leukocyte aggregation and adhesion to endothelium in vivo. Proc Natl Acad Sci USA 1994; 91:7688–7692.

77. Benedich A, Machlin LJ, Scandurra O, et al. The antioxidant role of vitamin C. Adv Free Radical Biol Med 1986; 2:419–444.

78. Chen LH, Chang HM. Effects of high level of vitamin C on tissue antioxidant status of guinea pigs. J Int Vitam Nutr Res 1979; 49:87–91.

79. Niki E, Tsuchiya J, Tanimura R, Kamiya Y. Regeneration of vitamin E from α-chromanoxy radical by glutathione and vitamin C. Chem Lett 1982; 789–792.

80. Packer JE, Slater TF, Wilson RL. Direct observation of a free radical interaction between vitamin E and vitamin C. Nature 1979; 278:737–738.

81. Reddy RC, Scholz RW, Thomas CE, Massaro EJ. Vitamin E dependent reduced glutathione inhibition of rat liver microsomal lipid peroxidation. Life Sci 1982; 31:571–576.

82. Wefers H, Sies H. The protection by ascorbate and glutathione against microsomal lipid peroxidation is dependent on vitamin E. Eur J Biochem 1988; 174:353–357.

83. Bridge KR, Hoffman KE. The effects of ascorbic acid on the intracellular metabolism of iron and ferritin. J Biol Chem 1986; 261:14273–14277.

84. Diliberto E Jr, Dean G, Carter C, Allen PL. Tissue, subcellular and submitochondrial distributions of semidehydroascorbate reductase: possible role of semidehydroascorbate reductase in cofactor regeneration. J Neurochem 1982; 39:563–568.

25

Vitamin C, Smoking, and Alcohol Consumption

RITVA JÄRVINEN
University of Kuopio, Kuopio, Finland

PAUL KNEKT
National Public Health Institute, Helsinki, Finland

INTRODUCTION

Recognition of the potential role of oxidative damage in the development of chronic disease has led to the search for protective antioxidant agents. Vitamin C is an effective reductant ubiquitously appearing in all tissue fluids, and thus it can provide protection against harmful effects of oxidative agents by directly trapping free radicals or other reactive oxygen species or by regenerating other antioxidants, e.g., vitamin E (1–4). There is much epidemiological evidence suggesting an inverse relation between the intake of vitamin C and the occurrence of a variety of chronic diseases (5–8), thus indicating that vitamin C could have importance beyond the role of preventing the deficiency of the vitamin. Poorer nutritional status of vitamin C has been associated with the increased risk of several hormone-unrelated cancers, especially those of the upper gastrointestinal tract (9–16); cardiovascular diseases (17–23); and age-related eye diseases, in particular, cataracts (24,25). However, inconclusive or contradictory data have also been reported.

In these studies vitamin C nutrition has been estimated on the basis of the measurement of dietary intake or determinations of ascorbic acid concentrations in serum, plasma, or leukocytes. In humans, the nutritional status of vitamin C is directly dependent on the intake of vitamin C, and significant associations have been demonstrated between the intake and concentrations of ascorbic acid in plasma, leukocytes, and other blood compartments (26–32). Although the concentration of ascorbic acid in leukocytes is more representative of the cellular vitamin C content, concentration in plasma or serum is much easier to determine (32), and it has been the most common method of assessment of body vitamin C status besides the measurement of dietary intake.

Several of the chronic diseases, in which the implicated effect of vitamin C is most evident, are known to be related to smoking and alcohol consumption. As a result of both behavioral and metabolic influences these factors are also associated with the intake and tissue level of vitamin C (33–43). Consequently, they may potentially confound or modify the association between vitamin C nutrition and the incidence of chronic diseases in epidemiological studies. Thus, the estimation of the health effects of vitamin C in such studies requires an understanding of the complex relationships among smoking, alcohol consumption, and vitamin C nutrition.

In the following, new data on dietary intake of vitamin C, smoking habits, and alcohol consumption in a large cohort of adult Finnish men are presented and the results are discussed together with earlier studies on the effects of smoking and drinking habits on vitamin C nutrition.

THE FINNISH MOBILE CLINIC HEALTH EXAMINATION SURVEY: DIETARY VITAMIN C, SMOKING, AND ALCOHOL INTAKE

Materials and Methods

The Mobile Clinic Health Examination Survey carried out multiphasic health examinations in 12 municipalities in four regions of Finland during 1973–1976 (44). A total of 19,518 men and women from rural, industrial, and semiurban populations participated in the examinations. In different regions about 15% to 25% of the examinees were interviewed for dietary habits. Altogether 2,244 men, 22–83 years of age, participated in the interview. Data on habitual food consumption over a 1-year period before the examination were collected using a modified dietary history method (45). The vitamin C content of food items was derived from the Finnish Food Composition Tables (46), which collect data on vitamin C from several sources, mainly from food composition tables of other European countries. The vitamin C intake represents amounts in raw foodstuffs. Alcohol consumption was estimated as ethanol intake calculated from the dietary history interview data.

A questionnaire with items concerning socioeconomic background, health behavior, and medical history was sent to the subjects together with the invitation to the medical checkup for completion before the examination. The answers to this self-administered questionnaire were checked and completed by a specially trained nurse at the examination. Education was classified as follows: only elementary school; basic education, including primary school (8 years); intermediate education, including junior high school (9–13 years); and higher education, including studies or degrees taken at institutes or universities (over 13 years). The categories of smoking history were as follows: never smoked; ex-smoker; current smoker of cigars and pipe, current smoker of fewer than 25 cigarettes per day; and current smoker of 25 or more cigarettes per day. Never smoked and ex-smokers were also combined to distinguish the group of nonsmokers, and all other smokers to distinguish the group of current smokers.

The age-adjusted mean levels of vitamin C in categories of demographic variables, smoking status, and alcohol intake were estimated using the general linear model (47). Models including all variables in Table 1 and interaction terms were also made. Tests for the significance of the associations between vitamin C intake and the different variables were based on the model.

Results

There was an inverse association between age and mean daily intake of vitamin C; younger men had a higher vitamin C intake than older (Table 1). Men from higher social classes or

Table 1 Mean Vitamin C Intake in Categories of Different Variables

Variable	Category	No. of persons	Mean vitamin C level (mg/day)	
			Age-adjusted	Simultaneous model[a]
Age (years)	22–39	333	86.2	83.7
	40–49	818	80.2	78.9
	50–59	675	72.0	72.6
	60–83	418	68.3	71.5
	p Value[b]		<0.001	<0.001
Social class	I (highest)	100	95.2	90.0
	II	1137	78.0	75.8
	III	590	75.6	76.5
	IV (lowest)	416	68.5	74.3
	p Value		<0.001	0.02
Education	Elementary	173	63.0	65.6
	Basic	1457	74.9	75.6
	Intermediate	505	83.0	81.9
	Higher	105	89.0	78.6
	p Value		<0.001	<0.001
Marital status	Unmarried	208	70.0	75.7
	Married	1940	77.5	76.9
	Widowed	50	64.7	63.6
	Divorced	45	69.7	70.1
	p Value		0.003	0.07
Type of region	Semiurban	683	76.1	74.8
	Rural	767	68.9	70.9
	Industrial	794	83.9	83.1
	p Value		<0.001	<0.001
Smoking	Never	578	80.3	80.8
	Ex	759	78.6	77.9
	Cigar or pipe	56	76.8	74.7
	Cigarettes <25/day	700	72.5	73.9
	Cigarettes ≥25/day	133	66.0	65.7
	p Value		<0.001	<0.001
Alcohol intake (g/day)	0	194	71.6	74.5
	1–5	860	74.0	74.5
	6–20	795	79.0	78.0
	21–35	266	77.6	77.8
	>35	129	78.7	78.9
	p Value		0.25	0.31

[a]Simultaneous model includes all variables in the table.
[b]p Value for difference between categories.

from industrial areas had a higher vitamin C intake than other men, whereas men with low education and widowed men had a low vitamin C intake.

Vitamin C intake was strongly associated with smoking habits. Those who had never smoked and ex-smokers had the highest levels of intake of the vitamin, whereas heavy smokers had the lowest intakes (Table 1). Alcohol consumption was not significantly associated with vitamin C intake. These results were also independent of differences in

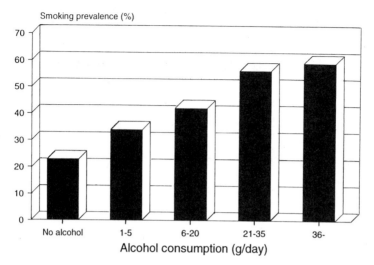

Figure 1 Age-adjusted prevalence of current smokers in categories of alcohol consumption.

other characteristics of the subjects. Nor were the associations of smoking and alcohol consumption with vitamin C intake modified by demographic variables (results not shown). Total energy intake was increased with increased alcohol consumption, but nonalcohol energy was similar in quartiles of alcohol intake (results not shown).

There was a strong association between current smoking and alcohol consumption (Fig. 1). About 20% of persons not using alcohol at all were current smokers, whereas almost 60% of the persons using over 35 g alcohol per day were current smokers. To study the possible interaction between smoking and alcohol consumption and vitamin C intake the three variables were studied simultaneously (Fig. 2). The different prevalence of smoking among men in different alcohol intake categories, however, did not change the relationship between alcohol consumption and vitamin C intake.

SMOKING AND VITAMIN C

Vitamin C Intake by Cigarette Smokers

We demonstrated a higher mean intake of vitamin C among nonsmokers than among smokers, and a lower intake among heavy smokers (25 cigarettes or more per day) than among moderate smokers in a large cohort of adult Finnish males studied in 1973–1976. Our results are in line with the findings of several previous studies from other countries (34,35, Table 2), and the results of an earlier report based on the same cohort investigated four-to-seven years earlier (67).

Hornig and Glatthaar (34) and Murata (35) have previously reviewed the effect of smoking on vitamin C nutrition. Table 2 presents a number of recent studies published during the eighties and nineties investigating the relationships between smoking habits and dietary vitamin C. The mean intakes of vitamin C vary considerably between populations, but the findings are uniform in that the smokers have lower dietary intake of vitamin than nonsmokers. Approximately four studies in five demonstrated significantly lower vitamin

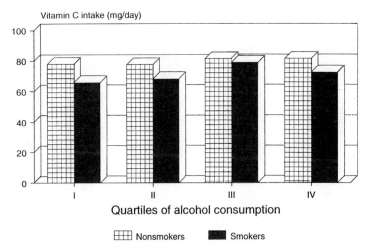

Figure 2 Age-adjusted mean vitamin C intake in categories of smoking status and alcohol consumption.

C intake in smokers. This relationship is evident in comprehensive investigations from the United States (39,40,49,55,56,65,68) and the United Kingdom (41,50,53,57,62) including men and women of different age, race, ethnicity, and socioeconomic position. Overall, the mean intake of vitamin C of smokers seems to be approximately 20% below that of smokers, and the largest difference was 45%. Lower vitamin C density in the diet of smokers compared to that of nonsmokers has also been reported (53,54,56,71), although the difference has not been seen in all studies (72). The decreased consumption of fruits by current smokers described in several studies from different countries (73–77) can also be taken to indicate lower vitamin C intake among smokers. Obvious consistency of the inverse relationship between dietary vitamin C intake and current smoking in studies from different circumstances suggests that dietary patterns of smokers do not reflect cultural influences but rather universal personal characteristics (73).

The inverse association between smoking and dietary vitamin C in the present study was independent of differences in alcohol intake and several other personal characteristics, as has also been demonstrated in other population-based studies (39,43,55,62). In Table 2 vitamin C intake figures refer mainly to vitamin C provided by foods. Because less frequent use of vitamin supplements has been observed in smokers, especially in heavy male smokers (43,68,78–81), the differences in total vitamin C intake between smokers and nonsmokers could be more pronounced. In some studies shown in Table 2, mainly comprising smaller groups of volunteers, no significant difference in dietary vitamin C intake between smokers and nonsmokers was observed, however. These discrepant results may indicate the different dietary habits of smokers in some subpopulations, but they may also reflect the inadequacies of dietary survey methods used to measure habitual long-term diet.

We found a lower intake of vitamin C among ex-smokers than among never smokers, but a higher intake than among smokers. Other studies showing the results of past smokers also suggest that their dietary intake of vitamin C falls in between those of current smokers and never smokers, or may approach that of never smokers, especially in women (39,43,55–57,60,63,65,67). These findings imply that persons who stop smoking change

Table 2   Studies on Associations Between Intake of Vitamin C and Smoking Status

Ref.	Population	Sample size	Sex	Age (years)	Diet survey method	Smoking category	Mean vitamin C intake (mg/day)	Comments
48	Healthy males; United States	22	M	25–38	3-Day food record	Nonsmoker Smoker	106.0 81.4 NS	
49	Random sample; noninstitutionalized adults; Alameda County, United States	3,119	M/F	≥16	Questions about intake of vitamin C pills, fruits, and vegetables			Cigarette smoking inversely related to vitamin C intake
50	Sample from general population; Caerphilly, South Wales	493	M	45–59	7-Day food record	Nonsmoker Smoker	57.5 44.7 $p < 0.001$[a]	Adjusted for social class
51	Pregnant women at delivery; New York, United States	12 14	F	Mean 28.5 Mean 29.5		Nonsmoker Smoker	87 76 NS	
52	Healthy elderly; Nagano City area, Japan	79	M	63–80	3-Day food record	Nonsmoker Smoker	158.4 126.3 $p < 0.05$	
39	National sample; white and black; NHANES II (1976–1980); United States	11,592	M/F	18–74	24-Hour food recall	Nonsmoker, never > 1 year < 1 year Smoker, < 1 pack/day 1 pack/day > 1 pack/day	111 105 92 97 78 79	Adjusted for age, sex, race, alcohol intake, monetary income, and body weight
53,54	Pregnant Caucasian women; attending prenatal booking clinic; London, England	206	F		7-Day food record	Nonsmoker Smoker	72 44 $p < 0.001$	Adjusted for height Significant inverse association between smoking and vitamin C intake persisted after adjustment for education, income, tenure, social class, and height

Ref.	Population	n	Sex	Age	Dietary method	Smoking status	Value	Comments
55	Cohort population; white males; upper Midwest area, United States	14,214	M		FFQ, 37 food items	Nonsmoker Ex-smoker Smoker, 1–19 cig./day 20–29 cig./day ≥30 cig./day	113 108 109 103 98 $p < 0.001$ (trend)	Adjustment for age, energy intake (vitamin C/1000 kcal), body mass, education, and alcohol intake did not materially change the results
56	National sample; CSFII (1985) United States	1,338	F	19–50	24-Hour food recall	Never smoked Ex-smoker Smoker	88 89 64 $p < 0.001$	Adjustment for physial activity, health status, and demographic variables did not change the results
40	National sample; black and white; NHANES II (1976–1980); United States	>10,000	M/F	19–74	24-Hour food recall	Mean vitamin C intake was higher among nonsmokers in all 12 age–race–sex categories		Negative association between smoking and vitamin C intake remained for both races after adjustment for age, sex, energy intake, and poverty index ratio
30	Random sample from general practitioners' registers; two towns, Scotland	196	M	Born in 1938–1947	FFQ, 50+ food items	Nonsmoker Smoker	61.1 49.4 $p < 0.001$	
57	Sample from general practitioners' registers; three towns, England	1,115	M	35–54	24-Hour food record	Nonsmoker Ex-smoker Current smoker	55.2 52.3 47.7 $p = 0.05$	Differences nonsignificant after adjustment for social class
		1,225	F			Nonsmoker Ex-smoker Current smoker	49.3 47.6 41.7 $p = 0.007$	Result persisted after adjustment for social class
58	Hospital employees, medical students; Lausanne, Switzerland	14 10	M	Mean 26 Mean 27	Diet history interview	Nonsmoker Smoker	107 116 NS	

Table 2   Continued

Ref.	Population	Sample size	Sex	Age (years)	Diet survey method	Smoking category	Mean vitamin C intake (mg/day)	Comments
59	Hospital controls for cancer study; Milan area, Italy	1,039	M	21–74	FFQ, 30 food items	Never smoked	120[b]	Adjusted for age
						Ex-smoker	117	
						Smoker,		
						<15 cig./day	117	
						≥15 cig./day	107	
							$p < 0.05$ (trend)	
		735	F			Never smoked	123	
						Exsmoker	123	
						Smoker,		
						<15 cig./day	123	
						≥15 cig./day	123	
							NS	
41,60	Random sample of middle-aged people; Scotland	4,343	M	40–59	FFQ, 50+ food items	Never smoked	56	Adjusted for age, social class, and body mass index
						Ex-smoker	53	
						Current smoker	49	
							$p < 0.001$	
		4,907	F			Never smoked	55	
						Ex-smoker	56	
						Current smoker	46	
							$p < 0.001$	
61	Randomly selected middle-aged adults; Scotland	95	M/F	45–69	7-Day food record	Never smoked	61	
						Ex-smoker	54	
						Current smoker	63	
							NS	

	Sample	N	Sex	Age	Method	Category	Value	Comments
62	National sample; subjects in private households; England, Wales, and Scotland	950	M	16–64	7-Day food record	Nonsmoker Smoker, <20 cig./day ≥20 cig./day	81.7 65.9 62.5 $p = 0.01$	Adjustment for age, sex, region, occupation group, alcohol intake, height, and weight did not notably alter differences between smokers and nonsmokers
		892	F			Nonsmoker Smoker, <20 cig./day ≥20 cig./day	82.8 57.5 45.9 $p < 0.001$	
63	Population-based controls for breast cancer cases; Adelaide, Australia	451	F	20–74	FFQ, 179+ food items	Never smoked Ex-smoker Smoker, <Median >Median	162.7 182.5 150.4 158.7 $p = 0.40$	Adjustment for age, energy intake, education, and alcohol intake did not change the results
64	Random sample; middle-aged men; two provinces, Sweden	174	M	40–49	FFQ, 49 food items	No tobacco Smokeless tobacco Smoker	61.1 52.8 48.7 NS	
65	National sample; white, black, Hispanic; NHIS (1987); United States	8,385	M	≥18	FFQ, 59 food items	Never smoked Ex-smoker Current smoker	124[c] 111 95	In current smokers, significant negative association ($p ≤ 0.001$) between cigarette consumption and vitamin C intake.
		11,758	F			Never smoked Ex-smoker Current smoker	107 103 86	
66	Premenopausal women; specific smoking exposure criteria; United States	141	F	25–45	FFQ, 98 food items	Nonsmoker Passive smoker Smoker	142[c] 104 113 NS	

Table 2   Continued

Ref.	Population	Sample size	Sex	Age (years)	Diet survey method	Smoking category	Mean vitamin C intake (mg/day)	Comments
67	Population-based; six regions (1967–1972); Finland	5,304	M	≥15	Diet history interview	Never smoked	80.9	Adjusted for age and geographical region
						Ex-smoker	80.7	
						Smoker,		
						<15 cig./day	78.4	
						≥15 cig./day	77.8	
							$p = 0.04$	
		4,705	F			Never smoked	82.7	
						Ex-smoker	93.2	
						Smoker,		
						<15 cig./day	85.4	
						≥15 cig./day	83.1	
							$p = 0.01$	
68	Random sample; two communities; New England, United States	632	M	18–64	FFQ, 61 food items	Nonsmoker	137.1	Adjusted for age
						Smoker	126.6	
							NS	
		976	F			Nonsmoker	139.0	
						Smoker	123.1	
							$p < 0.01$	
69	Healthy students; Bangladesh	88	M	22–28	7-Day food record	Nonsmoker	83.4	
						Smoker	70.4	
							$p = 0.19$	

Ref	Description	N	Sex	Age	Method	Category	Value	Notes
70	Volunteers; specific tobacco exposure criteria; United States	44	M	25–55	24-Hour food recall + 2-day food record	No tobacco Tobacco chewer Smoker	106.5[d] 81.0 84.8 NS	

43	Random sample; three towns; the Netherlands	1,916	M	20–59	FFQ, 80 food items	Never smoked
						Ex-smoker
						Smoker,
						  1–9 cig./day
						  10–19 cig./day
						  ≥20 cig./day
							118.0
							116.3
							
							119.0
							112.4
							95.8
							$p < 0.001$
								Adjusted for age, body mass index, education, town, total energy intake, and alcohol intake

		2,328	F			Never smoked
						Ex-smoker
						Smoker,
						  1–9 cig./day
						  10–19 cig./day
						  ≥20 cig./day
							131.5
							131.6
							
							129.9
							114.3
							115.1
							$p < 0.001$	

[a] p Value for difference unless stated otherwise.
[b] Calculated from original values given in grams per month.
[c] Median values.
[d] Vitamin C from supplements included. NS, nonsignificant difference; FFQ, food frequency questionnaire; NHANES, National Health and Nutrition Examination Survey; CSFII, Continuing Survey of Food Intake by Individuals; NHIS, National Health Interview Survey.
References are cited in the order of the year of publication.

their dietary habits so that vitamin C intake is increased. However, it cannot be concluded from these cross-sectional comparisons whether the demonstrated differences are due to the stopping of smoking or whether quitters represent persons whose dietary habits differ from those of continuing smokers. In prospective studies on small groups of quitters no significant differences were demonstrated in the dietary intake of vitamin C within an interval of 6–8 weeks (82) or during a follow-up period of 1 year (83). Accordingly, it may take longer than 1 year for implicated dietary changes of ex-smokers to be manifested. However, in cross-sectional comparisons the diet of ex-smoking women resembled that of never smokers more directly (60). In addition to differences in the diet, the vitamin C intake of the past smokers may also be increased as a result of their more frequent use of vitamin supplements (78,80,84).

Vitamin C Status of Cigarette Smokers

The impaired vitamin C status of smokers was first suggested in the late thirties and early forties, and during the following decades several reports were published showing decreased ascorbic acid concentrations in blood, plasma, serum, leukocytes, and urine in male and female cigarette smokers compared to nonsmokers, as reviewed by Hornig and Glatthaar (34) and by Murata (35). Table 3 shows findings from 28 recent studies comparing plasma vitamin C and smoking habits in populations from Europe, the United States, Japan, and some other countries. Four studies in five demonstrate the significant negative effect of smoking on plasma vitamin C concentration. In these studies the mean plasma vitamin C values of smokers appear to be 15% to 55% below those of nonsmokers. Lower plasma ascorbic acid concentrations have been observed in heavy smokers compared to lighter smokers (39,42,98,99); this finding suggests a dose–response effect between cigarette consumption and plasma vitamin C level. The risk of low plasma vitamin C values of smokers has been reported to be two to four times higher than that of nonsmokers (39,100). In general, ascorbic acid concentrations in other components of the blood of smokers and nonsmokers have been observed to behave similarly to plasma or serum (35). The increased content of ascorbic acid in bronchoalveolar lavage and in alveolar macrophages potentially reflects an adaptation to elevated levels of oxidant stress in smokers' lungs (58).

Although smokers frequently have a lower dietary intake of vitamin C (Table 2), differences in intake do not seem to explain fully their poorer vitamin C status. This has been demonstrated methodologically by stratification or adjustment for vitamin C intake in the analyses, or by presentation of similar vitamin C intake in the groups of smokers and nonsmokers. On the basis of findings from a national Canadian Nutrition Survey, Pelletier (98) reported that smokers had consistently lower serum ascorbic acid levels than non-smokers at different levels of vitamin C intake. Similarly, comparisons from a national cross-sectional survey in the United States demonstrated that at different levels of vitamin C intake plasma ascorbic acid concentrations maintained by smokers were approximately 0.2 mg/dL lower than those of nonsmokers (39,100). Schectman and coworkers (39) also reported that the increased risk for smokers of low plasma ascorbic acid values, suggesting hypovitaminosis of vitamin C, was only slightly reduced by adjustment for dietary vitamin C intake. With the exception of two studies (28,52) shown in Table 3, the inverse associations between smoking and plasma vitamin C values persisted after adjustment for the intake of vitamin C and other potential confounders (29,39,64,95,96). In addition, several studies demonstrate decreased plasma ascorbic acid values in smokers compared to nonsmokers despite approximately similar dietary intake of vitamin C. The inverse relationship between smoking and plasma vitamin C level seems to be independent of alcohol consumption (29,39,42,95,96).

Poorer plasma vitamin C concentration of current smokers was not, however, detected in all populations (58,72,85,93,94). Variable findings may be due to differences in the number of cigarettes smoked and in the intake of vitamin C and the accuracy of their measurements. It is possible that high intake levels of vitamin C may be adequate to supply enough vitamin to the smokers, and thus restore their plasma vitamin C concentrations. In agreement with that hypothesis, some studies reporting normal plasma levels of vitamin C in smokers were performed in groups with a relatively high dietary intake of vitamin C (58,72,93).

Mechanisms by Which Smoking Affects Vitamin C Status

Lower dietary intake of vitamin C gives only a partial explanation of the observed decreased tissue vitamin C concentrations of cigarette smokers. Thus, other mechanisms for poorer vitamin C status in smokers are obvious. Nicotine from cigarette smoke can destroy vitamin C in vitro (35). Cigarette smoke also contains remarkably high quantities of free radicals and substances that generate free radicals in the body (101,102). Since smoking induces inflammatory events, phagocyte-derived reactive oxygen species increase endogenous radical production (93,103). Vitamin C is an effective scavenger of superoxide anion, singlet oxygen, and hydroxyl and peroxyl radicals and may be consumed in the body's efforts to inactivate these harmful oxidants (1–4,35,104,105).

Kallner et al. (106) demonstrated increased metabolic turnover and diminished half-life of vitamin C in a kinetic study of smokers consuming 20 cigarettes or more per day. The metabolic turnover rate of vitamin C was approximately 40% higher in smokers compared to nonsmokers exhibiting a similar plasma ascorbic acid level. Increased utilization rather than urinary loss appeared to be responsible for this higher turnover rate. The mechanism of increased utilization is unknown, but it may include enhanced oxidation of ascorbic acid by cigarette smoke. Suggested decreased bioavailability of ascorbic acid in smokers (98,106, 107) potentially indicates the interference of cigarette smoking with vitamin C absorption. The effect of smoking on vitamin C status does not seem to be acute. Short-term exposure to cigarette smoke for 10 to 20 min (108) or up to 6 h (109) was not found to have immediate effects on tissue ascorbic acid concentrations.

Vitamin C Requirement by Cigarette Smokers

Smokers who take vitamin C supplements have higher plasma vitamin C concentrations than smokers who do not use vitamin supplements (34,35). Their values have been reported to correspond to those of nonsmokers not taking supplements (90). Among adult Americans the plasma vitamin C concentrations of smokers reporting daily use of vitamin supplements did not differ significantly from those of nonsmokers who regularly used vitamin supplements, with the exception of women aged 20–59 years (110). Approximately a similar percentage of subjects with marginal plasma vitamin C concentration were found among vitamin C–supplemented smokers and nonsmokers who did not use supplements (100). The risk of low plasma ascorbic acid values among smokers taking vitamin C supplements did not differ from that of unsupplemented nonsmokers consuming

Table 3   Studies on Associations Between Plasma Vitamin C Concentration and Smoking Status

Ref.	Population	Sample size	Sex	Age (years)	Smoking category	Plasma vitamin C (mg/dl)[a]	Comments
48	Healthy males; United States	22	M	25–38	Nonsmoker Smoker	0.88 0.69	Nonsignificant difference in mean vitamin C intake
85	Random sample; 20- to 40-year olds; Heidelberg, Germany	355	F	20–40	Nonsmokers Smokers	$p < 0.05$[b] 0.73 0.68 NS	
86	Healthy males from submarine crew; United States	28	M	19–36	Nonsmoker Smoker	1.12 0.53 $p < 0.01$	Nonsignificant difference in mean vitamin C intake
87	Healthy males; United States	83	M	18–29	Nonsmoker Smoker	0.73 0.54 $p = 0.01$	Nonsignificant difference in mean vitamin C intake
88	Smokers and age- and race-matched controls; United States	250	M	Mean 34.4 Mean 35.1	Nonsmoker Smoker	0.88 0.63 $p = 0.001$	
51	Pregnant women at delivery; New York, United States	12 14	F	Mean 28.5 Mean 29.5	Nonsmoker Smoker	0.89 0.40 $p < 0.01$	Nonsignificant difference in mean vitamin C intake
28	Healthy, elderly people; Boston area, United States	233 439	M F	60–98	Nonsmoker Smoker Nonsmoker Smoker	1.13 1.06 1.34 1.22	Nonsignificant differences after adjustment for total vitamin C intake
89	Women attending a family planning clinic; New York, United States	155	F	15–48	Nonsmoker Smoker	0.682 0.565 $p = 0.006$	
29	Self-sufficient elderly; Nancy, Metz, France	277	M/F	60–82			Significant inverse association ($p < 0.05$) between cigarette consumption and plasma vitamin C level after adjustment for vitamin C intake, sex, alcohol intake, ponderal index, and antibiotic use

Ref	Description	N	Sex	Age	Group	Value	Comments
52	Healthy elderly; Nagano City area, Japan	79	M	63–80	Nonsmoker Smoker	0.99 0.81 $p < 0.05$	Nonsignificant inverse association between cigarette consumption and serum vitamin C level after adjustment for vitamin C intake
90	University staff members; Japan	406	M	40–65	Nonsmoker, in 1983 in 1984 in 1985 Smoker, in 1983 in 1984 in 1985	0.72 0.84 0.86 0.49 0.56 0.52	Nonsignificant difference in fruit and vegetable consumption
39	National sample; white and black adults; NHANES II (1976–1980); United States	11,592	M/F	18–74	Nonsmoker, Never >1 year <1 year Smoker, <1 pack/day 1 pack/day >1 pack/day	$p < 0.001$ (smokers vs. nonsmokers) 1.12 1.11 1.03 0.99 0.88 0.89	Adjustment for vitamin C intake, age, sex, race, alcohol intake, body weight, and supplementation status
91	Smokers and age- and race-matched controls; United States	320	M		Nonsmoker Smoker	0.869 0.595 $p = 0.0001$	
	Sample from initial population studied 5 years later	120	M		Nonsmoker Smoker	1.123 0.854 $p \leq 0.01$	Nonsignificant difference in mean vitamin C intake
30	Random sample from general practitioners' registers; two towns, Scotland	196	M	Born in 1938–1947	Nonsmoker Smoker	0.65 0.32 $p < 0.001$	
92	Population based controls for angina pectoris cases; Edinburgh, Scotland	390	M	35–54	Never smoked Ex-smoker Pipe or cigar smoker Cigarette smoker	0.72 0.75 0.68 0.42 $p < 0.001$ (cigarette smokers vs. others)	
58	Hospital employees, medical students; Lausanne, Switzerland	14 10	M	Mean 26 Mean 27	Nonsmoker Smoker	1.53 1.60 NS	Nonsignificant difference in mean vitamin C intake

Table 3 Continued

Ref.	Population	Sample size	Sex	Age (years)	Smoking category	Plasma vitamin C (mg/dl)[a]	Comments
61	Randomly selected middle-aged adults; Scotland	242	M/F	45–69	Never smoked Ex-smoker Current smoker	0.79 0.62 0.48 $p < 0.001$	
93	Gold miners; Caucasians; South Africa	54 106	M	Mean 30 32	Nonsmoker Smoker	0.91 0.77 $p = 0.0012$	
	University personnel and students; Caucasians; South Africa	62 43	M	Mean 36 Mean 43	Nonsmoker Smoker	1.01 0.98 $p = 0.167$	
94	Caucasian healthy adults selected from different groups; Barcelona, Spain	114	M/F	18–82	Nonsmoker Smoker	0.895 0.818 NS	
64	Random sample; middle-aged men; two provinces, Sweden	97	M	40–49	No tobacco Smokeless tobacco Smoker	0.97 1.01 0.67 $p < 0.001$ (smokers vs. nontobacco users) $p = 0.011$ (smokers vs. snuff dippers)	Lower level of plasma vitamin C in smokers persisted after control for vitamin C intake
66	Premenopausal women; specific smoking exposure criteria; United States	141	F	25–45	Nonsmoker, nonexposed Passive smoker Smoker	1.23[c] 0.93 0.70 $p = 0.001$	Nonsignificant differences in mean vitamin C intake
95	Random sample; Paris area, France	837	M/F	>18			In women, significant inverse association ($p < 0.005$) between tobacco smoking and plasma vitamin C level after adjustment for dietary vitamin C density, alcohol intake, and use of oral contraceptives In men, nonsignificant association

Ref.	Description	N	Sex	Age	Group	Value	Comments
96	Random sample; healthy adults; West Germany	2,006	M/F	18–88			In men and women significant inverse association ($p = 0.001$) between cigarettes/day and plasma vitamin C level after adjustment for vitamin C intake, age, energy intake, body mass index, and alcohol intake
72	Patients attending outpatient clinics; low-income African-American women; United States	91	F	30–69	Nonsmoker	1.02	Adjusted for vitamin C intake, age, supplement intake, energy intake, alcohol intake, medications, and body mass index
					Smoker	0.99	
						$p = 78$	
97	Random sample of ≥16 year-olds; Northern Ireland	229	M	16–74	Nonsmoker	1.01	
					Smoker	0.79	
						$p = 0.01$	
		251	F		Nonsmoker	1.25	
					Smoker	0.98	
						$p < 0.001$	
69	Healthy students; Bangladesh	88	M	22–28	Nonsmoker	0.53	Nonsignificant difference in mean vitamin C intake
					Smoker	0.39	
						$p < 0.0004$	
70	Adult men with specific tobacco exposure criteria; United States	44	M	25–55			Smokers and tobacco chewers had significantly lower ($p < 0.01$) plasma vitamin C levels than nonsmokers
							Nonsignificant differences in mean vitamin C intake
42	Participants of a chemoprevention trial at study entry; Venezuela	646	M	35–69	Nonsmoker	0.849	Adjustment for age, alcohol intake, and month of examination did not change the results
					Smoker,		
					<10 cig./day	0.750	
					≥10 cig./day	0.703	
						$p < 0.001$ (trend)	
		718	F		Nonsmoker	0.973	
					Smoker,		
					<10 cig./day	0.828	
					≥10 cig./day	0.765	
						$p < 0.001$ (trend)	

[a] Multiply by 56.78 to convert values into micromoles per liter (μmol/L). Original values given in milligrams per deciliter (mg/dL), milligrams per liter (mg/L), μg/mL, or μmol/L.

[b] p Value for difference unless stated otherwise.

[c] Median values. NS, nonsignificant difference; NHANES, National Health and Nutrition Examination Survey.

References are cited in the order of the year of publication.

the recommended daily allowance of 60 mg of vitamin C (111). Thus the decreased tissue concentrations of smokers can be compensated by the increased intake of vitamin C. The restoration of the tissue vitamin C stores of smokers has been shown in experiments with vitamin C supplements (35,107).

On the basis of their kinetic study on ascorbic acid turnover Kallner et al. (106) suggested that smokers consuming more than 20 cigarettes per day would need to ingest at least 40 mg per day more vitamin C than nonsmokers in order to maintain their higher vitamin C turnover. Utilizing the data on intake and plasma values of vitamin C from the second National Health and Nutrition Examination Survey in the United States, Smith and Hodges (100) suggested that smokers would need an additional 59 to 65 mg per day of vitamin C to maintain equivalent serum levels to nonsmokers. In the recommended dietary allowances given in the United States in 1989 the authorities recommended a daily intake of at least 100 mg of vitamin C for smokers instead of 60 mg suggested to be adequate for nonsmokers (112). In France the recommendation for smokers has been set at 120 mg of vitamin C per day (35). However, a smoker's need for vitamin C may be even higher. On the basis of their analysis of the second National Health and Nutrition Examination Survey data Schectman and coworkers (111) estimated that smokers would need 200 mg or more of vitamin C to maintain a plasma vitamin C concentration comparable to that of nonsmokers whose average daily intake of vitamin C corresponded to the recommended dietary amount for healthy nonsmokers. Further studies are needed to illustrate more accurately the amount of dietary vitamin C necessary to increase the plasma vitamin C concentrations of smokers at different exposure levels comparable to those of nonsmokers.

Vitamin C Status of Other Groups Exposed to Tobacco Smoke

As stated, the depressed vitamin C status of heavy cigarette smokers seems to be obvious. In other tobacco user groups the associations are more variable, however. Plasma ascorbic acid concentrations of smokers of cigars or pipe tobacco have been suggested to be comparable to those of nonsmokers (92,98); that may be the effect of their different smoking habits' inducing lower exposure to tobacco smoke (113). Furthermore, the dietary intake of vitamin C of cigar or pipe smokers seems to approach that of nonsmokers, as demonstrated in the present and previous studies (55).

Decreased plasma vitamin C concentrations were observed in a group of individuals exposed to environmental tobacco smoke, although their vitamin C intake did not differ significantly from that of nonexposed nonsmokers (66). On the other hand, decreased intake of vitamin C among passive smokers compared to that of nonsmokers not exposed to tobacco smoke has been reported in other studies (71,114), but not in all studies (115). High serum levels of nicotine are produced by chewing tobacco (116). Whether tobacco chewing also impairs vitamin C status seems to be disputable. Two recent studies showing plasma vitamin C values in small groups of snuff dippers from Sweden and the United States resulted in contrary findings (64,70).

Former smokers appear to have higher plasma ascorbic acid concentrations compared to current smokers (36,61,92). The association obviously reflects their decreased exposure to cigarette smoke, since the difference persisted after adjustment for dietary vitamin C and several other variables (39). However, suggested higher vitamin C intake of ex-smokers demonstrated in the present and several previous studies (Table 2) could also contribute to improved vitamin C status of ex-smokers.

ALCOHOL CONSUMPTION AND VITAMIN C

Alcohol Consumption and Vitamin C Intake

In contrast to the effect of smoking we found no significant relationship between alcohol intake and dietary vitamin C in the present study. There was a strong association between alcohol consumption and current smoking. The lack of association was, however, not due to confounding by smoking habits or several other personal characteristics. In the present study population heavier alcohol consumption was associated with higher social standing and longer education, factors which have been found to predict better vitamin C nutrition (50,53,54,59,67,117–119). The relationship between alcohol consumption and vitamin C intake was not, however, modified by the socioeconomic position or the stage of education. In another Finnish study including middle-aged male smokers, differences in dietary intake of vitamin C according to alcohol consumption were small, but there was a trend for lower values in higher alcohol consumption categories (120).

In recent population-based studies from different countries the effect of alcohol consumption on the absolute intake of vitamin C seems to be small (Table 4). Although 7 of the 10 studies shown in Table 4 indicate lower mean vitamin C intake in drinkers compared to nondrinkers or in heavy drinkers compared to light drinkers, only 4 studies reported statistically significant difference (38,120,123,126). In other studies no significant association between alcohol consumption and vitamin C intake was observed. Some studies also reported vitamin C intake per energy intake unit (121,122,124,127). Their results indicate that vitamin C intake expressed per total energy intake may be decreased in the diets of heavy drinkers (124,127).

Le Marchand et al. (126) studied multiethnic populations in Hawaii and demonstrated a lower intake of vitamin C in male drinkers compared to abstainers, and the association was independent of smoking and other personal characteristics. The vitamin C intake of drinkers did not, however, differ according to the amount of alcohol consumed (126). Herbeth et al. (38) reported decreased dietary vitamin C to be associated with high alcohol consumption among French males. These men consumed less than 20 cigarettes per day, and their smoking habits did not differ in the alcohol intake categories. On the other hand, no significant differences were observed in the absolute intake of vitamin C according to drinking habits among French males and females from four areas, but vitamin C intake related to energy intake decreased among heavy drinkers (124). Nuttens et al. (77) demonstrated in middle-aged French males a significant inverse association between the intake of fruits and alcohol, when smoking and several other variables were controlled in the analysis. Although the lower nutrient density of vitamin C in the diet of users of alcoholic beverages was demonstrated in Italian females, the absolute intake of the vitamin was independent of the alcohol intake level (127). Population-based studies from the United States do not suggest a significant relationship between alcohol consumption and vitamin C intake estimated in absolute amounts or related to dietary energy (121,122,125), with the exception of selected groups with heavy alcohol consumption (123). Variable findings on different populations obviously reflect differences in the amounts and types of alcohol consumed, as well as differences in the sociocultural associations of alcohol consumption (38,128). The use of vitamin supplements is not suggested to be decreased by increasing alcohol consumption (78–80).

Alcoholic patients hospitalized for medical reasons form an extreme group of drinkers. Malnutrition and insufficient nutrient intake have been frequently described among these alcoholics (129–131). The lower dietary intake of vitamin C has also been reported in

Table 4 Studies on Associations Between Intake of Vitamin C and Alcohol Consumption in Normal Populations

Ref.	Population	Sample size	Sex	Age (years)	Diet survey method	Alcohol intake category	Mean vitamin C intake (mg/day)	Mean vitamin C intake (mg/1000 kcal)	Comments
121	Sample from a national survey; NFCS (1977–1978); United States	1,027	M/F	≥15	24-Hour food recall + 2-day food record	Nondrinker Drinker	89 91 NS	48 48 NS	Adjusted for age, sex, region, urbanization, day of the week, and body weight
122	National sample; NHANES I; United States	10,428	M/F	18–74	24-Hour food recall	Nondrinker Alcohol, <6 g/day Alcohol, 6–24 g/day Alcohol, >24 g/day		52.3[a] 55.4 54.7 52.3	All drinkers combined had significantly higher ($p \geq 0.05$) vitamin C density than nondrinkers
123	Middle-class males, without and with alcohol problem; United States	179	M		24-Hour food recall	Lowest tertile, <7.9 g/day Middle tertile, 7.9–35.4 g/day Highest tertile, >35.4 g/day	120 93 47 $p < 0.05$ (trend)		
124	Apparently healthy subjects; four regions, France	356	M	18–44	7-Day food record	Control, ≤43 g/day Moderate drinker, 44–87 g/day Heavy drinker, ≥88 g/day	75 66 68 NS	24.6 18.9 17.6 $p < 0.01$ (controls vs. drinkers)	
		196	F			Control, ≤21 g/day Moderate drinker, 22–43 g/day Heavy drinker, ≥44 g/day	74 73 64 NS	31.5 27.6 19.8 $p < 0.01$ (controls vs. heavy drinkers)	
38	Apparently healthy French men; Lorraine, France	216	M	18–44	7-Day food record	Control, ≤43 g/day Moderate drinker, 44–87 g/day Heavy drinker, ≥88 g/day	73 57 53 $p = 0.005$[b]		Adjustment for age or socio-professional status did not change the results
125	Nonalcoholic, noninstitutionalized elderly; Boston area, United States	586	M/F	60–100	3-Day food record	Alcohol, 0–4 g/day Alcohol, 5–14 g/day Alcohol, ≥15 g/day	369[c] 315 234 NS		Adjusted for age, sex, and energy intake

Ref	Population	N	Sex	Age	Assessment	Category	Vitamin C density	Comments
126	Random sample; five ethnic groups; Hawaii (1977–1979), United States	2,272	M	≥45	Diet history interview, 83 food items	Abstainer Drinker	108.5 99.2 $p = 0.009$[b]	Adjusted for age, ethnicity, income, and cigarette consumption
		2,337	F			Abstainer Drinker	107.3 100.7 NS	
127	Population-based controls for breast cancer; northwestern Italy	499	F	Mean 57.2	Diet history interview	Alcohol, <5 g/day Alcohol, 5–19 g/day Alcohol, 20–39 g/day Alcohol, ≥40 g/day	107 52.9 105 51.5 107 48.2 118 47.2 $p < 0.05$ (trend)	Significant inverse association ($p = 0.02$) between alcohol consumption and vitamin C density remained after adjustment for age, place of residence, occupation, and body mass index
59	Hospital controls for cancer study; Milan area, Italy	1,039	M	21–74	FFQ, 30 food items	Drinks, 0/day Drinks, <3/day Drinks, ≥3/day	117[d] 120 113 NS	Adjusted for age
		735	F			Drinks, 0/day Drinks, <3/day Drinks, ≥3/day	127 117 127 NS	
120	Trial subjects; middle-aged smokers, Finland	27,215	M	50–69	FFQ, 270 food items	Abstainer Alcohol, <15 g/day Alcohol, 15–29.9 g/day Alcohol, 30–59.9 g/day Alcohol ≥60 g/day	104 108 106 103 98 $p < 0.001$ (trend)	

[a]In this study of vitamin C density is vitamin C intake divided by total nonalcoholic energy intake and expressed per 1000 kcal. NS, nonsignificant difference; FFQ, food frequency questionnaire; NFCS, Nationwide Food Consumption Survey; NHANES, National Health and Nutrition Examination Survey.

[b]p Value for difference unless stated otherwise.

[c]Vitamin C from supplements included.

[d]Calculated from original values given in grams per month.

References are cited in the order of the year of publication.

alcoholic patients compared to nonalcoholic controls, although not all patients have insufficient vitamin C intake (33). The nutrition of alcoholic patients is, however, complex and
obviously depends on socioeconomic factors and severity of alcohol dependence (130–
132). Since most alcoholics are also heavy smokers (133), potential interference of smoking
is plausible. In a group of middle-class alcoholic patients in which alcohol accounted for on
average one-third of their energy intake, most patients were deemed to be adequately
nourished (134). Nevertheless, in approximately 30% of the patients the intake of some
vitamins including vitamin C was suggested to be low compared to the recommended
dietary allowance (134). In another group of alcoholic patients ingesting a great proportion
(65%) of their total energy through ethanol the mean intake of vitamin C remained far
below the recommendation for vitamin C (135). In employed male problem drinkers in
Finland the mean intake of vitamin C did not differ significantly from that of the controls
selected from regular occupational health examinations (136). In this study energy derived
from alcohol contributed on average 15% and 4% of the total energy intake of cases and
controls, respectively, and approximately 80% of drinkers and 30% of controls were
current smokers.

Mechanisms by Which Alcohol Affects Vitamin C Status

The role of alcohol in nutrition is complex and probably involves behavioral as well as
metabolic influences (132). Alcohol consumption may reduce the intake and bioavailability
of nutrients and thus enhance nutritional deficiencies (129–131). Alcoholic beverages
provide energy, but they are usually devoid of vitamins, minerals, and proteins (121,129,
131). In the general population, several studies, including the present one, agree that energy
derived from alcohol is added to that of the diet (38,120,124,127,137–139). However, some
studies reported decreased intake of nonalcoholic energy as alcohol intake increased
(122,123).

Bioavailability of vitamin C can be impaired as a result of the direct effects of ethanol or
in association with nutritional disorders caused by alcohol intake (129,130). In a small
number of healthy subjects the ingestion of 35 g ethanol with 2 g ascorbic acid resulted in
significantly lower plasma ascorbic acid concentrations than when no alcohol was ingested
during the following 24 h; the result may be due to the impaired absorption of vitamin C
(140). Enhanced urinary excretion of ascorbic acid was demonstrated after an acute alcohol
load administered as either whiskey or lager (141).

The requirement of vitamin C may be increased as a result of the hypothesized increased
free radical activity associated with ethanol metabolism (142–144). Vitamin C may also be
directly involved in the metabolism of ethanol (145–147). Studies in animals seem to
support the contention that a diet which is nutritionally adequate may no longer be so in the
presence of high ethanol intake, and that supplemental vitamin C ingestion may afford
protection against ethanol toxicity (148,149). Both short-term and long-term supplementation with vitamin C have been shown to increase the rate of ethanol clearance from blood in
healthy male subjects (145,150,151).

Alcohol Consumption and Vitamin C Status

Deficient vitamin C status has been frequently described in chronic alcoholics hospitalized
for medical reasons compared to nonalcoholic controls. Bonjour (33) reviewed several

studies that demonstrated significantly lower vitamin C status among alcoholic patients based on measurements of ascorbic acid in plasma, leukocytes, and urinary excretion of ascorbic acid. However, vitamin C status of alcoholic patients can be greatly variable. More than 90% of alcoholic patients were suggested to be vitamin C–deficient in some studies (153), whereas in other studies this proportion was considerably lower (13%–15%) (152), and some studies reported similar plasma vitamin C values in alcoholic patients and healthy controls (154). In patients with alcohol-related illness leukocyte ascorbic acid concentrations were poorly correlated with a plasma marker for alcohol consumption, indicating a complex relationship between alcohol intake and vitamin C status (155). In several cases lower vitamin C status has been associated with lower vitamin C intake, but exceptions to this rule indicate that insufficient dietary vitamin C intake only partially explains low plasma vitamin C values of alcoholic patients (33). Since most chronic alcoholics are also heavy smokers (133) the influence of alcohol consumption as opposed to smoking can hardly be distinguished among this group.

In a few population-based studies the relationship between alcohol consumption and vitamin C nutrition seems to be controversial. A significant inverse relationship between alcohol intake and plasma ascorbic acid concentration was demonstrated in a study on German adult females in multiple regression analysis, adjusting for vitamin C intake, energy intake, smoking, and body mass index (96), whereas in men the association was not significant. Plasma vitamin C values were also suggested to be lowered with heavier drinking among young adult females in another study from Germany (85). Two studies from France, one in 60- to 82-year-olds from Nancy (29) and the other in a random sample from the Paris area, including persons 18 years or older (95) did not reveal a significant effect of alcohol consumption on plasma ascorbic acid concentration when dietary vitamin C, smoking, and other potential confounding factors were taken into account. No significant differences in plasma ascorbic acid values according to alcohol consumption were found in a large general population-based survey on adult Americans (39), or in a group of older Americans when their plasma vitamin C values were adjusted for age, sex, and vitamin C intake (125). Murata and coworkers (90) reported in Japanese males almost the same plasma vitamin C levels between drinkers and nondrinkers regardless of their smoking status, indicating that moderate consumption of alcohol does not affect vitamin C status. In a recent study from Venezuela, women who were regular drinkers tended to have lower plasma vitamin C concentrations, but the association between plasma vitamin C and alcohol consumption was not significant in either men or women when age and cigarette smoking were controlled in the analysis (42). Though the conclusion is based on only a few studies, it appears that the generalizations over different populations made for smoking and vitamin C cannot be similarly made for alcohol consumption and vitamin C status in normal populations. It is suspected that the most probably undernourished indigent alcoholic patients seldom participate in health examination studies.

VITAMIN C, SMOKING, AND ALCOHOL CONSUMPTION

Alcohol consumption and smoking, especially heavy drinking and heavy smoking, are positively correlated, as demonstrated in the present and several other studies (39,43,50, 62,68,73,77,133,139). Thus, it is probable that persons who both smoke and heavily consume alcohol have a lower intake of vitamin C than persons who either smoke or use alcohol. Of special interest is whether there is an interaction between smoking and alcohol on vitamin C intake. Our results did not, however, suggest any interaction between current smoking and alcohol consumption level on the intake of dietary vitamin C among adult male Finns. This finding may be due to the fact that we found no association between alcohol intake and dietary vitamin C. Unfortunately, this potential interaction effect or the possible modifying effect of smoking and alcohol consumption on tissue vitamin C level has hardly been investigated in other studies. Because of suggested interaction in the effects of smoking and alcohol consumption on the occurrence of some cancers (156,157) where vitamin C may also be important, it should be investigated whether there is a greater demand for vitamin C among persons exposed to both cigarette smoke and alcohol.

SUMMARY

We observed decreased dietary intake of vitamin C among smokers in a large Finnish male cohort. Similar inverse associations between smoking and dietary vitamin C have also been demonstrated in several studies from other countries. In addition to the decreased intake of vitamin C in smokers, cigarette smoke can also directly impair vitamin C status, increasing the metabolic turnover rate of the vitamin. Thus there seems to be a clear adverse effect of smoking on vitamin C status, an effect which is not explained by differences in other personal characteristics.

There was no significant association between alcohol consumption and vitamin C intake in the present study. In most other population-based studies the impact of alcohol consumption on vitamin C nutrition is also suggested to be small, whereas low vitamin C intakes have been observed in chronic alcoholics. Alcohol consumption may adversely affect vitamin C status by decreasing bioavailability of the vitamin. Increased free radical activity associated with alcohol metabolism has also been implicated. Low plasma ascorbic acid concentrations have been described in alcohol abusers, but in nonalcoholic populations the independent effect of alcohol intake on plasma vitamin C level seems to be small. Accordingly, the relationship between alcohol consumption and vitamin C status appears to depend on the population under study.

Since alcohol consumption and smoking, especially heavy drinking and heavy smoking, are correlated behavior patterns, as demonstrated in the present and several other studies, their effects on vitamin C nutrition were expected to interfere with each other. Our results did not, however, reveal any interaction of smoking and the use of alcohol on the intake of dietary vitamin C. This issue and the possible modifying effect of smoking and alcohol consumption on tissue vitamin C have scarcely been studied so far. Further studies are thus needed on the complex relationships among vitamin C, smoking, and alcohol consumption until we can draw unconstrained conclusions about the association between vitamin C nutrition and risk of chronic diseases.

ACKNOWLEDGMENT

We gratefully recognize the contribution of Ritva Seppänen, Ph.D., and Jouni Maatela, M.D. (Social Insurance Institution, Turku, Finland), and Arpo Aromaa, M.D., Antti Reunanen, M.D., and Markku Heliövaara, M.D. (National Public Health Institute, Helsinki, Finland, and Social Insurance Institution, Helsinki, Finland) to the compilation of the baseline data of the Finnish Mobile Clinic Health Examination Survey.

REFERENCES

1. Bendich A, Machlin LJ, Scandurra O, et al. The antioxidant role of vitamin C. Adv Free Radical Biol Med 1986; 2:419–444.
2. Padh H. Cellular functions of ascorbic acid. Biochem Cell Biol 1990; 68:1166–1173.
3. Frei B. Ascorbic acid protects lipids in human plasma and low-density lipoprotein against oxidative damage. Am J Clin Nutr 1991; 54(suppl):1113S–1118S.
4. Niki E. Vitamin C as an antioxidant. World Rev Nutr Diet 1991; 64:1–30.
5. Byers T, Perry G. Dietary carotenes, vitamin C, and vitamin E as protective antioxidants in human cancers. Annu Rev Nutr 1992; 12:139–159.
6. Gershoff SN. Vitamin C (ascorbic acid): new roles, new requirements? Nutr Rev 1993; 51: 313–326.
7. Sauberlich HE. Pharmacology of vitamin C. Annu Rev Nutr 1994; 14:371–391.
8. Bendich A, Langseth L. The health effects of vitamin C supplementation: a review. J Am Coll Nutr 1995; 14:124–136.
9. Glatthaar BE, Hornig DH, Moser U. The role of ascorbic acid in carcinogenesis. Adv Exp Med Biol 1986; 206:357–377.
10. Block G. Vitamin C and cancer prevention: the epidemiologic evidence. Am J Clin Nutr 1991; 53(suppl):270S–282S.
11. Block G. Vitamin C status and cancer. Epidemiologic evidence of reduced risk. Ann NY Acad Sci 1992; 669:280–290.
12. Stähelin HB, Gey KF, Eichholzer M, et al. Plasma antioxidant vitamins and subsequent cancer mortality in the 12-year follow-up of the Prospective Basel Study. Am J Epidemiol 1991; 133:766–775.
13. Fontham ETH. Vitamin C, vitamin C-rich foods, and cancer: epidemiologic studies. In: Frei B, ed. Natural Antioxidants in Human Health and Disease. Orlando, FL: Academic Press, 1994:157–197.
14. Byers T, Guerrero N. Epidemiologic evidence for vitamin C and vitamin E in cancer prevention. Am J Clin Nutr 1995; 62(suppl):1385S–1392S.
15. Cohen M, Bhagavan HN. Ascorbic acid and gastrointestinal cancer. J Am Coll Nutr 1995; 14:565–578.
16. Flagg EW, Coates RJ, Greenberg RS. Epidemiologic studies of antioxidants and cancer in humans. J Am Coll Nutr 1995; 14:419–427.
17. Gey KF, Stähelin HB, Puska P, Evans A. Relationship of plasma level of vitamin C to mortality from ischemic heart disease. Ann NY Acad Sci 1987; 498:110–120.
18. Trout DL. Vitamin C and cardiovascular risk factors. Am J Clin Nutr 1991; 53(suppl):322S–325S.
19. Simon JA. Vitamin C and cardiovascular disease: a review. J Am Coll Nutr 1992; 11: 107–125.
20. Gey KF, Moser UK, Jordan P, et al. Increased risk of cardiovascular disease at suboptimal plasma concentrations of essential antioxidants: an epidemiological update with special attention to carotene and vitamin C. Am J Clin Nutr 1993; 57(suppl):787S–797S.
21. Gaziano JM, Manson JE, Hennekens CH. Natural antioxidants and cardiovascular disease: observational epidemiologic studies and randomized trials. In: Frei B, ed. Natural Antioxidants in Human Health and Disease. Orlando, FL: Academic Press, 1994:387–409.
22. Knekt P, Reunanen A, Järvinen R, et al. Antioxidant vitamin intake and coronary mortality in a longitudinal population study. Am J Epidemiol 1994; 139:1180–1189.
23. Hennekens CH, Gaziano JM, Manson JE, Buring JE. Antioxidant vitamin-cardiovascular disease hypothesis is still promising, but still unproven: the need for randomized trials. Am J Clin Nutr 1995; 62(suppl):1377S–1380S.
24. Jacques PF, Chylack LT Jr, Taylor A. Relationships between natural antioxidants and cataract

formation. In: Frei B, ed. Natural Antioxidants in Human Health and Disease. Orlando, FL: Academic Press, 1994:515–533.

25. Taylor A, Jacques PF, Epstein EM. Relations among aging, antioxidant status, and cataract. Am J Clin Nutr 1995; 62(suppl):1439S–1447S.

26. Bates CJ, Rutishauser IHE, Black AE, et al. Long-term vitamin status and dietary intake of healthy elderly subjects. 2. Vitamin C. Br J Nutr 1979; 42:43–56.

27. Mahalko JR, Johnson LK, Gallagher SK, Milne DB. Comparison of dietary histories and seven-day food records in a nutritional assessment of older adults. Am J Clin Nutr 1985; 42:542–553.

28. Jacob RA, Otradovec CL, Russell RM, et al. Vitamin C status and nutrient interactions in a healthy elderly population. Am J Clin Nutr 1988; 48:1436–1442.

29. Herbeth B, Chavance M, Musse N, et al. Dietary intake and other determinants of blood vitamins in an elderly population. Eur J Clin Nutr 1989; 43:175–186.

30. Bolton-Smith C, Casey CE, Gey KF, et al. Antioxidant vitamin intakes assessed using a food-frequency questionnaire: correlation with biochemical status in smokers and non-smokers. Br J Nutr 1991; 65:337–346.

31. Jacques PF, Sulsky SI, Sadowski JA, et al. Comparison of micronutrient intake measured by a dietary questionnaire and biochemical indicators of micronutrient status. Am J Clin Nutr 1993; 57:182–189.

32. Jacob RA, Skala JH, Omaye ST. Biochemical indices of human vitamin C status. Am J Clin Nutr 1987; 46:818–826.

33. Bonjour JP. Vitamins and alcoholism. I. Ascorbic acid. Int J Vitam Nutr Res 1979; 49:434–441.

34. Hornig DH, Glatthaar BE. Vitamin C and smoking: increased requirement of smokers. Int J Vitam Nutr Res 1985; (suppl 27):139–155.

35. Murata A. Smoking and vitamin C. World Rev Nutr Diet 1991; 64:31–57.

36. Preston AM. Cigarette smoking—nutritional implications. Prog Food Nutr Sci 1991; 15:183–217.

37. Thompson RL, Margetts BM, Wood DA, Jackson AA. Cigarette smoking and food and nutrient intakes in relation to coronary heart disease. Nutr Res Rev 1992; 5:131–152.

38. Herbeth B, Didelot-Barthelemy L, Lemoine A, le Devehat C. Dietary behavior of French men according to alcohol drinking pattern. J Stud Alcohol 1988; 49:268–272.

39. Schectman G, Byrd JC, Gruchow HW. The influence of smoking on vitamin C status in adults. Am J Public Health 1989; 79:158–162.

40. Subar AF, Harlan LC, Mattson ME. Food and nutrient intake differences between smokers and non-smokers in the US. Am J Public Health 1990; 80:1323–1329.

41. Bolton-Smith C. Antioxidant vitamin intakes in Scottish smokers and nonsmokers. Ann NY Acad Sci 1993; 686:347–358.

42. Buiatti E, Munoz N, Kato I, et al. Determinants of plasma anti-oxidant vitamin levels in a population at high risk for stomach cancer. Int J Cancer 1996; 65:317–322.

43. Zondervan KT, Ocke MC, Smit HA, Seidell JC. Do dietary and supplementary intakes of antioxidants differ with smoking status? Int J Epidemiol 1996; 25:70–79.

44. Knekt P. Serum Alpha-Tocopherol and the Risk of Cancer. Helsinki: Social Insurance Institution, Finland, Series ML:83, 1988.

45. Järvinen R, Seppänen R, Knekt P. Short-term and long-term reproducibility of dietary history interview data. Int J Epidemiol 1993; 22:520–527.

46. Rastas M, Seppänen R, Knuts L-R, et al., eds. Nutrient composition of foods. (In Finnish with English affiliations). Helsinki, Finland: Social Insurance Institution, 1989.

47. Cohen J, Cohen P. Applied Multiple Regression/correlation Analysis for the Behavioral Sciences. New York: John Wiley & Sons, 1975.

48. Keith RE, Driskell JA. Effects of chronic cigarette smoking on vitamin C status, lung function, and resting and exercise cardiovascular metabolism in humans. Nutr Rep Int 1980; 21:907–912.

49. Shapiro LR, Samuels S, Breslow L, Camacho T. Patterns of vitamin C intake from food and supplements: survey of an adult population in Alameda County, California. Am J Public Health 1983; 73:773–778.

50. Fehily AM, Phillips KM, Yarnell JWG. Diet, smoking, social class, and body mass index in the Caerphilly Heart Disease Study. Am J Clin Nutr 1984; 40:827–833.

51. Norkus EP, Hsu H, Cehelsky MR. Effect of cigarette smoking on the vitamin C status of pregnant women and their offspring. Ann NY Acad Sci 1987; 498:500–501.

52. Itoh R, Yamada K, Oka J, et al. Sex as a factor in levels of serum ascorbic acid in a healthy elderly population. Int J Vitam Nutr Res 1989; 59:365–372.

53. Haste FM, Brooke OG, Anderson HR, et al. Nutrient intakes during pregnancy: observations on the influence of smoking and social class. Am J Clin Nutr 1990; 51:29–36.

54. Haste FM, Brooke OG, Anderson HR, et al. Social determinants of nutrient intake in smokers and nonsmokers during pregnancy. J Epidemiol Community Health 1990; 44:205–209.

55. Gridley G, McLaughlin JK, Blot WJ. Dietary vitamin C intake and cigarette smoking. Am J Public Health 1990; 81:1526.

56. Larkin FA, Basiotis PP, Riddick HA, et al. Dietary patterns of women smokers and non-smokers. J Am Diet Assoc 1990; 90:230–237.

57. Cade JE, Margetts BM. Relationship between diet and smoking—Is the diet of smokers different? J Epidemiol Community Health 1991; 45:270–272.

58. Bui MH, Sauty A, Collet F, Leuenberger P. Dietary vitamin C intake and concentrations in the body fluids and cells of male smokers and nonsmokers. J Nutr 1992; 122:312–316.

59. La Vecchia C, Negri E, Franceschi S, et al. Differences in dietary intake with smoking, alcohol, and education. Nutr Cancer 1992; 17:297–304.

60. Bolton-Smith C, Woodward M, Brown CA, Tunstall-Pedoe H. Nutrient intake by duration of ex-smoking in the Scottish Heart Health Study. Br J Nutr 1993; 69:315–332.

61. Duthie GG, Arthur JR, Beattie JAG, et al. Cigarette smoking, antioxidants, lipid peroxidation, and coronary heart disease. Ann NY Acad Sci 1993; 686:120–129.

62. Margetts BM, Jackson AA. Interactions between people's diet and their smoking habits: the dietary and nutritional survey of British adults. Br Med J 1993; 307:1381–1384.

63. Midgette AS, Baron JA, Rohan TE. Do cigarette smokers have diets that increase their risks of coronary heart disease and cancer? Am J Epidemiol 1993; 137:521–529.

64. Stegmayr B, Johansson I, Huhtasaari F, et al. Use of smokeless tobacco and cigarettes—Effects on plasma levels of antioxidant vitamins. Int J Vitam Nutr Res 1993; 63:195–200.

65. Subar AF, Harlan LC. Nutrient and food group intake by tobacco use status: The 1987 National Health Interview Survey. Ann NY Acad Sci 1993; 686:310–321.

66. Tribble DL, Guiliano LJ, Fortmann SP. Reduced plasma ascorbic acid concentrations in nonsmokers regularly exposed to environmental tobacco smoke. Am J Clin Nutr 1993; 58:886–890.

67. Järvinen R, Knekt P, Seppänen R, et al. Antioxidant vitamins in the diet: relationships with other personal characteristics in Finland. J Epidemiol Community Health 1994; 48:549–554.

68. McPhillips JB, Eaton CB, Gans KM, et al. Dietary differences in smokers and nonsmokers from two southeastern New England communities. J Am Diet Assoc 1994; 94:287–292.

69. Faruque O, Rahman Khan M, Rahman M, Ahmed F. Relationship between smoking and antioxidant nutrient status. Br J Nutr 1995; 73:625–632.

70. Giraud DW, Martin HD, Driskell JA. Plasma and dietary vitamin C and E levels of tobacco chewers, smokers, and nonusers. J Am Diet Assoc 1995; 95:798–800.

71. Emmons KM, Thompson B, Feng Z, et al. Dietary intake and exposure to environmental tobacco smoke in a worksite population. Eur J Clin Nutr 1995; 49:336–345.

72. Pamuk ER, Byers T, Coates RJ, et al. Effect of smoking on serum nutrient concentrations in African-American women. Am J Clin Nutr 1994; 59:891–895.

73. Le Marchand L, Ntilivamunda A, Kolonel LN, et al. Relationship of smoking to other life-style factors among several ethnic groups in Hawaii. Asia Pacific J Public Health 1988; 2:120–126.

74. Whichelow MJ, Golding JF, Treasure FP. Comparison of some dietary habits of smokers and non-smokers. Br J Addict 1988; 83:295–304.

75. Hebert JR, Kabat GC. Differences in dietary intake associated with smoking status. Eur J Clin Nutr 1990; 44:185–193.

76. Morabia A, Wynder EL. Dietary habits of smokers, people who never smoked, and exsmokers. Am J Clin Nutr 1990; 52:933–937.

77. Nuttens MC, Romon M, Ruidavets JB, et al. Relationship between smoking and diet: The MONICA-France project. J Intern Med 1992; 231:349–356.

78. Klaukka T, Riska E, Kimmel U-M. Use of vitamin supplements in Finland. Eur J Clin Pharmacol 1985; 29:355–361.

79. Block G, Cox C, Madans J, et al. Vitamin supplement use, by demographic characteristics. Am J Epidemiol 1988; 127:297–309.

80. Subar AF, Block G. Use of vitamin and mineral supplements: demographics and amounts of nutrients consumed. Am J Epidemiol 1990; 132:1091–1101.

81. Dorant E, van den Brandt PA, Hamstra AM, et al. The use of vitamins, minerals and other dietary supplements in The Netherlands. Int J Vitam Nutr Res 1993; 63:4–10.

82. Rodin J. Weight change following smoking cessation: the role of food intake and exercise. Addict Behav 1987; 12:303–317.

83. Thompson RL, Pyke SDM, Scott EA, et al. Dietary change after smoking cessation: a prospective study. Br J Nutr 1995; 74:27–38.

84. Kim I, Williamson DF, Byers T, Koplan JP. Vitamin and mineral supplement use and mortality in a US cohort. Am J Public Health 1993; 83:546–550.

85. Arab L, Schellenberg B, Schlierf G, et al. Nutrition and health. A survey of young men and women in Heidelberg. Ann Nutr Metab 1982; 26(suppl 1):1–244.

86. Biersner RJ, Gilman SC, Thornton RD. Relationship of plasma vitamin C to the health and performance of submariners. J Appl Nutr 1982; 34:29–37.

87. Bazzarre TL. Effects of vitamin C supplementation among male smokers and non-smokers. Nutr Rep Int 1986; 33:711–720.

88. Chow CK, Thacker RR, Changchit C, et al. Lower levels of vitamin C and carotenes in plasma of cigarette smokers. J Am Coll Nutr 1986; 5:305–312.

89. Basu J, Vermund SH, Mikhail M, et al. Plasma reduced and total ascorbic acid in healthy women: effects of smoking and oral contraception. Contraception 1989; 39:85–93.

90. Murata A, Shiraishi I, Fukuzaki K, et al. Lower levels of vitamin C in plasma and urine of Japanese male smokers. Int J Vitam Nutr Res 1989; 59:184–189.

91. Bridges RB, Chow CK, Rehm SR. Micronutrient status and immune function in smokers. Ann NY Acad Sci 1990; 587:218–231.

92. Riemersma RA, Wood DA, Macintyre CCA, et al. Risk of angina pectoris and plasma concentrations of vitamins A, C, and E and carotene. Lancet 1991; 337:1–5.

93. Van Antwerpen L, Theron AJ, Myer MS, et al. Cigarette smoke-mediated oxidant stress, phagocytes, vitamin C, vitamin E, and tissue injury. Ann NY Acad Sci 1993; 686:53–65.

94. Fernández-Bañares F, Giné JJ, Cabré E, et al. Factors associated with low values of biochemical vitamin parameters in healthy subjects. Int J Vitam Nutr Res 1993; 63:68–74.

95. Hercberg S, Preziosi P, Galan P, et al. Vitamin status of a healthy French population: dietary intakes and biochemical markers. Int J Vitam Nutr Res 1994; 64:220–232.

96. Heseker H, Schneider R. Requirement and supply of vitamin C, E and β-carotene for elderly men and women. Eur J Clin Nutr 1994; 48:118–127.

97. Sharpe PC, MacAuley D, McCrum EE, et al. Ascorbate and exercise in the Northern Ireland population. Int J Vitam Nutr Res 1994; 64:277–282.

98. Pelletier O. Vitamin C and cigarette smokers. Ann NY Acad Sci 1975; 258:156–167.

99. Ritzel G, Bruppacher R. Vitamin C and tobacco. Int J Vitam Nutr Res 1977; (suppl 16):171–183.

100. Smith JL, Hodges RE. Serum levels of vitamin C in relation to dietary and supplemental intake of vitamin C in smokers and nonsmokers. Ann NY Acad Sci 1987; 498:144–151.

101. Church DF, Pryor WA. Free-radical chemistry of cigarette smoke and its toxicological implications. Environ Health Perspect 1985; 64:111–126.

102. Pryor WA, Stone K. Oxidants in cigarette smoke. Radicals, hydrogen peroxide, peroxynitrate, and peroxynitrite. Ann NY Acad Sci 1993; 686:12–27.

103. Ludvig PW, Hoidal JR. Alterations in leukocyte oxidative metabolism in cigarette smokers. Am Rev Respir Dis 1982; 126:977–980.

104. Frei B, Forte TM, Ames BN, Cross CE. Gas phase oxidants of cigarette smoke induce lipid peroxidation and changes in lipoprotein properties in human blood plasma. Protective effects of ascorbic acid. Biochem J 1991; 277:133–138.

105. Eiserich JP, van der Vliet A, Handelman GJ, et al. Dietary antioxidants and cigarette smoke-induced biomolecular damage: a complex interaction. Am J Clin Nutr 1995; 62(suppl):1490S–1500S.

106. Kallner AB, Hartman D, Hornig DH. On the requirements of ascorbic acid in man: steady-state turnover and body pool in smokers. Am J Clin Nutr 1981; 34:1347–1355.

107. Pelletier O. Vitamin C status of cigarette smokers and nonsmokers. Am J Clin Nutr 1970; 23: 520–524.

108. Yeung DL. Relationships between cigarette smoking, oral contraceptives, and plasma vitamins A, E, C, and plasma triglycerides and cholesterol. Am J Clin Nutr 1976; 29:1216–1221.

109. Calder JH, Curtis RC, Fore H. Comparison of vitamin C in plasma and leukocytes of smokers and non-smokers. Lancet 1963; 1:556.

110. Dickinson VA, Block G, Russek-Cohen E. Supplement use, other dietary and demographic variables, and serum vitamin C in NHANES II. J Am Coll Nutr 1994; 13:22–32.

111. Schectman G, Byrd JC, Hoffman R. Ascorbic acid requirements for smokers: analysis of a population survey. Am J Clin Nutr 1991; 53:1466–1470.

112. National Research Council. Recommended Dietary Allowances. 10th ed. Washington, DC: National Academy Press, 1989.

113. Kershbaum A, Bellet S, Hirabayashi M, et al. Effect of cigarette, cigar, and pipe smoking on nicotine excretion. The influence of inhaling. Arch Intern Med 1967; 120:311–314.

114. Matanoski G, Kanchanaraksa S, Lantry D, Chang Y. Characteristics of nonsmoking women in NHANES I and NHANES I Epidemiologic Follow-up Study with exposure to spouses who smoke. Am J Epidemiol 1995; 142:149–157.

115. Le Marchand L, Wilkens LR, Hankin JH, Haley NJ. Dietary patterns of female nonsmokers with and without exposure to environmental tobacco smoke. Cancer Causes Control 1991; 2:11–16.

116. Russell MAH, Jarvis MJ, West RJ, Feyerabend C. Buccal absorption of nicotine from smokeless tobacco sachets. Lancet 1985; 2:1370.

117. Bolton-Smith C, Smith WCS, Woodward M, Tunstall-Pedoe H. Nutrient intakes of different social-class groups: results from the Scottish Heart Health Study (SHHS). Br J Nutr 1991; 65:321–335.

118. Hulshof KFAM, Löwik MRH, Kok FJ, et al. Diet and other life-style factors in high and low socio-economic groups (Dutch Nutrition Surveillance System). Eur J Clin Nutr 1991; 45: 441–450.

119. Tucker K, Spiro A III, Weiss ST. Variation in food and nutrient intakes among older men: age, and other sociodemographic factors. Nutr Res 1995; 15:161–176.

120. Männistö S, Pietinen P, Haukka J, et al. Reported alcohol intake, diet, and body mass index in male smokers. Eur J Clin Nutr 1996; 50:239–245.

121. Windham CT, Wyse BW, Hansen RG. Alcohol consumption and nutrient density of diets in the Nationwide Food Consumption Survey. J Am Diet Assoc 1983; 82:364–370, 373.

122. Gruchow HW, Sobocinski KA, Barboriak JJ, Scheller JG. Alcohol consumption, nutrient intake and relative body weight among US adults. Am J Clin Nutr 1985; 42:289–295.

123. Hillers VN, Massey LK. Interrelationships of moderate and high alcohol consumption with diet and health status. Am J Clin Nutr 1985; 41:356–362.

124. Lemoine A, Le Devehat C, Herbeth B, et al. ESVITAF. Vitamin status in three groups of French adults: controls, obese subjects, alcohol drinkers. Ann Nutr Metabol 1986; 30(suppl 1):1–94.

125. Jacques PF, Sulsky S, Hartz SC, Russell RM. Moderate alcohol intake and nutritional status in nonalcoholic elderly subjects. Am J Clin Nutr 1989; 50:875–883.

126. Le Marchand L, Kolonel LN, Hankin JH, Yoshizawa CN. Relationship of alcohol consumption to diet: a population-based study in Hawaii. Am J Clin Nutr 1989; 49:567–572.

127. Toniolo P, Riboli E, Cappa APM. A community study of alcohol consumption and dietary habits in middle-aged Italian women. Int J Epidemiol 1991; 20:663–670.

128. Gex-Fabry M, Raymond L, Jeanneret O. Multivariate analysis of dietary patterns in 939 Swiss adults: sociodemographic parameters and alcohol consumption profiles. Int J Epidemiol 1988; 17:548–555.

129. Morgan MY. Alcohol and nutrition. Br Med Bull 1982; 38:21–29.

130. World MJ, Ryle PR, Thomson AD. Alcoholic malnutrition and the small intestine. Alcohol Alcoholism 1985; 20:89–124.

131. Feinman L, Lieber CS. Nutrition and diet in alcoholism. In: Shils ME, Olson JA, Shike M, eds. Modern Nutrition in Health and Disease. Vol. 2. 8th ed. Philadelphia: Lea & Febiger, 1994: 1081–1101.

132. Darnton-Hill I. Interactions of alcohol, malnutrition and ill health. World Rev Nutr Diet 1989; 59:95–125.

133. Istvan J, Matarazzo JD. Tobacco, alcohol, and caffeine use: a review of their interrelationships. Psychol Bull 1984; 95:301–326.

134. Hurt RD, Higgins JA, Nelson RA, et al. Nutritional status of a group of alcoholics before and after admission to an alcoholism treatment unit. Am J Clin Nutr 1981; 34:386–392.

135. Bunout D, Gattas V, Iturriaga H, et al. Nutritional status of alcoholic patients: its possible relationship to alcoholic liver damage. Am J Clin Nutr 1983; 38:469–473.

136. Rissanen A, Sarlio-Lähteenkorva S, Alftan G, et al. Employed problem drinkers: a nutritional risk group? Am J Clin Nutr 1987; 45:456–461.

137. Fisher M, Gordon T. The relation of drinking and smoking habits to diet: The Lipid Research Clinics Prevalence Study. Am J Clin Nutr 1985; 41:623–630.

138. Colditz GA, Giovannucci E, Rimm EB, et al. Alcohol intake in relation to diet and obesity in women and men. Am J Clin Nutr 1991; 54:49–55.

139. Veenstra J, Schenkel JAA, van Erp-Baart AMJ, et al. Alcohol consumption in relation to food intake and smoking habits in The Dutch National Food Consumption Survey. Eur J Clin Nutr 1993; 47:482–489.

140. Fazio V, Flint DM, Wahlqvist ML. Acute effects of alcohol on plasma ascorbic acid in healthy subjects. Am J Clin Nutr 1981; 34:2394–2396.

141. Faizallah R, Morris AI, Krasner N, Walker RJ. Alcohol enhances vitamin C excretion in the urine. Alcohol Alcoholism 1986; 21:81–84.

142. Kaplowitz N, Fernandez-Checa J, Ookhtens M. Glutathione, alcohol, and hepatotoxicity. In: Halsted CH, Rucker RB, eds. Nutrition and the Origin of Disease. San Diego, CA: Academic Press, 1989:267–283.

143. Nordmann R, Ribiere C, Rouach H. Implication of free radical mechanisms in ethanol-induced cellular injury. Free Radical Biol Med 1992; 12:219–240.

144. Nordmann R. Alcohol and antioxidant systems. Alcohol Alcoholism 1994; 29:513–522.

145. Krasner N, Moore MR, Dow J, Goldberg A. Ascorbic-acid saturation and ethanol metabolism. Lancet 1974; 2:693–695.

146. Yunice AA, Lindeman RD. Effect of ascorbic acid and zinc sulfate on ethanol toxicity and metabolism. Proc Soc Exp Biol Med 1977; 154:146–150.

147. Susick RL Jr, Zannoni VG. Ascorbic acid and alcohol oxidation. Biochem Pharmacol 1984; 33:3963–3969.

148.   Yunice AA, Hsu JM, Fahmy A, Henry S. Ethanol-ascorbate interrelationship in acute and chronic alcoholism in the guinea pig. Proc Soc Exp Biol Med 1984; 177:262–271.

149.   Susick RL Jr, Abrams GD, Zurawski CA, Zannoni VG. Ascorbic acid and chronic alcohol consumption in the guinea pig. Toxicol Appl Pharmacol 1986; 84:329–335.

150.   Susick RL Jr, Zannoni VG. Effect of ascorbic acid on the consequences of acute alcohol consumption in humans. Clin Pharmacol Ther 1987; 41:502–509.

151.   Chen MF, Boyce HW Jr, Hsu JM. Effect of ascorbic acid on plasma alcohol clearance. J Am Coll Nutr 1990; 9:185–189.

152.   Devgun MS, Fiabane A, Paterson CR, Zarembski P. Vitamin and mineral nutrition in chronic alcoholics including patients with Korsakoff's psychosis. Br J Nutr 1981; 45:469–473.

153.   Majumdar SK, Patel S, Shaw GK, et al. Vitamin C utilization status in chronic alcoholic patients after short-term intravenous therapy. Int J Vitam Nutr Res 1981; 51:274–278.

154.   Johansson U, Johansson F, Joelsson B, et al. Selenium status in patients with liver cirrhosis and alcoholism. Br J Nutr 1986; 55:227–233.

155.   Baines M. Vitamin C and exposure to alcohol. Int J Vitam Nutr Res 1982; (suppl 23):287–293.

156.   Saracci R. The interactions of tobacco smoking and other agents in cancer etiology. Epidemiol Rev 1987; 9:175–193.

157.   Blot WJ. Alcohol and cancer. Cancer Res 1992; 52(suppl):2119S–2123S.

26

Vitamin C, Lipid Peroxidation, and the Risk of Myocardial Infarction: Epidemiological Evidence from Eastern Finland

JUKKA T. SALONEN, KRISTIINA NYYSSÖNEN, and MARKKU T. PARVIAINEN

Research Institute of Public Health, University of Kuopio, Kuopio, Finland

LIPID PEROXIDATION, ATHEROSCLEROSIS, AND CARDIOVASCULAR DISEASES

Steinberg and coworkers formulated the hypothesis that oxidative modification increases the atherogenicity of low-density lipoprotein (LDL) (1). Several authors have suggested that some form of modification of LDL is involved in atherogenesis and in the progression of early atherosclerotic plaques (2–4). The original theory is based on the concept that oxidative modification promotes the uptake and retention of circulating LDL in the arterial wall. However, lipid peroxidation could also promote atherogenesis through other pathways. These include the oxidation of membrane lipids of thrombocytes as well as arterial wall endothelial cells and smooth muscle cells. These effects could enhance the intercellular interactions that promote atherogenesis.

There is evidence that supports the hypothesis concerning the role of lipid peroxidation in atherogenesis, but this evidence is indirect. Experiments in rabbits have shown that atherogenesis can be inhibited by the supplementation with antioxidants such as probucol (1,5), butylated hydroxytoluene (BHT) (6,7), and vitamin E (8). Epidemiological follow-up studies suggest that a high intake of vitamin E is associated with a reduced risk of coronary events (9,10). Elevated body stores of the transition metals iron and mercury, which catalyze lipid peroxidation, have been associated with excess risk of myocardial infarction (11,12).

We observed an association between a high titer of autoantibodies against oxidized LDL and accelerated progression of carotid atherosclerosis in a prospective nested case-control study (13). An Italian group reported an association between elevated titers of antibodies against oxidatively modified LDL and increased severity of atherosclerosis (14). Regnström and coworkers reported an association between reduced oxidation resistance of LDL and severity of coronary atherosclerosis (15).

VITAMIN C AND LIPID PEROXIDATION

The role of antioxidative vitamins in the prevention of coronary heart disease (CHD) has recently received a lot of attention (16). We have previously observed an association between low plasma vitamin C concentrations and enhanced progression of atherosclerosis (17).

Ascorbate has been hypothesized to be the most effective antioxidant in human blood plasma (18). Vitamin C has inhibited the oxidation of LDL in vitro (19–22). Ames and coworkers (18,19) and Frei (22) have reported that ascorbic acid is the first antioxidant consumed during lipid peroxidation in plasma and detectable lipid peroxidation starts only after all ascorbate has been consumed completely. They have even suggested that only ascorbate could prevent the initiation of lipid peroxidation. Also the oxidized form of vitamin C, dehydro-L-ascorbic acid (DHA), has been shown to protect LDL against oxidation, but through different chemical mechanisms (23).

Ascorbate is an important physiological antioxidant that functions in the regeneration of tocopheroxyl radical back to the reduced antioxidative tocopherol (24,25). Through this role ascorbate could theoretically also inhibit lipid peroxidation even though it is not lipid-soluble. Retsky and Frei have shown that in copper^{2+}-exposed LDL, vitamin C spares, rather than regenerates, alpha-tocopherol and other endogenous antioxidants and that ascorbic acid can terminate lipid peroxidation, thereby protecting partially oxidized LDL against further oxidative modification (26). The lipid peroxidation inhibiting effect of vitamin C in vivo has not, however, yet been confirmed in supplementation studies in humans.

Jialal and coworkers carried out a small clinical trial in which they supplemented 10 healthy smokers with 1000 mg of vitamin C daily and gave 9 subjects placebo for 4 weeks (27). In the ascorbate-supplemented group there was a reduction in LDL oxidative susceptibility as measured by thiobarbituric acid reactive substances and the formation of conjugated dienes. We supplemented 39 smoking men with 500 mg of vitamin C daily for 8 weeks in the Multiple Antioxidant Supplementation Intervention (MASI) trial. There were no significant differences in changes in either the oxidation resistance of VLDL + LDL to oxidation, in LDL-TRAP (total antioxidative capacity of LDL), or in the percentage of electronegatively charged LDL in the supplemented group, as compared to 20 randomized placebo subjects.

VITAMIN C AND CARDIOVASCULAR DISEASES

In a prospective population study, the National Health and Nutrition Examination Survey (NHANES I) Epidemiologic Follow-Up Study, men and women, respectively, with the highest vitamin C intakes (> 50 mg/day and regular vitamin C containing supplements) had 45% and 25% lower CHD mortality rates than subjects with the lowest vitamin C intake (28). In the Health Professionals' Follow-Up Study and in the Nurses Health Study, the use of vitamin C supplements was not significantly associated with the risk of coronary events (9,10), even though there was a nonsignificant trend toward reduced risk among supplement users.

In the 12-year follow-up evaluation of the Prospective Basel Study, a low level of both plasma vitamin C (< 22.7 μmol/L) and carotene (< 0.23 μmol/L) was associated with twofold risk of CHD ($p = 0.022$) (29,30). The excess CHD mortality associated with low plasma ascorbate concentration alone was, however, not statistically significant in this study in 2974 Swiss men with relatively high average antioxidant intake.

In the Finnish Mobile Clinic Study, a low dietary intake of vitamin C was associated with increased coronary mortality rate among women but not among men in a cohort of 5133 CHD-free Finnish men and women, followed for 14 years (31). In a 20-year follow-up study of 730 elderly men and women in Britain, free of major cardiovascular disease at baseline, the mortality from cerebrovascular stroke was highest in those with the lowest vitamin C intake (32). Persons in the highest third of vitamin C intake had 50% reduced risk of stroke compared to those in the lowest third, after adjusting for a number of cardiovascular risk factors. No association was found between vitamin C intake and mortality from CHD (32).

Riemersma and coworkers observed an association between low plasma levels of vitamin C and an increased risk of angina pectoris in a population-based case-control study (33). The unadjusted risk was 2.4-fold in the lowest quintile of plasma vitamin C (< 13.1 μmol/L). This odds ratio was weakened to 1.6 and became statistically not significant after adjustment for smoking and other coronary risk factors.

A major potential source of bias in studies concerning the association of supplement use or plasma vitamin levels with the risk of CHD are other differences, besides vitamin intake, between persons with a low and a high intake of vitamins. This bias is an even greater worry in studies in which vitamin status has been estimated on the basis of reported use of vitamin supplements. Vitamin supplement users are likely to be a very health-conscious group that has more healthy habits in many other ways as well. This potential bias has not been thoroughly excluded in any of the previous studies, as measurements of some of the relevant coronary risk factors have been lacking. Studies in which vitamin status is assessed by determining plasma concentration overcome this problem partly, as plasma concentration is an objective measure and it is determined, besides by supplement use, also by diet.

Common to all prospective studies in which the association between vitamin C intake or status and the risk of CHD or cardiovascular events has been weak or absent are a narrow range and a high overall population level of vitamin C. We have previously reported that the average plasma ascorbate level is relatively low in eastern Finnish men and in winter months falls below values considered sufficient (34). As the previous epidemiological evidence is inconsistent, we investigated the association of vitamin C deficiency with the risk of acute myocardial infarction (AMI) in CHD-free eastern Finnish middle-aged men, a population with a low average vitamin C intake. We found a strong and consistent association between low plasma levels of vitamin C and an increased risk of AMI.

We attempted to assess differences between subjects with low and high plasma ascorbate levels in every respect that was considered relevant with regard to the risk of CHD. We also repeated our analyses after the exclusion of vitamin C supplement users. The proportion of vitamin C supplement users was low (5.5%) in our study cohort. The association between vitamin C deficiency was, if anything, stronger among men who did not report vitamin C supplement use.

METHODS IN THE KUOPIO ISCHEMIC HEART DISEASE RISK FACTOR STUDY

Study Subjects

The Kuopio Ischemic Heart Disease Risk Factor Study (KIHD) is a population study to investigate risk factors for cardiovascular diseases, atherosclerosis, and related outcomes in eastern Finnish men (35), the population with the highest recorded incidence of and mortality from CHD. The baseline examinations were carried out between March 1984 and

December 1989. The study sample included 3235 Eastern Finnish men aged 42, 48, 54, or 60 years at the baseline examination. Of these 2682 (82.9%) participated. Men with prevalent symptomatic CHD ($n = 92$) or ischemia in a maximal exercise test ($n = 359$) or both ($n = 585$) were excluded from the present analyses. Symptomatic ischemic heart disease was defined as either a history of myocardial infarction or angina pectoris or a positive angina pectoris result on effort in a London School of Hygiene interview (36) or the use of nitroglycerin tablets once a week or more frequently. Asymptomatic CHD was determined in a maximal exercise tolerance test (37). Out of the remaining 1646 men, data on plasma ascorbate concentration at baseline were available for 1605 men.

Chemical Measurements

The examination protocol and measurements have been described in detail earlier (11–13). Subjects gave blood specimens between 8:00 and 10:00 AM on Tuesday, Wednesday, or Thursday after having been instructed to abstain from ingesting alcohol for 3 days, from smoking for 12 h, and from eating for 12 h. After the subject had rested in the supine position for 30 min, blood was drawn with Terumo Venoject vacuum tubes (Terumo Corp., Tokyo). No tourniquet was used.

Plasma ascorbate concentrations were determined by a high-performance liquid chromatography (HPLC) method from deep-frozen samples, which were stabilized in 5% metaphosphoric acid immediately after blood drawing (35,38). The freezing time of the samples was 1–3 months. The between-batch coefficient of variation was 7.2% ($n = 12$) (35,38).

Plasma ascorbate concentration was redetermined in a subsample of 403 hypercholesterolemic men in samples drawn 1–5 years after the KIHD baseline examination. The Pearson's correlation between the baseline and the remeasurement values was 0.27.

Serum ferritin concentrations were measured with a radioimmunoassay (Amersham International, Amersham, United Kingdom) using Multigamma Model 1261 gamma counter (LKB Wallac, Turku, Finland) (11). The method is based on a double-antibody technique. Blood hemoglobin was measured photometrically (Gilford Stasar III, Instrument Laboratories Inc., Ohio, United States) using the cyanmethemoglobin method within a few hours of blood sampling (11). Blood hematocrit was determined with a hematocrit centrifuge and leukocyte count with a cell counter (Coulter Counter model DN, Luton, United Kingdom).

The main lipoprotein fractions (VLDL, LDL, and HDL) were separated from fresh serum samples using ultracentrifugation and precipitation as described earlier in detail (39). The HDL_2 and HDL_3 subfractions were separated during a second ultracentrifugal spin at 108,000 for 62 h against a density of 1.125 g/cm^3 (39). The cholesterol contents of all lipoprotein fractions were measured enzymatically (CHOD-PAP method, Boehringer Mannheim, Mannheim, Germany) on the day after the last spin. Serum apolipoprotein B was determined by an immunoturbidimetric and triglycerides by an enzymatic method (KONE Oy, Espoo, Finland).

Blood glucose was measured by a glucose dehydrogenase method (Merck, Darmstadt, Germany) after precipitation of proteins by trichloroacetic acid. Diabetes was defined as either previous diagnosis of diabetes mellitus or fasting blood glucose > 8.0 mmol/L. Serum selenium and copper were determined with atomic-absorption spectrometric techniques (12,40). Plasma fibrinogen was determined on the basis of clotting of diluted plasma with excess of thrombin (12). Hair mercury content was measured (Flow Injection and Amalgam System [FIAS-200] in the Perkin Elmer Zeeman 5000 Spectrometer) (12).

Assessment of Dietary Intake of Foodstuffs and Nutrients

The consumption of foods was assessed at time of blood sampling with an instructed and interview-checked 4-day food recording by household measures (41). The intake of nutrients, including dietary vitamin C, was estimated using the Nutrica computer program for calculation of nutrient intake. The databank of Nutrica is compiled using mainly Finnish values for the nutrient composition of foods. The food recording was repeated approximately 12 months after the baseline examination in a random subsample of 50 men. The Pearson's correlation coefficient between the original and reassessment of vitamin C intake was 0.62. The use of vitamin C tablets and vitamin C–containing nutritional supplements was assessed by a self-administered questionnaire.

Other Risk Factor Measurements

The number of cigarettes, cigars, and pipefuls of tobacco currently smoked daily; the duration of regular smoking in years; history of myocardial infarction, angina pectoris, and other ischemic heart disease; the presence of hypertension and current antihypertensive medication were recorded by using a self-administered questionnaire, which was checked by an interviewer. Reinterviews to obtain medical history were conducted by a physician. The family history of CHD was defined to be positive if the biological father, mother, sister, or brother of the subject had CHD history. The history of hypertension in siblings was defined to be positive if any sisters or brothers was reported ever to have had hypertension.

A subject was defined as a smoker if he had ever smoked on a regular basis and had smoked cigarettes, cigars, or pipe within the past 30 days. The lifelong exposure to smoking (cigarette pack-years) was estimated as the product of years smoked and the number of tobacco products smoked daily at the time of examination. Years smoked were defined as the sum of years of smoking regardless of when smoking had started, whether the subject had stopped smoking, and whether it had occurred continuously or during several periods. The consumption of alcohol in the previous 12 months was assessed with the Nordic Alcohol Consumption Inventory, which contains 15 items. Leisure-time physical activity was assessed by a 12-month history method (42).

Resting blood pressure was measured between 8:00 and 10:00 AM in the first examination day by one nurse with a random-zero mercury sphygmomanometer. The measuring protocol included, after a supine rest of 5 min, three measurements in supine, one in standing, and two in sitting position with 5-min intervals. The mean of all six systolic pressure values was used in the present analyses as the systolic and the mean of all six diastolic measurements as diastolic blood pressure.

The respiratory gas exchange was measured breath by breath (with the MGC 2001 system, Medical Graphics Corp., Minneapolis, Minnesota, United States) during a symptom-limited exercise test. The testing protocol comprised a linear increase of work load by 20 W/min (37). Highest oxygen uptake (average of 8 s) during the test was defined as VO_2 max. Exercise electrocardiograms were coded manually by one cardiologist. The criteria for ischemia were (1) an ischemic electrocardiogram, defined as horizontal or down-sloping ST depression of 0.5 mm or more or up-sloping ST depression of 1.0 mm or more; (2) typical angina pectoris pain leading to discontinuation of exercise; or (3) maximal heart rate during exercise of 130 breaths/min or less.

Determination of Follow-Up Events

As a part of the multinational MONICA project (43,44), an AMI registry was established in the province of Kuopio in 1982. The registry collects detailed diagnostic information of all heart attacks in the population (which also includes the present study cohort) in a prospective manner. Heart attacks were classified either as definite AMI, possible AMI, no AMI, or insufficient data according to explicitly defined, uniform diagnostic criteria, described earlier in detail (12,43,44). The coverage of the AMI registry was checked against the national computerized death certificate register. We obtained diagnostic information and the date of onset of all heart attacks in our study cohort by record linkage based on the uniform Finnish personal identification code (social security number). No personal identification codes were missing either in our study cohort or in the AMI registry data. Therefore, the losses to follow-up evaluation were negligible, if any.

Between March 1984 and December 1992, a suspected fatal or nonfatal AMI was registered in 70 of the 1605 men at risk. In the case of multiple events during the follow-up period, the first one for each subject was taken as the endpoint for the present analyses. The follow-up period for individual subjects was up to 8 3/4 years and mean follow-up time approximately 5 years.

Statistical Methods

Associations between plasma ascorbate concentrations and risk factors for CHD were estimated with the Pearson's correlation coefficients adjusted simultaneously for age, season (August to October vs. other), and the year of the baseline examination (1985 vs. other, 1986 vs. other, 1987 vs. other, 1988 vs. other, 1989 vs. other) as these cofounders covaried with plasma ascorbate.

Risk factors were entered in SPSS Cox proportional hazards' models uncategorized (45,46). Different sets of fixed covariates were entered; AMIs were defined as events and deaths from other causes as losses. The fit of the proportional hazards models was examined by analyzing changes in the proportionality of hazards with time and with risk factor levels. The results indicated that the application of the models was appropriate. All tests of significance were two-sided. Risk factor–adjusted relative hazards were estimated as antilogarithm of a coefficient for independent variables. Their confidence intervals were estimated with a macro based on the assumption of the asymptotic normality of estimates.

PLASMA VITAMIN C AND CORONARY RISK FACTORS

Plasma ascorbate concentration ranged in our study subjects from 0.3 mg/L to 24.2 mg/L with a mean of 8.4 mg/L (47.7 μmol/L) and standard deviation (SD) of 4.1 mg/L. There was a slow average increase in the mean plasma ascorbate concentration over time during the 6 years of baseline examinations ($r = 0.12$, $p < 0.0001$ for linear trend). The means in consequent examination years were 8.1, 7.6, 7.7, 8.7, 10.0, and 8.5 mg/L. For this reason, the examination year was adjusted for in all statistical analyses. The mean daily estimated dietary intake of vitamin C was 96 mg (range 6.6 mg to 550 mg, SD 59 mg) (35).

Plasma ascorbate concentration decreased with increasing age ($r = 0.17$). The age-specific plasma ascorbate means were 9.8, 9.2, 7.8, and 8.2 mg/L for the age groups 42, 48, 54, and 60 years, respectively ($p < 0.0001$ for linear trend). Of all foodstuff intakes, only that of fruits and berries ($r = 0.276$) and vegetables ($r = 0.255$) had any notable adjusted correlations with plasma ascorbate concentration. Of all nutrients, plasma ascorbate correlated with the dietary intake of carotenes ($r = 0.159$) and the sum of C14 to C16 saturated fatty acids (-0.096). Plasma ascorbate concentration also had significant ($p < 0.05$) age-, season-, and examination-year-adjusted correlations with cigarette pack-years (-0.217), serum copper (-0.163), blood leukocyte count (-0.160), maximal oxygen uptake (0.156), conditioning leisure time physical activity (0.151), serum selenium (0.148), socioeconomic status in adulthood (0.138), plasma fibrinogen (-0.110), intake of alcohol (-0.095), and systolic blood pressure (-0.089).

Men with plasma vitamin C < 2.0 mg/L differed from men with higher plasma vitamin C in many respects (Table 1). Vitamin C–deficient men were older, had smoked more in their lifetime, and had lower socioeconomic status, lower maximal oxygen uptake, lower dietary carotene intake, higher blood leukocyte count, lower dietary iron intake, less conditioning leisuretime physical activity, higher systolic blood pressure, higher alcohol intake, and higher coffee consumption (35).

In out study subjects, men with vitamin C deficiency had lower leisure-time physical activity. Plasma ascorbate concentration also correlated with maximal oxygen uptake, an indicator of cardiorespiratory fitness. It is possible that persons who were health-conscious and exercised more also ate more fruits, berries, and vegetables. A low maximal oxygen

Table 1   Means (Standard Errors) of Major Coronary Risk Factors in Men With and Without Vitamin C Deficiency (35)

Characteristic	Plasma ascorbate ≤2.0 mg/L (n = 91)	Plasma ascorbate >2.0 mg/L (n = 1514)	p Value for difference in means[a]
Age (years)	54.7 (0.42)	52.1 (0.14)	<0.001
Pack-years of smoking	18.9 (2.2)	7.0 (0.4)	<0.001
Smokers (%)	63 (5)	28 (1)	<0.001
Adulthood socioeconomic status (0–26)[b]	9.92 (0.37)	7.76 (0.11)	<0.001
Maximal oxygen uptake (ml/min/kg)	29.5 (0.6)	32.6 (0.2)	<0.001
Dietary carotene (μg/day)	1226 (110)	2723 (86)	<0.001
Examination in August to October (%)	6 (3)	30 (1)	<0.001
Blood leukocytes (10^9/L)	6.2 (0.2)	5.6 (0.0)	0.001
Dietary iron (mg/day)	16.8 (0.7)	18.9 (0.1)	0.004
Conditioning leisure-time physical activity (kcal/day)	94 (15)	140 (4)	0.005
Systolic blood pressure (mm Hg)	139 (2)	133 (0)	0.021
Alcohol intake (g/week)	116 (18)	72 (3)	0.019
Coffee intake (g/day)	645 (34)	562 (7)	0.019
Serum LDL cholesterol (mmol/L)	4.18 (0.12)	3.98 (0.03)	0.099
Serum apolipoprotein B (g/L)	1.06 (0.03)	1.03 (0.01)	0.126
Diabetes (%)	6.6 (2.6)	2.9 (0.4)	0.168
Rural place of residence (%)	34 (5)	27 (1)	0.188
Hair mercury content (μg/g)	1.69 (0.16)	1.89 (0.05)	0.233
Dietary polyenes (g/day)	12.3 (0.6)	13.0 (0.1)	0.303
Dietary monoenes (g/day)	35.4 (1.1)	35.6 (0.3)	0.819
Serum triglycerides (mmol/L)	1.26 (0.07)	1.24 (0.02)	0.846
Serum HDL cholesterol (mmol/L)	1.31 (0.03)	1.32 (0.01)	0.941

[a]Based on t-tests allowing for unequal within-group variances.
[b]A high value denotes a low socioeconomic status.

uptake is also an indicator of existing cardiovascular disease. Most likely, vitamin C deficiency had preceded the development of prior atherosclerosis-based CHD.

Vitamin C deficiency was associated in our data with elevated blood pressure. There is some evidence in favor of a role of oxidative stress in causing hypertension (47). The function of the endothelium-derived relaxing factor, nitric oxide, is dependent on the redox balance in the arterial wall (48). We have observed in a cross-sectional population study an independent association between lowered plasma levels of ascorbic acid and elevated levels of resting blood pressure in both normotensive and in hypertensive men (49).

We earlier carried out a small clinical trial to investigate the effect of antioxidant supplementation on blood pressure (50). The subjects were 40 regularly smoking middle-aged men who were randomized either to supplementation with a combination of 200 mg of d-α-tocopherol, 400 mg of ascorbic acid, 30 mg of β-carotene, and 100 μg of organic selenium daily or to double-masked placebo for 3 months. The mean systolic blood pressure decreased by 12.5 mm Hg (SE 2.5) in the supplemented group and by 5.2 mm Hg (SE 1.9) in the placebo group. The difference between groups in the blood pressure change was statistically significant ($p = 0.027$ in t-test), and the blood pressure reduction correlated strongly with the increase of plasma ascorbic acid concentration. Our trial data provide some evidence suggesting that antioxidant supplementation can lower blood pressure, at least in regularly smoking men. There is supporting evidence from other population studies and small uncontrolled trials (51). There are, however, no previous major controlled trials concerning the specific effects of the reduction of oxidative stress by supplementation with vitamin C on blood pressure in humans. If vitamin C deficiency elevates blood pressure, this could be one mechanism through which vitamin C deficiency increases the risk of AMI.

A decreased plasma vitamin C concentration was associated in our data with elevated values of indicators of inflammation such as blood leukocyte count, serum copper, and plasma fibrinogen, which all were also predictors of AMI risk in our data. It is possible that elevated blood leukocyte, serum copper, and plasma fibrinogen were simply indicators of preexisting atherosclerotic disease, or that vitamin C deficiency truly increases the susceptibility to infections or stimulates inflammation-mediating cytokines. Infections and/or inflammation could in turn increase the risk of AMI. Either way, vitamin C deficiency would have an etiological role in coronary disease. Most likely, this is not the main pathway of the increase in CHD risk.

Our data provided no evidence in favor of any association between vitamin C status and HDL cholesterol, as suggested earlier (52).

PLASMA VITAMIN C AND THE RISK OF MYOCARDIAL INFARCTION IN THE KIHD STUDY

The strongest predictors of AMI, when adjusting only for age (in years), examination year (covariates for individual years), and season of the year (August to October vs. rest of the year), in the present study cohort were pack-years smoked, maximal oxygen uptake (inversely), blood leukocyte count, and low plasma ascorbate concentration (Table 2). Also serum apolipoprotein B, plasma fibrinogen, serum copper and triglyceride concentrations, hair mercury content, blood hemoglobin, systolic blood pressure, diabetes, conditioning leisure-time physical activity (inversely), serum HDL_2 cholesterol (inversely), family history of CHD, and low socioeconomic status had statistically significant associations with the risk of AMI. Dietary carotene intake had a nonsignificant inverse association with

Table 2 Strongest Risk Factors for Acute Myocardial Infarction in 1605 Coronary Heart Disease-Free Men from Eastern Finland (35)

Risk factor	Mean or proportion	Standard deviation	Range	Adjusted for age, season, examination year			Multivariate[a]		
				Relative risk	95% Confidence Interval	p Value	Relative risk	95% Confidence interval	p Value
Pack-years of smoking	7.6	15.5	0–144	1.03	1.02–1.04	<0.0001	1.001	1.0004–1.0016	0.0016
Maximal oxygen uptake (ml/min × kg)	32.5	7.0	6.4–65.4	0.92	0.89–0.96	<0.0001	0.94	0.90–0.99	0.0205
Blood leukocyte count (10^9/L)	5.6	1.6	2.4–18.9	1.30	1.18–1.43	<0.0001	1.09	9.95–1.25	0.2080
Plasma vitamin C (<2.0 mg/L vs. >2.0 mg/L)	5.7%	n.a.	n.a.	3.49	1.82–6.69	0.0002	2.32	1.16–4.66	0.0173
Serum apolipoprotein B (g/L)	1.0	0.2	0.01–1.9	5.72	2.21–14.77	0.0003	2.89	0.98–8.38	0.0545
Plasma fibrinogen concentration (g/L)	2.96	0.53	1.32–6.71	1.76	1.20–2.59	0.0038	0.99	0.59–1.64	0.9593
Serum copper concentration (mg/L)	1.10	0.17	0.50–1.91	5.37	1.55–18.58	0.0080	0.95	0.21–4.30	0.9461
Serum triglycerides (mmol/L)	1.24	0.74	0.18–10.93	1.33	1.06–1.68	0.0148	1.17	0.83–1.64	0.3617
Hair mercury (>2.0 µg/g vs. <2.0 µg/g)	33.6%	n.a.	0–1	1.78	1.10–2.87	0.0184	1.64	0.98–2.72	0.0582
Blood hemoglobin (g/L)	147	9	105–234	1.03	1.004–1.05	0.0219	1.02	0.99–1.05	0.2484
Systolic blood pressure (mm Hg)	134	16	88–213	1.02	1.002–1.03	0.0224	1.008	0.99–1.02	0.2860
Diabetes (yes vs. no)	3.1%	n.a.	0–1	2.81	1.12–7.08	0.0279	2.09	0.79–5.51	0.1372
Conditioning leisure-time physical activity (kcal/day)	137	170	0–2493	0.99	0.988–0.999	0.0289	0.997	0.991–1.002	0.2521
Serum HDL_2 cholesterol (mmol/L)	0.87	0.28	0.09–2.77	0.35	0.13–0.90	0.0298	0.87	0.28–2.71	0.8132
Family history of CHD (yes vs. no)	44.4%	n.a.	0–1	1.67	1.04–2.68	0.0326	1.85	1.14–3.01	0.0127
Low socioeconomic status in adulthood (0–26)	7.9	4.2	0–18	1.06	1.0002–1.12	0.0492	1.02	0.96–1.08	0.5831
Dietary carotene intake (g/day)	2.6	3.3	0.03–60.6	0.89	0.78–1.02	0.0835	0.98	0.87–1.10	0.7445
Body mass index (kg/m^2)	26.7	3.5	18.8–48.6	1.05	0.98–1.11	0.1545	0.99	0.92–1.07	0.8252

[a] All risk factors shown were entered simultaneously in the model.

the risk of AMI and body-mass index a weak nonsignificant direct association (Table 2). Men who had vitamin C deficiency (plasma ascorbate <2.0 mg/L) had a 3.5-fold (95% confidence interval [CI] 1, 8, 6.7, p = 0.0002) adjusted risk of AMI (Table 2) (35).

To estimate the independent impacts of risk factors, all factors shown in Table 2 were also entered simultaneously in a Cox proportional hazards model. In this multivariate model, only cigarette pack-years smoked, family history of CHD, low plasma vitamin C, and maximal oxygen uptake (in order of strength) had significant associations with AMI risk (Table 2). An insufficient statistical power due to the limited number of AMIs was probably the reason why other risk factors did not reach statistical significance in this analysis. When allowing for all risk factors shown in Table 2, men with plasma ascorbate of less than 2.0 mg/L had a 2.3-fold (95% CI 1.2, 4.7, p = 0.0173) risk-factor-adjusted risk of AMI compared to those with plasma ascorbate 2.0 mg/L or more (35).

Only 5.5% of our study subjects used vitamin C–containing supplements. The exclusion of these men did not materially change the results. In fact, among 1516 men who had not used vitamin C–containing supplements during the previous week, men with plasma vitamin C below 2.0 mg/L had a 3.7-fold (95% CI 1.9, 7.2, p = 0.0001) age-, season-, and examination-year-adjusted risk of AMI compared with men with higher plasma vitamin C levels. The respective risk-factor-adjusted relative risk of AMI was 2.4 (95% CI 1.2, 4.8, p = 0.0167). The use of vitamin C supplements had no significant association with the risk of AMI. There was no association between plasma vitamin C levels and AMI risk above very low values (35).

A lack of protective effect of high vitamin C intakes might be due to a number of reasons. First, ascorbic acid is a reducing agent that can reduce ferric iron to ferrous iron. This could, in theory, promote lipid peroxidation in vivo through Fenton–Haber–Weissman chemical reactions. Second, dietary vitamin C enhances the absorption of dietary nonheme iron. We and others have observed an association between high dietary iron intake and high serum ferritin levels with an excess risk of AMI (11,53–55). If this observation holds in repeated valid replications, the iron-absorption-facilitating effect of large doses of vitamin C could tend to increase the risk of AMI and at least in part negate other, beneficial effects of vitamin C.

CONCLUSIONS AND IMPLICATIONS

The present data provide empirical evidence in humans in favor of the role of vitamin C deficiency, as measured as low plasma ascorbate concentration, as a risk factor for CHD. The association appears strong, especially if one considers the weak tracking and the sizable regression toward the mean over time of plasma ascorbate concentrations.

In our study cohort, there was no association between plasma vitamin C and AMI risk at levels of vitamin C exceeding the limit of relative deficiency. Thus, on the basis of these data, high intakes of vitamin C or vitamin C supplements would not appear to reduce the risk of AMI. Our findings suggest, instead, that if a minimal necessary requirement of vitamin C is not met, there is an increased risk of AMI.

ANTIOXIDANT SUPPLEMENTATION IN ATHEROSCLEROSIS PREVENTION TRIAL

So far no results are available from clinical trials testing the effect of vitamin C in the prevention of atherosclerotic progression or cardiovascular events. The only ongoing trial, to our knowledge, is the Antioxidant Supplementation in Atherosclerosis Prevention (ASAP) trial, carried out by our team. This is double-masked, randomized, placebo-controlled clinical trial in over 500 men and women aged 45–69 to study the effect of either 250 mg of slow-release vitamin C twice daily or 100 mg of d-α-tocopheryl acetate twice daily, or both combined, on the progression of ultrasonographically assessed common carotic atherosclerosis, blood pressure, and eye lens opacities, as compared to these of placebo. The randomization of subjects was completed in October 1995, the 3-year treatment period will be completed for the last subject in October 1998, and the main findings will be available in 1999. This trial will provide the necessary additional information about the role of vitamin C supplements in the prevention of atherosclerotic progression and hypertension. If positive, the results will also have broader implications regarding the usefulness of vitamin C supplementation in the prevention of events due to atherosclerosis-based cardiovascular diseases.

ACKNOWLEDGMENTS

We are grateful to Rainer Rauramaa, M.D., Ph.D., for the participation of the Kuopio Research Institute of Exercise Medicine in data collection. We also thank Dr. Riitta Salonen, M.D., Ph.D., for clinical examinations, Ms. Merja Ihanainen, M.Sc., for food recordings, Dr. Jaakko Eränen for coding of exercise electrocardiograms, and Dr. Esko Taskinen, Dr. Juha Venäläinen, and Dr. Hannu Litmanen for their participation in the supervision of the maximal exercise tests, Mrs. Marjatta Kantola, M.Sc., Mrs. Sirpa Suntioinen, Ph.D., and Kari Seppänen, M.Sc., for some of the chemical analyses, and Kimmo Ronkainen, M.Ph., for carrying out the data analyses.

REFERENCES

1. Steinberg D, Parthasarathy S, Carew TE, et al. Beyond cholesterol: modifications of low-density lipoprotein that increase its atherogenicity. N Engl J Med 1989; 320:915–924.
2. Witztum JL. The oxidation hypothesis of atherosclerosis. Lancet 1994; 344:793–795.
3. Halliwell B. Free radicals, antioxidants, and human disease: curiosity, cause, or consequence? Lancet 1994; 344:721–724.
4. Shigenaga MK, Hagen TM, Ames BN. Oxidative damage and mitochondrial decay in aging. Proc Natl Acad Sci USA 1994; 91;10771–10778.
5. Carew TE, Schwenke DC, Steinberg D. Antiatherogenic effect of probucol unrelated to its hypocholesterolemic effect: evidence that antioxidants in vivo can selectively inhibit low density lipoprotein degradation in macrophage-rich fatty streaks slowing the progression of atherosclerosis in the WHHL rabbit. Proc Natl Acad Sci USA 1987; 84:7725–7729.
6. Björkhem I, Henriksson-Freyschuss A, Breuer, O, et al. The antioxidant butylated hydroxytoluene protects against atherosclerosis. Arterioscler Thromb 1991; 11:15–22.
7. Freyschuss A, Stiko-Rahm A, Swedenborg J, et al. Antioxidant treatment inhibits the development of intimal thickening after balloon injury of the aorta in hypercholesterolemic rabbits. J Clin Invest 1993; 91:1282–1288.
8. Williams RJ, Motteram JM, Sharp CH, Gallagher PJ. Dietary vitamin E and the attenuation of early lesion development in modified Watanabe rabbits. Atherosclerosis 1992; 94:153–160.
9. Stampfer MJ, Hennekens CH, Manson JE, et al. Vitamin E consumption and risk of coronary disease in women. N Engl J Med 1993; 328:1444–1449.
10. Rimm EB, Stampfer MJ, Ascherio A, et al. Vitamin E consumption and the risk of coronary heart disease in men. N Engl J Med 1993; 328:1450–1456.

11. Salonen JT, Nyyssönen K, Korpela H, et al. High stored iron levels are associated with excess risk of myocardial infarction in eastern Finnish men. Circulation 1992; 86:803–811.

12. Salonen JT, Seppänen K, Nyyssönen K, et al. Intake of mercury from fish, lipid peroxidation and the risk of myocardial infarction and coronary, cardiovascular and any death in Eastern Finnish men. Circulation 1995; 91:645–655.

13. Salonen JT, Ylä-Herttuala S, Yamamoto R, et al. Autoantibody against oxidised LDL and progression of carotid atherosclerosis. Lancet 1992; 339:883–887.

14. Maggi E, Finardi G, Poli M, et al. Specificity of autoantibodies against oxidized LDL as an additional marker for atherosclerotic risk. Coronary Artery Dis 1993; 4:1119–1122.

15. Regnström J, Nilsson J, Tornvall P, et al. Susceptibility to low-density lipoprotein oxidation and coronary atherosclerosis in man. Lancet 1992; 339:1183–1186.

16. Steinberg D and Workshop Participants. Antioxidants in the prevention of human atherosclerosis. Circulation 1992; 85:2337–2344.

17. Salonen JT, Salonen R, Seppänen K, et al. Interactions of serum copper, selenium, and low density lipoprotein cholesterol in atherogenesis. Br Med J 1991; 302:756–760.

18. Frei B, Stocker R, England L, Ames BN. Ascorbate: the most effective antioxidant in human blood plasma. Adv Exp Med Biol 1990; 264:155–163.

19. Frei B, England L, Ames BN. Ascorbate is an outstanding antioxidant in human blood plasma. Proc Natl Acad Sci USA 1989; 86:6377–6381.

20. Jialal I, Grundy SM. Preservation of the endogenous antioxidants in low density lipoprotein by ascorbate but not probucol during oxidative modification. J Clin Invest 1991; 87:597–601.

21. Harats D, Ben-Naim M, Dabach Y, et al. Effect of vitamin C and E susceptibility of plasma lipoproteins to peroxidation induced by acute smoking. Atherosclerosis 1990; 85:47–54.

22. Frei B. Ascorbic acid protects lipids in human plasma and low-density lipoprotein against oxidative damage. Am J Clin Nutr 1991; 54:1113S–1118S.

23. Retsky KL, Freeman MW, Frei B. Ascorbic acid oxidation product(s) protect human low density lipoprotein against atherogenic modification: anti-rather than pro-oxidant activity of vitamin C in the presence of transition metal ions. J Biol Chem 1993; 268:1304–1309.

24. Packer JE, Slater TF, Willson RL. Direct observation of a free radical interaction between vitamin E and Vitamin C. Nature 1979; 278:737–738.

25. Kagan VE, Servinava EA, Forte T, et al. Recycling of vitamin E in human low density lipoproteins. J Lipid Res 1992; 33:385–387.

26. Retsky KL, Frei B. Vitamin C prevents metal ion-dependent initiation and propagation of lipid peroxidation in human low-density lipoprotein. Biochim Biophys Acta 1995; 1257:279–287.

27. Fuller CJ, Grundy SM, Norkus EP, Jialal I. Effect of ascorbate supplementation on low density lipoprotein oxidation in smokers. Atherosclerosis 1995; 119:139–150.

28. Enstrom JE, Kanim LE, Lein MA. Vitamin C intake and mortality among sample of the United States population. Epidemiology 1992; 3:194–202.

29. Eichholzer M, Stahelin HB, Gey KF. Inverse correlation between essential antioxidants in plasma and subsequent risk to develop cancer, ischemic heart disease and stroke respectively: 12-year follow-up of the Basel Study. EXS 1992; 62:398–410.

30. Gey KF, Stahelin HB, Eichholzer M. Poor plasma status of carotene and vitamin C is associated with higher mortality from ischemic heart disease and stroke: Basel Prospective Study. Clin Invest 1993; 71:3–6.

31. Knekt P, Reunanen A, Järvinen R, et al. Antioxidant vitamin intake and coronary mortality in a longitudinal population study. Am J Epidemiol 1994; 139:1180–1189.

32. Gale CR, Martyn CN, Winter PD, Cooper C. Vitamin C and risk of death from stroke and coronary heart disease in cohort of elderly people. Br Med J 1995; 310:1563–1566.

33. Riemersma RA, Wood DA, MacIntyre CCA, et al. Risk of angina pectoris and plasma concentrations of vitamins A, C, and E and carotene. Lancet 1991; 337:1–5.

34. Parviainen MT, Salonen JT. Vitamin C status of 54-year old Eastern Finnish men throughout the year. Int J Vitam Nutr Res 1990; 60:47–51.

35. Nyyssönen K, Parviainen MT, Salonen R, Tuomilento J, Salonen JT. Vitamin C deficiency and increased risk of myocardial infarction: prospective population study in men in Eastern Finland. Br Med J, in press.

36. Rose GA, Blackburn H, Gillum RF, Prineas RJ. Cardiovascular Survey Methods. Geneva: World Health Organization, 1982:162–165.

37. Lakka TA, Venäläinen JM, Rauramaa R, et al. Relation of leisure-time physical activity and cardiorespiratory fitness to the risk of acute myocardial infarction in men. N Engl J Med 1994; 330:1549–1554.

38. Parviainen MT, Nyyssönen K, Penttilä IM, et al. A method for routine assay of plasma ascorbic acid using high-performance liquid chromatography. J Liquid Chromatogr 1986; 9:2185–2197.

39. Salonen JT, Salonen R, Seppänen K, et al. HDL, HDL_2, and HDL_3 subfractions, and the risk of acute myocardial infarction: a prospective population study in eastern Finnish men. Circulation 1991; 84:129–139.

40. Salonen JT, Salonen R, Korpela H, Tuomilehto J. Serum copper an the risk of acute myocardial infarction: a prospective population study in men in Eastern Finland. Am J Epidemiol 1991; 134:268–276.

41. Ihanainen M, Salonen R, Seppänen K, et al. Nutrition data collection in the Kuopio Ischaemic Heart Disease Risk Factor Study: nutrient intake of middle-aged Eastern Finnish men. Nutr Res 1989; 9:597–604.

42. Lakka T, Salonen JT. Physical activity and serum lipids: a cross-sectional population study in Eastern Finnish men. Am J Epidemiol 1992; 136:806–818.

43. WHO Monica Project. WHO Monica Project: assessing CHD mortality and morbidity. Int J Epidemiol 1989; 18:S38–S45.

44. Tuomilehto J, Arstila M, Kaarsalo E, et al. Acute myocardial infarction (AMI) in Finland: baseline data from the FINMONICA AMI register in 1983–1985. Eur Heart J 1992; 13: 577–587.

45. Cox DR. Regression models and life-tables. J R Stat Society 1972; 34:187–201.

46. SPSS Inc. SPSS for UNIX. Chicago, 1993.

47. Nakazono K, Watanabe N, Matsuno K, et al. Does superoxide underlie the pathogenesis of hypertension. Proc Natl Acad Sci USA 1991; 88:10045–10048.

48. Vane JR, Änggård EE, Botting RM. Regulatory functions of the vascular endothelium. N Engl J Med 1990; 323:27–36.

49. Salonen JT, Salonen R, Ihanainen M, et al. Blood pressure, dietary fats and antioxidants. Am J Clin Nutr 1988; 48:1226–1232.

50. Salonen R, Korpela H, Nyyssönen K, et al. Reduction of blood pressure by antioxidant supplementation: a randomised double-blind clinical trial. Life Chem Rep 1994; 12:65–68.

51. Salonen JT. Dietary fats, antioxidants and blood pressure. Ann Med 1991; 23:295–298.

52. Hallfrisch J, Singh VN, Muller DC, et al. High plasma vitamin C associated with high plasma HDL- and HDL_2 cholesterol. Am J Clin Nutr 1994; 60:100–105.

53. Salonen JT, Nyyssönen K, Salonen R. Body iron stores and the risk of coronary heart disease. New Engl J Med 1994; 331:1159.

54. Salonen JT. Role of iron as a cardiovascular risk factor. Curr Opin Lipidol 1993; 4:277–282.

55. Salonen JT. Epidemiological studies on LDL oxidation, pro- and antioxidants and atherosclerosis. In: Bellomo G, Finardi G, Maggi E, Rice-Evans C, eds. Free Radicals, Lipoprotein Oxidation and Atherosclerosis. London: Richelieu Press, 1995.

27

Vitamin C and Infectious Diseases

HARRI HEMILÄ
University of Helsinki, Helsinki, Finland

INTRODUCTION

In the early part of this century it was thought that low vitamin C intake may decrease resistance to infections (1–6). Nevertheless, the precise role of vitamin C in infectious diseases is still poorly understood. The purpose of this chapter is to review the literature relating vitamin C intake to the susceptibility to and severity of infections. Two exhaustive searches of the old literature on studies about vitamin C and infections have been carried out, but the data of the original publications were not thoroughly analyzed in either of these reviews (7,8).

VITAMIN C AND THE COMMON COLD

In the early 1970s Linus Pauling suggested that vitamin C supplementation may decrease the incidence and severity of common cold infections (9,10). His conclusions were based on earlier studies in which groups supplemented with vitamin C showed some benefit. Since Pauling has made the issue popular, a large number of studies have been carried out to examine whether vitamin C supplementation has an effect on colds (8,11–15).

Severity of Common Cold Episodes

There are eight published studies that have examined the effect of high-dosage (≥ 2 g/day) regular vitamin C supplementation on the duration and severity of common cold episodes (Table 1) (16–25). Each of these studies found a statistically significant decrease in at least one outcome. If the *p* values found in the eight studies are combined by the Fisher method (28,29), a very small combined *p* value results. Thus it is unlikely that the published differences in favor of vitamin C are caused by chance alone. All of the eight studies were placebo-controlled, double-blind studies and five of them were randomized (16,20,21

Table 1   Vitamin C and Common Cold Symptoms[a]

Ref.	Subjects, country	No. of episodes in vitamin C group	Dose (g/day)	Effect on duration or severity[b]	p (1 − t)	−2 × ln(p)
16	Military recruits, USA	37[c]	2	−72[d]	0.016	8.27
17	Adults, USA	4[e]	2	−50[f]	0.023	7.55
18	Adults, USA	11[e]	3	−30[g]	0.005	10.60
19	Schoolchildren, USA	16	2	−29	0.006[h]	10.23
20	Schoolchildren, Chile	38	2	−24	0.041	6.39
21,22	Adults, Canada	561	1 + 3[i]	−21[j] −5	0.008	9.66
23,24	Adults, USA	76	3 + 3[i]	−17	0.025	7.38
25	Military recruits, USA	600	2	−5[f] −3	0.012	8.85
	Total:	1343	Median	−26	χ^2 (16 df) = 68.9	
			Mean	−31	combined p(1 − t) =	
			Weighted mean	−15	0.00000001	

[a]Studies in which ≥2 g/day of vitamin C was regularly administered were selected. In the case of short-term studies supplementation was initiated before the symptoms started and continued after the symptoms ended. For a more comprehensive list of the original data see Table 1 in Ref. 14. Anderson's 1972 study (26) was included as the dose was 4 g/day during the episodes although the regular dose was 1 g/day. Anderson's 1974 study was excluded since there is bias in the distribution of subjects in the study groups (26,27). In the case of the studies by Anderson (21) and Pitt and Costrini (25) the days indoors and the severity of symptoms, respectively, were selected as outcomes in the calculations. The weighted mean was calculated using the number of episodes in the vitamin C groups as the weight. The p values were recalculated when appropriate data were available. The combined p value was calculated by the Fisher method (28,29).
[b]The outcome is the duration of cold symptoms except when otherwise indicated.
[c]The number of subjects; the number of episodes is not given in the report.
[d]Days of morbidity for sore throats.
[e]Induced rhinovirus infection.
[f]Severity of symptoms.
[g]Severity of symptoms at the fourth day after challenge.
[h]p Value for comparing the sickness days between the groups.
[i]At the onset of a cold episode an additional 3 g/day was given for 3–5 days.
[j]Days indoors due to a cold episode.

23,25). Consequently it is unlikely that biases between the study groups or the placebo effect would cause the consistent differences in favor of vitamin C.

From the published studies it is clear that vitamin C has physiological effects on common cold symptoms. Nevertheless, there have been great quantitative differences in the effects (Table 1; 14,15), and it is not clear what the practical significance of vitamin C supplementation in the treatment of colds is. Most of the controlled studies have administered vitamin C regularly, whereas in the treatment of symptoms it would appear more reasonable to start supplementation immediately after the first symptoms, but it is not clear whether the effects of therapeutic supplements are comparable to those found with regular supplements (Table 1).

Incidence of the Common Cold

If high vitamin C doses decreased common cold incidence substantially, the most convincing evidence should be seen in studies using large vitamin doses and recording large numbers of cold episodes. However, none of the four largest studies using ≥ 1 g/day of vitamin C found a significant decrease in cold incidence (Table 2; 21,25,30,31). Furthermore, the pooled estimate does not suggest any real difference between vitamin C and placebo groups. Consequently, high-dose vitamin C supplementation has no meaningful preventive effect on cold episodes in subjects comparable to those used in the four major studies.

Nonetheless, although the major studies show that a high vitamin C dose per se does not prevent colds to any meaningful extent in large segments of the general population, this should not be interpreted as definite evidence that vitamin C intake can have no effects on cold incidence in any conditions. A number of smaller studies have found a statistically significant decrease in cold incidence in subjects supplemented with vitamin C. It is possible that some of the positive results are caused by the use of different kinds of subjects or by other differences in the experimental conditions compared to the major studies in Table 2. In a recent metaanalysis of three studies using subjects under acute heavy physical stress it was calculated that the pooled risk ratio (RR) of cold episodes in vitamin C groups was 0.50 (90% confidence interval [CI]: 0.37, 0.66; $p(1 - t) = 0.00003$), suggesting that vitamin C intake can affect cold incidence in certain specific conditions (33).

Furthermore, it is possible that some of the positive results are not due to the high vitamin C dose used, but to the correction of marginal deficiency in the control group. In this respect the randomized double-blind study by Baird et al. (34) is particularly interesting as the dietary vitamin C intake was rather low, 50 mg/day, and the supplement dose was also small, 80 mg/day. This study is relevant to the question of whether marginally low intake in the control group (50 mg/day) increases susceptibility to colds compared to the

Table 2 Vitamin C and Common Cold Incidence[a]

Ref.	Subjects, country	Vitamin C dose (g/day)	Duration (months)	No. of episodes Vitamin C	Placebo	RR	90% CI
21	Adults, Canada	1	3	561	609	0.93	0.84, 1.03
30	Women, UK	1	3	627	690	0.93	0.85, 1.03
25	Military recruits, USA	2	2	600	619	1.00	0.91, 1.10
31	Schoolchildren, Sweden	1	3	657	622	1.08	0.98, 1.19
		Totals:		2,445	2,540	RR_{Pool}: 0.99	0.94, 1.03

[a]Studies in which ≥ 1 g/day of vitamin C was regularly administered and >300 cold episodes were recorded were selected. The smaller studies using ≥ 1 g/day of vitamin C excluded from this table contain approximately 1500 episodes in all (cf. Table 1 in Ref. 14) and thus their weight is small compared to that of the studies included. Anderson's 1974 study is excluded since there is bias in the distribution of subjects in the study groups (26,27). The RR and CI values were calculated with the normal approximation of the Poisson distribution and the pooled values were calculated using the inverses of variances as weights (32). RR, relative risk; CI, confidence interval.

somewhat higher intake (130 mg/day). There were 184 and 135 cold episodes among the 133 and 61 male subjects administered vitamin C and placebo, respectively. Thus, among Baird's male subjects receiving higher vitamin C intake (130 mg/day) the RR of cold episodes was 0.63 (90% CI: 0.52, 0.75; $p(1-t) = 0.00002$). A few other studies are also consistent with the suggestion that low vitamin C intake increases the susceptibility to colds (34a). Even if the association of vitamin C intake and common cold susceptibility were largely limited to the marginal deficiency region, this could be of great importance globally. For example, vitamin A supplementation has been shown to decrease the mortality rate of children in several developing countries in which dietary vitamin A intakes are low (35); in developed countries vitamin A supplementation has no comparable effects.

Subgroup Differences in the Effects of Vitamin C on Cold Severity

Some of the common cold studies have compared the effects of vitamin C supplementation on different subgroups (Table 3; 21,36,37). Anderson et al. (21,36) carried out two studies with adults, both of which compared various subgroups. However, the experimental protocols of his studies differed considerably. In the first, subjects were given 1 g/day of vitamin C regularly over the entire study period and 3 g/day extra for 3 days during cold episodes (21). In the other study 1.5 g was administered on the first day of the cold episode and 1 g/day on 4 consecutive days (36); these subjects were also administered a regular dose of 0.5 g per week (i.e., 0.07 g/day), which is such a small dose that it should not affect the results. Thus the former study (21) may be considered one with regular supplementation (1–4 g/day), whereas the latter (36) may be considered one with therapeutic supplementation (1–1.5 g/day), i.e., supplementation starting only after the onset of cold symptoms.

In both studies Anderson found that vitamin C supplementation was more beneficial for subjects who had a low intake of fruit juices, which are a major dietary source of vitamin C (Table 3). This finding is biologically reasonable as supplementation should be most beneficial for people with low dietary intake. The effect of vitamin C status on cold duration was also studied by Coulehan, who determined the plasma vitamin C level in selected subjects administered placebo or vitamin C and divided the subjects of both study groups into three subgroups on the basis of vitamin C plasma levels (Table 4). Coulehan found that the duration of colds gradually decreased while the vitamin C level in plasma increased; however, the subjects with the highest plasma levels had the longest colds (Table 4; 38). Thus it appears possible that 1 g/day of vitamin C supplementation produced plasma levels that were too high for a subgroup of subjects. Still, there are no other data indicating that excessive vitamin C intakes or plasma levels could increase the duration of colds. Two studies comparing two different vitamin C doses found a greater decrease in the duration of colds in the group given the higher vitamin dose (19,23,24). The significance of Coulehan's puzzling observation thus remains unclear.

Children are an important source of common cold infections in the community (39), and therefore Anderson's observation in both studies that vitamin C is more beneficial to adults having contact with children is noteworthy (Table 3). Anderson also found other subgroup differences, but these were not consistent between the studies. For example, regular supplementation was more beneficial to people frequently in crowds, but this subgroup difference was not found in the therapeutic study (Table 3). It is possible that some of the further subgroup differences are caused by chance; however, different protocols in the two

Table 3   Effect of Vitamin C Supplementation on Colds in Certain
Subgroups

	Effect on the "total days indoors"	
	1972 Study (21) regular supplement	1975 Study (36) therapeutic supplement
Anderson et al. studies (21,36)		
Daily juice		
0–3 oz	−48%	−33%
4+ oz	−22%	−22%
Contact with young children		
Yes	−46%	−40%
No	−17%	−13%
Frequently in crowds		
Yes	−34%	−25%
No	−17%	−29%
Smoker		
Yes	−30%	−31%
No	−31%	−22%
Sex		
Male	−36%	−25%
Female	−26%	−27%
Age (years)		
<25	−30%	<30 −37%
≥25	−31%	≥30 −15%
Student		
No	−39%	—
Yes	−18%	—
Usual colds		
2+	−43%	—
0–1	−13%	—
	Effect on the symptom	
	"Duration"	"Severity"
Carr et al. study (37)		
Twins living		
Together	+1%	+6%
Apart	−35%	−35%

studies (regular/therapeutic) can also determine which groups show the greatest benefits from supplements.

Carr et al. found that vitamin C had a considerable effect on twins living apart, but no effect on twins living together (Table 3). An obvious explanation of the difference is that twins living together exchanged their tablets to great extent. Two other studies with children found an increase in plasma (19) and urine (40) vitamin C levels in the placebo [sic!] groups, a finding which even more directly shows that tablet exchange may take place among playful children under study conditions. It is also noteworthy that in Carr's study

Table 4   Plasma Vitamin C Level and the Duration
of Colds

Vitamin C level in plasma	Episodes (no.)	Mean duration (days)	Difference from low-placebo
Placebo group			
Low	20	5.6	0%
Middle	18	4.5	−20%
High	10	4.4	−21%
Vitamin C group (1 g/day)			
Low	22	4.0	−29%
Middle	15	2.7	−52%
High	13	6.8	+21%

Source: Ref. 38.

(37) the average duration of colds in both groups of twins living together (5.4 days) was intermediate between that of the vitamin C (4.9 days) and placebo (7.5 days) groups of twins living apart, also consistent with the notion that tablets were exchanged by twins living together. Carr's subgroup analysis is important in suggesting that in some studies with children the mischief of the subjects may have confounded the results and the observed difference may underestimate the true physiological effect.

Some Problems in the Interpretation of the Common Cold Studies

Many people have drawn more or less inappropriate conclusions about the vitamin C–common cold studies. From the studies published so far it is clear that Pauling (9,10) was correct in his general conclusion that vitamin C has effects on colds, on both their severity and incidence. Nevertheless, quantitatively he was substantially overoptimistic. Pauling based his quantitative conclusions (10) on the study by Ritzel on schoolchildren in a skiing school in the Swiss Alps (41,42), but such children are not a good representative sample of the general population. Thus, when Pauling implicitly extrapolated the results to all people (i.e., children at school and adults), he took a bold step and went wrong. Furthermore, Pauling's conclusion (10) that the 45% decrease in cold incidence in the vitamin group in Ritzel's study was caused by the high vitamin C dose (1 g/day) per se was also hasty. It is possible that the effect was due to the correction of marginal vitamin C deficiency in the control group, in which case a much smaller dose could have produced a similar effect. This interpretation is supported, for example, by Baird's study (34), as noted. The lack of effect of high vitamin C doses in the major studies (Table 2) also suggests that if the vitamin affects cold incidence it is in the low-intake range rather than in the high-intake range.

Several reviewers have drawn quite different conclusions about the effects of vitamin C on colds than Pauling. However, there are profound problems in many reviews of the topic. In one major review (43) there were data inconsistent with the original publications and the data were analyzed improperly (27,44). In another major review (45) some data were misrepresented and some other relevant data were not presented at all (44,46,47). In a brief review of vitamin C and colds in a major medical journal (48) a few explicit statements were gravely inconsistent with the data in the original reports (44). Furthermore, the vitamin C–common cold trial carried out at the National Institutes of Health (NIH) in the middle of the 1970s (23), which appears to be the most influential study so far, was interpreted inappropriately (24). However, overtly negative conclusions from the original data are not a problem that appeared after Pauling made the issue popular, since in some earlier studies the authors' conclusions were much more negative than objective interpretation of the findings would have permitted (13).

It appears quite clear that the great quantitative variation in the results (Table 1; 14,15) has been an important factor hampering the conclusion that vitamin C has real effects on the severity of colds. However, it seems that there are also much deeper conceptual reasons for prejudice against vitamin C at the paradigm level, to use Thomas Kuhn's terminology (44,49–51).

There is a widespread belief that the sole physiological role of vitamin C is to prevent scurvy, and evidently this belief has generated strong prejudices against all other observed physiological effects of the vitamin (44,49,50). Nevertheless, vitamin C participates in the function of several enzymes that are unrelated to connective tissue metabolism (52–55), and as a major physiological antioxidant it can have numerous nonspecific biochemical effects. Consequently, there are no biochemical reasons to assume that the physiological effects of vitamin C are strictly limited to the prevention of overt scurvy. None of the three major reviews (43,45,48) discussed the possible effects of vitamin C on the immune system to provide a background to the examination of whether the effects of vitamin C on the common cold make any sense biologically. This is important as the evaluation of the effectiveness of a therapeutic method usually depends greatly on the possibility of rationalizing the method biologically, and not just on the interpretation of experimental results (56,57).

Furthermore, if a treatment bypasses the medical establishment and is marketed directly to the public there may be a temptation in the medical community to accept the first bad news that comes along uncritically without considering the entire body of relevant data (57). Vitamin C is of great interest among nonprofessionals and therefore such psychological effects may be pertinent. Finally, there are numerous obviously erroneous claims about the effects of vitamin C supplementation and a vast commercial exploitation of such claims. In the minds of critical people not engaged with vitamin C in particular, this kind of background may lead to a biased view of vitamin C in general.

VITAMIN C AND THE IMMUNE SYSTEM

The common cold studies suggest implicitly that vitamin C intake affects the immune system. There are many experimental data indicating that vitamin C has effects on the immune system, but experimental data have been inconsistent to a large extent (58–61). Although the role of vitamin C in the immune system still is not clear, there are certain effects that may be physiologically relevant.

Protection Against Oxidants Produced During Infection

Phagocytes have an enzyme system which produces superoxide, hypochlorite, and other oxidants with the purpose of killing viruses and bacteria. Many of these oxidants may be harmful to the host cells if they are released into the extracellular medium (62,63).

Moreover, oxidants produced during viral infections may play some role in the appearance of symptoms (64–69). Vitamin C is an efficient reducing agent (antioxidant), and it may protect various kinds of cells against harmful oxidants (14,70–76).

Functions of the Phagocytes

The concentration of vitamin C in the phagocytes and lymphocytes is over 10 times higher than in plasma (77–83), suggesting that the vitamin has functional roles in these immune system cells. A decrease in the intracellular concentration of vitamin C occurs when phagocytes are activated in vitro (84,85) and during common cold infections (86).

Low vitamin C intake has been reported to decrease the phagocytic activity in guinea pigs (87–93) and monkeys (94), although no changes in phagocytosis were found in some studies (85,95,96). Vitamin C may also affect the chemotactic responsiveness of phagocytes (92–94,96–106). It seems possible that the effects of vitamin C on the phagocytes are mediated by antioxidant effects (107), as oxidants have been shown to suppress phagocyte functions (108–110). Furthermore, vitamin C has been reported to decrease neutrophil dysfunctions caused by corticosteroids (111–113).

The physiological significance of vitamin C intake to the function of human phagocytes in vivo is not clear. In certain pathological conditions vitamin C supplementation has been reported to normalize the functions of phagocytes (114–134), suggesting that vitamin C intake may be important in some situations. However, some of these effects could not be repeated (135), and in one study the ability of phagocytes to kill *Escherichia coli* in vitro was decreased when a healthy subject was administered 2 g/day of the vitamin (136).

Proliferation of T Lymphocytes

A number of studies have found that a higher vitamin C concentration increases the proliferative responses of T lymphocytes in vitro (124,137–144). Vitamin C supplementation has increased T-cell proliferative responses in some animal species (145–148). Some studies with human subjects administered vitamin C have reported an increase in lymphocyte proliferative responses (120,124,138,149–153), while some others found no changes (135,137,138,141,154,155). It seems possible that there are real effects of vitamin C supplementation, but they may be quantitatively relevant only in some specific groups of people.

The effect of vitamin C on T cells can be a nonspecific antioxidant effect, as some other reducing agents also increase the proliferative responses of lymphocytes (156–159). Moreover, it has been suggested that physiological oxidants suppress lymphocyte proliferation (160–162), providing a biological rationale for the effects of antioxidants.

Production of Interferon

Vitamin C has been reported to increase the induced production of interferon in cell culture (163–166) and in mice (167,168). However, vitamin C had no effect on interferon production in two lymphoblastoid cell lines induced by Sendai virus (165) and in mouse embryo cells induced by Semliki Forest virus (169).

Other Possible Effects on the Immune System

A few reports have suggested that vitamin C status may affect the production of antibodies and complement components, but the data are conflicting (58,59,145–147,170–175).

In one study with hospital patients a significant positive correlation was observed between natural killer (NK) cell activity and vitamin C concentration in leukocytes (176). In a study with healthy subjects vitamin C supplementation first led to a slight suppression of NK cell activity and thereafter to a significant enhancement (177). In patients with Chédiak–Higashi syndrome NK cell activity normalized during vitamin C supplementation (138). In normal mice vitamin C supplementation did not affect NK cell activity (178).

Several studies have found that vitamin C suppresses the replication of viruses in cell cultures (163,179–184), but the mechanism of this effect is not known. D-Isoascorbic acid also caused suppression of replication (180), suggesting a mechanism based on a non-specific antioxidant effect. It is not clear whether the effect is physiologically relevant. In one study vitamin C did not affect the replication of selected respiratory viruses in cell culture (185).

Under in vitro conditions vitamin C has been found to inactivate viruses and bacteria directly and to break deoxyribonucleic acid (DNA) (186–190), but the physiological significance of this effect is doubtful. Vitamin C is easily oxidized under in vitro conditions in the presence of transition metals (e.g., iron), causing the generation of reactive radicals. However, in healthy subjects the concentration of free iron ion in plasma is extremely low (191), so that such radical-forming reactions apparently do not occur to any significant extent. Furthermore, there is a problem with the nonspecificity of the reaction as the radicals produced should be as harmful to the host tissues as to the infecting agents.

Vitamin C participates in the synthesis of carnitine (52–54), and there are some data suggesting that carnitine affects the immune system (192). This may be a further way vitamin C intake affects the immune system.

In the intensive search for proteins and smaller molecules efficiently and specifically defending the body against viruses and bacteria vitamin C has not been of any particular interest. Still, it is possible that as an efficient reducing agent vitamin C has nonspecific effects on the immune system, similarly to the nonspecific effects of pH or temperature on various biological systems. If the major role of vitamin C in the immune system is that of a physiological antioxidant protecting various cells against oxidants released during an infection, it could have quantitatively meaningful effects even though the mechanisms may be nonspecific. Finally, it is also possible that there are substantial individual differences in the effects of vitamin C in humans, as has been found in the guinea pig (193–195).

INFECTIONS IN ANIMALS

If vitamin C affects the immune system in a nonspecific manner as an antioxidant, it is probable that the effects are not strictly limited to the respiratory viruses, which in fact consist of half a dozen unrelated viruses with over 100 serotypes. Consequently, it is possible that vitamin C intake affects susceptibility to and severity of infections by some of the nonrespiratory viruses and possibly by some bacteria as well.

Most mammals synthesize vitamin C in the liver. The guinea pig is one of the rare species that have lost the capability to synthesize vitamin C (196,197), and therefore it provides a good experimental model for studies dealing with the effects of low vitamin C levels on susceptibility to infections. Low vitamin C intake has been found to decrease the resistance of guinea pigs to *Mycobacterium tuberculosis* (198–205), other bacteria (2,95,206–211), Rickettsiae (212), *Endamoeba histolytica* (213), and *Candida albicans* (214). Supplementation of guinea pigs with vitamin C has been reported to increase resistance to the rabies virus (215–217). In some studies vitamin C supplementation had no effects on bacterial infections (218–220), but there is such a large number of experimental variables of potential importance that discrepancies in results are not surprising.

In guinea pigs infected with *M. tuberculosis* vitamin C supplementation slightly increased the hemoglobin level (221). In histological studies fewer caseonecrotic lesions, more collagenous tissue within and around the tuberculous centers, and less dispersion of tubercle bacilli were observed in vitamin C–supplemented animals (202,203,222). Furthermore, in guinea pigs infected with *M. tuberculosis* there was a decrease in vitamin C level in the adrenals, the liver, and urine (223,224).

Primates lack the ability to synthesize vitamin C (196,197). In some studies with rhesus monkeys vitamin C was reported to decrease the incidence of poliomyelitis (225,226), while in one study no effect was observed (227). Nonetheless, in the latter study it was noted that many rhesus monkeys on a scorbutic diet died of spontaneous infections, chiefly pneumonia and enterocolitis, while those receiving adequate amounts of vitamin C remained well (227). In rhesus monkeys vitamin C intake affects the bacterial flora in the oral cavity (228,229). In marmosets vitamin C supplementation decreased the rates of morbidity and mortality due to parainfluenza infection (230). In macaque monkeys malarial infection decreased the vitamin C level in plasma (231).

Fishes require exogenous vitamin C (196,232). In catfish (232) and rainbow trout (233,234) vitamin C supplementation decreased the mortality rate of bacterial and parasitic infections.

Rats and mice synthesize vitamin C in the liver and consequently cannot be used to study the effects of low vitamin C intakes. However, the effect of vitamin C supplementation and the effect of infections on vitamin C metabolism can be studied in these species and in others that synthesize vitamin C. In mice infected with *Pseudomonas aeruginosa* (235) and *Candida albicans* (135) vitamin C supplementation increased the proportion of surviving animals. In mice infected with rodent malaria parasites, vitamin C depressed parasitemia and extended the mean survival time of the infected mice (236). Vitamin C inhibited the multiplication of *Mycobacterium lepra* in mouse foot pads (237). In mice infected with *Streptococcus pneumoniae* vitamin C supplementation enhanced the clearance of bacteria from the lungs, apparently through an increased influx of neutrophils to the lungs; however, the survival rate was not significantly changed in the vitamin C group (238). In rats infected with *Trypanosoma hippicum* there was a decrease in the vitamin C concentration in the liver, spleen, and adrenals, but the level of vitamin C in plasma was doubled (239). In cats vitamin C supplementation decreased the duration of rhinotracheitis (240). In chickens vitamin C supplementation increased the resistance to *Salmonella gallinarum* (241), *E. coli* (242), and viral bronchitis (243).

It is possible that the amount of the infecting agent affects the role of vitamin C intake. If vitamin C has only moderate effects on the immune system it is possible that it shows effects when the infectious dose is rather small, whereas there may be no effect when the infectious dose is very large. In rhesus monkeys vitamin C provided moderate protection when quite a small dose of polio virus was used, while it was without effect when a large dose was used (226), but the number of animals was so small that the conclusion is not strong. In a study with guinea pigs infected with bacteria, it was also pointed out that the infectious dose seemed to affect the role of vitamin C intake (206).

From the studies examining the effects of vitamin C on the immune system and on various animal infections it seems possible that vitamin C intake may have effects on the susceptibility of humans to infections other than the common cold.

INFECTIONS IN HUMANS

Most of the placebo-controlled studies that have examined the effects of vitamin C on infections have dealt with the common cold. There are few controlled studies of the role of vitamin C on other infections, although quite a large number of uncontrolled reports have suggested that vitamin C may have beneficial effects on various infections. In this section the review is restricted to studies of vitamin C and infections in which some kind of control group has been used. The type of the control group is indicated in the tables; in most cases the control group was not administered placebo. A few uncontrolled reports are briefly commented on in the next section.

Incidence of Infections

The results of all studies known to us that have reported quantitative data on the incidence of infections in two groups differing in vitamin C intake are listed in Tables 5 and 6. Table 5 contains intervention studies and Table 6, observational studies.

In Tables 5 and 6 the odds ratio (OR) is used as the measure of the effect of the difference in the vitamin C intake. When the incidence is low ($< 20\%$) the OR is a good approximation of the RR (32). Furthermore, the exact confidence interval (CI) of the OR is much more easily calculated than the exact CI of the RR, making the OR a more practical measure of an effect when there are only a few cases per group (32). The one-tailed p value was calculated since the question being considered in the present analysis was whether higher vitamin C intake decreases the incidence of infections or not; there is no theoretical or experimental reason to assume that a higher vitamin C intake would increase the incidence of infections.

Several studies have reported much lower incidence of infections in the study group receiving a larger amount of vitamin C compared to the corresponding control group. However, all of these studies are small and the results are inaccurate; i.e., the confidence intervals are wide. Furthermore, in several cases the studies have been poorly planned and/ or reported, and thus it is possible that there are serious biases between the study groups. Some important aspects of the studies are listed in the tables, but for more specific technical details the reader is referred to the original references.

Three intervention studies have analyzed the relation between vitamin C intake and posttransfusion hepatitis. Morishige and Murata reported a lower frequency of hepatitis among subjects administered vitamin C (244), but the validity of this poorly described study is questionable. Nevertheless, on the assumption that the groups are comparable the difference in favor of vitamin C is significant. Banic and Kosak found only one case of hepatitis among subjects administered vitamin C but seven cases among controls not administered placebo (245). Knodell et al. found a small decrease in the incidence of hepatitis in the vitamin C group, but the confidence interval is wide because of the small number of cases (246). Furthermore, in Knodell's study the vitamin C group was transfused on average 1.29 times as much blood as the placebo group. Assuming that the risk is directly proportional to the amount of blood given there was a 45% decrease in the incidence of hepatitis (247). Accordingly, all three intervention studies are consistent with the conclusion that vitamin C supplementation decreases the incidence of posttransfusion hepatitis, but as a result of the various technical shortcomings in the studies the conclusion is not strong.

Three intervention studies and one observational study have reported on the relation of vitamin C intake and the incidence of pneumonia. Pitt and Costrini carried out a ran-

Table 5 Vitamin C Intake and the Incidence of Infections: Intervention Studies

Ref.	Vitamin C dose (g/day)	Control type[a]	Cases/Total subjects Vitamin C	Cases/Total subjects Control	OR (90% CI)[b]	p (1 − t)	Subjects/notes
Posttransfusion hepatitis							
244	2–6	C	3/1367	12/170	0.03 (0.009, 0.082)	<0.001	See text
245	3–10	C	1/141	7/155	0.15 (0.013, 0.78)	0.025	See text
246,247,248	3.2	P, DB	6/90	8/85	0.69 (0.26, 1.8)	0.26	See text
Pneumonia							
25	2	P, DB	1/331	7/343	0.15 (0.013, 0.74)	0.022	Military recruits
249	0.05–0.3	F	0/335	17/1100	0.00 (0, 0.32)	0.005	Schoolchildren
249a	0.3	C	2/114	10/112	0.18 (0.03, 0.77)	0.009	Military recruits
Tuberculosis							
250	0.02–0.37[c]	C	1/644[d]	10/1096[d]	0.17 (0.015, 0.81)[d]	0.026	Blacks
Bronchitis							
41,42	1	P, DB	8/139	13/140	0.60 (0.27, 1.3)	0.14	Schoolchildren in a skiing camp
Pharyngitis, laryngitis, or tonsillitis							
41,42	1	P, DB	7/139	14/140	0.48 (0.21, 1.1)	0.062	Schoolchildren in a skiing camp
Tonsillitis							
249	0.05–0.3	F	29/335	94/1100	1.01 (0.70, 1.5)	—	Schoolboys
249	0.05–0.3	F	1/60	7/90	0.20 (0.018, 1.06)	0.057	New recruits to the school
Secondary bacterial infections after a common cold episode							
251	6	C	6/45	15/45	0.31 (0.12, 0.75)	0.014	From Table 1 in Ref. 251. See text
Rheumatic fever							
252	0.1	P	14/28	10/28	1.8 (0.72, 4.5)	—	From Table 1 in Ref. 252.
249	0.05–0.3	F	0/335	16/1100	0.0 (0, 0.34)	0.007	Schoolboys

[a]Type of control: C, placebo not used; F, vitamin C added to the food; P, placebo-controlled; DB, double-blind.
[b]p Values are 1-tailed mid-p values and 90% CI are mid-p confidence intervals (32). The p values and the CIs were calculated with the StatXact program (Cytel Software Co., Cambridge, MA). OR, odds ratio; CI, confidence interval.
[c]Vitamin C doses: 0.02–0.075 g/day to children under 4 years, C.05–0.22 g/day to children 5–12 years, and 0.075–0.375 g/day to those over 13 years. In addition to vitamin C certain other essential nutrients were administered: niacin, thiamin, riboflavin, vitamin A, Ca, Fe.
[d]The denominator is the number of person-years in the group; the OR and CI are calculated from the figures shown.

Table 6 Vitamin C Intake and the Incidence of Infections: Observational Studies

Ref.	Plasma vitamin C limit (μmol/L)	Cases/total Vitamin C levels High	Low	OR	(90% CI)[a]	p^a $(1 - t)$	Subjects/notes
Tuberculosis							
253	34 (6 mg/L)	0/117	27/896	0	(0, 0.46)	0.017	Mostly blacks (85%); cohort study
Acute necrotizing ulcerative gingivitis							
254	70	—	—	0.14 1.00[c]	(0.06, 0.33)[b]	<0.001 —	Case-control study; 60 matched pairs
Postoperative pneumonia							
255	11 (2 mg/L)	10/74	7/35	0.62	(0.25, 1.6)	0.20	Hospital patients; cohort study

[a]For calculation of OR, 90% CI, and p value, see Table 5. OR, odds ratio; CI, confidence interval.
[b]Unadjusted OR from logistic regression analysis calculated in the reference.
[c]OR from logistic regression adjusted for social class calculated in the reference.

domized double-blind study with military recruits in a training camp (25). Their trial was primarily concerned with the role of vitamin C in relation to the common cold (cf. Tables 1 and 2), but they also reported a dramatic decrease in the incidence of pneumonia in the vitamin C group. Glazebrook and Thomson studied schoolboys in an institution and found no cases of pneumonia in the vitamin C group (249). In their study vitamin C was added to the food in the kitchen. Kimbarowski and Mokrow (249a) examined the effect of vitamin C supplementation in military recruits having upper respiratory symptoms at the start of the study, and observed a substantially lower incidence of pneumonia in subjects administered the vitamin. In an observational study with surgical patients Lund and Crandon (255) found a slightly increased risk of pneumonia in patients with the lowest vitamin C levels, but the difference is not statistically significant. Moreover, in Lund and Crandon's study there were three fatalities due to pneumonia and all of these were among subjects with high vitamin C levels, pointing out the difficulty of drawing conclusions from small studies and particularly from small observational studies.

In a placebo-controlled study Ritzel reported a decrease in the incidence of bronchitis, pharyngitis, laryngitis, and tonsillitis in schoolchildren in a skiing camp with vitamin C supplementation (41). Glazebrook and Thomson found a decrease in tonsillitis with vitamin C in schoolboys newly recruited to the school, but not in those who had remained in the school for a longer time (249). Asfora compared vitamin C to some other medications in the same subjects and reported a lower number of secondary infections after common cold episodes when vitamin C was administered (251). However, the number of cold episodes was not disclosed and it appears indirectly that the number is not the same for the two treatments, hampering the interpretation of the available data.

Glazebrook and Thomson found no cases of rheumatic fever, a complication of streptococcal infection, among the schoolboys administered vitamin C, but 16 cases in the control group (249). In contrast, an older study by Schultz showed no preventive effect of vitamin C on rheumatic fever (252). Nevertheless, there are considerable differences between the two studies. Schultz selected as subjects children who had previous episodes of rheumatic fever, whereas Glazebrook and Thomson had no such selection. Also, the dietary vitamin C intake was particularly low in Glazebrook and Thomson's subjects at 10–15 mg/day. Schultz did not estimate the dietary intake of his subjects, but possibly it was much higher.

Two studies have reported a lower incidence of tuberculosis in subjects with higher vitamin C intake. In an intervention study by Downes (250) there was only one case of tuberculosis among subjects administered vitamin C. However, some other nutrients were also given, and therefore the difference between the groups is not specifically attributable to vitamin C (250). In a prospective cohort study Getz et al. found no cases of tuberculosis among subjects with high plasma vitamin C levels (253).

In an observational study on acute necrotizing ulcerative gingivitis caused by anaerobic oral bacteria high vitamin C intake was associated with lower risk of infection (254). However, when the social classes were included in the logistic regression model no association with vitamin C intake remained. Vitamin C intake is a strong life-style indicator, and therefore in observational studies the associations with vitamin C intake may be caused indirectly by some other life-style factors. For this reason intervention studies provide much more reliable information about the effects of vitamin C intake. It is also clear that in the case of observational studies the potential confounding factors should be carefully considered.

Two studies have reported an association between vitamin C intake and the prevalence of hemolytic streptococcus in the tonsils (Table 7; 38,256). Although the association is consistent with vitamin C's having physiological effects on the immune system, its clinical significance is not clear. For example, Coulehan (38) did not find a lower rate of secondary infections after common cold episodes in the group supplemented with vitamin C.

From the statistical point of view the studies discussed leave the role of vitamin C intake on the incidence of infections other than the common cold largely unresolved. In several studies no placebo was used nor were subjects randomly allocated to the study groups. Consequently, it is possible that there are substantial biases in the study groups. Further-

Table 7   Vitamin C Intake and the Colonization of Tonsils with Hemolytic Streptococci

| | Cases/total | | | | |
| | Vitamin C levels | | OR | p^a | |
Ref.	High	Low	(90% CI)[a]	(1 − t)	Subjects/notes
Intervention study: supplementation: 1 g/day					
38	6/57	13/57	0.40 (0.16, 0.97)	0.043	Children
Observational study: limit: 49 μmol/L (8.6 mg/L) in blood					
256	4/32	30/64	0.16 (0.06, 0.42)	<0.001	From table 1 in Ref. 256. Children referred to tonsillectomy

[a]For calculation of OR, 90% CI, and p value, see Table 5. OR, odds ratio; CI, confidence interval.

more, in many studies the number of cases was so small that the studies had no reasonable statistical power. For example, it is quite amazing that in two intervention studies the incidence of hepatitis (245) and pneumonia (25) was >80% lower in the vitamin C group, yet the differences between the vitamin C and control groups are barely statistically significant when employing the conservative two-tailed test. Such lack of statistical power has been a persistent problem in medical studies. The number of subjects are sometimes so small that the results are practically meaningless. Freiman et al. (257) surveyed 71 studies published in the medical literature that had reported a "negative result." They calculated that 50 of the studies would, from the statistical point of view, have missed a 50% improvement from the therapy tested. Still, such an effect can often be clinically relevant if it is real.

Pauling (247) explicitly pointed out the lack of statistical power in the study of Knodell et al. on posttransfusion hepatitis (246), which was presented by the authors as definitely proving that vitamin C has no effect on patients undergoing blood transfusion. However, the 90% CI of Knodell's results is also consistent with an OR as low as 0.26. It is clear that Knodell's data do not support the conclusion that vitamin C intake has no physiological effect on the incidence of posttransfusion hepatitis. Nevertheless, it is a question of subjective interpretation whether the study provides weak evidence for benefit from vitamin C supplementation, or whether such a small-scale study lacking any reasonable statistical power should simply be disregarded. We prefer to see Knodell's study and many other small-scale studies in Table 5 as consistent with the hypothesis that vitamin C has effects on infections other than the common cold. However, because of various technical shortcomings the conclusion is not strong. Neither is it clear what the specific infections on which vitamin C intake may have the greatest effects are. In any case, as regards the great apparent reduction in the incidence of various infections as reported in several studies in Table 5, it would seem worthwhile carrying out well-planned studies that do not suffer from a similar lack of statistical power and other experimental defects as many studies in the table do.

Vitamin C Metabolism During Infections

A large number of studies have reported a decrease in vitamin C levels in plasma, white blood cells, or urine during infections. Tuberculosis has been studied most extensively (258–272), but low levels have also been reported in patients with other infections (271, 273–282). Several reports have noted that more severe forms of tuberculosis (263–272) and other infections (280) are often associated with lower vitamin C levels than the milder forms. It is noteworthy that plasma, leukocyte, and urine vitamin C levels are also decreased in the common cold (18,86,283–285).

The reasons for the lower vitamin C status in patients with infections have been considered in some of the papers. The dietary vitamin C intake of the patients may have been rather low in some studies (261,274,275). However, in some other studies the dietary vitamin C intake was comparable for the infectious patients and the healthy controls, suggesting that low dietary intake cannot be the only cause of reduced vitamin C levels in the patients (258,264,265,268). Furthermore, several studies have found differences in the metabolism of vitamin C test doses in patients compared to healthy control subjects (258,264,266–268,270,274,277,280).

Banerjee et al. reported that the decrease in the reduced vitamin C (ascorbate) level in plasma and urine is associated with a concomitant increase in the oxidized form (dehydroascorbate) (259,271,279). Their assay method found that in normal healthy people 5%–10% of the vitamin C is in the dehydroascorbate form, while 65%–80% was in the oxidized form in patients who later died of meningococcal meningitis, tetanus, pneumonia, or typhoid fever (271). This observed increase in dehydroascorbate level is consistent with the idea that the role of vitamin C in infections is particularly that of a reducing agent (antioxidant) protecting against oxidants produced during an infection. Furthermore, the change in the oxidation level also indicates that the low levels of reduced vitamin C in patients with infections are not caused by poor diet alone, but are partially caused by physiological changes resulting from the infections.

The decrease in vitamin C levels in infected patients is no proof that supplementation would benefit the patients. Nonetheless, the consistent benefit of vitamin C supplementation on the severity of the common cold, along with the changes in the vitamin C metabolism in various infections including the common cold, provides a sound reason to wonder whether large doses of vitamin C might also have beneficial effects on other infections than the common cold.

The Severity of Infections

A number of studies have directly or indirectly assessed the effects of vitamin C supplementation on the severity of various infections (Table 8; 246–249,270,286–293). The severity of a disease is a much more poorly defined variable than the incidence of the disease. Various measures of severity yield numerical values that are not meaningfully comparable. For example, changes in the red blood cell sedimentation rate (RBC SR) or in the numbers of various blood cells may indicate true physiological effects of vitamin C, but such changes are not easy to interpret as a real benefit to the patient. Consequently, an estimate of the effect was not calculated in Table 8, but the original results in the two study groups and the p value for the difference are presented.

There are great experimental differences among the studies in Table 8. Some of the observations come from therapeutic studies in which vitamin C administration was commenced only after the onset of the disease. In some other studies vitamin C was administered regularly and the episodes occurring were affected by regular vitamin administration. As regards the question of whether vitamin C intake has any real physiological effects on the severity of the infections, both types of studies can yield relevant information. Nevertheless, it is possible that the quantitative effects of regular and therapeutic supplementation are not similar, and this is a further reason for not calculating any explicit estimates of benefit. In this analysis the primary interest is in the question of whether the level of vitamin C intake has any physiological effects on the severity of infections, rather than on the quantitative estimate of its potential effects.

In a double-blind placebo-controlled study Terezhalmy et al. (286) observed a significant decrease in the duration of herpes labialis infections among subjects administered 0.6–1.0 g/day of vitamin C and a similar amount of bioflavonoids. A significant decrease in the formation of vesicles was also found.

In a double-blind placebo-controlled study with elderly patients admitted to hospital with bronchitis or bronchopneumonia, Hunt et al. (286a) found a significantly greater decrease in respiratory symptoms in subjects admnistered vitamin C.

Glazebrook and Thomson (249) did not observe any marked effect of vitamin C on the incidence of tonsillitis (cf. Table 5); however, significantly fewer tonsillitis cases in the vitamin C group were sent to a hospital, suggesting that on average the infections were milder (Table 8). Furthermore, among the children who were sent to a hospital the stay was significantly shorter among those who had been administered vitamin C.

Ganguly and Waldman (287,288) studied the effect of orange juice on the symptoms of an experimental infection with attenuated rubella virus. They found a significant decrease in the number of subjects in whom respiratory symptoms developed in the orange juice group using nasal inoculation. Also, the antibodies against the rubella virus developed more rapidly in the subjects administered orange juice. In subjects inoculated subcutaneously no significant effect on respiratory symptoms or on the emergence of antibodies was observed. The control group was administered placebo tablets as part of a double-blind study evaluating an antiviral drug, so that the control group thought that they might receive an effective antiviral substance and accordingly the placebo effect is not an obvious explanation of the difference between the groups. Orange juice is an important source of vitamin C and while the observed benefit may be due to vitamin C, there are other substances in the orange juice as well.

Knodell et al. (246) administered vitamin C for 2 weeks to patients undergoing blood transfusion, while the hepatitis infections occurred on average 7 weeks after blood transfusion. The mean serum glutamic-oxaloacetic transaminase (SGOT) level was lower in the hepatitis cases administered vitamin C, and there were fewer cases of chronic hepatitis among the vitamin C group. Furthermore, the incubation period was longer in the vitamin C–supplemented group. Although none of Knodell's observations was significant statistically, the consistency in the results is striking and the pattern is not easy to interpret as purely a result of chance.

Several studies have reported that vitamin C has some effects on subjects with tuberculosis. All of these studies are old and technically more or less deficient. In some reports there are no data that allow calculation of the p value corresponding to the reported mean differences. A number of the tuberculosis studies have reported statistically significant differences between the vitamin C and control groups, but it is likely that the differences are caused at least in part by the placebo effect and biases between the study groups.

A few German and Swiss studies suggested that vitamin C supplementation may decrease the duration of epidemic hepatitis and poliomyelitis (294–298). There are various shortcomings in these controlled studies and they do not have much weight in considering whether vitamin C intake affects the severity of infections.

In a cohort study with human immunodeficiency virus (HIV)–infected subjects the relative hazard of progression to acquired immunodeficiency syndrome (AIDS) was 0.55 in subjects with the highest level of vitamin C intake (299).

In the case of common cold severity there are some data suggesting that the effect of vitamin C is not saturated by 1 g/day (15,19,24). In this respect most of the studies in Table 8 used rather small doses. Nonetheless, Terezhalmy et al. (286) found that 0.6 and 1.0 g/day produced comparable effects on herpes infections, indicating that the effect of vitamin C may reach saturation with doses of 0.6 g/day or lower. Nevertheless, 10 mg/day of vitamin C prevents scurvy and 60 mg/day is the recommended dietary allowance (RDA) recommendation for vitamin C (300); thus Terezhalmy's results are not trivial even though the effect could be reproduced with doses somewhat smaller than 600 mg/day.

In the treatment of infections one factor that may be important is the promptness of initiating vitamin C supplementation. In the case of the common cold Asfora (251) reported that the greatest benefit from therapeutic vitamin C (6 g/day) was obtained when the treatment was initiated within 24 h of the onset of symptoms. Terezhalmy et al. also found time dependency in the case of herpes labialis (286). In their study in 6 of 26 subjects (23%) herpes vesicles developed when supplementation was initiated within 24 h of the onset of the symptoms, whereas vesicles developed in 8 of 12 subjects (67%) with later initiation. It is unlikely that the difference is caused by chance ($p(2 - t) = 0.02$).

In therapeutic studies the observer bias and the placebo effect may be much greater

Table 8 Vitamin C Intake and the Severity of Infections

Ref.	Vitamin C (g/day)	Control type[a]	No. of cases		Outcome value		p^b (1 − t)	Outcome[c]
			Vitamin C	Control	Vitamin C	Control		
Herpes labialis								
286	0.6[d]	P, DB	19	10	1.7 ± 0.6	3.5 ± 0.8 (SD)	<0.001	Pain (days)
					4.2 ± 1.7	9.7 ± 2.8 (SD)	<0.001	Healing (days)
	1.0[d]	P, DB	19	10	1.3 ± 0.6	3.5 ± 0.8 (SD)	<0.001	Pain (days)
					4.4 ± 3.9	9.7 ± 2.8 (SD)	<0.001	Healing (days)
	0.6–1[d]	P, DB	38	10	37% (14)	100% (10)	<0.001	PCTG with vesicle formation
Bronchitis								
286a	0.2	PL, DB	28	29	3.4 ± 1.8	2.3 ± 2.5 (SD)	0.027	Decrease in respiratory clinical scores in four weeks
Tonsillitis								
249	0.05–0.3	F	29	94	62% (18)	88% (83)	0.002	PCTG admitted to hospital
249	0.05–0.3	F	18	83	10.1 ± 7.0	16.7 ± 11.9 (SD)	0.013	Stay in hospital (days)
Rubella infection, inoculated by nose drops								
287,288	0.3[e]	P	11	13	27% (3)	77% (10)	0.011	PCTG with respiratory symptoms
					100% (11)	31% (4)	<0.001	PCTG with antibody appearing <28 days after inoculation
Rubella infection, inoculated subcutaneously								
287,288	0.3[e]	P	22	9	32% (7)	22% (2)	—	PCTG with respiratory symptoms

Posttransfusion hepatitis								
246,247,248	3.2[f]	P, DB	6	8	474 ± 386	759 ± 907 (SD)	0.25	SGOT (unit)
					33% (2)	62% (5)	0.17	PCTG with chronic liver disease
					7.6 ± 2.0	6.9 ± 2.1 (SD)	0.27	Incubation period
Tuberculosis								
289	0.2–1.0	C	19	6	42% (8)	0% (0)	0.035	RBC SR decreased at least 5 mm
270,290	0.25	C	28[g]	57[g]	70%	53%	—	PCTG with decrease in RBC SR at 3 months
291	0.2	C	101	101	79% (80)	65% (65)	0.010	PCTG feeling better
					49% (49)	33% (33)	0.012	PCTG with decrease in sputum
292	0.15	P	82	77	58% (48)	48% (37)	0.10	PCTG clinically improved
292	0.15	P	45	37	51% (23)	30% (11)	0.028	PCTG with improved mucous membrane lesions in tuberculous tracheobronchitis
293	0.2	C	37[g]	37[g]	90%	25%	—	PCTG feeling better
					72%	25%	—	PCTG with increase in hemoglobin

[a]Type of control: C, placebo not used; F, vitamin C added to food; P, placebo-controlled; DB, double-blind.
[b]For dichotomous data the mid-p value was calculated (cf. Table 5) and for continuous variables the t-test was used.
[c]PCTG, percentage of patients with the characteristic indicated. RBC SR, red blood cell sedimentation rate. SGOT, serum glutamic-oxaloacetic transaminase. Not all outcomes from the studies are listed.
[d]Terezhalmy et al. also gave their patients bioflavonoids (0.6–1 g/day).
[e]Vitamin C was given as orange juice.
[f]Vitamin C was administered for 2 weeks after the blood transfusion, i.e., it was terminated before the occurrence of the episodes.
[g]The approximate numbers are deduced from the total number of subjects given in the publication; the precise number per group was not published.

problems than in studies on incidence. An observer or a patient faithfully believing in a new method of treatment may easily form the impression that the severity of a disease is slightly decreased even if there are no real physiological effects. In contrast, for an initially healthy person it may be much more difficult to prevent an episode of illness merely by wishing. Therefore, the lack of the double-blind placebo-control method is a much more dangerous shortcoming in the therapeutic studies (Table 8) than in studies on incidence (Table 5). Nevertheless, the differences between the vitamin and control groups have been so great in some studies listed in Table 8 that they justify further work with better experimental features.

UNCONTROLLED REPORTS ON THE USE OF VITAMIN C

Case reports and experience of individual physicians are not good evidence when considering whether a method of treatment has any real physiological effects. It is clear that for a better understanding of the role of vitamin C on various infectious diseases well-planned studies are required. However, placebo-controlled studies are a rigid means of seeking the best modifications of a treatment. They are at their best when testing whether there is any physiological effect at all, but in a double-blind study the treatment cannot easily be adjusted individually if there are substantial individual differences or if the treatment should be modified depending on the response to it.

The reports by physicians who have been interested in vitamin C may provide worthwhile information on the various possible ways of using vitamin C in the treatment of infectious diseases. Nevertheless, the literature on uncontrolled reports on vitamin C and infections is not thoroughly reviewed in this section apart from a few of the more interesting papers. Previously Stone (7) and Briggs (8) carefully surveyed the literature on vitamin C and infections and provided much longer lists of references on the uncontrolled reports.

Cathcart suggested that for the treatment of various infections the optimum oral vitamin C dose should be determined individually for each patient (301,302). He reported that patients with severe bacterial and viral diseases can ingest over 100 g/day of vitamin C without problems, while healthy people usually have diarrhea or other gastrointestinal symptoms with 4–15 g/day. Cathcart's approach is to increase the dose to a level causing mild gastrointestinal discomfort and thereafter use somewhat lower doses for the treatment. This approach is a good example of treatments that are not easy to test rigorously by the double-blind method.

Some other physicians have administered large doses of vitamin C to their patients by intravenous (IV) infusion (303–306). The vitamin C level in plasma increases instantaneously and there is no loss of vitamin C in the intestines, and in this respect the IV infusion may be more efficient than oral administration. Vitamin C has also been used in the form of nose drops in the treatment of the common cold (307).

Some physicians studying the effects of vitamin C supplementation on immunological parameters have reported clinical benefit for patients (117–123,126,128,133a). Although there are no control groups in these studies, the immunological changes observed give greater weight to the reported benefits.

CONCLUSIONS

The role of vitamin C in infections was studied quite extensively in the first part of this century but much less actively thereafter. Several of the studies reported highly favorable results but had various technical deficiencies. The topic was not ignored because of carefully conducted studies showing no effects from vitamin C. Rather, there appear to be two major reasons for the general disregard of the early studies. Antibiotics were introduced in the 1940s and because of their highly specific effects on microbes they have obviously been a much more rational choice of drugs for patients with infections than vitamin C. A second reason for the rejection of the issue apparently was the notion that the true physiological effect of vitamin C is simply the prevention of scurvy. Evidently it has not been reasonable to think that a substance that participates in the synthesis of collagen would have effects on infections. However, the biochemical characteristics of vitamin C are complex. It participates in the function of several enzymes unrelated to collagen metabolism (52–55), and as one of the major biological antioxidants it can have a large number of nonspecific effects that may be physiologically important. Although vitamin C is not a specific agent against any infection it possibly has moderate effects on general resistance to infections.

The effect of vitamin C supplementation on the common cold has been most extensively studied, and it is the only case in which certain unequivocal conclusions can be drawn, although it is unknown what the best dosage, the maximal effect, and the characteristics of subjects who benefit most are. Nevertheless, the role of vitamin C in colds was not studied for any specific biological reason, but because of the wide publicity aroused by Pauling. Apparently some people wanted to show that he was either right or wrong, while still others just wanted to study a topic on which a Nobel Prize winner had put his credibility on the line.

From the conflicting results from controlled studies published so far, it seems clear that vitamin C is no panacea against infections, in either prevention or therapy. Nevertheless, a few intervention studies have found such considerable effects that the issue should be investigated in more detail. Furthermore, vitamin C is a safe nutrient (13,308,309) costing only pennies per gram, so that even quite modest effects may be worth exploitation.

ACKNOWLEDGMENT

This work was supported by the Academy of Finland.

REFERENCES

1. Hess AF, Infantile scurvy. V. Am J Dis Child 1917; 14:337–353.
2. Höjer JA. Studies in scurvy: scurvy and infection. Acta Paediatr 1924; 3(suppl):115–122.
3. Hess AF. Diet, nutrition and infection. N Engl J Med 1932; 207:637–644.
4. Clausen SW. The influence of nutrition upon resistance to infection. Physiol Rev 1934; 14: 309–350.
5. Robertson EC. The vitamins and resistance to infection: vitamin C. Medicine 1934; 13: 190–206.
6. Perla D, Marmorston J. Role of vitamin C in resistance. Arch Pathol 1937; 23:543–575, 683–712.
7. Stone I. The Healing Factor: Vitamin C Against Disease. New York: Grosset & Dunlap, 1972.
8. Briggs M. Vitamin C and infectious disease. In: Briggs MH, ed. Recent Vitamin Research. Boca Raton, FL: CRC Press, 1984:39–81.
9. Pauling L. Vitamin C and the Common Cold. San Francisco: Freeman, 1970.
10. Pauling L. The significance of the evidence about ascorbic acid and the common cold. Proc Natl Acad Sci USA 1971; 68:2678–2681.

11. Kleijnen J, Riet G, Knipschild PG. Vitamin C and the common cold. Ned Tijdschr Geneeskd 1989; 133:1532–1535.

12. Kleijnen J, Knipschild P. The comprehensiveness of Medline and Embase computer searches. Pharmaceutisch Weekblad Scientific edition 1992; 14:316–320.

13. Pauling L. How to Live Longer and Feel Better. New York: Freeman, 1986.

14. Hemilä H. Vitamin C and the common cold. Br J Nutr 1992; 67:3–16.

15. Hemilä H. Does vitamin C alleviate the symptoms of the common cold? A review of current evidence. Scand J Infect Dis 1994; 26:1–6.

16. Elliott B. Ascorbic acid: efficacy in the prevention of symptoms of respiratory infection on a Polaris submarine. Int Res Commun Syst Med Sci 1973; 1(3):12.

17. Mink KA, Dick EC, Jennings LC, Inhorn SL. Amelioration of rhinovirus colds by vitamin C supplementation (abstr). Med Virol 1988; 7:356.

18. Schwartz AR, Togo Y, Hornick RB, et al. Evaluation of the efficacy of ascorbic acid in prophylaxis of induced rhinovirus 44 infection in man. J Infect Dis 1973; 128:500–505.

19. Coulehan JL, Reisinger KS, Rogers KD, Bradley DW. Vitamin C prophylaxis in a boarding school. N Engl J Med 1974; 290:6–10.

20. Bancalari A, Seguel C, Neira F, et al. Prophylactic value of vitamin C in acute respiratory infections of schoolchildren. Rev Med Chile 1984; 112:871–876.

21. Anderson TW, Reid DB, Beaton GH. Vitamin C and the common cold. Can Med Assoc J 1972; 107:503–508.

22. Anderson TW, Reid DB, Beaton GH. Vitamin C and the common cold (correction). Can Med Assoc J 1973; 108:133.

23. Karlowski TR, Chalmers TC, Frenkel LD, et al. Ascorbic acid for the common cold. JAMA 1975; 231:1038–1042.

24. Hemilä H. Vitamin C, the placebo effect, and the common cold: a case study of how preconceptions influence the analysis of results. J Clin Epidemiol 1996; 49:1079–1084, 1087.

25. Pitt HA, Costrini AM. Vitamin C prophylaxis in marine recruits. JAMA 1979; 241:908–911.

26. Anderson TW, Suranyi G, Beaton GH. The effect on winter illness of large doses of vitamin C. Can Med Assoc J 1974; 111:31–36.

27. Hemilä H, Herman ZS. Vitamin C and the common cold: a retrospective analysis of Chalmers' review. J Am Coll Nutr 1995; 14:116–123.

28. Fisher RA, Statistical Methods for Research Workers. 7th ed. London: Oliver & Boyd, 1938:104–106.

29. Wolf FM. Meta-Analysis: Quantitative Methods for Research Synthesis. London: Sage, 1986.

30. Elwood PC, Lee HP, Leger AS, et al. A randomized controlled trial of vitamin C in the prevention and amelioration of the common cold. Br J Prev Soc Med 1976; 30:193–196.

31. Ludvigsson J, Hansson LO, Tibbling G. Vitamin C as a preventive medicine against common colds in children. Scand J Infect Dis 1977; 9:91–98.

32. Rothman KJ. Modern Epidemiology. Boston: Little, Brown, 1986.

33. Hemilä H. Vitamin C and common cold incidence: a review of studies with subjects under heavy physical stress. Int J Sports Med 1996; 17:379–383.

34. Baird IM, Hughes RE, Wilson HK, et al. The effects of ascorbic acid and flavonoids on the occurrence of symptoms normally associated with the common cold. Am J Clin Nutr 1979; 32:1686–1690.

34a. Hemilä H. Vitamin C intake and susceptibility to the common cold. Br J Nutr 1997; 77:59–72.

35. Fawzi WW, Chalmers TC, Herrera MG, Mosteller F. Vitamin A supplementation and child mortality. JAMA 1993; 269:898–903.

36. Anderson TW, Beaton GH, Corey PN, Spero L. Winter illness and vitamin C. Can Med Assoc J 1975; 112:823–826.

37. Carr AB, Einstein R, Lai LYC, et al. Vitamin C and the common cold. Acta Genet Med Gemellol 1981; 30:249–255.

38. Coulehan JL, Eberhard S, Kapner L, et al. Vitamin C and acute illness in Navajo school-children. N Engl J Med 1976; 295:973–977.

39. Monto AS. Studies of the community and family. Epidemiol Rev 1994; 16:351–373.

40. Miller JZ, Nance WE, Norton JA, et al. Therapeutic effect of vitamin C. JAMA 1977; 237:248–251.

41. Ritzel G. Critical analysis of the role of vitamin C in the treatment of the common cold. Helv Med Acta 1961; 28:63–68.

42. Ritzel G. Ascorbic acid and the common cold (letter). JAMA 1976; 235:1108.

43. Chalmers TC. Effects of ascorbic acid on the common cold: an evaluation of the evidence. Am J Med 1975; 58:532–536.

44. Hemilä H. Vitamin C supplementation and common cold symptoms: problems with inaccurate reviews. Nutrition 1996; 12:804–809.

45. Dykes MHM, Meier P. Ascorbic acid and the common cold: evaluation of its efficacy and toxicity. JAMA 1975; 231:1073–1079.

46. Pauling L. Ascorbic acid and the common cold: evaluation of its efficacy and toxicity. Part I. Med Tribune 1976; 17(12):18–19.

47. Pauling L. Ascorbic acid and the common cold. Part II. Med Tribune 1976; 17(13):37–38.

48. Truswell AS. Ascorbic acid (letter). N Engl J Med 1986; 315:709.

49. Hemilä H. Nutritional need versus optimal intake. Med Hypotheses 1984; 14:135–139.

50. Hemilä H. A re-evaluation of nutritional goals: not just deficiency counts. Med Hypotheses 1986; 20:17–27.

51. Kuhn TS. The Structure of Scientific Revolutions. 2d ed. Chicago: University of Chicago Press, 1970.

52. Englard S, Seifter S. The biochemical functions of ascorbic acid. Annu Rev Nutr 1986; 6:365–406.

53. Padh H. Cellular functions of ascorbic acid. Biochem Cell Biol 1990; 68:1166–1173.

54. Rebouche CJ. Ascorbic acid and carnitine biosynthesis. Am J Clin Nutr 1991; 54:1147S–1152S.

55. Eipper BA, Mains RE. The role of ascorbate in the biosynthesis of neuroendocrine peptides. Am J Clin Nutr 1991; 54:1153S–1156S.

56. Goodwin JS, Goodwin JM. Failure to recognize efficacious treatments: a history of salicylate therapy in rheumatoid arthritis. Perspect Biol Med 1981; 25:78–92.

57. Goodwin JS, Goodwin JM. The tomato effect: rejection of highly efficacious therapies. JAMA 1984; 251:2387–2390.

58. Bourne GH. Vitamin C and immunity. Br J Nutr 1949; 2:341–347.

59. Thomas WR, Holt PG. Vitamin C and immunity. Clin Exp Immunol 1978; 32:370–379.

59a. Gross RL, Newberne PM. Role of nutrition in immunologic function: vitamin C. Physiol Rev 1980; 60:255–260.

60. Beisel WR. Single nutrients and immunity: vitamin C. Am J Clin Nutr 1982; 35(suppl):423–428.

61. Leibovitz B, Siegel BV. Ascorbic acid and the immune system. Adv Exp Med Biol 1981; 135:1–25.

62. Weiss SJ. Tissue destruction by neutrophils. N Engl J Med 1989; 320:365–376.

63. Smith JA. Neutrophils, host defence, and inflammation. J Leukocyte Biol 1994; 56:672–686.

64. Oda T, Akaike T, Hamamoto T, et al. Oxygen radicals in influenza-induced pathogenesis and treatment with pyran polymer-conjugated SOD. Science 1989; 244:974–976.

65. Akaike T, Ando M, Oda T, et al. Dependence on O_2^- generation by xanthine oxidase of pathogenesis of influenza virus infection in mice. J Clin Invest 1990; 85:739–745.

66. Christen S, Peterhans E, Stocker R. Antioxidant activities of some tryptophan metabolites. Proc Natl Acad Sci USA 1990; 87:2506–2510.

67. Maeda H, Akaike T. Oxygen free radicals as pathogenic molecules in viral diseases. Proc Soc Exp Biol Med 1991; 198:721–727.

68. Hennet T, Peterhans E, Stocker R. Alterations in antioxidant defenses in lung and liver of mice infected with influenza A virus. J Gen Virol 1992; 73:39–46.

69. Buffinton GD, Christen S, Peterhans E, Stocker R. Oxidative stress in lungs of mice infected with influenza A virus. Free Radical Res Comm 1992; 16:99–110.

70. Hemilä H, Roberts P, Wikström M. Activated polymorphonuclear leucocytes consume vitamin C. FEBS Lett 1984; 178:25–30.

71. Theron A, Anderson R. Investigation of the protective effect of ascorbate on the phagocyte-mediated oxidative inactivation of human alpha-1-protease inhibitor. Am Rev Respir Dis 1985; 132:1049–1054.

72. Anderson R, Lukey PT. A biological role for ascorbate in the selective neutralization of extracellular phagocyte-derived oxidants. Ann NY Acad Sci 1987; 498:229–247.

73. Halliwell B, Wasil M, Grootveld M. Biologically significant scavenging of the myelo-peroxidase-derived oxidant hypochlorous acid by ascorbic acid. FEBS Lett 1987; 213:15–18.

74. Frei B, Stocker R, Ames BN. Antioxidant defenses and lipid peroxidation in human blood plasma. Proc Natl Acad Sci USA 1988; 85:9748–9752.

75. Thomas EL, Learn DB, Jefferson MM, Weatherred W. Superoxide-dependent oxidation of extracellular reducing agents by isolated neutrophils. J Biol Chem 1988; 263:2178–2186.

76. Hu ML, Louie S, Cross CE, et al. Antioxidant protection against hypochlorous acid in human plasma. J Lab Clin Med 1993; 121:257–262.

77. Crandon JH, Lund CC, Dill DB. Experimental human scurvy. N Engl J Med 1940; 223:353–369.

78. Vitamin C requirement of human adults. Lancet 1948; 254:853–858.

79. DeChatelet LR, McCall CE, Cooper MR, Shirley PS. Ascorbic acid levels in phagocytic cells. Proc Soc Exp Biol Med 1974; 145:1170–1173.

80. Evans RM, Currie L, Campbell A. The distribution of ascorbic acid between various cellular components of blood, in normal individuals, and its relation to the plasma concentration. Br J Nutr 1982; 47:473–482.

81. Washko P, Rotrosen D, Levine M. Ascorbic acid transport and accumulation in human neutrophils. J Biol Chem 1989; 264:18996–19002.

82. Bergsten P, Amitai G, Kehrl J, et al. Millimolar concentrations of ascorbic acid in purified human mononuclear leukocytes. J Biol Chem 1990; 265:2584–2587.

83. Washko PW, Wang Y, Levine M. Ascorbic acid recycling in human neutrophils. J Biol Chem 1993; 268:15531–15535.

84. Winterbourn CC, Vissers MCM. Changes in ascorbate levels on stimulation of human neutrophils. Biochim Biophys Acta 1983; 763:175–179.

85. Stankova L, Gerhardt HB, Nagel L, Bigley RH. Ascorbate and phagocyte function. Infect Immun 1975; 12:252–256.

86. Hume R, Weyers E. Changes in leucocyte ascorbic acid during the common cold. Scott Med J 1973; 18:3–7.

87. Cottingham E, Mills CA. Influence of environmental temperature and vitamin-deficiency upon phagocytic functions. J Immunol 1943; 47:493–502.

88. Nungester WJ, Ames AM. The relationship between ascorbic acid and phagocytic activity. J Infect Dis 1948; 83:50–54.

89. Merchant DJ. The effect of serum on the activity of the polymorphonuclear leukocytes of the guinea pig. J Infect Dis 1950; 87:275–284.

90. Chatterjee GC, Majumder PK, Banerjee SK, et al. Relationships of protein and mineral intake to L-ascorbic acid metabolism, including considerations of some directly related hormones. Ann NY Acad Sci 1975; 258:382–400.

91. Shilotri PG. Glycolytic, hexose monophosphate shunt and bactericidal activities of leukocytes in ascorbic acid deficient guinea pigs. J Nutr 1977; 107:1507–1512.

92. Ganguly R, Waldman RH. Macrophage functions in aging: effects of vitamin C deficiency. Allerg Immunol 1985; 31:37–43.

93. Goldschmidt MC, Masin WJ, Brown LR, Wyde PR. The effect of ascorbic acid deficiency on leukocyte phagocytosis and killing of Actinomyces viscosus. Int J Vitam Nutr Res 1988; 58:326–334.

94. Alvares O, Altman LC, Springmeyer S, et al. The effect of subclinical ascorbate deficiency on periodontal health in nonhuman primates. J Periodontal Res 1981; 16:628–636.

95. Werkman CH, Nelson VE, Fulmer EI. Immunologic significance of vitamins. J Infect Dis 1924; 34:447–453.

96. Ganguly R, Durieux MF, Waldman RH. Macrophage function in vitamin C-deficient guinea pigs. Am J Clin Nutr 1976; 29:762–765.

97. Goetzl EJ, Wasserman SI, Gigli I, Austen KF. Enhancement of random migration and chemotactic response of human leukocytes by ascorbic acid. J Clin Invest 1974; 53:813–818.

98. Sandler JA, Gallin JI, Vaughan M. Effects of serotonin, carbamylcholine, and ascorbic acid on leukocyte cyclic GMP and chemotaxis. J Cell Biol 1975; 67:480–484.

99. Anderson R, Theron A. Effects of ascorbate on leucocytes. I. S Afr Med J 1979; 56:394–400.

100. Boxer LA, Vanderbilt B, Bonsib S, et al. Enhancement of chemotactic response and microtubule assembly in human leukocytes by ascorbic acid. J Cell Physiol 1979; 100:119–126.

101. Dallegri F, Lanzi G, Patrone F. Effects of ascorbic acid on neutrophil locomotion. Int Arch Allergy Appl Immunol 1980; 61:40–45.

102. Gatner EMS, Anderson R. An in vitro assessment of cellular and humoral immune function in pulmonary tuberculosis. Clin Exp Immunol 1980; 40:327–336.

103. Patrone F, Dallegri F, Lanzi G, Sacchetti C. Prevention of neutrophil chemotactic deactivation by ascorbic acid. Br J Exp Pathol 1980; 61:486–489.

104. Anderson R, Jones PT. Increased leucoattractant binding and reversible inhibition of neutrophil motility mediated by the peroxidase/H_2O_2/halide system. Clin Exp Immunol 1982; 47:487–496.

105. Pryzwansky KB, Schliwa M, Boxer LA. Microtubule organization of unstimulated and stimulated adherent human neutrophils in Chediak-Higashi syndrome. Blood 1985; 66:1398–1403.

106. Johnston CS, Huang S. Effect of ascorbic acid nutriture on blood histamine and neutrophil chemotaxis in guinea pigs. J Nutr 1991; 121:126–130.

107. Nath J, Gallin JI. Effect of vitamin C on tubulin tyrosinolation in polymorphonuclear leukocytes. Ann NY Acad Sci 1987; 498:216–228.

108. Baehner RL, Boxer LA, Allen JM, Davis J. Autooxidation as a basis for altered function by polymorphonuclear leukocytes. Blood 1977; 50:327–335.

109. Nelson RD, McCormack RT, Fiegel VD, et al. Chemotactic deactivation of human neutrophils. Infect Immun 1979; 23:282–286.

110. Stendahl O, Coble BI, Dahlgren C, et al. Myeloperoxidase modulates the phagocytic activity of polymorphonuclear neutrophil leukocytes. J Clin Invest 1984; 73:366–373.

111. Chretien JH, Garagusi VF. Correction of corticosteroid-induced defects of polymorphonuclear neutrophil function by ascorbic acid. J Reticuloendothel Soc 1973; 14:280–286.

112. Olson GE, Polk HC. In vitro effect of ascorbic acid on corticosteroid-caused neutrophil dysfunction. J Surgical Res 1977; 22:109–112.

113. Roth JA, Kaeberle ML. In vivo effect of ascorbic acid on neutrophil function in healthy and dexamethasone-treated cattle. Am J Vet Res 1985; 46:2434–2436.

114. Boxer LA, Watanabe AM, Rister M, et al. Correction of leukocyte function in Chediak-Higashi syndrome by ascorbate. N Engl J Med 1976; 295:1041–1045.

115. Foster CS, Goetzl EJ. Ascorbate therapy in impaired neutrophil and monocyte chemotaxis. Arch Ophthalmol 1978; 96:2069–2072.

116. Boxer LA, Albertini DF, Baehner RL, Oliver JM. Impaired microtubule assembly and polymorphonuclear leucocyte function in the Chediak-Higashi syndrome correctable by ascorbic acid. Br J Haematol 1979; 43:207–213.

117. Anderson R, Theron A. Effects of ascorbate on leucocytes. III. S Afr Med J 1979; 56:429–433.

118. Anderson R, Dittrich OC. Effects of ascorbate on leucocytes. IV. S Afr Med J 1979; 56: 476–480.

119. Friedenberg WR, Marx JJ, Hansen RL, Haselby RC. Hyperimmunoglobulin E syndrome. Clin Immunol Immunopathol 1979; 12:132–142.

120. Anderson R, Hay I, Wyk H, et al. The effect of ascorbate on cellular humoral immunity in asthmatic children. S Afr Med J 1980; 58:974–977.

121. Anderson R. Assessment of oral ascorbate in three children with chronic granulomatous disease and defective neutrophil motility over a 2-year period. Clin Exp Immunol 1981; 43:180–188.

122. Weening RS, Schoorel EP, Roos D, et al. Effect of ascorbate on abnormal neutrophil, platelet, and lymphocyte function in a patient with the Chediak-Higashi syndrome. Blood 1981; 57:856–865.

123. Rebora A, Dallegri F, Patrone F. Neutrophil dysfunction and repeated infections. Br J Dermatol 1980; 102:49–56.

124. Anderson R. Ascorbate-mediated stimulation of neutrophil motility and lymphocyte transformation by inhibition of the peroxide/H_2O_2/halide system in vitro and in vivo. Am J Clin Nutr 1981; 34:1906–1911.

125. Saitoh H, Komiyama A, Norose N, et al. Development of the accelerated phase during ascorbic acid therapy in Chediak-Higashi syndrome and efficacy of colchicine on its management. Br J Haematol 1981; 48:79–84.

126. Corberand J, Nguyen F, Fraysse B, Enjalbert L. Malignant external otitis and polymorphonuclear leukocyte migration impairment: improvement with ascorbic acid. Arch Otolaryngol 1982; 108:122–124.

127. Anderson R, Hay I, Wyk HA, Theron A. Ascorbic acid in bronchial asthma. S Afr Med J 1983; 63:649–652.

128. Patrone F, Dallegri F, Bonvini E, et al. Disorders of neutrophil function in children with recurrent pyogenic infections. Med Microbiol Immunol 1982; 171:113–122.

129. Thorner RE, Barker CF, MacGregor RR. Improvement of granulocyte adherence and in vivo granulocyte delivery by ascorbic acid in renal transplant patients. Transplantation 1983; 35:432–436.

130. Yegin O, Sanal O, Yeralan O, et al. Defective lymphocyte locomotion in Chediak-Higashi syndrome. Am J Dis Child 1983; 137:771–773.

131. Boura P, Tsapas G, Papadopoulou A, et al. Monocyte locomotion in anergic chronic brucellosis patients. Immunopharmacol Immunotoxicol 1989; 11:119–129.

132. Vohra K, Khan AJ, Telang V, et al. Improvement of neutrophil migration by systemic vitamin C in neonates. J Perinatol 1990; 10:134–136.

133. Johnston CS, Martin LJ, Cai X. Antihistamine effect of supplemental ascorbic acid and neutrophil chemotaxis. J Am Coll Nutr 1992; 11:172–176.

133a. Levy R, Shriker O, Porath A, et al. Vitamin C for the treatment of recurrent furunculosis in patients with impaired neutrophil functions. J Infect Dis 1996; 173:1502–1505.

134. Maderazo EG, Woronick CL, Hickingbotham N, et al. A randomized trial of replacement antioxidant vitamin therapy for neutrophil locomotory dysfunction in blunt trauma. J Trauma 1991; 31:1142–1150.

135. Gallin JI, Elin RJ, Hubert RT, et al. Efficacy of ascorbic acid in Chediak-Higashi syndrome. Blood 1979; 53:226–234.

136. Shilotri PG, Bhat KS. Effect of mega doses of vitamin C on bactericidal activity of leukocytes. Am J Clin Nutr 1977; 30:1077–1081.

137. Delafuente JC, Panush RS. Modulation of certain immunological responses by vitamin C. II. Int J Vitam Nutr Res 1980; 50:44–51.

138. Panush RS, Delafuente JC, Katz P, Johnson J. Modulation of certain immunologic responses by vitamin C. III. Int J Vitam Nutr Res 1982; (suppl 23):35–47.

139. Manzella JP, Roberts NJ. Human macrophage and lymphocyte responses to mitogen stimulation after exposure to influenza virus, ascorbic acid, and hyperthermia. J Immunol 1979; 123:1940–1944.

140. Joffe MI, Sukha NR, Rabson AR. Lymphocyte subsets in measles: depressed helper/inducer subpopulation reversed by in vitro treatment with levamisole and ascorbic acid. J Clin Invest 1983; 72:971–980.

141. Delafuente JC, Prendergast JM, Modigh A. Immunologic modulation by vitamin C in the elderly. Int J Immunopharmacol 1986; 8:205–211.

142. Oh C, Nakano K. Reversal by ascorbic acid of suppression by endogenous histamine of rat lymphocyte blastogenesis. J Nutr 1988; 118:639–644.

143. Smit MJ, Anderson R. Inhibition of mitogen-activated proliferation of human lymphocytes by hypochlorous acid in vitro. Agents Actions 1990; 30:338–343.

144. Standefer JC, Vanderjagt D, Anderson RE, et al. Protective effect of ascorbate on radiation-sensitive thymidine uptake by lymphocytes. Ann NY Acad Sci 1987; 498:519–521.

145. Siegel BV, Morton JI. Vitamin C and the immune response. Experientia 1977; 33:393–395.

146. Anthony LE, Kurahara CG, Taylor KB. Cell-mediated cytotoxicity and humoral immune response in ascorbic acid-deficient guinea pigs. Am J Clin Nutr 1979; 32:1691–1698.

147. Fraser RC, Pavlovic S, Kurahara CG, et al. The effect of variations in vitamin C intake on the cellular immune response of guinea pigs. Am J Clin Nutr 1980; 33:839–847.

148. Kristensen B, Thomsen PD, Palludan B, Wegger I. Mitogen stimulation of lymphocytes in pigs with hereditary vitamin C deficiency. Acta Vet Scand 1986; 27:486–496.

149. Yonemoto RH. Vitamin C and immune responses in normal controls and cancer patients. Int J Vitam Nutr Res 1979; (suppl 19):143–154.

150. Anderson R, Oosthuizen R, Maritz R, et al. The effects of increasing weekly doses of ascorbate on certain cellular and humoral immune functions in normal volunteers. Am J Clin Nutr 1980; 33:71–76.

151. Kennes B, Dumont I, Brohee D, et al. Effect of vitamin C supplements on cell-mediated immunity in old people. Gerontology 1983; 29:305–310.

152. O'Brien BC, McMurray DN. Human plasma lipid and immunologic responses to eggs and ascorbic acid. Nutr Res 1988; 8:353–366.

153. Penn ND, Purkins L, Kelleher J, et al. The effect of dietary supplementation with vitamins A, C and E on cell-mediated immune function in elderly long-stay patients. Age Aging 1991; 20:169–174.

154. Kay NE, Holloway DE, Hutton SW, et al. Human T-cell function in experimental ascorbic acid deficiency and spontaneous scurvy. Am J Clin Nutr 1982; 36:127–130.

155. Goodwin JS, Garry PJ. Relationship between megadose vitamin supplementation and immunological function in a healthy elderly population. Clin Exp Immunol 1983; 51:647–653.

156. Heidrick ML, Albright JW, Makinodan T. Restoration of impaired immune functions in aging animals. Mech Ageing Dev 1980; 13:367–378.

157. Furukawa T, Meydani SN, Blumberg JB. Reversal of age-associated decline in immune responsiveness by dietary glutathione supplementation in mice. Mech Ageing Dev 1987; 38:107–117.

158. Bendich A, Gabriel E, Machlin LJ. Dietary vitamin E requirement for optimum immune responses in the rat. J Nutr 1986; 116:675–681.

159. Meydani SN, Barklund MP, Liu S, et al. Vitamin E supplementation enhances cell-mediated immunity in healthy elderly subjects. Am J Clin Nutr 1990; 52:557–563.

160. Metzger Z, Hoffeld JT, Oppenheim JJ. Macrophage-mediated suppression. J Immunol 1980; 124:983–988.

161. Zoschke DC, Messner RP. Suppression of human lymphocyte mitogenesis mediated by phagocyte-released reactive oxygen species. Clin Immunol Immunopathol 1984; 32:29–40.

162. El-Hag A, Clark RA. Immunosuppression by activated human neutrophils. J Immunol 1987; 139:2406–2413.

163. Schwerdt PR, Schwerdt CE. Effect of ascorbic acid on rhinovirus replication in WI-38 cells. Proc Soc Exp Biol Med 1975; 148:1237–1243.

164. Siegel BV. Enhancement of interferon production by poly(rI)·poly(rC) in mouse cell cultures by ascorbic acid. Nature 1975; 254:531–532.

165. Dahl H, Degre M. The effect of ascorbic acid on production of human interferon and the antiviral activity in vitro. Acta Pathol Microbiol Scand 1976; 84B:280–284.

166. Karpinska T, Kawecki Z, Kandefer-Szerszen M. The influence of ultraviolet irradiation,

L-ascorbic acid and calcium chloride on the induction of interferon in human embryo fibro-blasts. Arch Immunol Ther Exp 1982; 30:33–37.

167. Siegel BV. Enhanced interferon response to murine leukemia virus by ascorbic acid. Infect Immun 1974; 10:409–410.

168. Geber WF, Lefkowitz SS, Hung CY. Effect of ascorbic acid, sodium salicylate, and caffeine on the serum interferon level in response to viral infection. Pharmacology 1975; 13:228–233.

169. Versteeg J. Effects of ascorbic acid on virus replication, and production and activity of interferon in vitro. Proc Koninkl Nederl Akad Wetensch (Biol Med) 1969; 72:207–212.

170. Prinz W, Bortz R, Bregin B, Hersch M. The effect of ascorbic acid supplementation on some parameters of the human immunological defence system. Int J Vitam Nutr Res 1977; 47: 248–257.

171. Bates CJ, Levene CI, Oldroyd RG, Lachmann PJ. Complement component C1q is insensitive to acute vitamin C deficiency in guinea pigs. Biochim Biophys Acta 1978; 540:423–430.

172. Feigen GA, Smith BH, Dix CE, et al. Enhancement of antibody production and protection against systemic anaphylaxis by large doses of vitamin C. Res Commun Chem Pathol Pharmacol 1982; 38:313–333.

173. Johnston CS, Kolb WP, Haskell BE. The effect of vitamin C nutriture on complement component C1q concentrations in guinea pig plasma. J Nutr 1987; 117:764–768.

174. Johnston CS. Complement component C1q unaltered by ascorbate supplementation in healthy men and women. J Nutr Biochem 1991; 2:499–501.

175. Tanaka M, Muto N, Gohda E, Yamamoto I. Enhancement by ascorbic acid 2-glucoside or repeated additions of ascorbate of mitogen-induced IgM and IgG productions by human peripheral blood lymphocytes. Jpn J Pharmacol 1994; 66:451–456.

176. Dowd PS, Kelleher J, Walker BE, Guillou PJ. Nutrition and cellular immunity in hospital patients. Br J Nutr 1986; 55:515–527.

177. Vojdani A, Ghoneum M. In vivo effect of ascorbic acid on enhancement of human natural killer cell activity. Nutr Res 1993; 13:753–764.

178. Siegel BV, Morton JI. Vitamin C and immunity. Int J Vitam Nutr Res 1983; 53:179–183.

179. Atherton JG, Kratzing CC, Fisher A. The effect of ascorbic acid on infection of chick-embryo ciliated tracheal organ cultures by coronavirus. Arch Virol 1978; 56:195–199.

180. Bissell MJ, Hatie C, Farson DA, et al. Ascorbic acid inhibits replication and infectivity of avian RNA tumor virus. Proc Natl Acad Sci USA 1980; 77:2711–2715.

181. Morigaki T, Ito Y. Intervening effect of L-ascorbic acid on Epstein-Barr virus activation in human lymphoblastoid cells and its comparison with the effect of retinoic acid. Cancer Lett 1982; 15:255–259.

182. Harakeh S, Jariwalla RJ, Pauling L. Suppression of human immunodeficiency virus replication by ascorbate in chronically and acutely infected cells. Proc Natl Acad Sci USA 1990; 87:7245–7249.

183. Harakeh S, Jariwalla RJ. Comparative study of the anti-HIV activities of ascorbate and thiol-containing reducing agents in chronically HIV-infected cells. Am J Clin Nutr 1991; 54:1231S–1235S.

184. Schwartz RI. Ascorbate stabilizes the differentiated state and reduces the ability of Rous sarcoma virus to replicate and to uniformly transform cell cultures. Am J Clin Nutr 1991; 54:1247S–1251S.

185. Walker GH, Bynoe ML, Tyrrell DAJ. Trial of ascorbic acid in prevention of colds. Br Med J 1967; 1:603–606.

186. Klein M. The mechanism of the virucidal action of ascorbic acid. Science 1945; 101: 587–589.

187. Miller TE. Killing and lysis of gram-negative bacteria through the synergistic effect of hydrogen peroxide, ascorbic acid, and lysozyme. J Bacteriol 1969; 98:949–955.

188. Drath DB, Karnovsky ML. Bactericidal activity of metal-mediated peroxide-ascorbate systems. Infect Immun 1974; 10:1077–1083.

189. Samuni A, Aranovitch J, Godinger D, et al. On the cytotoxicity of vitamin C and metal ions. Eur J Biochem 1983; 137:119–124.

190. Wang Y, Ness BV. Site-specific cleavage of supercoiled DNA by ascorbate/Cu(II). Nucleic Acids Res 1989; 17:6915–6926.

191. Halliwell B. Free radicals, reactive oxygen species and human disease. Br J Exp Pathol 1989; 70:737–757.

192. Famularo G, Simone CD. A new era for carnitine? Immunol Today 1995; 16:211–213.

193. Williams RJ, Deason G. Individuality in vitamin C needs. Proc Natl Acad Sci USA 1967; 57:1638–1641.

194. Yew MS. Recommended daily allowances for vitamin C. Proc Natl Acad Sci USA 1973; 70:969–972.

195. Yew MS. Biological variation in ascorbic acid needs. Ann NY Acad Sci 1975; 258:451–457.

196. Chatterjee IB. Evolution and the biosynthesis of ascorbic acid. Science 1973; 182:1271–1272.

197. Sato P, Udenfriend S. Studies on ascorbic acid related to the genetic basis of scurvy. Vitam Horm 1978; 36:33–52.

198. Höjer JA. Studies in scurvy: scurvy and tuberculosis. Acta Paediatr 1924; 3(suppl):140–171.

199. McConkey M, Smith DT. The relation of vitamin C deficiency to intestinal tuberculosis in the guinea pig. J Exp Med 1933; 58:503–517.

200. DeSavitsch E, Steward JD, Hanson L, Walsh EN. The influence of orange juice on experimental tuberculosis in guinea pigs. Natl Tuberc Assoc Transact 1934; 30:130–135.

201. Greene MR, Steiner M, Kramer B. The role of chronic vitamin C deficiency in the pathogenesis of tuberculosis in the guinea pigs. Am Rev Tuberc 1936; 33:585–624.

202. Steinbach MM, Klein SJ. Vitamin C in experimental tuberculosis. Am Rev Tuberc 1941; 43:403–414.

203. Russell WO, Read JA, Rouse ET. Morphologic and histochemical study of the effect of scurvy on tuberculosis in guinea pigs. Arch Pathol 1944; 38:31–39.

204. Boyden SV, Andersen ME. Diet in experimental tuberculosis in the guinea pig. Acta Pathol Microbiol Scand 1955; 37:201–204.

205. Boyden SV, Andersen ME. Diet and experimental tuberculosis in the guinea pig. Acta Pathol Microbiol Scand 1956; 39:107–116.

206. Findlay GM. The relation of vitamin C to bacterial infection. J Pathol Bacteriol 1923; 26:1–19.

207. Grant AH. Effect of the calcium, vitamin C, vitamin D ratio in diet on the permeability of intestinal wall to bacteria. J Infect Dis 1926; 39:502–508.

208. Rinehart JF, Mettier SR. The heart valves and muscle in experimental scurvy with superimposed infection. Am J Pathol 1934; 10:61–79.

209. Rinehart JF, Connor CL, Mettier SR. Further observations on pathologic similarities between experimental scurvy combined with infection, and rheumatic fever. J Exp Med 1934; 59:97–114.

210. McCullough NB. Vitamin C and resistance of the guinea pig to infection with Bacterium necrophorum. J Infect Dis 1938; 63:34–53.

211. Witt WM, Hubbard GB, Fanton JW. Streptococcus pneumoniae arthritis and osteomyelitis with vitamin C deficiency in guinea pigs. Lab Anim Sci 1988; 38:192–195.

212. Zinsser H, Castaneda MR, Seastone CV. Studies on typhus fever. VI. J Exp Med 1931; 53:333–338.

213. Sadun EH, Bradin JL, Faust EC. Effect of ascorbic acid deficiency on the resistance of guinea pigs to infection with Endamoeba histolytica of human origin. Am J Trop Med 1951; 31:426–437.

214. Rogers TJ, Adams-Burton K, Mallon M, et al. Dietary ascorbic acid and resistance to experimental renal candidiasis. J Nutr 1983; 113:178–183.

215. Banic S. Prevention of rabies by vitamin C. Nature 1975; 258:153–154.

216. Banic S. Prophylactic effect of vitamin C on the incidence of rabies in guinea pigs inoculated with fixed rabies virus. Int J Vitam Nutr Res 1977; (suppl 16):235–244.

217. Banic S. The effect of vitamin C on the efficiency of immunization with cell culture rabies vaccine in guinea-pigs. Int J Vitam Nutr Res 1979; (suppl 19):35–39.

218. Heise FH, Martin GJ. Supervitaminosis C in tuberculosis. Proc Soc Exp Biol Med 1936; 35:337–338.

219. Heise FH, Steenken W. Vitamin C and immunity in tuberculosis of guinea pigs. Am Rev Tuberc 1939; 39:794–795.

220. Peck MD, Alexander JW. Survival in septic guinea pigs is influenced by vitamin E, but not by vitamin C in enteral diets. J Parent Enter Nutr 1991; 15:433–436.

221. Birkhaug KE. The role of vitamin C in the pathogenesis of tuberculosis in the guinea pig. III. Acta Tuberc Scand 1938; 12:359–372.

222. Birkhaug KE. The role of vitamin C in the pathogenesis of tuberculosis in the guinea pig. V. Acta Tuberc Scand 1939; 13:52–66.

223. Birkhaug KE. The role of vitamin C in the pathogenesis of tuberculosis in the guinea pig. I and II. Acta Tuberc Scand 1938; 12:89–104.

224. Harris LJ, Passmore R, Oxon BM, et al. Vitamin C and infection. Lancet 1937; 2:183–186.

225. Jungeblut CW. Further observations on vitamin C therapy in experimental poliomyelitis. J Exp Med 1937; 66:459–477.

226. Jungeblut CW. A further contribution to vitamin C therapy in experimental poliomyelitis. J Exp Med 1939; 70:315–333.

227. Sabin AB. Vitamin C in relation to experimental poliomyelitis. J Exp Med 1939; 69:507–515.

228. Kelly FC. Bacteriology of artifically produced necrotic lesions in the oropharynx of the monkey. J Infect Dis 1944; 74:93–108.

229. Goldschmidt MC. Reduced bactericidal activity in neutrophils from scorbutic animals and the effect of ascorbic acid on these target bacteria in vivo and in vitro. Am J Clin Nutr 1991; 54:1214S–1220S.

230. Murphy BL, Krushak DH, Maynard JE, Bradley DW. Ascorbic acid and its effects on parainfluenza type III virus infection in cotton-topped marmosets. Lab Anim Sci 1974; 24: 229–232.

231. McKee RW, Geiman QM. Studies on malarial parasites. V. Proc Soc Exp Biol Med 1946; 63:313–315.

232. Li Y, Lovell RT. Elevated levels of dietary ascorbic acid increase immune response in channel catfish. J Nutr 1985; 115:123–131.

233. Wahli T, Meier W, Pfister K. Ascorbic acid induced immune-mediated decrease in mortality in Ichthyophthirius mulfiliis infected rainbow-trout. Acta Trop 1986; 43:287–289.

234. Waagbo R, Sandnes K, Glette J, et al. Dietary vitamin B_6 and C. Ann NY Acad Sci 1992; 669:379–382.

235. Rawal BD, McKay G, Blackhall MI. Inhibition of Pseudomonas aeruginosa by ascorbic acid acting singly and in combination with antimicrobials. Med J Aust 1974; 1:169–174.

236. Bourke GC, Coleman RM, Rencricca NJ. Effect of ascorbic acid on host resistance in virulent rodent malaria (abstr). Clin Res 1980; 28:642A.

237. Hastings RC, Richard V, Christy SA, Morales MJ. Activity of ascorbic acid in inhibiting the multiplication of M. leprae in the mouse foot pad. Int J Lepr 1976; 44:427–440.

238. Esposito AL. Ascorbate modulates antibacterial mechanisms in experimental pneumococcal pneumonia. Am Rev Respir Dis 1986; 133:643–647.

239. Nyden SJ. Changes in ascorbic acid metabolism of the rat during infection with Trypanosoma hippicum. Proc Soc Exp Biol Med 1948; 69:206–210.

240. Edwards WC. Ascorbic acid for treatment of feline rhinotracheitis. Vet Med Small Anim Clin 1968; 63:696–698.

241. Hill CH, Garren HW. The effect of high levels of vitamins on the resistance of chicks to fowl typhoid. Ann NY Acad Sci 1955; 63:186–194.

242. Gross WB. Effect of environmental stress on the responses of ascorbic acid treated chickens to E. coli challenge infection. Avian Dis 1988; 32:432–436.

243. Davelaar FG, Bos J. Ascorbic acid and infectious bronchitis infections in broilers. Avian Pathol 1992; 21:581–589.

244. Morishige F, Murata A. Vitamin C for prophylaxis of viral hepatitis B in transfused patients. J Int Acad Prev Med 1978; 5(1):54–58.

245. Banic S, Kosak M. Prevention of post-transfusion hepatitis by vitamin C. Int J Vitam Nutr Res 1979; (suppl 19):41–44.

246. Knodell RG, Tate MA, Akl BF, Wilson JW. Vitamin C prophylaxis for posttransfusion hepatitis: lack of effect in a controlled trial. Am J Clin Nutr 1981; 34:20–23.

247. Pauling L. Vitamin C prophylaxis for posttransfusion hepatitis. Am J Clin Nutr 1981; 34:1978–1979.

248. Sutnick MR. Vitamin C prophylaxis for posttransfusion hepatitis. Am J Clin Nutr 1981; 34:1980–1981.

249. Glazebrook AJ, Thomson S. The administration of vitamin C in a large institution and its effects on general health and resistance to infection. J Hyg 1942; 42:1–19.

249a. Kimbarowski JA, Mokrow NJ. Farbige Ausfällungsreaktion des Harns nach Kimbarowski, als index der Wirkung von Ascorbinsäure bei Behandlung der Virusgrippe. Dtsch Gesundheitsw 1967; 22:2413–2418.

250. Downes J. An experiment in the control of tuberculosis among Negroes. Milbank Mem Fund Q 1950; 28:127–159.

251. Asfora J. Vitamin C in high doses in the treatment of the common cold. Int J Vitam Nutr Res 1977; (suppl 16):219–234.

252. Schultz MP. Studies of ascorbic acid and rheumatic fever. II. J Clin Invest 1936; 15:385–391.

253. Getz HR, Long ER, Henderson HJ. A study of the relation of nutrition to the development of tuberculosis. Am Rev Tuberc 1951; 64:381–393.

254. Melnick SL, Alvarez JO, Navia JM, et al. A case-control study of plasma ascorbate and acute necrotizing ulcerative gingivitis. J Dent Res 1988; 67:855–860.

255. Lund CC, Crandon JH. Human experimental scurvy and the relation of vitamin C deficiency to postoperative pneumonia and to wound healing. JAMA 1941; 116:663–668.

256. Kaiser AD, Slavin B. The incidence of hemolytic streptococci in the tonsils of children as related to the vitamin C content of tonsils and blood. J Pediatr 1938; 13:322–333.

257. Freiman JA, Chalmers TC, Smith H, Kuebler RR. The importance of beta, the type II error and sample size in the design and interpretation of the randomized control trial. N Engl J Med 1978; 299:690–694.

258. Bumbalo TS, Jetter WW. Vitamin C in tuberculosis. J Pediatr 1938; 13:334–340.

259. Banerjee S, Sen PB, Guha BC. Urinary excretion of combined ascorbic acid in pulmonary tuberculosis. Nature 1940; 145:706–707.

260. Pijoan M, Sedlacek B. Ascorbic acid in tuberculous Navajo indians. Am Rev Tuberc 1943; 48:342–346.

261. Bumbalo TS. Urinary output of vitamin C of normal and of sick children. Am J Dis Child 1938; 55:1212–1220.

262. Getz HR, Koerner TA. Vitamin nutrition in tuberculosis. Am Rev Tuberc 1943; 47:274–283.

263. Heise FH, Martin GJ. Ascorbic acid metabolism in tuberculosis. Proc Soc Exp Biol Med 1936; 34:642–644.

264. Martin GJ, Heise FH. Vitamin C nutrition in pulmonary tuberculosis. Am J Dig Dis Nutr 1937; 4:368–374.

265. Jetter WW, Bumbalo TS. The urinary output of vitamin C in active tuberculosis in children. Am J Med Sci 1938; 195:362–366.

266. Chang CE, Lan TH. Vitamin C in tuberculosis. Am Rev Tuberc 1940; 41:494–506.

267. Abbasy MA, Hill NG, Harris LJ. Vitamin C and juvenile rheumatism, with some observations on the vitamin C reserves in surgical tuberculosis. Lancet 1936; 2:1413–1417.

268. Abbasy MA, Harris LJ, Ellman P. Vitamin C and infection. Excretion of vitamin C in pulmonary tuberculosis and in rheumatoid arthritis. Lancet 1937; 2:181–183.

269. Getz HR, Koerner TA. Vitamin A and ascorbic acid in pulmonary tuberculosis. Am J Med Sci 1941; 202:831–847.

270. Sweany HC, Clancy CL, Radford MH, Hunter V. The body economy of vitamin C in health and disease. JAMA 1941; 116:469–474.

271. Chakrabarti B, Banerjee S. Dehydroascorbic acid level in blood of patients suffering from various infectious diseases. Proc Soc Exp Biol Med 1955; 88:581–583.

272. Awotedu AA, Sofowora EO, Ette SI. Ascorbic acid deficiency in pulmonary tuberculosis. East Afr Med J 1984; 61:283–287.

273. Harde E, Rothstein IA, Ratish HD. Urinary excretion of vitamin C in pneumonia. Proc Soc Exp Biol Med 1935; 32:1088–1090.

274. Bullowa JGM, Rothstein IA, Ratisch HD, Harde E. Cevitamic acid excretion in pneumonias and some other pathological conditions. Proc Soc Exp Biol Med 1936; 34:1–7.

275. Rinehart JF, Greenberg LD, Christie AU. Reduced ascorbic acid content of blood plasma in rheumatic fever. Proc Soc Exp Biol Med 1936; 35:350–353.

276. Faulkner JM, Taylor FHL. Vitamin C and infection. Ann Intern Med 1937; 10:1867–1873.

277. Rinehart JF, Greenberg LD, Olney M, Choy F. Metabolism of vitamin C in rheumatic fever. Arch Intern Med 1938; 61:552–561.

278. Abt AF, Hardy LM, Farmer CJ, Maaske JD. Relation of vitamin C to scarlet fever, rheumatic infections and diphtheria in children. Am J Dis Child 1942; 64:426–442.

279. Banerjee S, Belavady B. Dehydroascorbic acid level of blood in health and in typhoid fever. Lancet 1953; 2:912–913.

280. Abbasy MA, Harris LJ, Hill NG. Vitamin C and infection: excretion of vitamin C in osteomyelitis. Lancet 1937; 2:177–180.

281. Sayed SM, Roy RB, Acharya PT. Leucocyte ascorbic acid and wound infection. J Indian Med Assoc 1975; 64:120–123.

282. Sinha SN, Gupta SC, Bajaj AK, et al. A study of blood ascorbic acid in leprosy. Int J Lepr 1984; 52:159–162.

283. Abbasy MA, Harris LJ, Ray SN, Marrack JR. Diagnosis of vitamin C subnutrition by urine analysis. Lancet 1935; 2:1399–1405.

284. Wilson CWM. Vitamin C metabolism and the common cold. Eur J Clin Pharmacol 1974; 7:421–428.

285. Davies JEW, Hughes RE, Jones E, et al. Metabolism of ascorbic acid in subjects infected with common cold viruses. Biochem Med 1979; 21:78–85.

286. Terezhalmy GT, Botomley WK, Pelleu GB. The use of water-soluble bioflavonoid-ascorbic acid complex in the treatment of recurrent herpes labialis. Oral Surg 1978; 45:56–62.

286a. Hunt C, Chakravorty NK, Annan G, et al. The clinical effects of vitamin C supplementation in elderly hospitalised patients with acute respiratory infections. Int J Vitam Nutr Res 1994; 64:212–219.

287. Ganguly R, Waldman RH. Effect of orange juice on attenuated rubella virus infection. Indian J Med Res 1977; 66:359–363.

288. Ganguly R, Khakoo R, Spencer JC, Waldman RH. Immunoenhancing agents in prevention and treatment of influenza and other viral respiratory infections. Dev Biol Stand 1977; 39: 363–372.

289. Heise FH, Martin GJ, Schwartz S. Vitamin C and blood sedimentation. Br J Tuberc 1937; 31:23–31.

290. Radford M, DeSavitsch E, Sweany HC. Blood changes following continuous daily administration of vitamin C and orange juice to tuberculous patients. Am Rev Tuberc 1937; 35: 784–793.

291. Kaplan A, Zonnis ME. Vitamin C in pulmonary tuberculosis. Am Rev Tuberc 1940; 42: 667–673.

292. Bogen E, Hawkins L, Bennett ES. Vitamin C treatment of mucous membrane tuberculosis. Am Rev Tuberc 1941; 44:596–603.

293. Babbar IJ. Therapeutic effect of ascorbic acid in tuberculosis. Indian Med Gaz 1948; 83: 409–410.

294. Baur H, Staub H. Therapy of hepatitis with ascorbic acid infusions. Schweiz Med Wochenschr 1954; 84:595–597.

295. Kirchmair H, Kirsch B. Treatment of epidemic hepatitis in children with high doses of ascorbic acid. Med Monatschrift 1957; 11:353–357.

296. Kirchmair H. Epidemic hepatitis in children and its treatment with high doses of ascorbic acid. Dtsch Gesundheitsw 1957; 12:1525–1536.

297. Baetgen D. Results of the treatment of epidemic hepatitis in children with high doses of ascorbic acid in the years 1957–1958. Med Monatschrift 1961; 15:30–36.

298. Baur H. Poliomyelitis therapy with ascorbic acid. Helv Med Acta 1952; 19:470–474.

299. Tang AM, Graham NMH, Kirby AJ, et al. Dietary micronutrient intake and risk of progression to AIDS in HIV-1-infected homosexual men. Am J Epidemiol 1993; 138:937–951.

300. National Research Council. Recommended Dietary Allowances. 10th ed. Washington, DC: National Academy Press, 1989.

301. Luberoff BJ. Symptomectomy with vitamin C: a chat with Robert Cathcart. Chemtech 1978; 8:76–86.

302. Cathcart RF. Vitamin C, titrating to bowel tolerance, anascorbemia, and acute induced scurvy. Med Hypotheses 1981; 7:1359–1376.

303. Klenner FR. Virus pneumonia and its treatment with vitamin C. South Med Surg 1948; 110: 36–38, 46.

304. Klenner FR. Massive doses of vitamin C and the virus diseases. South Med Surg 1951; 113: 101–107.

305. Klenner FR. Observations on the dose and administration of ascorbic acid when employed beyond the range of a vitamin in human pathology. J Appl Nutr 1971; 23:61–88.

306. Dalton WL. Massive doses of vitamin C in the treatment of viral diseases. J Indiana State Med Assoc 1962; 55:1151–1154.

307. Gotzsche AL. Pernasal vitamin C and the common cold (letter). Lancet 1989; 2:1039.

308. Rivers JM. Safety of high-level vitamin C ingestion. Ann NY Acad Sci 1987; 498:445–454.

309. Bendich A, Langseth L. The health effects of vitamin C supplementation: a review. J Am Coll Nutr 1995; 14:124–136.

28

Ascorbic Acid and Periodontal Disease

OLAV ALVARES
University of Texas Health Science Center, San Antonio, Texas

INTRODUCTION

The impact of an adequate intake of ascorbic acid on oral health can be traced back to ancient times. While today scurvy has no impact on society in industrialized countries, it is interesting to note that there was a time when this nutritional deficiency shaped the outcome of military campaigns and naval explorations (1). In 1747, the Scottish naval surgeon James Lind undertook the classical experiment on board the H.M.S. *Salisbury* (2). He demonstrated that lemons and oranges that we now know today as a good source for ascorbic acid were the best cure for scurvy. More recently, studies in humans and experimental animals have shown that diets deficient in ascorbic acid produce profound changes in the supporting structures of the tooth, i.e., the periodontal tissues (3–7). Thus, historically, ascorbic acid deficiency came to be associated with the clinical features of periodontal disease such as gingival bleeding, loss of attachment of the periodontal tissues, and tooth mobility. This chapter will be devoted to the role of ascorbic acid (vitamin C) in the maintenance of periodontal health and the pathogenesis of periodontal disease.

PERIODONTAL DISEASES

This section will present a brief overview of periodontal diseases. Today, more individuals are maintaining and retaining their natural dentition primarily because of better control of dental caries. However, these teeth are vulnerable to destruction of their supporting structures in a variety of ways collectively referred to as periodontal diseases. These diseases are endemic in the U.S. population and are the major cause of tooth loss after the age of 35. The expenditures (estimated in millions of dollars) incurred and the time lost by the labor force in the course of its treatment and management have drawn attention to the tremendous socioeconomic impact of periodontal diseases.

The common forms of periodontal diseases may be broadly classified into the inflammatory involvement of the gingiva, or gingivitis, and that of the supporting tooth structures (periodontal ligament), or periodontitis. A national survey conducted by the National Institute of Dental Research (8) showed that 47% of males and 39% of females aged 18–64 exhibited gingivitis. This same survey showed that 70% of adults aged 35–44 years and >90% aged 55–64 exhibited some degree of periodontitis, with advanced periodontitis affecting approximately 15% of the individuals between the ages of 60 and 64. The studies by Loe and coworkers (9) on Sri Lankan tea workers (14–46 years old) provide insights into the natural progression of periodontal disease in humans as this study population never had any dental care. In this group of individuals, 11% exhibited gingivitis only. Thus, while gingivitis usually precedes periodontitis, it does not inevitably progress to periodontitis. Further, in the Sri Lankan study population, 8% showed severe periodontitis; 81%, moderate periodontitis. These data for gingivitis and periodontitis suggest that in humans there are differences in the susceptibility to this disease process. Experimental animal and human studies have altered the long held perception of chronic adult periodontitis as a slowly creeping, progressive disease. What has emerged from these studies is that in spite of significant accumulations of dental plaque and its attendant gingivitis, the destructive consequences may vary greatly not only between individuals, but also between sites in the same mouth (10). More importantly, Socransky et al. have proposed models according to which the pattern of progress of adult periodontitis is characterized by "bursts" of tissue destruction rather than by a continuous progressive destruction (11). These bursts of destructive disease are of relatively short duration, are followed by varying periods of quiescence, and may occur asynchronously in different sites in the same mouth. Local or systemic factors (discussed later) which decrease host resistance or increase the virulence of plaque-associated organisms may act as a trigger for setting off an episode of tissue destruction (12).

The primary causative factor of gingivitis and periodontitis is the complex mass of bacteria that constitutes "dental plaque"—a material that is omnipresent in the dentogingival area. There is an ecological shift in the resident bacteria in the progression from healthy to diseased sites. The former harbor primarily gram-positive organisms; the latter, largely anaerobic gram-negative organisms and spirochetes (13–15). Of the vast number (200–300 species) of bacteria that reside in the oral cavity only a few appear to be responsible for the tissue destruction that characterizes periodontal disease. The putative periodontal pathogens include *Porphyromonas gingivalis, Prevotella intermedia, Fusobacterium intermedium, Campylobacter rectus, Eikenella corodens, Actinobacillus actinomycetemcomitans*, and spirochetes (16). This list of periodontal pathogens keeps changing as a result of increased sophistication in cultural techniques and diagnostic probes. Suffice it to say for now that, beginning with pioneering work of Keyes and Jordan (17), there is enough evidence to regard the common forms of periodontal diseases as infections. Three decades ago, Loe and coworkers (18) showed that if individuals refrained from the practice of oral hygiene there was an accumulation of dental plaque which subsequently led to the development of gingivitis. When oral hygiene was reintroduced, the gingival tissues returned to health. These studies led to the recognition that dental plaque is the primary causative factor of periodontal disease. However, secondary factors, both local and systemic, may also play a role in the initiation and progression of periodontal disease. Notable secondary local factors include poorly fabricated dental appliances and restorations, badly broken down teeth, and smoking. Secondary systemic factors that can impact on periodontal health include altered nutritional and hormonal levels, diabetes, and a compromised immune system.

Clinically, chronic gingivitis is characterized by varying degrees of redness and loss of contour of the gingiva and possibly bleeding when a probe is inserted into the naturally occurring space between the gingiva and the tooth. Histologically, chronic gingivitis exhibits proliferation of the gingival epithelium facing the tooth, loss of collagen, and a chronic inflammatory infiltrate.

There are several clinical presentations of periodontitis. These include localized early onset or juvenile periodontitis, generalized early onset or rapidly progressive periodontitis, and adult periodontitis (19). The discussion in this chapter will be limited to adult periodontitis. The clinical appearance of plaque-associated chronic adult periodontitis also varies considerably. The two most consistent features are the increase in the depth of the space between the gingiva and tooth, i.e., pocket formation, and radiographic evidence of loss of tooth supporting bone. The pathogenesis of chronic periodontitis is not fully understood but is likely to be the outcome of a complex interaction between the causative organisms and host defense mechanisms (20). It is not readily apparent to what extent the destruction of the supporting tooth structures can be attributed to bacterially derived toxic products and the host's reactions to these environmental insults. Bacteria-derived collagenase, neutral and acid proteases, and activation of the inflammatory–immune system by the host coupled with release of prostaglandins and activation of cytokines, such as interleukin-1β, all appear to contribute to and interact in a complex manner in the connective tissue and bone destruction that characterizes chronic adult periodontitis (16,20,21). The period of active tissue destruction is followed by repair and healing. During healing, the negative regulators of inflammation, including transforming growth factor-β, γ-interferon, interleukin-4, and interleukin-1 receptor antagonists, prevail (16). It is clear that the host defense (the inflammatory–immune response) mechanisms play a critical role during both the destructive and healing phases of periodontitis. Further, these host defense components require a steady and adequate supply of nutrients, including ascorbic acid, in order to function efficiently.

HOST DEFENSE, PERIODONTAL DISEASE, AND ASCORBIC ACID

During the last few decades, experimental studies have failed to demonstrate a significant causative relationship between ascorbic acid status and periodontal diseases (22). These studies can be faulted for study design and were undertaken when our understanding of the nature of periodontal diseases was relatively meager. Epidemiological studies carried out by Russell (23,24) in developing societies also failed to demonstrate an association between ascorbic acid deficiency and periodontal disease. This finding does not come as a surprise because in these developing countries the practice of oral hygiene is minimal and therefore the dental plaque–induced inflammatory process could easily have masked the effects of an underlying nutritional deficiency including that of ascorbic acid. In the United States, Ismail et al. (25) have shown that, at best, there is weak correlation between ascorbic acid status and periodontal health. More recently, Vaananen et al. (26) examined the relationship between plasma ascorbic acid level and the severity of periodontal disease. Periodontal disease in subjects with a low (≤ 25 μmol/L) plasma ascorbic acid level was compared with that of control subjects (≥ 50 μmol/L) matched for age, sex, and number of teeth. The dietary intake of ascorbic acid in the study subjects was 52 mg $\pm$ 24.9; that of controls, 77 mg $\pm$ 43.2. These investigators found more severe periodontal disease in the study group as compared to controls. Taken together, the foregoing seems to suggest that the role of ascorbic acid in periodontal health and disease is clouded over with some degree of uncertainty. Conceptually, however, this uncertainty can be resolved.

One can trace back to antiquity that inadequate nutrition is invariably accompanied by an increase in susceptibility to a wide variety of infections. Invariably this increased susceptibility to infections has been due to a compromise in host defense systems (27). Given the fact that periodontal diseases are infectious in nature it seems reasonable to propose that periodontal health may be compromised by an inadequate intake of ascorbic acid via a compromise in host defense systems that are of relevance to periodontal health. This section will examine this proposition.

The Barrier Function of Oral Epithelium

The barrier function of the oral epithelium, and by implication its permeability, is an expression of the cumulative integrity of the intraepithelial barrier, basement membrane, and plasma membrane of the epithelial cells (28,29). With respect to the periodontal tissues, an increase in the permeability of the gingival sulcular epithelium would facilitate the passage of dental plaque bacterial toxins into the gingival connective tissue and trigger an inflammatory–immune response.

Employing an in vitro system, Alfano et al. (30) showed that the oral epithelium of guinea pigs exhibits significantly greater permeability on an ascorbate-deficient diet of a period of 2 weeks or greater. Furthermore, tissue permeability was inversely related to oral tissue level of ascorbate, and this level dropped sooner and faster than blood ascorbate levels. When the deficient animals were rehabilitated for 2 weeks after being on the ascorbate-deficient diet for 3 weeks, the permeability of the oral epithelium declined slightly, thereby revealing that the effect of ascorbate deficiency on the epithelial barrier function is not rapidly reversible. The next logical step was the demonstration of the existence of a link between a compromise in the barrier function and increased susceptibility to periodontal disease in the circumstance of inadequate dietary ascorbic acid. Alvares and Siegel (31) showed that in young adult nonhuman primates typical scorbutic gingivitis develops when the animals are maintained on an inadequate dietary ascorbic acid level for a period of 12 weeks. Interestingly, 2–3 weeks prior to the clinical manifestation of the scorbutic gingivitis, the experimental animals exhibited a significant increase in the in vivo permeability of the gingival sulcular epithelium. This increase in permeability could have played a role in the pathogenesis of the scorbutic gingivitis by facilitating the penetration of bacterial toxins into the gingival tissues. The mechanism whereby ascorbic acid deficiency leads to an increase in epithelial permeability is not fully understood. It is known that scorbutic guinea pigs exhibit a reduced capacity to synthesize oral epithelia basement membrane collagen (30). This defect is accompanied by a compromise in basement membrane integrity and, by implication, its permeability. Alfano et al. (30) have suggested that these changes may represent the mechanism by which capillary fragility and subsequent gingival bleeding are induced in scurvy.

Just as ascorbic acid deficiency can increase epithelial permeability, conversely the supplementation of this vitamin may also strengthen this host defense component. There are some interesting data in humans to support this notion. In humans subsisting on a mean daily dietary intake of ascorbic acid above the U.S. RDA of 60 mg/day, ascorbate supplementation (1 g/day for 4 weeks) resulted in an increase in gingival tissue concentration of the vitamin (32). This increase in gingival tissue level was associated with increased collagen synthesis and decreased permeability of the gingival sulcular epithelium. Recently, in two well-controlled studies on humans, Leggott et al. (33,34) showed that ascorbic acid depletion led to increased gingival bleeding, a clinical finding that was not related to pathogenic periodontal microflora. More importantly, when compared to the control group (60 mg/day), individuals receiving 10× (600 mg/day) the U.S. recommended dietary allowance (RDA) for ascorbic acid exhibited significantly fewer gingival bleeding sites despite the fact that dental plaque (primary causative factor) levels were similar in both groups. One could infer that the improvement in the gingival health in the ascorbate-supplemented groups may, in part, be due to a strengthening of the barrier function of the gingival sulcular epithelium. Other investigators (35,36) have reported biochemical and morphological evidence to support the beneficial effects of ascorbate supplementation on oral mucosa.

The foregoing results on ascorbate supplementation bring into focus the fact that conventional indices of nutritional status may not always reveal a true picture of nutriture at the tissue or organ level. Conceptually, an "end-organ" deficiency may exist in the gingival and periodontal tissues despite an adequate intake (RDA level) of the nutrient. Such a deficiency may arise from an increased nutrient requirement dictated by factors (host–parasite interactions, a continuous need for epithelial and connective tissue repair, an adequate inflammatory–immune response) that are continuously operational in the dento-gingival area.

Neutrophil Function

The role of the white blood cell, polymorphonuclear neutrophil (PMN), in host defense is well documented. Optimal PMN function is critical to the maintenance of periodontal health. In the healthy state, PMNs have been shown to emigrate continuously from the gingival connective tissue into the gingival pocket in response to a chemical gradient elaborated by dental plaque microorganisms (37). In the gingival pocket the PMNs interpose themselves between the organisms and the gingival tissues, and they have been shown to ingest and digest microorganisms (38). Individuals with agranulocytosis, cyclic neutropenia, Chédiak–Higashi syndrome, and insulin-dependent diabetes exhibit impaired PMN function, and this impairment is associated with an increased risk for periodontal disease (39). This finding suggests that the PMN plays a protective role in the human periodontium.

Human neutrophils serve as a rich reservoir for ascorbic acid, and the level of this vitamin in PMNs is 25-fold greater than that in plasma (40,41). There appears to be an association between intracellular level of ascorbate in PMNs, altered PMN function, and increased frequency of infection (42). Ascorbic acid has been shown to stimulate PMN chemotaxis, oxidative metabolism and glycolysis, and microtubule assembly (43–46). Ascorbic acid, along with other antioxidants, serves as a scavenger of free oxygen radicals and in the prevention of cell membrane lipid peroxidation (47). In addition, ascorbic acid has an important role in neutralizing histamine (48). All of these functions of ascorbic acid are likely to play an important role in modulating the initiation, progression, and resolution of the inflammatory process in chronic periodontitis.

Neutrophils obtained from scorbutic guinea pigs exhibited a marked depletion of ascorbate and a significant impairment in phagocytic and chemotactic functions (49). It is also noteworthy that chronic subclinical ascorbate deficiency in nonhuman primates is associated with an increased susceptibility to dental plaque–associated periodontal disease (50). This increased susceptibility to periodontal disease was accompanied by an impairment in PMN chemotactic and phagocytic activities. While this latter study draws attention to the possible role of leukocyte defects in subclinical ascorbic acid deficiency–induced periodontal disease, one cannot overlook the significance of other factors. Conceivably, these other factors could include an impairment of collagen synthesis, an increase in gingival tissue levels of histamine, and a depletion in the complement component, Clq, a protein regarded as essential for host defense against pathogens (51). In contrast to these studies in experimental animals, Vogel et al. (52) did not notice a significant effect of vitamin C supplementation (1500 mg daily for 4 months) on PMN chemotaxis and experimental gingivitis in adult humans. It should be noted that the volunteers in this study were already consuming twice the recommended daily allowance of vitamin C. It may well be that dietary ascorbic acid beyond a certain threshold level, albeit at present an unknown one, may not have a further beneficial effect on neutrophil function.

Hormonal Balance

Altered hormonal levels impact on gingival and periodontal health. Examples of hormonal influences on these tissues include the increased risk for gingivitis in some pubescent and pregnant individuals and users of oral contraceptives (53,54). Sex hormone receptors have been demonstrated in human gingiva, thereby implying that it is a target tissue for hormones (55,56). Indeed, high plasma progesterone levels have been associated with periodontitis. It is also noteworthy that Kornman and Loesche (57) observed a strong correlation between plasma levels of estrogen and progesterone and putative periodontal pathogens, although this finding disagrees with those of other studies (58).

Ascorbic acid is present in high concentration in the major salivary glands, suggesting that this vitamin may play a role in the physiological function of these glands (59,60). In a recent study, Sawiris et al. (61) showed that scorbutic guinea pigs exhibited a significant reduction in salivary output (xerostomia) via an impairment in a transmembrane signaling system. This xerostomia, in turn, deprives the oral cavity of crucial salivary host defense molecules (secretory immunoglobulin A [sIgA], antimicrobial and antifungal agents, etc.) that are essential for the maintenance of oral health (62). The xerostomia in scorbutic guinea pigs is also accompanied by a 4.0- and 2.5-fold increase in plasma and salivary cortisol levels, respectively (63). The increase in salivary cortisol levels could facilitate an increase in the bacterial load of periodontal pathogens (57). In addition, the antiinflammatory nature of steroids could dampen the host inflammatory response to periodontal pathogen antigens and thereby compromise periodontal health. Enwonwu (64) has suggested that the elevated salivary steroid levels "may be an important and unexplored mechanism by which ... ascorbic acid deficiency serves as an important risk factor" for a form of periodontal disease referred to as acute necrotizing ulcerative gingivitis.

POPULATION GROUPS AT RISK FOR PERIODONTAL DISEASE VIA A COMPROMISE IN ASCORBIC ACID METABOLISM

Diabetes

Diabetes mellitus is a chronic disorder that affects several million individuals in the United States. The American Diabetic Association now recognizes that periodontal disease is one of the forgotten complications of poorly controlled diabetes (65). From a clinical standpoint, it is important to recognize that chronic dental plaque–associated periodontal diseases are infectious in nature. If undiagnosed (because of its generally symptomatic presentation, lack of concern for oral health, etc.) and therefore untreated, this hidden infection could represent a significant stress factor in the glycemic control in a diabetic individual. This subsection will summarize the periodontal findings in experimental animal models of diabetes and in human diabetics. This will be followed by a discussion of the possible role of altered ascorbic acid metabolism as a risk factor for periodontal disease in diabetes.

Experimentally induced diabetes in rats leads to (1) a decrease in the migration of PMNs into the gingival sulcus in response to chemoattractants; this represents a breach in host defense and parallels the findings seen in human diabetics with severe periodontal disease (66,67); (2) a marked reduction in the activities of the key enzymes (prolyl- and lysyl-hydroxylase activities) involved in gingival collagen synthesis (68); this is clinically significant since optimal collagen synthesis is fundamental to the repair process that must follow the connective tissue destruction that is so characteristic of periodontitis; (3) an increase in gingival collagenase (69) which could conceivably contribute to collagen destruction; (4) a decrease in gingival and PMN ascorbic acid level (70). It is noteworthy that the diabetes-induced depletion of gingival and PMN ascorbic acid and the impairment in collagen synthesis can be reversed by dietary supplementation of ascorbic acid (70,71).

While some investigators have not shown a relationship between insulin-dependent diabetes mellitus (IDDM) and periodontal disease (72), others have reported an increase in the severity of gingivitis and periodontitis in IDDM and non-insulin-dependent diabetes mellitus (NIDDM) (73,74). These conflicting findings may be related to the realization that diabetes mellitus is a syndrome with a broad range of clinical manifestations. The extent to which blood glucose control is achieved as well as certain other factors, e.g., genetic predisposition, may influence the clinical manifestations of this disorder, including the susceptibility to periodontal diseases. It has been suggested that the increased susceptibility to periodontal diseases in diabetics may be due to an altered microbial flora of dental plaque or to an altered host defense. There are data to support both of these possibilities. Mashimo et al. (75) have reported higher proportions of a putative periodontal pathogen, i.e., *Capnocytophaga* sp. and other gram-negative organisms, in dental plaque of IDDM subjects. Still other have found higher proportions of *Bacteroides gingivalis* and *Bacteroides intermedius* in the plaque of individuals who have NIDDM (76). With respect to host defense, there are reports of defects in PMN chemotaxis in diabetic subjects exhibiting periodontal disease (67). In an assessment of risk factors for periodontal disease, Grossi et al. (74) reported that diabetics are twice as likely to exhibit loss of tooth support due to periodontal disease than nondiabetics.

Previous sections have discussed the role of ascorbic acid as it impacts on host defenses that are relevant to periodontal health. It would be intriguing to examine the evidence for an altered ascorbic acid metabolism in diabetics which might explain their predisposition to periodontal diseases via a compromise in host defense. Ascorbic acid levels are reduced in various tissues of animals with experimental diabetes (77,78). This alteration has also been noted in the gingival tissues of diabetic animals, and, further, some of the gingival changes in the diabetic rat can be reversed with dietary ascorbic acid supplementation. Reduced tissue ascorbic acid levels have also been reported in diabetic patients (79). A reduction in mononuclear leukocyte ascorbic acid content has been observed even in diabetic patients subsisting on more than an adequate intake of the vitamin (80). This finding has been ascribed to an inhibition in the transport of ascorbic acid across the cell membrane. Indeed hyperglycemia interferes with the transport of ascorbic acid in a number of cell systems, including lymphocytes and mononuclear and polymorphonuclear leukocytes (81,82).

Along with a reduction in ascorbic acid content in mononuclear and polymorphonuclear leukocytes there is a concomitant reduction in chemotaxis. The impairment in the chemotactic function of these cells was significantly correlated with their ascorbic acid content (82). It is tempting to postulate that an impairment in function of PMN, a cell that is regarded as vital for periodontal health, may represent a mechanism that increases the diabetic's susceptibility to periodontal disease. It is not known whether there is an impairment in the uptake of ascorbic acid by the oral epithelium and salivary glands under conditions of hyperglycemia. From the previous discussion (see the sections The Barrier Function of Oral Epithelium and Hormonal Balance), an impairment in the oral epithelial barrier function, altered salivary gland physiological characteristics, and decrease in collagen synthesis by fibroblasts could be additional modes that could compromise periodontal health in the diabetic. Long-term clinical trials to assess the possible beneficial effect of ascorbic acid supplementation on periodontal health in diabetics would seem to be in order.

Smokers

While dental plaque, and its attendant microorganisms, is the primary causative factor of periodontal diseases, secondary local (e.g., defective restorations) and systemic (e.g., compromise in the immune system) factors may also modulate the initiation and progression of periodontal diseases. Over the years, a number of studies have examined the effect of smoking on periodontal health (83). While there is no universal agreement in the findings of these past studies, more recent and well-controlled investigations seem to make a strong case for smoking as a risk factor for loss of tooth support due to periodontal disease (84,85). The odds of periodontal disease in smokers as compared to nonsmokers range from approximately 2.0 for light smokers to 4.75 for heavy smokers (74). More significantly, the combined odds for periodontal disease in an individual who is older than 45 years, a diabetic, and a moderate or heavy smoker and whose periodontal tissues are infected with two periodontal pathogens, *P. gingivalis* and *B. forsythus*, are 30 times higher than in an individual who has none of these traits (74). In addition to their systemic effects, nicotine and its by-products have a vasoconstrictive effect on gingival blood vessels (86). Smoking has also been reported to reduce oxygen levels in dental plaque; that reduction, in turn, is associated with a decrease in PMN mobility and an increase in the proportion of anaerobic bacteria in dental plaque (87). The major metabolite of nicotine, cotine, is present in saliva, gingival crevicular fluid, and the root surfaces of periodontally involved teeth of smokers (88,89). Grossi et al. (74) have postulated that cotine on the root surfaces may interfere with periodontal wound healing and alter the host response in periodontal disease. Finally, the impairment of chemotaxis and phagocytosis in PMNs of smokers could deprive the host of the protective phagocytic response to periodontal pathogens.

A number of investigators have reported low ascorbate levels in blood, plasma, and leukocytes in smokers as compared to nonsmokers (90). The reduced levels do not appear to be due to reduced dietary intake of the vitamin. Rather, an impairment in the absorption of the vitamin and/or its higher metabolic turnover may explain the reduced ascorbic acid levels in tissue and cells (91,92). It has been suggested that the vitamin C requirement of smokers may be twice that of nonsmokers (90).

The abundance of free radicals in cigarette smoke, an impairment in PMN function due to a lower ascorbic acid level, and a decrease in the level of the antioxidant function of ascorbic acid may all conspire to place the smoker at a greater risk for periodontal disease.

CONCLUDING REMARKS

There are still some significant unanswered questions. For example, conventional wisdom states there is a demographic shift in the age structure of our population as reflected in the increase in the number of older individuals. These older individuals are retaining their natural dentition for a longer period because of better control of dental caries. However, these teeth are vulnerable to a destruction of their supporting structures due to periodontal diseases. The RDAs for nutrients in the 55+ years age group have not been established. In these older individuals, might a compromise in ascorbic acid metabolism (due to inadequate dietary intake, malabsorption arising from gastrointestinal problems, drug–nutrient interactions) play a role in the loss of tooth supporting structures due to periodontal disease? The clinical feature of bleeding gums in ascorbic acid deficiency was noted more than 300 years ago. But we still have a long way to go in improving our understanding of the role of ascorbic acid at the molecular level, in the homeostasis of the periodontal tissues, and in the modulation of the initiation and progression of periodontal disease.

ACKNOWLEDGMENT

The author thanks Dr. Eleanor Young for reviewing this manuscript.

REFERENCES

1. Hodges RE, Baker EM. Ascorbic acid. In: Goodhart RS, Shils ME, eds. Modern Nutrition in Health and Disease. Philadelphia: Lea & Febiger, 1973:245–255.
2. Blockley CH, Baenziger PE. An investigation into the connection between vitamin C content of the blood and periodontal disturbances. Br Dent J 1942; 3:57–62.
3. Crandon JH, Lund CC, Dill DB. Experimental human scurvy. New Engl J Med 1940; 223: 353–369.
4. Linghorne WJ, McIntosh WG, Tice JW, et al. The relation of ascorbic acid intake to gingivitis. Can Med Assoc J 1946; 54:106–112.
5. Glickman I. Acute vitamin C deficiency and periodontal disease. I. The periodontal tissues of the guinea pig in acute vitamin C deficiency. J Dent Res 1948; 27:9–23.
6. Werhaug J. Effect of C-avitaminosis on the supporting structure of the teeth. J Periodontol 1958; 29:87–97.
7. Hodges RE, Baker EM, Hood J, et al. Experimental scurvy in man. Am J Clin Nutr 1969; 22:535–548.
8. US Public Health Service, National Institute of Dental Research. Oral Health of United States Adults: National Findings. NIH Publication # 87-2868. Bethesda, MD: NIDR, 1987.
9. Loe H, Anerud A, Boysen H, Morrison E. Natural history of periodontal disease in man: Rapid, moderate and no loss of attachment in Sri Lankan laborers 14 to 46 years of age. J Clin Periodontol 1986; 13:431–445.
10. Taichman N, Lindhe J. Pathogenesis of plaque-associated periodontal disease. In: Lindhe J, ed. Textbook of Clinical Periodontology. Copenhagen: Munksgaard, 1989:153–190.
11. Socransky SS, Hafajee AD, Goodson JM, Lindhe J. New concepts of destructive periodontal disease. J Clin Periodontol 1984; 11:21–32.
12. Listgarten MA. Nature of periodontal diseases: pathogenic mechanisms. J Periodont Res 1987; 22:172–178.
13. Listgarten MA. Structure of microbial flora associated with periodontal health and disease in man: a light and electron microscopic study. J Periodontol 1976; 47:1–18.

14. Genco RJ, Zambon JJ, Christerson LA. The origin of periodontal infections. Adv Dent Res 1986; 2:245–249.

15. Tanner AC, Dzink JL, Socransky SS, Des roches CL. Diagnosis of periodontal disease using rapid identification of "activity-related" gram-negative species. J Periodont Res 1987; 22:207–208.

16. Genco RJ. Host responses in periodontal diseases: current concepts. J Periodontol 1992; 63: 338–355.

17. Keyes PH, Jordan HV. Periodontal lesions in the syrian hamster. III. Findings related to an infectious and transmissible component. Arch Oral Biol 1964; 9:377–400.

18. Loe H, Theilade E, Jensen SB. Experimental gingivitis in man. J Periodontol 1965; 36:177–187.

19. Lindhe J, Slots J. Periodontal disease in children and young adults. In: Lindhe J, ed. Textbook of Clinical Periodontology. Copenhagen: Munksgaard, 1989: 193–220.

20. Williams RC. Periodontal Disease. N Engl J Med 1990; 322:373–382.

21. Ranney RR. Immunologic mechanisms of pathogenesis in periodontal diseases: an assessment. J Periodont Res 1991; 26:243–254.

22. Vogel RI, Alvares O. Nutrition and periodontal diseases. In: Pollack RL, Kravitz E, eds. Nutrition in Oral Health and Disease. Philadelphia: Lea & Febiger, 1985:136–150.

23. Russell AL. International nutrition surveys: a summary of preliminary dental findings. J Dent Res 1963; 42:233–244.

24. Russell AL, Leatherwood EC, Consolazio CF. Van reen R. Periodontal disease and nutrition in South Vietnam. J Dent Res 1965; 44:775–782.

25. Ismail AI, Burt BA, Eklund SA. Relations between ascorbic acid and periodontal disease in the United States. J Am Dent Assoc 1983; 107:927–935.

26. Vaananen MK, Markkanen HA, Tuovinen VJ, et al. Periodontal health related to plasma ascorbic acid. Proc Finn Dent Soc 1993; 89:51–59.

27. Gontzea I. Nutrition and anti-infectious defense. New York: Karger, 1974:49–53.

28. Squier CA, Johnson NW. The permeability of oral mucosa. Br Med Bull 1975; 31:169–175.

29. Alfano MC, Drummond JF, Miller SA. Localization of rate-limiting barrier to penetration of endotoxin through non-keratinized oral mucosa in vitro. J Dent Res 1975; 54:1143–1148.

30. Alfano MC, Miller SA, Drummond JF. Effect of ascorbic acid deficiency on the permeability and collagen biosynthesis of oral mucosal epithelium. Ann NY Acad Sci 1975; 258: 253–263.

31. Alvares O, Siegel I. Permeability of gingival sulcular epithelium in the development of scorbutic gingivitis. J Oral Pathol 1981; 10:40–48.

32. Mallek H. The role of ascorbic acid and iron in human gingivitis. PhD dissertation, Massachusetts Institute of Technology, Boston, 1978.

33. Leggott PJ, Robertson PB, Rothman DL, et al. The effect of controlled ascorbic acid depletion and supplementation on periodontal health. J Periodontol 1986; 57:480–485.

34. Leggott PJ, Robertson PB, Jacob RA, et al. Effects of ascorbic acid depletion and supplementation on periodontal health and subgingival microflora in humans. J Dent Res 1991; 70:1531–1536.

35. Buzina R, Aurer-Kozelj J, Srdak-Jorgic K, et al. Increase of gingival hydroxyproline and proline by improvement of ascorbic acid status in man. Int J Vitam Nutr Res 1986; 56:367–371.

36. Aurer-Kozelj J, Kralj-Klobucar N, Buzina R, Bacic M. The effect of ascorbic acid supplementation on periodontal tissue ultrastructure in subjects with progressive periodontitis. Int J Vitam Nutr Res 1982; 52:333–341.

37. Helden L, Lindhe J. Enhanced emigration of crevicular leukocytes mediated by factors in human dental plaque. Scand J Dent Res 1973; 81:123–129.

38. Garant PR. Plaque-neutrophil interaction in monoinfected rats as visualised by transmission electron microscopy. J Periodontol 1976; 47:132–138.

39. Van Dyke TE, Levine MJ, Genco RJ. Neutrophil function and oral disease. J Oral Pathol 1985; 14:95–120.

40. Evans RM, Currie L, Campbell C. The distribution of ascorbic acid between various cellular components of blood in normal individuals and its relation to the plasma concentration. Br J Nutr 1982; 47:473–482.

41. Bergsten P, Amitai G, Kehri J, et al. Millimolar concentrations of ascorbic acid in purified human mononuclear leukocytes: depletion and reaccumulation. J Biol Chem 1990; 265:2584–2587.

42. Rebora A, Dallegri F, Patrone F, Neutrophil dysfunction and repeated infections: influence of levamisole and ascorbic acid. Br J Dermatol 1980; 102:49–56.

43. Dallegri F, Lanzi GF, Patrone F. Effects of ascorbic acid on neutrophil locomotion. Int Arch Allergy Appl Immunol 1980; 61:40–45.

44. Patrone F. Effects of ascorbic acid on neutrophil function: studies on normal and chronic granulomatous disease neutrophils. Acta Vitaminol Enzymol 1982; 4:163–168.

45. Anderson R, Theron A. Effect of ascorbate on leukocytes. Part 1. Effects of ascorbate on neutrophil motility and intracellular cyclic nucleotide levels in vitro. S Afr Med J 1979; 56:394–400.

46. Boxer LA, Vanderbilt S, Bonsib R, et al. Enhancement of chemotactic response and microtubule assembly in human leukocytes by ascorbic acid. J Cell Physiol 1979; 199:119–126.

47. Padh H. Vitamin C: newer insights into its biochemical function. Nutr Rev 1991; 49:65–70.

48. Clemetson CAB. Histamine metabolism. In: Clemetson CAB, ed. Vitamin C. Vol III. Boca Raton, FL: CRC Press, 1989:1–13.

49. Goldschmidt MC. Reduced bactericidal activity in neutrophils from scorbutic animals and the effects of ascorbic acid on these target bacteria in vivo and in vitro. Am J Clin Nutr 1991; 54(Suppl):1214–1220.

50. Alvares O, Altman LC, Springmeyer S, et al. The effect of subclinical ascorbate deficiency on periodontal health in nonhuman primates. J Periodont Res 1981; 16:628–636.

51. Johnston CS, Kolb WP, Haskell BE. The effect of vitamin C nutriture on complement component Clq concentrations in guinea pig plasma. J Nutr 1987; 117:764–768.

52. Vogel RI, Lamster IB, Wechsler SA, et al. The effects of megadoses of ascorbic acid on PMN chemotaxis and experimental gingivitis. J Periodontol 1986; 57:472–479.

53. Lindhe J, Attstrom R, Bjorn AL. The influence of progestogen on gingival exudation during the menstrual cycle. J Periodont Res 1969; 4:97–102.

54. Kalkwarf KL. Effect of oral contraceptive therapy on gingival inflammation in humans. J Periodontol 1978; 49:560–563.

55. Vittek J. Hernandez MR, Wenk EJ, et al. Specific estrogen receptors in human gingiva J. Clin Endocrinol Metab 1982; 54:608–612.

56. Vittek J, Munnangi PR, Gordon GG, et al. Progesterone "receptors" in human gingiva. IRCS Med Sci 1982; 10:381.

57. Kornman KS, Loesche WJ. The subgingival microbial flora during pregnancy. J Periodont Res 1980; 15:111–122.

58. Jonsson R, Howland BE, Bowden GH. Relationship between periodontal health, salivary steroids and *Bacteroides intermedius* in males, pregnant and non-pregnant women. J Dent Res 1988; 67:1062–1069.

59. Hornig D. Distribution of ascorbic acid, metabolites and analogues in man and animals. Ann NY Acad Sci 1975; 258:103–117.

60. von Zastrow M, Tritton TR, Castle JD. Identification of L-ascorbic acid in secretion granules of the rat parotid gland. J Biol Chem 1984; 259:11746–11750.

61. Sawiris P, Chanaud N, Enwonwu CO. Impaired inositol triphosphate generation in carbachol-stimulated submandibular gland acinar cells from ascorbate deficient guinea pigs. J Nutr Biochem 1995; 6:557–563.

62. Mandel ID. The functions of saliva. J Dent Res 1987; 66:623–627.

63. Enwonwu CO, Sawiris P, Chanaud N. Effect of marginal ascorbic acid deficiency on saliva cortisol level in the guinea pig. Arch Oral Biol 1995; 40:737–742.

64. Enwonwu CO. Cellular and molecular effects of malnutrition and their relevance to periodontal diseases. J Clin Periodontol 1994; 21:643–657.

65. American Diabetic Association (personal communication), 1996.

66. Golub L, Nicoll GA, Iacono VJ, Ramamurthy N. In vivo crevicular leukocyte response to a chemotactic challenge: inhibition by experimental diabetes. Infect Immun 1982; 37:1013–1020.

67. Manouchehr-Pour M, Spagnulo PJ, Rodman HM, Bissada NF. Comparison of neutrophil

chemotactic response in diabetic patients with mild and severe periodontal disease. J Periodontol 1981; 52:410–415.

68. Ramamurthy NS, Greenwald RA, Schneir M, Golub LM. The effect of alloxan diabetes on prolyl and lysyl hydroxylase activities in uninflamed and inflamed gingiva. Arch Oral Biol 1985; 30:679–683.

69. Ramamurthy NS, Golub LM, Diabetes increases collagenase activity in extracts of rat gingiva and skin. J Periodontol Res 1983; 18:23–30.

70. Ramamurthy NS, Lee HM, Lehrer G, et al. Ascorbic acid levels in gingiva and PMN leukocytes of rats with "acute" or "chronic" diabetes. J Dent Res 1983; 62:A119.

71. Schneir M, Ramamurthy NS, Golub LM, Dietary ascorbic acid normalizes diabetes-induced under hydroxylation of nascent Type I collagen molecules. Collagen Rel Res 1985; 5:415–422.

72. Goteiner D, Vogel R, Deasy M, Goteiner C. Periodontal and caries experience in children with insulin-dependent diabetes mellitus. J Am Dent Assoc 1986; 113:277–279.

73. Cianciola LJ, Park BH, Bruck E, et al. Prevalence of periodontal disease in insulin-dependent diabetes mellitus (juvenile diabetes). J Am Dent Assoc 1982; 104:653–660.

74. Grossi SG, Zambon JJ, Ho AW, et al. Assessment of risk for periodontal disease. I. Risk indicators for attachment loss. J Periodontol 1994; 65:260–267.

75. Mashimo PA, Yamamoto Y, Slots J, et al. The periodontal microflora of juvenile diabetes. Culture, immunofluorescence and serum antibody studies. J Periodontol 1983; 54:420–430.

76. Genco RJ, Shlossman M, Zambon J. Immunologic studies of periodontitis patients with Type II diabetes mellitus. J Dent Res 1987; 66:A1200.

77. Yew MS. Effect of streptozotocin diabetes on tissue ascorbic acid and dehydroascorbic acid. Horm Metab Res 1983; 15:158.

78. Rikans LE. Effect of alloxan diabetes on rat liver ascorbic acid. Horm Metab Res 1981; 13:123.

79. Som S, Basu S, Mukherjee D, et al. Ascorbic acid metabolism in diabetes mellitus. Metabolism 1981, 30:572–577.

80. Cunningham JJ, Ellis SL, McVeigh KL, et al. Reduced mononuclear leukocyte ascorbic acid content in adults with insulin-dependent diabetes mellitus consuming adequate dietary vitamin C. Metabolism 1991; 40:146–149.

81. Davies KA, Lee WYL, Labbe RF. Energy dependent transport of ascorbic acid into lymphocytes. Fed Proc 1983; 42:2011.

82. Pecoraro RE, Chen MS. Ascorbic acid metabolism in diabetes mellitus. Ann NY Acad Sci 1987; 498:248–258.

83. Rivera-Hidalgo F. Smoking and periodontal disease. J Periodontol 1986; 57:617–624.

84. Holm G. Smoking as an additional risk factor for tooth loss. J Periodontol 1994; 65:996–1001.

85. Linden GJ, Mullally BH. Cigarette smoking and periodontal destruction in young adults. J Periodontol 1994; 65:718–723.

86. Baab DA, Oberg PA. The effect of cigarette smoking on gingival blood flow in humans. J Clin Periodontol 1987; 14:418–424.

87. Palmer RM. Tobacco smoking and oral health: review. Br Dent J 1988; 164:258–260.

88. McGuire JR, Mcquade MJ, Rossmann JA, et al. Cotine in saliva and gingival crevicular fluid of smokers with periodontal disease. J Periodontol 1989; 60:176–181.

89. Cuff MJ, McQuade MJ, Scheidt MJ, et al. The presence of nicotine on root surfaces of periodontally diseased teeth. J Periodontol 1989; 60:564–569.

90. Murata A. Smoking and vitamin C. World Rev Nutr Diet 1991; 64:31–57.

91. Kallner AB, Hartmann D, Hornig D. On the requirement of ascorbic acid in man: steady state turnover and body pool in smokers. Am J Clin Nutr 1981; 34:1347–1355.

92. Pelletier O. Vitamin C and tobacco. Int J Vit Nutr Res 1977; 16(suppl):147–169.

29

Topical Vitamin C

DOUGLAS J. DARR
*North Carolina Biotechnology Center, Research Triangle Park,
North Carolina*

ROY M. COLVEN
University of Washington, Seattle, Washington

SHELDON R. PINNELL
*Department of Medicine, Duke University Medical Center, Durham,
North Carolina*

The skin is doubly in need of adequate levels of vitamin C: first, the collagen-rich connective tissue component of this tissue requires this vitamin for its proper production—this through vitamin C's role as an enzymatic cofactor in important hydroxylation reactions; second, skin is clearly one of the most abused organs in terms of exposure to noxious agents (particularly ultraviolet radiation), many of which generate reactive oxygen species. Here vitamin C should be presumed to be a very important protectant via its well-known antioxidant properties.

At first blush, delivery of vitamin C to the skin via topical application would seem to be a desirable prophylactic treatment. However, formulation problems due to this molecule's inherent instability has slowed research into the effects topical application of this antioxidant vitamin might have in various skin conditions. Relatively recent advances in understanding how best to deliver vitamin C to the skin, i.e., formulation of stable compositions which allow penetration into the various cell layers, should now allow for further research.

Details of the chemical/biochemical characteristics of vitamin C and the mechanisms of its well-known antioxidant properties are excellently presented in other chapters and will not be reiterated here. Also, there is a reasonable body of literature documenting beneficial effects of other antioxidants on the skin and the reader is directed to several recent reviews (1–3). In the next few pages, we will briefly describe what is known about skin levels of vitamin C, factors which influence those levels, and the results of several studies investigating the utility of topical vitamin C in preventing oxidative damage to the skin.

SKIN LEVELS OF VITAMIN C

The human body's store of vitamin C at steady state is approximately 20 mg/kg body weight, corresponding to a plasma ascorbate level of 0.9 mg/dl (4). With increasing doses, intestinal absorption decreases; maximal absorptive capacity is reached when 3 g is taken as a single dose. Plasma levels peak at 3.5 mg/dl 3 h after this dose. Leukocyte levels, considered a more precise reflection of tissue levels, do not increase significantly with high-dose (up to 12 g) supplementation.

The half-life of ascorbate is 10–20 days and is dependent on plasma levels (4). Signs of scurvy take approximately 4 weeks to develop after cessation of vitamin C intake when starting with saturated body stores. Interestingly, body stores appear to deplete faster after cessation of high-dose supplementation (5). Rebound scurvy has been reported in those who abruptly stop supplementation (6).

Shindo et al. have recently determined dermal and epidermal levels of vitamin C, as well as various other antioxidants (7). Homogenized samples of separated epidermis and dermis were analyzed with high-performance liquid chromatography (HPLC). Epidermal ascorbate levels measured 3.8 mol/g skin (669 mg/kg skin), more than five times the level in the dermis (0.72 mol/g skin). This difference is much greater than that found in murine skin (8). One may speculate that these differential levels reflect differential activities of antioxidants in the dermis and epidermis.

The response of cutaneous levels of vitamin C to oral supplementation is not known. However, these measurements in normal skin help establish a baseline from which differences in oxidative stress, aging, and cutaneous disorders can be compared.

Generation of Reactive Oxygen Species and Depletion of the Antioxidant System in Skin

While again deferring to other chapters for comprehensive discussion of reactive oxygen species (ROS) generation, it is important to understand some of the known conditions where skin, particularly, is prone to oxidative stress and the consequences of this on the antioxidant defenses.

Cutaneous inflammation, regardless of cause, can lead to the formation of ROS. Neutrophils are well-known producers of O_2^- and other cytotoxic compounds—useful in bacterial killing through this "oxidative burst." This added ROS burden, however, can lead to untoward tissue damage in situ. A number of neutrophil-associated dermatoses, including cutaneous vasculitis, Behcet's disease, acne/rosacea, and psoriasis, have been implicated in just such cases.

ULTRAVIOLET LIGHT–GENERATED FREE RADICALS IN SKIN

Harkening back to work done 30 years ago, it is known that ultraviolet (UV) irradiation of intact skin generates a free radical signal measurable by electron spin resonance (ESR) spectroscopy (9,10). This first observation was seen to be due to the generation of a stabilized melanin radical. Subsequent work has confirmed these results. The use of spin traps has allowed a somewhat more definitive characterization of the UV-elicited free radical species. Thus UV irradiation of skin extracts or whole skin leads to the generation of the ascorbate radical (consistent with its antioxidant function) and carbon-centered radicals thought to be derived from lipid alkoxyl radicals. The UV-induced increases in the ESR signal from epidermis were oxygen-dependent, and superoxide dismutase (SOD)-inhibitable (11). Both ultraviolet B (UVB) and UVA wavelengths are implicated. Thus (while not certain to be the natural chromophore in skin), riboflavin irradiated with UVA generates copious amounts of hydrogen peroxide, which is cytocidal (12). It thus appears quite irrefutable that UV exposure of skin leads to the generation of a host of free radical species by as yet incompletely characterized mechanisms. Most work on the responses of skin's antioxidant system to oxidative stress has been carried out with UV radiation. In vitro and in vivo irradiation of murine skin leads to significant inhibition of superoxide dismutase and catalase activities (glutathione peroxidase effects were more variable) (8,13–17). More importantly, activities of these enzymes did not return to normal for hours or even days after irradiation. Nonenzymatic antioxidants are not spared. The lipophilic antioxidants (vitamin E and ubiquinol) are dramatically reduced after UVB irradiation (8). Vitamin C is markedly lost and this has been seen in murine (particularly epidermis) and porcine skin (18). Again, many of these changes can be seen in UVA-irradiated cells/tissues (19–21), raising concerns over the continued exposure of people to these wavelengths.

The depletion of nonenzymatic antioxidants bespeaks an ongoing attempt of the skin to combat the UV—mediated oxidative stress. Indeed this is a reasonable marker for the existence of just such a stress. As lipid membranes are a primary target for radical damage and vitamin E is the most important inhibitor of this damage, it would seem reasonable that levels of this vitamin would be maintained preferentially at the expense of more sacrificial antioxidants. This indeed has been shown. Thus, irradiation of skin homogenates generate a clear ascorbate radical ESR signal, which is to be expected as again, one of ascorbate's known roles is the reduction of the tocopherol radical to regenerate vitamin E. The ascorbyl radical signal persists until depletion of the vitamin C is complete, at which time the ESR signal characteristic of the vitamin E radical appears (22). Besides vitamin C, several other molecules thought to be important in regenerating vitamin E have been shown to be UV-depleted, sparing vitamin E. Ubiquinols completely disappear during UV irradiation, helping to recycle vitamin E. Again, glutathione, while presumably not directly reacting with vitamin E radical, can recycle vitamin C, extending the series of sacrificial antioxidants. Glutathione depletion has been noted in UV-irradiated skin (13). Other cutaneous inflammatory states lead to depressed antioxidant systems; e.g., lesional skin psoriasis has been shown to be characterized by decreased levels of SOD.

Aging—the ultimate disease—is thought by many to be free radical–mediated. One study of skin showed that while the overall antioxidant capacity was similar in skin from young vs. old mice, there was evidence for low-level oxidative stress in the older tissue manifested by a modest increase in levels of oxidized glutathione (23). It would be of interest to assess the known changes in the antioxidant system in response to UV/oxidative stress, i.e., the significant diminution, as a function of age. It has been shown that while absolute levels of antioxidants do not differ much with age, older animals routinely respond functionally to a lesser degree to stress. Perhaps the functional decrement in antioxidant homeostasis is greater in older animals and the time to return to normal longer, leading to increased tissue abnormality.

The use of topically applied vitamin C is not a recent development. Capitalizing on the long-known effects of ascorbate on collagen, the cosmetic industry has produced stable ascorbate products which can penetrate the skin and attempt to deliver L-ascorbate to the epidermis and dermis (24). Ascorbyl palmitate and ascorbyl phosphate have been formulated in cosmetics and marketed for the treatment of hyperpigmentation. The latter product has the commercial advantage of aqueous solubility, allowing a wide variety of cosmetic product formulations, and is stable for at least 6 months. Ascorbyl phosphate is hydrolyzed to L-ascorbate by phosphatases present in skin. Ascorbyl palmitate, an amphipathic molecule with a polar head and long hydrophobic tail, is touted as being easily compounded in water creams, lotions, and oils and having potential anticancer properties (25). The activity of lipophilic esters of ascorbate is critically tied to position of esterification. Locating the lipid moiety at the 2 or 3 position would not allow electron donation by ascorbate.

Unlike that of vitamin E (26), oral supplementation of vitamin C is not thought to increase skin levels of the vitamin in healthy, vitamin C–sufficient animals significantly. Thus investigators have looked to topical application to increase skin levels of this antioxidant. Levels of L-ascorbate, and its palmitate esters, have been measured in vitro in murine and human skin after topical application (27). Twenty-four hours post-application, the level of L-ascorbate was 15% that of the ascorbate-palmitate. The vitamin C in these studies was in the form of the ascorbate anion, which would hinder its penetration. In porcine skin (measured by HPLC), skin levels of ascorbic acid increased 25-fold compared to those of vehicle-treated sites (18). This represents about 15% of the applied dose resident in the skin. The vitamin C in this formulation was maintained at an acidic pH below ascorbic acid's pKa (4.2) to maintain it in an unionized form. Using either porcine or murine skin in vitro, considerably more vitamin C is percutaneously absorbed at pH 2.5 than at pH 5.1 or even pH 4 (unpublished). Again, though not specifically tested, these levels are assumed to be much higher than those obtainable with oral supplementation. Unexpectedly (fortuitously because of ascorbic acid's pKa of slightly over 4) these formulations are entirely nonirritating to the skin.

PROTECTIVE EFFECTS OF TOPICAL VITAMIN C

Again, ultraviolet radiation causes the most well-studied of cutaneous damage. In the past, UVB has been utilized in a far greater number of studies than those exploring UVA photodamage. But with very recent work confirming the pathological potential of UVA, e.g., connective tissue damage brought about by even suberythemogenic doses (28,29), as well as implications for skin cancer, more research will undoubtedly follow. As mentioned earlier, both UVB and UVA (perhaps to a greater extent) produce some of their damaging effects through the production of ROS. For reasons presented, it seems investigations using topical vitamin C to combat this cutaneous damage are warranted.

To date, few data are published showing the UV photoprotective effect of vitamin C applied to human skin. Murray et al. demonstrated that reduced post–UVB irradiation erythema in healthy volunteers' skin was reduced in those pretreated with topical vitamin C (30). In a separate study using 11 healthy volunteers, topical vitamin C attenuated a UVA-mediated immediate pigment response from modest to marked in all 11 (31).

Animal models do provide insight into topical vitamin C's photoprotective effect. In the porcine model, 10% aqueous vitamin C was applied several times to the animals' skin, which was then irradiated with 400 mJ/cm^2 UVB (narrow band, 311–312 nm) and sampled 24 h later (18). This source was used to eliminate any possible "sunscreen" effect of vitamin C. Both sunburn cell numbers, determined histologically, and UVB-induced erythema, determined by laser-Doppler velocimetry, were significantly reduced in vitamin C–treated skin compared with untreated skin. Using topically applied 8-methoxypsoralen with a UVA dose of 500 mJ/cm^2 (PUVA) and sampling after 48 h, topical vitamin C–treated skin had less than half the number of sunburn cells per sample than untreated skin.

In a separate study, topical vitamin C in combination with a UVB sunscreen (para-aminobenzoic acid [PABA]) produced a significant additive reduction in sunburn cell numbers in porcine skin. This was enhanced further with the addition of vitamin E in the formulation. Vitamin E was quite effective alone (better than vitamin C). In PUVA-exposed skin, vitamin C was the more effective, slightly enhanced by vitamin E and comparable to a low-concentration UVA/UVB sunscreen (oxybenzone), which was used. However, the combination of both antioxidants with oxybenzone produced a more than additive effect, nearly completely protecting the skin from phototoxicity (32) (see Table 1). These studies are particularly pertinent as recent research has confirmed that sunscreen use alone does not protect against the formation of melanoma, presumably by leading to increased exposure to unfiltered (UVA) wavelengths (33,34).

In the hairless mouse model, potential photoprotection by various topical antioxidants was studied (27). A freshly prepared 5% solution of ascorbate was applied 2 h prior to exposure (three times weekly for UVB and five times weekly for UVA). As the pH of this solution was 6–7, ascorbate was applied as the monovalent anion, limiting percutaneous absorption. Previously established visible, physical, and histological parameters for photoaging in this animal were used in this study (35). Both topical ascorbate and α-tocopherol reduced UVB-induced skin wrinkling and delayed onset of skin tumors to a similar degree. α-Tocopherol had an advantage of compound stability, as ascorbate was seen to lose its effectiveness if the solution was not freshly prepared. When compared to these antioxidants' lipophilic esters, UVB photoprotection induced by topical L-ascorbic acid and α-tocopherol occurred despite relatively lower levels obtained in the skin. Ultraviolet–induced skin sagging was not prevented by topical antioxidants. The difference between this and the preceding studies could be due to differences in pH which would limit penetration (and UVA penetrates deeper into the skin) or to the model used (skin sagging vs. PUVA-induced inflammation). Interestingly, mice orally supplemented with α-tocopherol, ascorbic acid, or β-carotene experienced no reduction in photodamage.

Table 1 Increased Protection from Ultraviolet A–Induced Phototoxicity by a Combination of Antioxidant Vitamins and Sunscreen[a]

Experimental condition	Number of "sunburn cells"/ 4 mm biopsy
Vehicle-treated (4)	TMTC
Vitamin C–vitamin E–treated (4)	59.5 ± 16.7
Oxybenzone-treated (4)	31.2 ± 11.9[b]
VC/VE- + oxybenzone-treated (4)	4.3 ± 1.1[c,d]

[a]Experimental sites (10 cm²) were treated for 3 days with 0.1 ml of the antioxidant, antioxidant/sunscreen, or vehicle in a cream base. Sixty minutes before UVA exposure, 0.1 ml of a 0.1% (w/v in ethanol) 8-MOP solution was applied to all sites. Thirty minutes later the last antioxidant treatment application was made. Triplicate 4 mm biopsy specimens were taken from all sites 48 h after UVA exposure, processed for histological characteristics, H & E stained, and sunburn cells enumerated, averaged, and normalized to the 4 mm biopsy specimen diameter. Vitamin C concentration, 10% (w/v); vitamin E, 2% (w/v); oxybenzone, 0.25% (w/v); TMTC, too many to count (>100 SBCs, epidermal necrosis).
[b]Not significantly different from VC/VE treated ($p > 0.1$).
[c]$p < 0.05$ compared to oxybenzone treated.
[d]$p < 0.01$ compared to VC/VE treated. Numbers in parentheses indicate animal number. Values given are the mean ± standard error of averaged values for the four animals.

To investigate topical vitamin C's potential for preventing radiation-induced skin damage, Halperin et al. carried out a double-blinded, prospective, randomized, placebo-controlled trial, using aqueous vitamin C (10%) applied to the scalp of patients undergoing external beam radiation therapy for intracranial tumors (36). No measurable reduction in radiation dermatitis was seen between skin treated with ascorbate and skin treated with vehicle alone. Skin levels of vitamin C were not measured so it is not known to what extent there was any increase in situ. Also, a combination with vitamin E might prove more effective.

Few published data exist studying the use of topical vitamin C for antiinflammatory effects. Perricone studied 12 patients with psoriasis in an unblinded trial comparing the effect of ascorbyl palmitate and vehicle versus vehicle alone on symmetric psoriatic plaques. Erythema, scale, and thickness of the plaques improved in lesions treated with the ascorbate ester, while only scale improved in the vehicle-only treated lesions (37).

When ultraviolet light is applied to skin, a temporary immunosuppression can be demonstrated (38); skin may be difficult to sensitize in irradiated areas. Moreover, a temporary tolerance is induced so that skin cannot be sensitized even in unirradiated areas. This phenomenon appears to be related to depletion of dendritic antigen presenting cells (39). Ultraviolet immunosuppression has been closely linked to the tendency to develop skin cancer in humans (38) and to acceleration of the metastatic potential of melanoma in animals (40). Most studies have been done with UVB, but UVA may also contribute to the phenomenon. Ultraviolet immunosuppression is a problem as it may not be completely prevented by sunscreens (41). In studies carried out with mice, topical vitamin C prevented UV immunosuppression (42), suggesting a cause related to reactive oxygen species. Moreover, topical vitamin C was also able to prevent UV-induced tolerance.

Despite its role in reducing reactive oxygen species and stimulating collagen synthesis, and despite an abundance of evidence that ROS induce both acute and chronic damage to the skin, no clinical trials have been carried out evaluating what would seem an obvious role for topical vitamin C—the treatment of photoaging.

In conclusion, on the basis of solid theoretical grounds and increasing amounts of experimental data, antioxidants (particularly vitamins C and E) should prove to be safe and effective skin protectants—this against varied cutaneous abnormalities, ranging from psoriasis to photoaging. Vitamin C's additional role in maintaining skin's connective tissue (collagen) homeostasis makes cutaneous supplementation of this vitamin even more desirable.

REFERENCES

1. Gilchrest BA. Photodamage. Cambridge: Blackwell Scientific, 1995.
2. Miyachi Y. Photoaging from an oxidative standpoint. J Dermatol Sci 1995; 9(2):79–86.
3. Pentland AP. Active oxygen mechanisms of UV inflammation. Adv Exp Med Biol 1994; 366:87–97.
4. Hornig D. Metabolism and requirements of ascorbic acid in man. S Afr Med J 1981; 60: 818–823.
5. Omaye ST, Skala JH, Jacob RA. Plasma ascorbic acid in adult males: effects of depletion and supplementation. Am J Clin Nutr 1986; 44:257–264.
6. Rhead WJ, Schrauzer GN. Risks of long term ascorbic acid overdosage. Nutr Rev 1971; 29: 262–263.
7. Shindo Y, Witt E, Han D, et al. Enzymic and non-enzymic antioxidants in epidermis and dermis of human skin. J Invest Dermatol 1994; 102:122–124.

8. Shindo Y, Witt E, Packer L. Antioxidant defense mechanisms in murine epidermis and dermis and their responses to ultraviolet light. J Invest Dermatol 1993; 100:260–265.
9. Pathak MA, Stratton K. Free radicals in human skin before and after exposure to light. Arch Biochem Biophys 1968; 123:468–476.
10. Jurkiewicz BA, Buettner GR. UV light induced free radical formation in skin: an electron paramagnetic resonance study. Photochem Photobiol 1994; 59(1):1–4.
11. Ogura R, Sugiyama M, Nishi J. Haramaki N. Mechanisms of lipid radical formation following exposure of epidermal homogenate to ultraviolet light. J Invest Dermatol 1991; 94:1044–1047.
12. Sato K, Taguchi H, Maeda T, et al. The primary cytotoxicity in ultraviolet-A-irradiated riboflavin solution is derived from hydrogen-peroxide. J Invest Dermatol 1995; 105:608–612.
13. Fuchs J, Huflejt ME, Rothfuss LM, et al. Impairment of enzymic and nonenzymic antioxidants in skin by UVB irradiation. J Invest Dermatol 1989; 93:769–773.
14. Pence BC, Naylor ME. Effects of single dose ultraviolet radiation in skin superoxide dismutase, catalase and xanthine oxidase in hairless mice. J Invest Dermatol 1990; 95:213–216.
15. Miyachi Y, Imamura S, Niwa Y. Decreased skin superoxide dismutase activity by a single exposure of ultraviolet radiation is reduced by liposomal superoxide dismutase pretreatment. J Invest Dermatol 1987; 89:111–112.
16. Iizawa O, Kato T, Tagami H, et al. Long term follow-up study of changes in lipid peroxide levels and the activity of superoxide dismutase catalase and glutathione peroxidase in mouse skin after acute and chronic UV irradiation. Arch Dermatol Res 1994; 286:47–52.
17. Shindo Y, Witl E, Han D, Packer L. Dose-response effects of acute ultraviolet irradiation on anti-oxidants and molecular markers of oxidation in murine epidermis and dermis. J Invest Dermatol 1994; 102:470–475.
18. Darr D, Combs S, Dunston S, et al. Topical vitamin C protects porcine skin from ultraviolet radiation-induced damage. Br J Dermatol 1992; 127:247–253.
19. Fuchs J, Huflejt ME, Rothfuss LM, et al. Acute effects of near ultraviolet and visible light on the cutaneous antioxidant defense system. Photochem Photobiol 1989; 50:729–744.
20. Punnonen K, Puntala A, Ahotupa M. Effects of ultraviolet A and B irradiation on lipid peroxidation and activity of the anti-oxidant enzymes in keratinocytes in culture. Photodermatol Photoimmunol Photomed 1991; 8:3–6.
21. Moysan A, Marquis I, Gaboriau F, et al. Ultraviolet A-induced lipid peroxidation and anti-oxidant defense systems in cultured human skin fibroblasts. J Invest Dermatol 1993; 100: 692–698.
22. Kagan V, Witt E, Goldman R, et al. Ultraviolet radiation induced generation of vitamin E radicals and their recycling: a possible photosensitizing effect of vitamin E in skin. Free Radical Res Commun 1992; 16:51–64.
23. Lopez-Torres M, Shinido Y, Packer L. Effect of age on antioxidants and molecular markers of oxidative damage in murine epidermis and dermis. J Invest Dermatol 1994; 102:476–480.
24. Takashima H, Nomura H, Imai Y, Mima H. Ascorbic acid esters and skin pigmentation. Am Perfumer Cosmetics 1971; 86:29.
25. Smart RC, Huang M-T, Han ZT, et al. Inhibition of 12-O-tetradecanoylphorbol-13-actate induction of ornithine decarbxxylase activity, DNA synthesis, and tumor promotion in mouse skin by ascorbic acid and ascorbyl palmitate. Cancer Res 1987; 47:6633–6638.
26. Packer L. Ultraviolet radiation (UVA, UVB) and skin antioxidants. In: Rice-Evans CA, Burdon RH, eds. Free Radical Damage and It's Control. New York: El Sevier Press, 1994:239–255.
27. Bissett DL, Chatterjee R, Hannon DP. Photoprotective effect of superoxide-scavenging antioxidants against ultraviolet radiation-induced chronic skin damage in the hairless mouse. Photodermatol Photoimmunol Photomed 1990; 7:56–62.
28. Lavker RM, Gerberick GF, Veres D, et al. Cumulative effects from repeated exposures to suberythemal doses of UVB and UVA in human skin. J Am Acad Dermatol 1995; 32:53–62.
29. Lowe N, Meyers D, Wieder JM, et al. Low doses of repetitive ultraviolet A induce morphologic changes in human skin. J Invest Dermatol 1995; 105:739–743.

30. Murray J, Darr D, Reich J, et al. Topical vitamin C treatment reduces ultraviolet B radiation-induced erythema in human skin (abstr). J Invest Dermatol 1991; 96:587.

31. Murray J, Darr D, Reich J, Pinnell SR. Photoprotection of human skin by topical vitamin C. Clin Res 1992; 40(20):143A.

32. Darr C, Combs S, Dunston S, et al. Effectiveness of antioxidants (vitamin C and E) with and without sunscreens as topical photoprotectants. 1996; Acta Dermatol Venereol (Stockh) 76:264–268.

33. Westerdahl J, Olsson H, Masback A, et al. Is the use of sunscreens a risk factor for malignant melanoma? Melanoma Res 1995; 5:59–65.

34. Autier P, Dore JF, Schiffers E, et al. Melanoma and use of sunscreens: an EORTC case-control study in Germany, Belgium and France. Int J Cancer 1995; 61:749–755.

35. Bissett DL, Hannon DP, Orr TV. An animal model of solar-aged skin: histological, physical, and visible changes in UV-irradiated hairless mouse skin. Photochem Photobiol 1987; 46:367–378.

36. Halperin EC, Gaspar L, Darr D, et al. A double-blind, randomized, prospective trial to evaluate topical vitamin C solution for the prevention of radiation dermatitis. Int J Radiat Oncol Biol Phys 1993; 26:413–416.

37. Perricone N. The photoprotective and anti-inflammatory effects of topical ascorbyl palmitate. J Geriatr Dermatol 1993; 1:5–10.

38. Streilein JW, Taylor JR, et al. Immune surveillance and sunlight-induced skin cancer. Immunol Today 1994; 15:174–179.

39. Cooper KD, Oberhelman L, et al. UV exposure reduces immunization rates and promotes tolerance to epicutaneous antigens in humans: Relationship to dose, CD1a-DR$^+$ epidermal macrophage induction, and Langerhans cell depletion. Proc Natl Acad Sci USA 1992; 89:8497–8501.

40. Wolf P, Donawho CK, Kripke ML. Effect of sunscreens on UV radiation-induced enhancement of melanoma growth in mice. J Natl Cancer Inst 1994; 86:99–105.

41. Ho KK-L, Halliday GM, Barnetson R. Sunscreens protect epidermal Langerhans cells and Thy-1$_+$ cells but not local contact sensitization from the effects of ultraviolet light. J Invest Dermatol 1992; 98:720–724.

42. Nakamura T, Pinnell SR, Streilein JW. Antioxidants can reverse the deleterious effects of UVB radiation on cutaneous immunity. J Invest Dermatol 1995; 104:600.

Index

About the Editors

LESTER PACKER is Professor of Molecular and Cell Biology, Division of Cell and Developmental Biology, University of California, Berkeley. Dr. Packer is the author of over 500 published articles and coeditor of the *Handbook of Antioxidants*, *Oxidative Stress in Dermatology*, *Vitamin E in Health and Disease*, *Retinoids: Progress in Research and Clinical Applications*, *Biothiols in Health and Disease*, and the *Handbook of Synthetic Antioxidants* (all titles, Marcel Dekker, Inc.). He is President of the Oxygen Club of California, President of the International Society of Free Radical Research, and a member of the Oxygen Society, the American Society of Biochemistry and Molecular Biology, and the American Institute of Nutrition, among others. Dr. Packer received the B.S. (1951) and M.S. (1952) degrees in biology and chemistry from Brooklyn College, Brooklyn, New York, and the Ph.D. degree (1956) in microbiology and biochemistry from Yale University, New Haven, Connecticut.

JÜRGEN FUCHS is Research Associate and clinical faculty member, Department of Dermatology, Johann Wolfgang Goethe University, Frankfurt, Germany. The author of over 100 published articles and the coeditor, with Lester Packer, of *Vitamin E in Health and Disease* and *Oxidative Stress in Dermatology* (both titles, Marcel Dekker, Inc.), he is a member of the Society for Investigative Dermatology, the International Society of Free Radical Research, and the Society for Electron Resonance Paramagnetic Tomography in Biomedicine, among other organizations. Dr. Fuchs received the Ph.D. degree (1985) in biology and the M.D. degree (1986) from the Unversity of Frankfurt, Germany.